NURSING

From Concept to Practice

SECOND EDITION

NURSING

From Concept to Practice

SECOND EDITION

NURSING

From Concept to Practice

SECOND EDITION

Janet-Beth McCann Flynn, R.N., M.S.N.
Ph.D. Candidate, School of Education
The Catholic University of America
Research Associate
American Association of Colleges of Nursing
Washington, D.C.

Phyllis Burroughs Heffron, R.N., M.S.N.
Education Specialist
Office of Academic Affairs
Veterans Administration
Washington, D.C.
Formerly, Assistant Professor
The Catholic University School of Nursing
Washington, D.C.
Lecturer, The University of Maryland School of Nursing
Baltimore, Maryland

APPLETON & LANGE
Norwalk, Connecticut/San Mateo, California

0-8385-7003-8

88 89 90 91 92 / 10 9 8 7 6 5 4 3 2 1

Prentice-Hall of Australia, Pty. Ltd., Sydney
Prentice-Hall Canada, Inc.
Prentice-Hall Hispanoamericana, S.A., Mexico
Prentice-Hall of India Private Limited, New Delhi
Prentice-Hall International (UK) Limited, London
Prentice-Hall of Japan, Inc., Tokyo
Prentice-Hall of Southeast Asia (Pte.) Ltd., Singapore
Whitehall Books Ltd., Wellington, New Zealand
Editora Prentice-Hall do Brasil Ltda., Rio de Janeiro

Library of Congress Cataloging-in-Publication Data

Nursing, from concept to practice.

   Includes bibliographies and index.
   1. Nursing.   I. Flynn, Janet-Beth McCann, 1944–
II. Heffron, Phyllis Burroughs, 1941–   . [DNLM:
1. Nursing Process. WY 100 N97515]
RT41.N883   1987   610.73   87–30628
ISBN 0-8385-7003-8

Production Editor: Elizabeth C. Ryan
Designer: M. Chandler Martylewski

PRINTED IN THE UNITED STATES OF AMERICA

Contributors

Sister Rose Therese Bahr, R.N., Ph.D.,
F.A.A.N.
Professor of Nursing
School of Nursing
The Catholic University of America
Washington, D.C.

Bertram Bandman, Ph.D.
Professor of Philosophy
Brooklyn Campus of Long Island University
New York, New York

Elsie L. Bandman, R.N. Ed.D., F.A.A.N.
Professor of Nursing
Hunter-Bellevue School of Nursing
Hunter College of the City University of New
    York
New York, New York

RoAnne Dahlen-Hartfield, R.N., D.N.Sc.
Coordinator of Nursing Research
Department of Nursing
The George Washington University Medical
    Center
Washington, D.C.

Sister Rosemary Donley, Ph.D., R.N.,
F.A.A.N.
Executive Vice President
The Catholic University of America
Washington, D.C.

Joann M. Eland, M.A., Ph.D., R.N.
Associate Professor
The University of Iowa College of Nursing
Iowa City, Iowa

Janet-Beth McCann Flynn, R.N., M.S.N.
Ph.D. Candidate, School of Education
The Catholic University of America
Research Associate
American Association of Colleges of Nursing
Washington, D.C.

Helen Foerst, R.N., B.S., M.A.
Project Officer
Refugee Mental Health Program
National Institute of Mental Health
Rockville, Maryland

Edna M. Fordyce, R.N., M.N., Ed.D., C.S.
Associate Professor
Department of Nursing
Towson State University
Towson, Maryland

Cathie Guzzetta, R.N., Ph.D., C.C.R.N.,
F.A.A.N.
Associate Professor and Chair
Graduate School of Nursing

Phyllis Burroughs Heffron, R.N., M.S.N.
Education Specialist
Office of Academic Affairs
Veterans Administration
Washington, D.C.
Formerly, Assistant Professor,
The Catholic University School of Nursing
Washington D.C.
Lecturer, The University of Maryland
School of Nursing
Baltimore, Maryland
The Catholic University of America
Washington, D.C.

Marion R. Johnson, R.N., Ph.D.
Assistant Professor
College of Nursing
University of Iowa
Iowa City, Iowa

Carol N. Knowlton, R.N., M.S.N.
Assistant Dean
School of Nursing
The Catholic University of America
Washington, D.C.

Rose Kurz-Cringle, R.N., Ph.D., C.S.
Research Associate
Maryland Psychiatric Research Center
Catonsville, Maryland

Sally Laliberté, C.N.M., M.S.N.
Nurse-Midwife
Group Health Association
Washington, D.C.

Linda Manglass, R.N., M.S.N., C.S.
Clinical Nurse Specialist
Private Practice
Washington, D.C.

Elizabeth A. McFarlane, R.N., D.N.Sc.
Associate Professor
Assistant Dean for Graduate Studies
The Catholic University of America
Washington, D.C.

Nancy S. McKelvey, R.N., M.S.N.
Medical Wellness Coordinator
American Red Cross Headquarters
Washington, D.C.

Cynthia E. Northrop, R.N., M.S., J.D.
Nurse-Attorney
Member, Maryland Bar
New York, New York

Nancie H. Pardue, R.N., D.N.Sc., C.C.R.N.
Assistant Professor
School of Nursing

Georgetown University
Washington, D.C.

Marie Rawlings, R.N., M.S.N.
Certified Clinical Specialist in Psychiatric/
    Mental Health Nursing
Washington, D.C.

Joan M. Roche, M.S.N., Ph.D.
Director, Nursing Education and Research
Fairfax Hospital
Falls Church, Virginia

M. Gaie Rubenfeld, R.N., M.S.
Assistant Professor
School of Nursing
Eastern Michigan University
Ypsilanti, Michigan

Mary Ann Schroeder, R.N., D.N.Sc.
Associate Professor
Community Health Nursing
The Catholic University of America
Washington, D.C.

Mary B. Walsh, R.N., M.S.N., F.A.A.N.
Associate Professor, Retired
School of Nursing
The Catholic University of America
Washington, D.C.

Eliza M. Wolff, R.N., Dr.P.H.
Staff Assistant
Office of Quality Assurance
Veterans Administration
Washington, D.C.

Helen Yura, R.N., Ph.D., F.A.A.N.
Eminent Professor and Graduate Program
    Director
School of Nursing
Old Dominion University
Norfolk, Virginia

Contents

Preface and Acknowledgments ix

Part I. Professional Aspects of Nursing and Health Care 1

1. Historical Perspectives in Nursing
   Janet-Beth McCann Flynn and Phyllis B. Heffron 3

2. Contemporary Nursing
   Phyllis B. Heffron 35

3. Theory, Concept, and Process
   Janet-Beth McCann Flynn and Phyllis B. Heffron 61

4. Theorists in Nursing
   Edna M. Fordyce 69
   A Comparison of Selected Nurse-authors and their Theories 88

5. Systems Theory and Adaptation
   Phyllis B. Heffron 99

6. The Health-care System
   Sister Rosemary Donley 115

Part II. Nursing as a Process 135

7. The Nursing Process
   Helen Yura and Mary B. Walsh 137

8. Nursing Diagnosis
   Cathie Guzzetta 169

9. Health Assessment
   M. Gaie Rubenfeld and Elizabeth A. McFarlane 181

10. Legal Aspects
    Cynthia E. Northrop. 205

11. Accountability
    Helen Foerst 229

12. Ethical Aspects of Nursing
    Elsie L. Bandman and Bertram Bandman. 261

Part III. Concepts Related to Communication 281

13. Culture, Health, and Illness
    Joan M. Roche and Janet-Beth McCann Flynn 283

14. Communication
    Rose Kurz-Cringle. 307

15. The Teaching and Learning Process
    Janet-Beth McCann Flynn 329

16. Change Theory
    Janet-Beth McCann Flynn 351

17. Nursing Research
    RoAnne Dahlen-Hartfield and Janet-Beth McCann Flynn 359

Part IV. The Human Perspective 393

18. Theories of Personhood
    Mary Ann Schroeder. 395

19. Self-concept
    Linda Manglass. 409

20. Human Sexuality
    Carol N. Knowlton 419

21. Perspectives on Aging
    Sister Rose Therese Bahr 433

Part V. Concepts Related to the Care of Individuals 457

22. Sensory Alterations
    Janet-Beth McCann Flynn 459

23. Sleep
    Janet-Beth McCann Flynn 477

24. Immobility
    Nancie H. Pardue 489

25. Pain
    Marion R. Johnson and Joann M. Eland 519

26. Anxiety, Fear, and Stress
    Marie Rawlings 543

27. Loss
    Sally Laliberté 559

28. Crisis Intervention and Suicide
    Linda Manglass 581

Part VI. Social Systems, the Environment, and Nursing 599

29. Group Concepts
    Nancy S. McKelvey, Sally Laliberté, and Phyllis B. Heffron 601

30. Family Systems Concepts
    Phyllis B. Heffron and Eliza M. Wolff 619

31. Community Concepts
    Eliza M. Wolff 653

32. Environmental Concepts
    Phyllis B. Heffron and Janet-Beth McCann Flynn 675

Index 699

Preface and Acknowledgments

This book is designed as an introduction to selected concepts that have contributed to the foundation of professional nursing. This foundation encompasses various philosophies, theories, concepts, and frameworks that give nurses the ability to provide quality nursing care. Once acquired and understood, this type of knowledge enables nurses to analyze situations, draw conclusions, make decisions, and solve problems.

The concepts chosen for this text represent selected topics that are fundamental to professional nursing practice. The principal goal in planning for and writing this book has been to consolidate these broad, widely applicable concepts into one text, and present them theoretically using a systems theory and adaptation approach as they relate to the nursing process.

This second edition contains four new chapters: Ethical Aspects of Nursing, Nursing Diagnosis, Nursing Research, and Perspectives on Aging. In addition, the third chapter from the first edition has been refined and divided into two separate chapters, Historical Perspectives in Nursing and Contemporary Nursing. The chapters in this second edition are divided into six major sections:

Part I   Professional Aspects of Nursing and Health Care
Part II   Nursing as a Process
Part III   Concepts Related to Communication
Part IV   The Human Perspective
Part V   Concepts Related to the Care of Individuals
Part VI   Social Systems, the Environment, and Nursing

Part I has been designed to give the reader an understanding of the nursing profession today as it relates to history, education, professional roles, theory, and the health-care system. Part II begins with a comprehensive discussion of the nursing process as the basic working framework for the application of nursing knowledge. Nursing diagnosis and health assessment are introduced as primary functions of nursing practice and as distinct, integral parts of the contemporary nursing role. The ethical and legal considerations that today's nurse must understand and incorporate into practice are presented, along with accountability, in terms of the client, the nurse, and the overall nursing and health-care professions.

In Part III, culture, health, and illness provide a necessary background of information to assist nurses in appreciating individuality and communicating more effectively with clients. Communication, a basic skill in nursing intervention, is discussed in depth, with emphasis on establishing trust and facilitating a therapeutic relationship. The principles of communication are carried through in the succeeding chapters in which the teaching–learning process and change theory are discussed as concepts significant to accomplishing nursing goals and objectives. Research is included here because publishing and presenting findings from studies are important aspects of communication.

Part IV explores the concept of personhood and human development as they relate to self-concept, sexuality, and the aging process. Part V focuses on seven additional concepts that are universal and relate personally to individual needs and circumstances. These fundamental concepts were chosen because of their applicability across a wide range of client situations and health conditions. Concepts related to specific body systems, pathologies, or specialized levels of care are not included. Suicide, however, is presented within the crisis chapter because of its significance as a national problem and as a developing trend in such groups as adolescents, the elderly, and individuals facing severe health problems. The last section, Part VI, contains four global concepts: family, groups, community, and environment. These concepts are presented as integral components of nursing and health care.

Distributive and episodic health care are discussed in Chapter 2 within the traditional model, i.e., outpatient setting versus inpatient setting. However, an effort has been made in this textbook to present each concept in such a way that it can be applied in either setting. For example, the importance of understanding family communication patterns is highlighted as important for acute-care nurses as well as community health nurses. Throughout the book, the authors have sought to reflect nursing's present-day professional achievements and accompanying changes in roles and responsibilities.

All of the chapters contain content outlines, behavioral objectives, glossaries, study questions, and annotated bibliographies. In addition some chapters contain assessment tools to enhance clinical practice. Most of the chapters offer a comprehensive, definitive overview of the concept, and a nursing process approach for applying the concept to practice. The four-step nursing process structure (assessment, planning, implementation, and evaluation) is used consistently, and examples of nursing diagnoses are presented where appropriate.

While not presented in a step-by-step procedural format, technical skills are identified in the appropriate chapters within the framework of the nursing process sections. Likewise, growth and development is not addressed as a separate entity but discussed as a part of selected chapters.

Acknowledgments

We gratefully acknowledge the help of those who have encouraged and supported us: our nursing colleagues and former teachers; our contributing authors for their excellent work and continued faith in us; and our families, in particular, who have continued to give us strength, perseverence, and confidence.

We thank our editor, Marion Kalstein-Welch, for her enthusiasm about the book and for her help and encouragement in planning for this second edition.

The reception of the first edition by the nursing community inspired us in many ways and enabled us to begin work on the revision with renewed spirits. We have gained an even greater appreciation for the vast changes taking place in the health-care environment and the resiliency and creativity of the nursing profession in responding to them.

Part I

Professional Aspects of Nursing and Health Care

The practice of nursing has evolved through the ages along with cultures, societies, and countries. American nursing has undergone profound changes, particularly in recent times, as women have attained greater credibility and authority and science and technology have advanced our way of life and given rise to changing health care needs and delivery.

This section focuses on the state of the art in professional nursing today. It provides a historical perspective of early American nursing leaders and significant events that have been instrumental in the long process of attaining professional status. Contemporary nursing is presented and discussed in terms of present-day educational programs and their diversities, nursing roles, and settings for practice.

The importance of theory building in nursing and the need for nurses to understand current theories and concepts are addressed separately as are specific nursing theories. Systems theory and the concept of adaptation provide theories applicable to nursing and give a comprehensive knowledge base of each of the theories as well.

The health-care system is presented as a complex and rapidly changing structure that influences nurses and nursing practice and contributes to social change. Conversely, nurses are challenged more than ever to exert their own influence and changes on the system and continue their advocacy for humanistic health care and equal access for all.

Chapter 1

Historical Perspectives in Nursing

Janet-Beth McCann Flynn
Phyllis B. Heffron

Chapter Outline

- Objectives
- History of Nursing
  Early History
  The Eighteenth Century
  The Nineteenth Century
- History of Nursing in America
  Early Leaders in American Nursing
- Historic Landmark Studies in Nursing
  The Goldmark Report
  The Grading Committee Report
  Nursing for the Future (The Brown Report, 1948)
- American Nursing in the Twentieth Century
  World War I (1914–1918)
  Post-World War I
  The Depression
  World War II
  Post-World War II
  The Korean War
  The Vietnam War
- Nursing Education
  Hospital Diploma Schools
  Collegiate Education in Nursing
- Summary
- Study Questions
- References
- Annotated Bibliography

Objectives

At the completion of this chapter, the reader will be able to:

▶ Discuss the historic development of nursing
▶ Describe Florence Nightingale's impact on modern nursing
▶ Discuss the roles played by early leaders in nursing in the United States
▶ Discuss how nursing was advanced by wars
▶ Compare and contrast the Landmark studies
▶ Identify and describe the different types of nursing education programs

HISTORY OF NURSING

Early History

Health Care in Antiquity. The history of caring for the sick is as old as humandkind. Methods of care were based on what people believed caused disease and injury and on what they believed about life. Over the years, technology changed what people believed and practiced. As these changes occurred, changes in the care of the sick followed.

In the earliest records, there is little evidence that nursing existed as a separate occupation, but it was often integrated as part of the practice of medicine men, priests, and priestesses, midwives, and wise women.[1,2]

Care of the sick in the home was primarily delegated to women, but it was probably the duty of all the adults to offer advice about care and treatment.

Nursing originally developed to fulfill the needs of society, and to care for the sick and weak members of the group. Early nursing can be viewed as an early form of community service related to the preservation of the group.

Nursing has its origins in the concept of mother-care of infants. The term nursing is derived from the Latin *nutrire,* meaning to nourish. The Latin noun *nutrix,* meaning nursing mother, was frequently used to describe a woman who suckled a child who was not her own. As time went on, the term *nutrix* was used to identify persons who provided care for weak or ill persons.

Medicine and health care developed in ancient civilizations. In India, sacred books, *The Vedas,* provided guidelines for religious, moral, and medical behavior. These books were written approximately 3500 years ago. Supplemental Vedas were also prepared. *The Ayur-Veda,* or *Science of Life,* contained eight sections that dealt with such topics as children's health, sanitation, medicine, and surgery and stressed prevention of illness. Indian surgery was most skilled. Hindu surgeons removed tonsils, performed amputations, excised tumors, removed bladder stones, repaired hernias and harelips, restructured noses, and performed Cesarean sections. Hindu surgeons also used drugs and hyponosis to provide anesthesia. Medical doctors diagnosed such conditions as tuberculosis, typhoid fever, leprosy, hepatitis, neurological disorders, diabetes mellitus, and cholera. Immunizations were performed. Many transmitters of disease were known, such as mosquitoes. The first hospitals known to have existed were in India, built during the reign of King Asoka (337–269 B.C.). Perhaps because of this, ancient Indian literature provides a complete description of nursing principles and practices.

In India it was believed that prevention of disease was more important than cure. It is here that a team concept of health care emerged. The ancient book *Charaka-Samhita*[3] describes the team as an aggregate of four and lists their attributes:

- *Physician:* mastery of scriptures, large experience, cleverness, and purity (of body and mind) are the principal qualities of the physician
- *Drugs:* virtue, adaptability to the disease under treatment, the capacity of being used in diverse ways, and lack of deterioration are attributes of drugs

- *Nurse:* knowledge of the manner in which drugs should be prepared or compounded for administration, cleverness, devotion to the patient, and purity (of both mind and body) are the principal qualities of the nurse
- *Patient:* memory, obedience to direction, fearlessness, and communicativeness (with respect to all that is experienced internally and done by him during the intervals between visits) are the qualities of the patient

The *Charaka-Samhita* further explains the interdependence among the members of the health care team, "Like clay, stick, in the absence of the potter . . . the three others, viz., drugs, nurse, and patient, cannot work out a cure in the absence of the physician."[4]

This book was the first to describe the role of the nurse in health care. In most instances, nurses in India were male, but occasionally old women served as nurses. The specific requirements of nurses included: good behavior, cleanliness, knowledge, kindness, skill in services that patients might require, competence in drug preparation and administration, pleasantness, indefatigability, obedience (to physician and patient).[5] Women also served in the Indian healthcare system as midwives.

Health care in China focused on prevention. Health was considered to be a state of harmony within an individual and the universe. This state of equilibrium was established by the balance of: yin (female principle) and yang (male principle). Any imbalance in the yin and yang were thought to produce illness. Four diagnostic methods were used: history, observation, palpation, auscultation. Treatment included: curing the spirit, nourishing the body, administering medications, treating the whole body, and performing acupuncture. Surgery was limited because of the religious belief that body mutilation would remain in evidence in life after death. There is little evidence of the existence of hospitals in this ancient society, but Halls of Healing were described. These consisted of sections of temples where the sick prayed for recovery. There is a lack of reference to nurses and nursing in the ancient literature of China. Perhaps this is related to the religious belief that diseases were caused by evil spirits taking up residence in the sick person's body. Fear that the evil spirits could enter anyone who touched a sick person would prevent people from caring for the sick.

Highly developed pre-Christian societies of Ceylon, Babylon, Assyria, and Egypt made substantial contributions to health care. Medicine and caring for the sick were advanced by the ancient Egyptians. Imhotep was so successful at healing the sick that he was elevated to the status of god of medicine and healing. The ancient Egyptians established public hygiene and sanitation.[6] When Egypt came under Greek influence, the Greek and Egyptian philosophies of care for the sick blended and advanced.

Asklepios (called Aesculapius in Rome), the son of Apollo and a human mother, was the greatest physician in Greek history. He may have been a mortal of great healing skill who grew famous and was raised to the rank of a god. Asklepios was represented holding the wand of Mercury, a staff entwined with serpents of wisdom. Today this symbol is known as a caduceus and is the symbol of medicine.

Epigone, the wife of Asklepios, was revered as "the soothing one." Of their six daughters, the two most noted were Hygeia, the goddess of health, and Panacea, the restorer of health.

The myth of Asklepios developed into a highly complex set of beliefs, and a cult of worshipers evolved. The priests of Asklepios provided religious healings and offered a blend of natural and supernatural remedies. Hippocrates (460–370 B.C.), a member of a branch of Asklepiades, and perhaps a direct descendent of Asklepios, was credited with establishing rational thought in medicine, changing medicine from a collection of magical concepts into a more concrete science. He encouraged physicians to use assessment skills to gather data rather than to use older methods based on myth and superstition. Hippocrates was considered to be one of the greatest physicians who ever lived and has become known as the father of medicine.

Greek literature contains many references to nurses, but most of these references pertain to nurses who were wet-nurses, children's nurses, and midwives. This is probably because Greek women were confined to the home by custom.

Greek medical practices spread to the Roman Empire around the year 200 B.C. when captive Greek physicians spread their practices throughout the Empire. Romans provided hospitals for the military, and a class of orderlies served as nurses. Other hospitals were built for slaves. Chief roles played by nurses were still as children's nurses and as midwives. These nurses were generally the slaves of the wealthy.

The Early Christian Era (A.D. 1–500). The Judeo-Christian tradition brought the view that care of the sick was a priority. The history of nursing becomes continuous with the events occurring with the beginning of Christianity. Nursing the sick was seen as a direct response to the teachings of Christ and care of the sick was considered an act of mercy. Service to others was considered a duty of all Christians, both men and women. This contributed heavily to the entry of women into nursing. Factors that aided this transition included: the rise in social position of women; the concept that men and women were equal; and the Christian ethic of mercy and compassion.[7] A number of the early Christians were highly educated. Many of these individuals were members of the clergy, and the Christian church assumed the care of the sick, poor, and helpless. Thus, those trained as nurses were likened to those who accepted a religious vocation. Many times nurses were thought of as having received a special "calling" to give service to humankind and to God.

Lay deaconesses, appointed by bishops of the early Christian church, visited the sick, much like today's visiting nurse. Hospitals, almshouses, orphanages, and homes for the aged were also founded during this time and supported by the Christian church. Appointments as lay deaconesses were highly esteemed and given to women of high social standing, who provided nursing care as part of their humanitarian responsibilities. No formal education was expected or provided for these nurses. It was assumed that the women used the skills they had previously acquired as wives and mothers. Gradually, the care of the sick and poor was assumed by a variety of religious orders.

The Middle Ages (A.D. 500–1000). During the Middle Ages, there were three classes of people: serfs (the majority); the aristocrats; and the clergy. The role of women had returned to one of subordination, but women could still acquire dignity in society by becoming nuns. During this time medicine in Europe was divided into two areas: lay medicine and ecclesiastical medicine; the latter centered around monasteries. As the Middle Ages advanced, the concept of nursing was identified, and nursing became an organized service. Three groups provided nursing services: military orders, regular orders, and secular orders. All of these groups worked under the auspices of the Roman Catholic church, which profoundly influenced their activities.

The regular orders of both men and women of God established monasteries where they organized hospices to care for orphans, the poor, and the sick. The uncertainty and insecurity of the Middle Ages caused people to seek protection behind moats and walls in the monsteries. Thus, nurses of this period cared for the institutionalized sick.

During the early Middle Ages, the first hospitals were established in Europe. These included the Hotel Dieu (God's house) in Lyons, France, in A.D. 542, Hotel Dieu in A.D. 650–651 in Paris, and Santo Spirito Hospital, established in Rome by the Pope in A.D. 717.[8] Both of the Hotel Dieu hospitals were established as almshouses and additionally provided shelter for pilgrims, orphans, the infirm, and the sick. Hotel Dieu in Lyons was staffed initially by women penitents, widows, and male servants. Hotel Dieu of Paris was originally staffed by a group of laywomen, but were organized into a religious order, the order of St. Augustine, by Pope Innocent IV. Religious brothers belonged to this strict order as well. These nurses received no formal training (except for their apprenticeship), worked long hours, and were permitted no recreational activities. They provided basic care for the sick.

The Late Middle Ages (A.D. 1000–1500). During the late Middle Ages, there was a redistribution of the population, many inland cities were established, and trade increased. A middle class formed of merchants, bankers, shopkeepers, and craftsmen arose. There was an upsurge in religious fervor, reforms within the Catholic Church, crusades, and pilgrimages to the Holy Land. Health care was affected by these happenings because crowded living conditions and poor santitation resulted in the spread of disease. Nursing underwent a reorganization during this period. Nurses tended to leave the monasteries and institutions and return to the home.[9] Great numbers of men entered nursing. Many military nursing orders were established to travel with and assist the crusaders. The nursing knights were as skilled in the use of bandages as swords. These knights were men from the Knights of St. John (later the Knights of Malta), the Teutonic Knights, and the Knights of St. Lazarus. There were three corresponding orders for women.

The female nurses did not travel with the crusaders but began hospitals in Europe and the Holy Land to care for those crusaders who fell ill while enroute to the Holy Wars. The Crusaders gained knowledge about illness and cures from the Arabs, who had an advanced knowledge of this subject.

At the same time that the orders of military knights were forming, groups of people banded together to form semireligious orders. These orders were not bound by vows of monastic life. These were *secular orders,* developed for the primary purpose of delivering nursing services to the ill and indigent. Individuals who entered these orders did not have to give up social standing, personal ties, relationships, or take vows of chastity. They primarily devoted their lives to a religious order in their home community without giving up rights as a citizen. One of the duties of these men and women was to provide nursing services in hospitals and homes. Many of the nurses were from wealthy or noble families and were highly educated in scriptures, philosophy, and language. At the end of a designated time, they could rededicate, resign, or take up another occupation. This secularization of nursing made a significant step for the advancement of nursing.

During the late Middle Ages, Pope Innocent III encouraged the foundation of hospitals in Europe. Clergy and wealthy individuals were invited to Santo Spirito Hospital to study and return to their own community to begin a simular project.

Because the concept of cure was not well developed, medieval hospitals were thought of as places to keep sick people. Therefore, these hospitals were custodial in nature. Nursing care was provided by monks and nuns. The hospitals were crowded and understaffed. Many times there was more than one patient in a bed. Physical care declined. Hospital administrators were forced to augment nursing staff with individuals of low character.

As hospitals were being built in Europe, universities were establishing medical schools. The beginning of the association between physician and hospital occurred. Unfortunately, much of the medical knowledge at that time was faulty or based on superstition. Astrology and alchemy were accepted practices. The philosophy of humoral therapy was still a basis for medical treatment.

Many societal changes took place in the last centuries of the Middle Ages. The feudal system declined, a middle class arose, large cities grew larger, knowledge increased. Many new needs arose and reforms were needed.

The Renaissance and Reformation. The *Renaissance* began in Italy about A.D. 1400 and swept across Western Europe. It brought a burst of intellectual growth, a great era of enlightenment. People quested for knowledge and beauty. The search for truth and knowledge produced the intellectual movement known as the Renaissance (rebirth). This same movement eventually produced the split within the Church that eventually divided it.

During the Renaissance, medicine underwent a period of enlightenment, a great bursting forth of new knowledge. The scientific method of inquiry or research was introduced. Leonardo da Vinci began a study of human anatomy. Many of his discoveries dispelled myths about illness; thus care of the sick took a new direction. During this time, nursing reached a high level of organization in the religious, lay, and military orders.

The *Reformation* (Protestant revolt) began in 1517 as a reform but ended in revolt. It was a religious movement caused by widespread abuses of the Church and doctrinal conflicts. The revolt against the Church was lead by Martin Luther, who broke away from the Roman Catholic Church. Those who followed him were called Protestants (those who protested). This led to the establishment of many separate Christian groups, such as the Anabaptists, Anglicans,

Calvinists, Lutherans, Presbyterians, and Puritans.

The Reformation had no direct effects on health care in nations where Catholicism remained the state religion, but in those countries where Catholicism was no longer the state religion, the religious orders were disbanded and the churches destroyed. Many religious leaders, monks, and nuns were driven out of the religious institutions in the Protestant countries, thereby causing a shortage of people prepared to care for the sick. Hospitals suffered from lack of staff when religious orders were disbanded because there was no group qualified to take their place. This was particularly true in England, where Henry the VIII suppressed Roman Catholicism and appropriated the property of approximately 600 religious charitable organizations.

Without people to provide health care, women from the jails were assigned nursing duties in lieu of jail sentences, producing a rapid decline in the level of nursing care. This period between 1550 and 1850 is known as the Dark Ages of Nursing. When the demand for health care became too great, hospitals were reopened under the direction of lay persons. Hospitals were built to be utilitarian. Large wards housed 50 to 100 patients. These wards were small, dark, and unsanitary. There was no form of isolation for patients with contagious diseases. Also, it was still common for several patients to share the same bed. Beds were close together, making it next to impossible to clean between or under them. Bed baths were not given, and bed linens were changed infrequently (once every two weeks) and hospital gowns once every four days.[10] The women who were assigned to care for the sick had no education or preparation in nursing.

There was little opportunity for advancement; work hours were long (sometimes extending to 48 hours at a time), the work hard, and the wages low. Nurses had no commitment to their patients, and no commitment to advancing the profession.

One final factor in the decline of the nursing profession during the age of Reformation was the social structure and the status of women within that structure. Under the auspices of the Church, women had been given freedom to move about in society and were permitted to create careers for themselves. Nursing was seen as a noble occupation through which to contribute to society.

With the Reformation came a different view. A woman's place was seen as in the home, and nothing was felt to be more fulfilling than being a wife and a mother. Any designated women's work, such as care of the sick, would have been unthinkable to most women because of the social status of nursing. Another factor keeping women at home was the great amount of work required to obtain food and clothing and maintain a household. This left little free time for education or work outside the home. Those women who were forced to work outside the home usually entered domestic services. Because nursing was left to those who could not receive employement elsewhere, nursing remained very much in the dark in the Protestant countries, not emerging again until the eighteenth century.

The Eighteenth Century

Social changes in the eighteenth century, caused primarily by the industrial revolution, brought about many needed changes in nursing. New lands were being settled during this time, and people began to emigrate to the European colonies in the new world.

Cities were built around manufacturing centers, and large numbers of workers were needed to build houses and factories and to work in the factories. As a result, large hospitals were required to accommodate the increased number of injuries and illnesses.

Prior to this period, society was more or less divided into the extremes of an upper and a lower class, with few individuals in between. As industrialization continued, a large middle class developed. With the rise of this middle class came a new social consciousness directed toward helping poor and lower class individuals who had great needs and few resources. As a result, the upper and middle classes began to carry out charitable acts, such as caring for the sick. The emancipation of women emerged along with general trends for personal freedom during the industrial revolution, and this movement greatly assisted the evolution of nursing professionally.

The emancipation of women had four main facets: judicial, political, educational, and occupational. First, in order to be emancipated, women had to be equal with men in the eyes of the law. Second, women needed to be able to vote. Third, they needed to be able to be admitted to and educated in professional schools in order to enter the work force as professionals. Last, women needed access to the work force. These four phases could not have been carried out prior to the industrial revolution, which gave individuals more free time for pursuits beyond food gathering and basic family maintenance. Nursing might well have remained a task-oriented craft without the strength and opportunity for advancement this movement provided.

The Nineteenth Century

During the nineteenth century, as a result of advances in medicine, social outcry regarding nursing, and the emancipation of women, nursing began to advance. The era of modern nursing began. In the British Isles, Ireland can be credited with the first systematic nursing institutions. These were the Irish Sisters of Charity, started by Mary Aikenhead, and the Sisters of Mercy, founded by Catherine M. Auley.

The need for better nurses was also identified in Germany around the same time. Theodore Fliedner, a minister, recognized the need for systematic training of nurses to care for the sick. In 1836, he bought a large house and established the Deaconess Institute at Kaiserworth. By 1842 the hospital had expanded to 200 beds with 120 nurses.

To be admitted to the Fliedner program, the prospective student had to be 18, in good health, and of high moral character. The course of study took three years to complete, and this program is considered to be the first of the systematically organized nursing schools. Kaiserworth became the most significant organization of Protestant deaconesses for nursing and is credited with creating the prototype of modern nursing.

The school and hospital flourished, and in 1846 Fliedner established nursing schools in London and, in 1850, Pittsburgh, Pennsylvania, and Milwaukee, Wisconsin. These schools were instrumental in advancing the idea of organized nursing education, and their excellent training programs did much to raise the level of nursing care and contribute to the respectability of nursing as a profession. Consequently, the profession of nursing was able to begin recruiting capable students from the middle and upper classes.

Florence Nightingale. One of the foremost nurses in all recorded history is Florence Nightingale, who is often referred to as the mother of modern nursing. Her contribution to nursing was profound, especially considering the status of nursing during her lifetime and the hardships of the time. She promoted health and hygiene, made reforms in military and civilian hospitals, and developed a philosophy of nursing based on wellness and health promotion.[11]

Born in Florence, Italy, in 1820, of wealthy parents, Florence Nightingale grew up in England. She was a gifted, precocious, and strong-minded individual with a strong religious and social conscience.[12] Biographies differ as to when she decided to enter nursing, but all agree on the factors that appear to have had the most influence on her. First, "she became conscious of the harder side of life—of suffering, pain, and deprivation."[13] By 1843, she was caring for the sick and poor, much to the distress of her family. Her mother's reaction was, "Are you sure you would not like to be a kitchen maid?"[14] and her sister "declared that she was dying . . . and Florence's behavior was killing her."[15] The second influence on Nightingale was her Oxford-educated father, who encouraged her and educated her as well as the highly educated men of her day. By the time she was 17 she had received an education in the classics, ancient and modern languages, literature, natural and social sciences, politics, economics, mathematics, and statistics. This education was actually much like the curriculum in many colleges today and was a good basis for her later nursing practice. It also set her apart from the wealthy ladies of her era and as a consequence, she was bored with them and the passive role of women in Victorian England. In a monograph entitled *Cassandra,* Miss Nightingale wrote a description of women as "sitting around a table in a drawing room, looking at paintings, doing worsted work and reading little books, or taking a little drive."

When night comes Cassandra states "women suffer—even physically . . . from the accumulation of nervous energy, which having had nothing to do during the day, makes them feel . . . as if they were going mad."[16]

The third influence was the visits she made with her mother to the sick. These sojourns initiated an unsatiable yearning in Nightingale to pursue this work in depth.[17]

In 1846, Nightingale learned of the Kaiserworth Deaconess Institute, the widely regarded health-care institution in Germany, and she decided to devote herself to nursing. Aware that she lacked clinical education, she looked for a place to study that would be acceptable to her family. Finally, in 1851 at age 31, she received parental consent for a period of three months' study at the Kaiserworth Deaconess Institute in Germany under the supervision of Pastor Fleidner and his wife. She was impressed with the organization and the purpose of this agency, but she felt that her three-month education was not enough. In 1853 she enrolled with the Sisters of Charity in Paris but became ill and had to leave. After this brief stay with the sisters, she accepted the charge position in a private nursing home for sick governesses.

Her genius for nursing, politics, and organization became evident at once; she reorganized the nursing home. As soon as she had it running smoothly, Nightingale again visited hospitals, and at this point she became interested in reforming nursing. She realized that before nursing reform could begin, some type of school for educating reliable and qualified nurses was needed. At the same time, she was being consulted by social reformers and physicians who were also beginning to see the need for qualified nurses. In 1854 a cholera epidemic broke out in England, and Florence Nightingale volunteered to care for the sick and dying. It was during this epidemic that she learned a great deal about epidemiology.

The same year, war in the Crimea broke out. The British, French, and Turks were fighting against the Russians over possession of the Crimean Peninsula and access to the Black Sea. As the war progressed, it became apparent that the British military had organizational difficulties and was deficient in providing for the wounded.

Nightingale wrote to the Minister of War, Sidney Herbert, and volunteered her services. In October, 1854, Florence Nightingale was appointed Superintendent of the Female Nursing Establishment of the English General Hospitals in Turkey. She had 38 nurses in her charge when they landed in Scutari (New Istanbul) in November, 1854.[18] The hospital there was overcrowded. It was designed to hold 1700 patients but between 3000 to 4000 patients were packed in. Wounded soldiers were lying on the floor, still in their bloody uniforms. Supplies were virtually nonexistent, food was scarce, and plumbing and sewage disposal were inadequate. Lighting was supplied by candles.

The nurses initially were refused admission to the wards by the physicians, but as the number of wounded and dying increased, the doctors turned to Nightingale and her nurses for assistance. Nursing and sanitary reforms initiated by Nightingale brought the death rate down from 42 to 2 percent within six months.[19]

She set up diet kitchens, established a laundry and a laboratory, and procured medical supplies and beds. She further reorganized the army service by starting a post office, so that soldiers and their families could communicate. She also began a savings fund for the men. She provided for rest and recreation, instituted care for the soldiers' families who had followed them to the war, and established convalescent camps. Once these units were thriving, Nightingale went to the front lines, where she contracted "Crimean fever" (probably typhus or typhoid) and almost died. During her slow recovery, she consistently refused to leave the Crimea and left only when the last contingent of nurses left Scutari.

One of the important outcomes of the Crimean war was the conviction that nurses needed organized education. Nightingale's work was respected widely, and in 1855, the Duke of Cambridge set up the Nightingale Fund for the purpose of educating nurses. Due to another illness, it was several years before she actually established the first school of nursing. She never did fully recover from this undisclosed illness and apparently spent the rest of her life in self-imposed isolation but worked unceasingly on nursing reform. In 1859 she published *Notes on Nursing,* to orient thinking on the meaning of nursing. Finally, in 1860, a Nightingale Training School for Nurses was opened in conjunction with St. Thomas' Hospital in London. It was financed by the Nightingale Fund. Students were to be women of good character. The objective of the school was to educate nurses for hospital nursing, home visiting, and to produce nurses who were able to educate other nurses.

The educational aims of the Nightingale school were to train hospital nurses, nursing educators, and district nurses for the care of the poor. The entire program of education lasted one year and included medical and nursing lectures and supervised practice. Some of the concepts taught were revolutionary at the time and included mental health, family and community health, nutrition, hygiene, and general health promotion. Nightingale recognized pain and suffering as harmful to health, made observations about the value of sleep, and encouraged the use of color and flowers in hospitals.

Finally, Nightingale influenced modern nursing by developing a philosophy of nursing, that nursing is an art that requires an organized, practical, and scientific basis for practice. She also felt that nurses are the "skilled servant in medicine, surgery, and hygiene, *not* the skilled servant of physicians. . . ."[20]

Through a life dedicated to nursing, Florence Nightingale set the stage for the evolution of modern nursing. Much of her basic philosophy has been incorporated into modern practice, and many of her principles are today's nursing goals: maintain health, maintain nutrition, observe accurately, provide a healthful environment, consider each person as an individual, and practice nursing as an art, not as a servant to others on the health care team.

HISTORY OF NURSING IN AMERICA

The social changes that occurred in Britain and Europe were reflected in America. The period of the Reformation was a period of great discovery and immigration to America. The early settlements in America held close ties to their motherlands. Therefore, health-care needs were met in the different colonies by the customs of the homeland. The Catholic colonies tended to be better prepared because they had not suffered from the Reformation. The religious orders followed the colonists to the New World. In the British colonies, however, English settlers lacked the religious organizations of the convent and mission, and the experience of the priests and nuns. Consequently, there were no hospitals. Most of the nursing care delivered to the sick was carried on in the home by the women of the household. Some areas of the colonies had more organized nursing services, but details of their role are unclear. In New York City, "nurses" sought out the sick and provided comfort measures.[21] These so-called nurses had no formal education, primarily because no formal nursing schools existed in the American colonies.

During the seventeenth and eighteenth centuries, colonial hospitals began to open, as either almshouses or pesthouses for contagious diseases.[22] These pesthouses were built in most of the major cities in order to reduce the spread of disease.

As a rule, most physicians received their training as apprentices of practicing physicians, not in colleges or hospitals. At the end of the period of apprenticeship, the person was able to open his own practice. A few physicians, however, were educated in Europe, and by the close of the colonial days, two medical schools had been established in the colonies: The Medical College of Philadelphia in 1765, and the medical department of King's College in 1767.

Wars helped to advance the credibility of nursing services and the role of nursing. Usually, women followed the men into battle and performed services, such as cooking, binding wounds, and helping with the ill. The idea of women as nurses, providing skilled nursing care on the battlefield, did not arise until the Crimean War, when Florence Nightingale took to the field with her group of nurses.

In 1751 the first real hospital was founded in Philadelphia, and other general hospitals soon followed. By 1850, many hospitals had been established but were thought of as agencies solely for the care of the sick and the poor. They were viewed as places for delivering care, not cures; infections and cross contamination were common occurrences. Nurses in these early hospitals were usually lower-class women who re-garded nursing the sick as drudgery rather than as a professional calling.[23]

In the period before the Civil War, medical standards declined as a result of a fast-growing population, urbanization, poor sanitation, and few adequately educated physicians. At the outbreak of the Civil War, the Union had no Army nurse corps, ambulance service, field hospitals, or medical corps. There was no group of formally educated nurses. By this time, Americans began to hear about Florence Nightingale and her work in the Crimea. Within three weeks of the outbreak of the Civil War on April 14, 1861, 100 women had been selected to take a short nursing course to be able to assist the wounded.

Dorothea Lynde Dix (1803–1887), already well known for her work on behalf of the mentally ill, was appointed as superintendent of the nurses. Although not a nurse, she earned this position by unceasing humanitarianism. She established the first Nurse Corps of the United States Army. An allowance of $12 per month was paid to these nurses, who came mostly from either Protestant or Catholic orders.[24] Eventually 10,000 nurses participated in the Civil War, but not all of them were employed by the Army. Only about 3,000 of them served in this official capacity. Approximately 600 sisters from twelve orders participated as nurses during this time. Another group consisted of women hired to do menial hospital chores. A fourth group consisted of those wives, mothers, and sisters who initially became involved because they wished to take an active part in the conflict. This latter group served throughout the war and were unpaid. Other groups consisted of black nurses employed by the U.S. Government for $10 a month and women employed by various relief agencies. Harriet Tubman and Sojourner Truth were prominent black women who served as nurses during the Civil War.

In the South, there was no organized effort to obtain nurses; therefore most nursing duties were performed by infantrymen, who were detailed against their wishes to this type of duty.[25]

In the North, the nursing system had its defects, and physicians did not approve of women in hospitals or on the battlefield. The Civil War clearly established the need for nurses in the health-care system and the need for organized nursing schools in the United States.

After the Civil War, nurses led a movement to establish nursing schools. During the postwar years, hospital schools of nursing began to develop. The instructors were usually physicians, and instruction generally took place at the bedside. Based on the guidelines of the Nightingale Schools, the first American school for nurses' training was established in 1872 at the New England Hospital for Women and Children in Boston, Massachusetts. The students worked from 5:30 A.M. until 9:00 P.M., and their rooms were located near the wards, so they could be called at night if they were needed. In October, 1873, the first diploma of nursing in the United States was awarded.

During the 1870s, other schools of nursing opened in New York, New Haven, and Boston. It was during this time that nurses adopted a standard nursing uniform consisting of a long dress of a somber color, white collar, cuffs, apron, and cap. By 1890 uniforms were an established custom, and each training school had a distinctive uniform, cap, and pin. Patients and physicians began to recognize these and to equate them with the various schools. The distinctive cap and pin became a symbol of pride for nurses for the high standards of nursing education in their schools.[26] Today not all nurses wear caps, but many proudly wear their nursing school pin.

In 1893, the superintendent of nursing at the Farrand Training School at Harper Hospital, in Detroit, felt that nurses needed something beyond a uniform to direct their pride to nursing.[27] She led the committee that composed "The Florence Nightingale Pledge" (Fig. 1–1). It was first used in 1893 by the graduating class. This pledge remains a part of nursing today, and many nurses recite it at a capping ceremony, dedication to nursing ceremony, or graduation. Although written nearly 100 years ago, it still conveys many of the ideals of nursing today.

The Spanish-American War began in April, 1898, and ended in August of the same year. The United States was unprepared for this war with Spain and had an army of only 28,000. The President sought congessional authorization to increase the Army's numbers to over 200,000. The Army, unable to supply trained

I solemnly pledge myself before God, and the presence of this assembly: to pass my life in purity and to practice my profession faithfully. I will abstain from whatever is deleterious and mischievous, and will not take or knowingly administer any harmful drug. I will do all in my power to maintain and elevate the standard of my profession and will hold in confidence all personal matters committed to my keeping and all family affairs coming to my knowledge in the practice of my calling. With loyalty will I endeavor to aid the physician in his work and devote myself to the welfare of those committed to my care.

Figure 1–1. The Nightingale pledge. *(From Deans, A.G. et al., 1936, p 58, with permission.[28])*

hospital corpsmen so quickly, was forced to look elsewhere. At that time, a plan to organize a nurse corps was established. Thousands of applications were received from young and old, trained and untrained. Each application was processed and filed. Only those educated in a school of nursing were formally sought to fill positions as Army nurses. More than 1,500 were accepted and were paid $30 a month plus a ration allowance.

The Spanish naval squadron was defeated and the short war formally ended on August 12, 1898. The majority of soldiers were discharged; therefore, the Army nurses were no longer needed. By 1900, only 202 nurses remained, but through the actions of influential women and prominent nurses, legislation was passed to establish the Army Nurse Corps permanently.[29] In 1908, the Navy established a Nurses Corps in much the same way.

During the early twentieth century, millions of immigrants flooded America. Many settled in the cities and took low-paying industrial jobs. This led to many public health problems. The health-care system for the poor was taxed beyond belief, as were sanitary facilities and municipal services. Crowded areas of cities degenerated into slums. Epidemics of typhus, scarlet fever, smallpox, and typhoid fever were rampant, and many died as a result of these communicable diseases.

Health conditions and historic happenings of this period gave rise to many new roles for nurses, and many nurses who would later become famous contributed during this time to nursing's struggle toward professionalism.

Early Leaders in American Nursing

During the nineteenth and early twentieth centuries, nursing began to emerge as a profession. Attention was paid to social welfare, and traditional roles of women were changing. Industry was growing, and cities were expanding. America was now ripe for the development of nursing education and nursing service.

A number of farsighted early nursing leaders struggled to make nursing a recognized and honored profession. These courageous women selflessly dedicated their lives and their careers to advancing nursing.

Sojourner Truth (1797–1881) was born a slave in New York State and later freed by the New York State Emancipation Act of 1827. In addition to being a nurse during the Civil War, she was an abolitionist, underground railroad agent, preacher, lecturer, women's rights worker, and a humanitarian.

During and following the Civil War, newly freed slaves flocked to Washington, D.C. Many were sick, decrepit, mentally and emotionally exhausted, and destitute. Because of this, the War Department created the Freedmen's Bureau and an emergency facility.

Sojourner Truth worked as a nurse and as a counselor for the Freedmen's Relief Association during the Reconstruction in the Washington, D.C. area. She spent much time in the Freedmen's Village providing care to people in hospitals. She also organized a corps of women to clean the Freedmen's Hospital because she felt that the sick could never get well in dirty surroundings.

Harriet Tubman (1820–1913) was an abolitionist and an unofficial conductor of the Underground Railroad. She is credited with making 19 trips to the South to assist over 300 slaves to freedom. Harriet Tubman also served as a nurse in the Sea Islands of South Carolina. Because of her outstanding work as a nurse, she was awarded a pension, but like all Civil War nurses, she did not receive it for almost 30 years, and then by an act of Congress. In addition to the pension as a nurse, she was awarded a pension for her work as a spy and scout for the Union.

Melinda (Linda) Richards (1841–1930) graduated in 1873 from a hospital-based school designed to provide nursing education, rather than the care of patients. Because of this, she is known as "America's first trained nurse." She was deluged with job offers and accepted a position as a night superintendent at Bellevue Hospital in New York City. She made many significant contributions to nursing, including: use of gaslights during the night; institution of written case histories and nurses' notes; identification of the mortality of puerperal fever. She went to England in 1877 to study nursing methods and to Japan (1885–1890) as a missionary. After returning to the United States, she pioneered nursing of psychiatric patients. Linda Richards spent a half century of her life to establish programs that provided nurses with a strong educational basis for nursing practice. She was also the first stockholder in the *American Journal of Nursing*.

Mary Eliza Mahoney (1845–1926) completed her nursing education in 1879 at the New England Hospital for Women and Children. Thus, she is considered America's first black professional nurse. She gave the welcoming address in 1909 at the first convention of the National Association of Colored Graduate Nurses (NACGN). Throughout her life she worked for the acceptance of blacks in nursing. After her death, NACGN established the Mary Mahoney Award. This award is presented at the American Nurses' Association's convention to an individual who has been instrumental in promoting equal opportunities to minorities in nursing.

Isabel Adams Hampton Robb (1860–1910) was born in Ontario, Canada, where she attended public school. Later she began her career as a teacher.

This career did not satisfy her, however. She was restless and ambitious. At one point she told her sister that if she were a man, she would be premier of Canada.[30]

She went to nursing school at Bellevue Hospital Training School, in New York City, in 1881 and was more interested in the academics related to nursing than the clinical application. After graduation, she worked for a short time as a supervisor of nursing and then spent about a year and a half as a staff nurse in Rome, caring for English and American travelers.

It was during this time that Hampton became convinced that nurses needed a firm foundation on which to build a clinical practice. After her return to the United States, she set as her goal the raising of standards of nursing education. She accepted a position as superintendent of the Illinois Training School for Nurses, where she introduced two important reforms. First, she planned the curriculum in graduated steps so that nursing students began with simple concepts and practices and advanced to complex. Second, she arranged for the students to affiliate with other hospitals to gain more experience.

When the Johns Hopkins Training School of Nurses was founded in Baltimore, Maryland, in 1889, she was appointed as its principal. There, she organized the work so that the students' day was limited to 12 hours, including two hours for recreation.[31]

In 1893, her reputation earned her the chairmanship of the nursing section of the Congress of Hospitals and Dispensaries. Within this organizational body, nursing leaders worked toward the formation of nursing associations. At the close of the Congress, she invited the superintendents of the training schools to join her in the formation of a nursing organization. This group called itself the American Society of Superintendents of Training Schools for Nurses and was chaired by Miss Hampton, who subsequently served on the executive board.[32] This group became known as the National League for Nurses in 1912.

In July of 1894, Isabel Hampton married Dr. Hunter Robb.[33] Although her colleagues thought her marriage would interfere with her contribution to nursing, she continued to work actively for the future of nursing.

Robb believed that staff nurses needed their own organization, and since the goals of the superintendents were quite different, she organized a new group at the national level. In 1896, she became the first president of the new nursing organization, the Nurses Associated Alumnae of the United States and Canada. This organization was renamed the American Nurses' Association in 1911. After the birth of her son, she helped establish university affiliation for nursing education.

At the turn of the century, Robb made another valuable contribution to nursing when she became one of the founders of the *American Journal of Nursing.* In 1910, Isabel Hampton Robb died at age 50 in a street accident. She

had been active in nursing for almost 30 years and made a great contribution in assisting nursing to emerge into a profession.

Mary Adelaide Nutting (1858–1948) was a graduate of the first class of the Johns Hopkins Training School for Nurses. Later, as superintendent of this school, she carried out many of the reforms begun by her predecessor. In 1896, she established the three-year curriculum, the eight-hour day for student nurses and abolished the monthly allowance they received.[34]

Miss Nutting firmly believed that nursing education needed two major reforms: provision of financial support for schools of nursing, and separation of the nursing schools from the hospital nursing service department.

Mary Adelaide Nutting's contributions to nursing were diverse. She is remembered in particular for her collection of historical works of nursing, *The History of Nursing,* a four-volume work coauthored with Lavinia Dock. She was instrumental in the creation of the Department of Nursing and Health at Teachers College, Columbia University, the first university-based school of nursing in the world. Her interest in nursing organizations throughout the world and the development of the International Council of Nurses made her known worldwide.

Lillian D. Wald (1867–1940) was a pioneer in the field of public health nursing and a champion of the urban poor. She was born in Ohio. In 1889, she entered the New York Hospital School of Nursing and graduated two years later. She worked in nursing for a short time and then entered medical school but later dropped out of school to help the destitute sick. She related the following story:

> A little girl led me . . . between . . . reeking houses . . . past odorous fishstands for the streets were a marketplace . . . unclean, . . . past evil-smelling, uncovered garbage cans, . . . where so many little children played. The child led me through a tenement hallway . . . and . . . into the sickroom. All the maladjustments of our [society] . . . seemed epitomized in this . . . journey and what was found at the end of it. Although the sick woman lay on a wretched, unclean bed, soiled with a hemorrhage two days old, they were not deranged human beings . . . That morning's experience was a baptism

of fire. Deserted were the laboratory and the academic work of the calling. I never returned to them . . . [C]onditions such as these were allowed because people did not know, and for me there was a challenge to know and tell . . . [S]uch horrors would cease to exist.[35]

In 1893 Lillian Wald, along with her classmate Mary Brewster, founded the Henry Street Settlement in the tenement district of New York. Henry Street eventually evolved into the Visiting Nurse Service of New York City. The purpose of the settlement was to improve the lives of the poor. The nurses who worked out of the house on Henry Street visted the sick, concerned themselves with living conditions, and sought to keep school children healthy.

Lillian Wald was also a public crusader and an avid fund-raiser. She was an accomplished speaker and was interested in the election of political officials who would assist the poor with legislation geared toward correcting those problems she, as a nurse, perceived. Wald helped initiate revision of child labor laws, supported enactment of pure food laws, and passage of enlightened immigration laws. Her interest and influence led to the development of courses in public health at Columbia University.

Wald had many ideas about how nurses could help people stay well, and the development of the nursing service of the Metropolitan Life Insurance Company and the Town and Country Nursing Service of the American Red Cross are both credited to her. She also introduced the concept of school nursing.

In 1912, Wald founded the National Organization of Public Health Nursing and was its first president. She encouraged the federal government to promote child health. Wald was a truly farsighted woman who did much to improve the health of the people and promote the concept of public health nursing.

Lavinia Lloyd Dock (1858–1956), another important nurse leader, was born in 1858 in Pennsylvania. Both of her parents were well educated, and they educated all of their children equally. When she chose to enter nursing, the community in which she lived was shocked. One person exclaimed "but I always thought the Dock girls were ladies."[36]

In 1886, after graduation from the Bellevue Training School for Nurses in New York City, she became the night supervisor there. She observed the difficulties that student nurses had with drugs and solutions and wrote one of the first pharmacology texts for nurses, *Materia Medica for Nurses*.[37] The book was extremely successful, selling over 100,000 copies.[38]

Lavinia Dock met Isabel Hampton during her years at Bellevue, and when Hampton became superintendent at Johns Hopkins, she asked Dock to be her assistant. Later she joined Lillian Wald in the Henry Street Settlement. She was highly committed to social reform and had a strong feeling for the poor in the New York slums. Miss Dock confronted legislators but became disillusioned when she found that women had little power and, consequently, little influence. She concluded that only the vote would bring power to women, and she devoted more than 20 years to this cause.

Miss Dock was a pacifist. She was the editor of the *American Journal of Nursing's* Foreign Department during World War I and never mentioned the war, to demonstrate her protest.

As she grew older she retired from nursing but always remained alert. She fell and fractured her hip in March, 1956, when she was 98, and died one month later. She campaigned during her life for the benefit of nurses, women, and humankind. She was one of the great women leaders in the early part of this century.

Martha M. Franklin (1870–1968) was the only black graduate in her class at Women's Hospital Training School for Nurses in Philadelphia. She was one of the first to campaign for racial equality in nursing. With her encouragement, 52 black nurses assembled to form the National Association of Colored Graduate Nurses (NACGN) in 1908. Martha Franklin was elected its president. The following year, the NACGN determined that black nurses must meet the same standards required for all nurses, so that the existing double standard based on race could be eliminated. By 1951, the NACGN determined that its mission had been met and NACGN merged with the American Nurses' Association (ANA).

Clara Louise Maass (1876–1901) graduated from the Christina Trefz Training School for Nurses of the Newark German Hospital in

1895. After working at the Newark German Hospital for three years, she volunteered to become a nurse with the U.S. Army during the Spanish-American War. She served in Florida, Cuba, and the Philippines. Then she volunteered to be a nurse in Havana, Cuba, where medical researchers were conducting studies on yellow fever. She cared for individuals who had contracted yellow fever. On June 4, 1901, she volunteered to be bitten by a mosquito. She suffered an attack of yellow fever, recovered, and was bitten again on August 14; she died ten days later. She was the last human subject to be used for a yellow fever experiment. In 1976, the United States commemorated her on a stamp, the first ever honoring an individual nurse.

Annie W. Goodrich (1876–1955) graduated in 1892 from the New York Hospital Training School for Nurses. In 1910 she became a state inspector of nurse training schools in New York City, and in 1914, an assistant professor at Teachers College, Columbia University.

During those years she worked with other nursing leaders in national and international nursing organizations to develop nursing into a profession. Internationally recognized for her excellence in nursing, she served as president of the International Council of Nurses (ICN) from 1912–1915.

In 1916 she became the director of the visiting nurses service of the Henry Street Settlement. During these years she worked closely with both Adelaide Nutting and Lillian Wald. The three women were known as "The Great Trio," because of their deep involvement with the movement of nursing toward professionalism.

In 1918, Goodrich was granted a leave of absence from Henry Street to make a survey of U.S. Army military hospitals with nursing departments. Later that year, when the U.S. Army organized a nursing school, she was appointed its first dean.

The need for nurses was great during World War I and an appeal was sent out to college women to assist in the war effort; Vassar College offered its facilities. The two-year program with a 12-week preclinical summer session was influenced by Adelaide Nutting. Students were then assigned to general hospitals as students. Four hundred and thirty women participated in this initial program. Their enthusiasm made it extremely successful and created an interest in nursing in colleges and universities throughout the country.

After World War I, Annie Goodrich returned to Henry Street and to nursing education. She was appointed dean at the Yale University School of Nursing and remained there until her retirement in 1934. In that year she was also elected president of the newly formed Association of Collegiate Schools of Nursing.

Isabel Maitland Stewart (1878–1963) was born in Canada. She taught in local schools before entering nursing at the Winnipeg General Hospital Training School. She graduated in 1903 and practiced as a private duty nurse, district nurse, and nursing supervisor.

She was attracted to the United States by an article in the *American Journal of Nursing* written by Adelaide Nutting. She entered a curriculum in hospital economics at Teachers College, Columbia University, in 1908, and in 1913, she was the first nurse to receive a master's degree from that institution. She remained at Columbia throughout her career, finally succeeding Adelaide Nutting as the Helen Hartley Foundation Professor of Nursing Education and as director of the department in 1925. She retained this position for 22 years. During her career at Teachers College, she participated in many nursing research studies.

She was interested in new developments in nursing and nursing education, and her greatest contribution to nursing was as an educator. She felt that students should receive some formal nursing education before entering the clinical area.

Isabel Stewart was a member and officer of many professional organizations. The idea of the Association of Collegiate Schools of Nursing (ACSN) is credited to her. She was active in the National League for Nursing Education (NLNE) and the ICN.

Isabel Stewart was interested in developing a standard curriculum for nursing and did much of the NLNE work that produced the Curriculum Guide in 1917 (later revised in 1927 and 1937). This guide was used during World War I to develop the Army Training School for Nurses. She served as chairperson of the Vassar

Training Camp Program throughout World War I.

During World War II, she chaired several important committees of the National Nursing Council for War Service and was quite forceful in bringing about the Cadet Nursing Corps.

During these years she wrote several books and pamphlets and, in 1916, became the first editor of the Department of Nursing Education of the *American Journal of Nursing*.

In her honor, the Department of Nursing Education at Teachers College, Columbia University, established the Isabel Stewart Professional Chair in Nursing Research.

Julie Catherine Stimson (1881–1948) was born in New England. She received a B.A. from Vassar in 1902 and then continued her studies in biology at the University of California. She entered the New York Hospital Training School in 1908. In 1917, Stimson received an M.A. in sociology, biology, and education at Washington University in St. Louis, Missouri.

Stimson's first nursing job was as the Superintendent of Nurses at Harlem Hospital. There she became aware of the health needs of the poor, and developed a social service department.

She went on to become the Superintendent of Nurses at Barnes and Children's Hospital in New York from 1913 to 1917, where she also established social services departments.

In 1917, Julia Stimson became an Army nurse and was sent to France to work with the English forces, where she became the Chief Red Cross nurse in France. After World War I ended, Annie Goodrich, Dean of the Army Training School, asked Stimson to take over that position. She did and held the position until 1933, when the school closed. In addition to this role, she became the Superintendent of the Army Nurse Corps.

With the help of legal advisors, military advisors, the public, and the Nineteeth Amendment to the Constitution (women's vote) in 1920, the Army nurses appealed to Congress for a change in status. They were victorious and were accorded officer rank. Miss Stimson received the rank of major. It was not until World War II, however, that nurses received full rank privileges and salaries on the same basis as the men.

Stimson did much to raise the public image of the nurse and played an important role in recruiting college-educated women for the Army Nurse Corps.

After retiring from the Army she was active in both the National League for Nursing and the ANA. With the outbreak of World War II she returned to serve as a recruiter for the Army Nurse Corps and was the first woman to receive the rank of colonel.

Mary May Roberts (1877–1959) entered the Jewish Hospital Training School for Nursing in Cincinnati, Ohio, and graduated in 1899.

Her early career was spent in a variety of positions: clinic nurse, assistant superintendent, and private duty nurse. During World War I she joined the American Red Cross and recruited nurses and later served as chief nurse at the Army School of Nursing at Camp Sherman, Ohio.

She obtained a B.S. degree from Teachers College at Columbia University. After graduation in 1921 she was appointed as coeditor of the *American Journal of Nursing*. In 1923, she was named editor, a position she retained until 1949. Under her watchful eye the *Journal* weathered the storms of the depression and World War II, increasing its circulation from 20,000 to 100,000.

Her goal was to produce a high-quality, literate journal for nurses to keep them abreast of the latest developments in science and in the profession. She used the *Journal* to publish and support the Goldmark Report of 1923 (see Historic Landmark Studies). After her retirement she wrote a book on the history of American nursing. She died in 1959 while at work on an editorial in the *Journal* offices.

Stella Goostray (1886–1969) entered nursing school during World War I, hoping to be assigned to Europe. She began her studies in Boston but contracted typhoid fever and had to drop out; she was strong enough to re-enter in 1917 and graduated in 1920.

She entered Teachers College, Columbia University, and earned a B.S. degree. During the years that she was completing her degree requirements at Teachers College, she took a position as an instructor at the Philadelphia General Hospital (PGH) School of Nursing.

She returned to Boston in 1926, to Children's Hospital, where she assumed the position of superintendent of both the school of nursing and the nursing service of the hospital, and where she remained until 1946.

Her contributions to nursing included improving the quality of nursing education and nursing services by hiring more qualified nurses and introducing auxiliary workers into the health-care system.

Nationally, Stella Goostray was on the NLNE's education committee, the board of directors of the ANA and a member of the board of directors of the *American Journal of Nursing.* She also served as chair for the Subcommittee on Nursing at the White House Conference on Child Health and Protection (1930).

She was interested in the accreditation of schools of nursing and served on the Committee on the Grading of Nursing Schools. In 1933 her master's thesis dealt with the significance of accreditation. From 1942 until 1946 she chaired the National Council for War Services, which planned nursing services during World War II.

In addition to all of her other roles she contributed to nursing literature by writing at least seven books with content ranging from mathematics, pharmacology, and chemistry to histories of nursing.

Helen Lathrop Bundge (1906–1969) studied at the University of Wisconsin, receiving a B.A. in sociology in 1928. In 1930 she received a Graduate Nurse Certificate from the same institution.

At graduation she became head nurse at Wisconsin General Hospital and later taught at the School of Nursing at the University of Wisconsin, where she became assistant director.

She earned an M.A. in 1936 and an Ed.D. in 1949 from Teachers College, Columbia University.

Helen Bundge's major contribution to nursing was in the area of nursing research. In 1952 the Rockefeller Foundation established the Institute of Research and Service in Nursing Education, and she was appointed as its director. She believed that it was every nurse's role to contribute to nursing's body of knowledge through research.[39,40]

It was through her interest in informing nurses about nursing research that the prestigious journal *Nursing Research* came into being

in 1952. She became its first editor and chairman of the 23-member editorial board. This journal continues to remain a well-respected publication in today's nursing literature.

Lydia Williams Hall (1906–1969) graduated in the 1920s from the York (Pennsylvania) School of Nursing, and later earned a B.S. in public health nursing and an M.A. in natural science from Teachers College, Columbia University.

She later held a position as instructor at the York School of Nursing and as a pediatric supervisor. After moving to New York she worked as a staff nurse, head nurse, and supervisor at both St. Mark's Hospital and the Visiting Nurse Service of New York.[41]

Although an administrator and an educator, she was most noted for her interest in nursing theory. She began her theory development in the 1950s when there were no known or published nursing theorists. Her colleagues at Columbia, Hildegard Peplau, Dorothy Johnson, Ida Orlando, and Martha Rogers continued theory development.

Mrs. Hall believed that nursing practice should be based on a theoretical framework. She also believed that nurses should develop their own theories and not have another discipline define a framework for them. Both of these ideas are widely accepted and supported by nurses today.

She developed her theory and implemented it at the Loeb Center for Nursing and Rehabilitation of Montefiore Hospital and Medical Center in New York in 1963. One of the major features of her framework is nursing autonomy.

These nursing leaders are but a few of the women who dedicated their lives to bringing nurses and nursing into the arena of professionalism. Others have worked within their various places of employment, within the professional organizations, and through the political process to strengthen and advance the state of nursing. Every hospital and every school of nursing has had behind it a nurse who strove to upgrade the professional status of nursing and bring it into the twentieth century as an autonomous profession.

It is also important to mention that great numbers of women who chose to work as staff nurses made their professional contributions within hospitals and the community. Throughout the first half of the century these nurses often worked under difficult employement conditions and societal prejudices, yet they continued to maintain a hopeful and growth-inspiring spirit toward their profession.

HISTORIC LANDMARK STUDIES IN NURSING

Evaluation is an important aspect of the activities of any professional group or occupation. Around the turn of the century, there began what was to become a series of landmark evaluation studies in nursing and nursing education. With the coming of industrialization, the demand for adequate health care increased rapidly, as social, political, and economic changes affected people's values and life-styles in the twentieth century. The early work of Florence Nightingale and her philosophy of patient care had enlightened people as to the realities and possibilities of better health care, particularly within the hospital setting. Nurses, as a group, were becoming more visible, and they began to distinguish themselves as an essential part of the health-care system.

There have been numerous efforts to examine the practice of nursing and to evaluate the methods of nursing education. Unfortunately, relatively few studies have come to the attention of the nation or had a significant impact on the development of the profession. Those that have generally are referred to as landmark nursing studies.

The Goldmark Report

Prior to World War I, nursing had been criticized by medical groups, who believed that nurses were either undertrained or overtrained and that the profession was failing to produce nurses prepared to provide quality patient care.[42] Nursing leaders, however, identified the need for broader educational programs to prepare nurses for roles in the expanding health-care system. In 1911, several nurses appealed to the Carnegie Foundation to conduct an impartial, scientific study of the system of nursing education similar to the Carnegie Foundation's study of medical education (the Flexner Report)

completed the year before.[43] In 1912, Adelaide Nutting reported poor education practices and substandard living and working conditions in nursing schools throughout the country.[44] Her report had little impact at the time, but it brought attention to the plight of nursing education.

In 1918, Nutting brought her concerns about nursing and nursing education to the Rockefeller Foundation, highlighting the lack of nurses to provide adequate nursing. This meeting brought about the establishment of the Committee for the Study of Nursing Education, made up of doctors, nurses, and individuals interested in health. The final report of this committee was prepared by a social researcher, Josephine Goldmark and became known as the Goldmark Report. Originally, the committee had been established to study the educational requirements of pubic health nursing, but because of the complexity of nursing, it was expanded in 1920 to include all of nursing. The committee was given the charge to

> suvey the entire field occupied by the nurse and other workers of related type; to form a conception of the tasks to be performed and the qualifications necessary for their execution and on the basis of such a study . . . to establish sound minimum educational standards for each type of nursing service for which there appears to be a vital social need.[45]

Owing to the constraints of time and money, only 23 representative hospital schools of nursing and 49 public health agencies were analyzed. The results of this first landmark study were published in 1923, and many conclusions were drawn from the findings[46]:

- Public health was a neglected subject
- Public health was an attractive field and efforts should be made to attract young women of high credentials
- Attempts to lower educational standards would bring danger to the public
- Steps should be taken for the definition and licensure of a subsidiary level of nursing service, possibly to assist under the direction of the trained nurse
- Hospital training schools were not organized

on a basis conforming to the standards accepted in other fields, and nursing education was frequently sacrificed for hospital services

- It was possible to reduce the period of hospital training to 28 months if students had to meet the criteria of a high school diploma for admission into nursing school, therefore attracting students of high quality
- Leaders in nursing should receive additional training beyond basic nursing courses
- Strengthening university schools of nursing for training leaders was important to further nursing education
- When licensure of a subsidiary grade of nursing was provided, schools for training should be established
- Development of adequate nursing service was dependent on securing funds for the development of nursing education

These conclusions encompassed all of nursing practice, and although the suggestions were constructive, the report criticized all phases of nursing. The committee's findings were not widely published, so the pubic remained uninformed as to the conditions in nursing and the need for change.

Although the report failed to initiate changes in nursing, it led to endowment of the Yale University School of Nursing by the Rockefeller Foundation.

The Grading Committee Report

The Committee on the Grading of Nursing Schools was established in 1926 in conjunction with the National League for Nursing Education, the American Nurses' Association, the National Organization for Public Health Nursing, the American Medical Association, the American College of Surgeons, the American Hospital Association, and the American Public Health Association.

The stated purpose of the committee was to "study the ways and means for ensuring an ample supply of nursing services, of whatever type and quality needed for an adequate care of the patient, at a price within his reach."[47] This included grading nursing schools, studying the work of nurses, defining the duties falling within the realm of nursing practice, identifying supply and demand for nursing service, and the problems of public health nursing.

The original purpose of the committee, the grading of nursing schools

> meant that certain minimum standards agreed to by the Committee had to be met by the school if they were to be considered qualified to prepare graduates for the nursing profession. It was impossible to decide minimum standards until it was known what abilities graduate nurses should possess, and those abilities could not be determined until it was understood what the graduate would be called on to do in practice.[48]

Therefore, grading had to be based on a careful study of nursing education and nursing practice.

The committee planned to divide its goals into three projects: a study of supply and demand for graduate nurses, an analysis of what nurses did and how they should be prepared, and the grading of schools of nursing. The committee planned to carry each goal to completion and publish the findings in separate reports. The committee worked for seven years and produced three reports: *Nurses, Patients, and Pocketbooks,* in 1928, *An Activity Analysis of Nursing,* in 1934, and *Nursing Schools Today and Tomorrow,* also in 1934.

In the process of gathering data on the nursing schools, the committee found that requirements for entry into nursing school were minimal, many not even requiring a high school diploma; the dropout rate was quite high; many schools were small and associated with hospitals that were too small to provide an adequate clinical experience; the student workday was long and the workweek longer than in other professions; and the number of qualified instructors was extremely low. These findings demonstrated that nursing schools existed to staff hospitals and not to educate nurses.[49] Furthermore, the study found a tremendous number of undereducated nurses. Salaries were low, hours long, and working conditions poor. Complaints of a nursing shortage were based on maldistribution of nurses, and nurses not qualified to meet the identified health care needs.[50]

Recommendations of the committee presented in *Nurses, Patients, and Pocketbooks* included:

- Reduce and improve the number of nurses

- Replace students with graduate nurses in the hospitals
- Help hospitals meet the costs of employing graduate nurses
- Get public support for the above

The results of this report were well received by nursing, medicine, and the public, because of the variety of groups represented on the committee and the large number and distribution of nursing schools that were surveyed.

The second report, *An Activity Analysis of Nursing* (1934), found that job analysis was essential before nursing schools could be graded. The committee wanted to learn what nurses actually did and the knowledge base necessary for performance in order to improve and standardize the educational programs in schools across the nation.

In 1934, the final report, *Nursing Schools Today and Tomorrow,* was published. This work, the grading of schools, was based on the information gathered in the two preceding reports. Once the essentials that constituted a good school of nursing were determined, schools were contacted for information concerning their curricula. Then they were ranked, based on their response to a self-report questionnaire. This enabled the committee to be objective, because the score was based on statistical data. The final grade received by each school was based on each school's comparative standing on each item studied, indicating where it stood in relation to the top school.[51] Three separate gradings were done on nursing schools nationwide, but school participation was strictly voluntary. A school was only graded at its own request. The committee did not so much desire the assigning of a rank to the school but to stimulate a desire in the schools to seek improvements where they were needed.[52] Because the committee hoped that schools would improve, each school grading was actually a series of gradings over a period of years, so that it was possible for schools to build stronger programs over time. The purpose was to reward good schools and to help poor schools recognize their limitations and correct them. Any reforms were made voluntarily, since the committee had no enforcing power.

The first report on grading was complete in 1929, the second in 1933, and the final survey in 1934. Between the first and second study, most schools improved their standing in 75 percent of the items on the questionnaires. The third survey showed even more improvement, which was really promising, given the economic depression of the era.[53]

Nursing for the Future (The Brown Report, 1948)

The Brown Report, considered to be the third landmark study of the status of nursing in the United States, was prompted by conditions inside and outside the field that had caused nurse shortages.[54] Social legislation of the 1930s and World War II gave rise to public demands for quality health care, while nursing schools continued to have difficulty attracting qualified students. Nursing leaders concluded that there was something chronically wrong with the system of nursing education. Findings from the two earlier reports had not been used effectively, and nursing leaders were determined to correct this with the results of a third study.[55]

The Brown Report was funded by a grant to the National Nursing Council from the Carnegie Corporation in 1947. Esther Lucille Brown, a distinguished social anthropologist, was appointed as director of the study. Its purpose was to learn who should organize, finance, administer, and control professional nursing to meet the needs of the community, not the profession.[56] The committee also considered the probable nature of nursing in the second half of the twentieth century and set the stage for research in nursing itself and in nursing as a part of overall health programs.[57]

Dr. Brown gathered data by making two major trips across the United States, visiting 50 representative schools in all parts of the country; held conferences in Washington, D.C., Chicago, and San Francisco with 1200 directors of nursing schools; and met with nurses, doctors, administrators, trustees, and university members about the current status and future prospects of nursing.[58]

The report pointed out the following needs: a study of nursing functions; building integrated nursing service teams; use of nonprofessional teams; mandatory licensing of practical nurses; expanded and improved inservice education; establishment of procedures and standards for state accreditation of nursing schools; establishment of a system for recognizing excellence in nursing practice to raise the status of the profession; and adequate financing of nursing education.[59]

The study recommended: that the term "professional education" be restricted to schools that furnish professional education (universities, colleges, or hospitals with institutions of higher learning), and that the term "professional nurse" be applied only to nurses who graduate from such a school. The study also recommended an increase in the social contributions of hospitals to nursing education; that financial structure and organization, adequate in facilities and faculties, be distributed to serve the nursing needs of the nation; a variety of other recommendations directed toward reorganizing nursing education and service.

No other publication had aroused such interest, and such alarm from those who felt threatened by the findings and recommendations.

AMERICAN NURSING IN THE TWENTIETH CENTURY

This century has seen the rise of the professional organizations, advances in nursing education, landmark studies, expansion of the nurse's role, the creation of nursing publications, the expansion of science and technology, and the women's movement. All of these factors have had an enormous positive impact on modern nursing and promise to do so in the future. In addition, a number of specific historic events had effects on the professional evolution of nursing during this time frame.

World War I (1914–1918)

Wars often provide the impetus for change and growth in science, technology, and medicine. This has been true for nursing as well. The United States became involved in World War I in 1917. Members of the American Nurses' Association and the National League for Nursing Education met to establish the role that American nurses would take in the war and sent President Woodrow Wilson information about the support of American nurses in the war effort.[60]

At the beginning of World War I, about 400 nurses were in the Army Nurse Corps. In the next 1½ years, this number increased to 21,000[61] through recruitment and participation of the reserves from the American Red Cross, under the direction of Jane Delano. Of these, 10,000 served overseas. They did not have military rank as officers but were subject to military law and had some of the privileges to the military.

During World War I, the United States experienced a shortage of nurses, so the Army opened schools of nursing at all of the major camp hospitals. There, students gained their clinical experiences. Annie Goodrich served as dean of the first school. Because of her philosophy of nursing, the students received more classroom instruction and less clinical experience.[62] By 1921, this program had graduated 500 students. By 1932, these schools were closed because of the financial pressures of the great depression.

The Vassar Training School was another federally funded nursing education program during World War I. Four hundred and thirty college graduates enrolled in this intensive three-month theoretical training program. At the completion of this program the graduates entered affiliated schools of nursing for a two-year-and-three-month program. Stimulated by this interest, another 50 colleges were planning similar programs when the war ended.[63] As the war ended, so did the desire to found such schools.

Another project created by the Red Cross to improve the nursing shortage situation was the training of nurses' aides. Over 2000 women were recruited, but only 250 of these eventually served overseas.[64] Courses were designed to prepare the average housewife to care for the homebound sick and taught hygiene and simple nursing procedures. Nursing organizations were against this program, however, feeling that this reinforced the public's image of nursing as women's work, requiring little education, instead of that of an emerging profession, requiring extensive education and preparation.

Post-World War I

Nurses began to recognize their impact as a group during the postwar years. Emphasis on health increased, and the field of public health

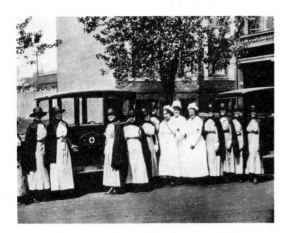

Figure 1–2. Public health nursing in Detroit, Michigan, in 1918.

nursing developed (Fig. 1–2). Nursing services were established in the Hospital Division of the United States Public Health Service in 1919, the Veterans Bureau in 1922, and the Indian Bureau in 1924. Red Cross nurses also were developing public health projects in areas where local resources were deficient.

Also, because of the war, public attention and interest were directed to nursing. During these years, we see the rise of universities sponsoring nursing courses, the endowment of schools (Yale, Western Reserve), the development of the Association of Collegiate Schools of Nursing, the employment of nurses in industry, nursing service in the federal government, and the landmark studies.

The Depression

The stock market crash of 1929 created widespread unemployment across the nation, and nurses were no exception. Although the need for qualified nurses increased, employers did not have the financial resources to hire them. Up to this time, a great numer of nurses had been employed as private duty nurses, but now potential clients no longer had the means to employ them. Hospitals continued to use students for service because they were cheaper than graduate nurses. Consequently, many nurses were without jobs.

Nursing organizations set aside their vested interests and formed the Joint Committee on the Distribution of Nursing Services to find solutions to the problems facing professional nursing. The government, through the establishment of the National Recovery Act (NRA) and the Works Progress Administration (WPA), was able to provide some jobs for nurses.

Nursing organizations decided on several ways to ease the unemployment situation. One strategy was to close small, inferior schools, which reduced the number of graduating nurses each year and stimulated increased interest in standards of care. It also created a need for graduate nurses to fill the positions previously filled by students. Another strategy was to reduce the workday from 12 to 8 hours. In addition, new government health programs were generated.[65,66]

Additional benefits for nurses came with the passage of the Social Security Act in 1935, which provided pensions to the aged, unemployment insurance, payments to the disabled, dependent mothers, and children, and an expanded health program. This newly established program was administered through the U.S. Public Health Service and the Children's Bureau and provided job opportunities in public health for nurses.[67] Another development that occurred simultaneously involved the epidemiology of chronic disease. Chronic illness began to be associated with advanced age and to replace communicable diseases as the leading cause of death. This, coupled with the growth of hospital insurance programs, brought more patients into hospitals, which in turn provided many more jobs in nursing and helped to change the focus of professional nursing from private duty to hospital nursing.

World War II

The United States officially entered World War II after the attack on Pearl Harbor on December 7, 1941. Hospital nurses were in great demand as were nurses for the war industry and the military. This was also the time of the baby boom in the United States, and nurses were needed to care for mothers, infants, and children in the community and in the schools. The nursing shortage during this time reached critical dimensions. Training of volunteers and teaching refresher courses for inactive nurses, the federal funding (Bolton Nurse Training Act) of nurse scholarship, and the development of the Cadet

Nurse Corps[68] all were suggested as solutions to the nursing shortage.

Students admitted into the Cadet Nurse Corps attended one of the 1125 participating schools and had all of their expenses—tuition, books, maintenance, uniforms, and monthly stipend—paid for by the United States Public Health Service.[69] In order to qualify for the Cadet Corps, candidates had to be between the ages of 17 and 35, in good health, and have good academic records from high school. Once the program ended, they had to work actively in nursing at either civilian health care agencies or in the military.

The Bolton Nurse Training Act, which established the Cadet Nurse Corps, allowed selected nursing programs to graduate students six months earlier than the traditional 36-month-long course. In order to meet state board requirements, however, another six-month period of education was needed. To meet this requirement, three levels of cadets were established: precadets, junior cadets and senior cadets. Precadets were those students in the first nine months in school. They spent this time learning the basic sciences and fundamentals of nursing. The next 15 to 21 months were spent as junior cadets, and they advanced through an accelerated curriculum. Senior cadets had finished their formal education and, in order to meet state board requirements, were assigned a practice assignment in a civilian, military, or federal health-care agency.[70,71]

The government spent $184 million in direct federal aid from 1942 to 1948. This expenditure allowed for great achievements in nursing. Eighty-seven percent of all nursing schools across the nation participated in the corps. Student enrollment ranged from 85,000 in 1940, to 129,000 in 1946, and dropped to 89,000 in 1949, as government support was phased out.[72]

Many nurse educators were concerned that the quality of nursing education would suffer because of the acceleration of these educational programs. On the contrary, it turned out that nursing schools were forced to re-evaluate and improve nursing curriculum, resulting in overall improvement of nursing education.

In addition, the Division of Nursing Education encouraged changes in students' working experience. They saw to it that the students workweek, including classroom education and clinical experience, was reduced to 48 hours per week from 55 to 75 hours per week.

Nursing during World War II was quite different from the way it had been in other wars. The introduction of more sophisticated firepower increased the number of military and civilian casualties, but improved medical care and transportation reduced mortality associated with injury, infection, and disease.

Also during World War II, the Army had demonstrated a need for a new type of battle hospital close to the front lines, the Mobile Army Surgical Hospital (MASH). This type of hospital would see much use in future wars.

Many changes and innovations in the delivery of health care came about as a direct result of World War II. Attempts at risky or radical surgery for war injuries were acceptable practices and led to advances in surgical techniques. The collection and storage of donated blood for battle casualties became common, creating the prototype for the blood banking system. The need for hospital beds promoted the likelihood of early discharge of patients, confirming notions of the hazards of immobility and actually improving recovery. Loss of limbs of war victims facilitated innovative mechanical and rehabilitation developments for those who would previously have been confined to bed or wheelchairs. Advances in drug therapy included the introduction of sulfonamides and antibiotics.

By the time the war ended, 100,000 nurses had volunteered and 76,000 served in the Army or Navy nurse corps.[73] By the end of the war, nurses had served in 50 countries around the world and had varied experiences. In the Philippines, 66 nurses remained behind after evacuation and became Japanese prisoners; 37 months later they were freed when Americans recaptured the area.[74]

During World War II, military nurses saw both their status and rank change. In 1920, Army nurses had been given equal rank to men, but not equal salary. In 1942, Navy nurses were given equal status and rank, and both Navy and Army nurses were granted equal pay. In 1947, full commissioned status was granted. The segregation of black nurses also ended. Later, in 1954, the last evidence of segregation was dropped by the Army, and male nurses were admitted to the service with full officer rank.[75–78]

The war also led to more freedom for women. When the men were serving overseas, many women supported the war industry by assuming jobs and roles traditionally held by men. Nurses served at the front and were wounded and killed. Nurses received a great deal of favorable publicity and were heroines.

Civilian nurses at home rose to meet the needs of the country. In some instances, because of lack of adequate staff, they had to assume roles beyond the traditional nursing role. To alleviate this situation, the Red Cross developed a program to train volunteer nurses' aides. By the end of 1945, 212,000 women had been certified as aides and contributed millions of hours of service in hospitals.[79] Nurses, to use the services of these aides effectively, were forced to define which nursing actions were skilled and which were not.

Post-World War II

Some changes brought about by the war resulted in definite gains for nursing. Schools improved and educators were more highly educated. Federal scholarships were made available for nurses, and salaries were raised. As integration of the races in nursing schools increased, black nurses were commissioned in the armed services. Men and married students were admitted into nursing schools. Use of nonprofessional workers became accepted.

The changes mentioned above were expected to increase the number of nurses practicing in hospitals and in public health, but this was not the case. The nursing shortage grew worse instead of better because of a drop in the number of students entering nursing school, attrition of nurses in the field, marriage, childbirth, retirement, etc., and a reduction in the number of nursing aides. Hospitals were forced to reduce their admissions primarily because of the lack of adequate nursing staff. But at the same time, public health needs for medical care were increasing.

Further complicating the shortage, was a reorganization of the general hospital into specialized units, such as recovery rooms, surgical units, and medical units. This concept eliminated the traditional pattern of separating clients by clinical diagnosis, sex, or economic status. Furthermore, each new type of unit required varying nurse–client ratios and specialized nursing care.

Because of the shortage of nurses, practical nurse education and licensing were promoted by the National Association for Practical Nurse Education, formed during World War II with the backing of the public, doctors, and many nurses. By the close of 1947, half of the states had established procedures for licensing practical nurses (L.P.N.). Professional nurses recognized their responsibility for assisting in teaching and supervising L.P.N.s and designed courses and standards for them. Another outcome of the nursing shortage was the hiring of nurses from other countries by some agencies. Use of nursing aides and volunteers also increased during the postwar years.

The concept of team nursing developed as a means of providing quality nursing care for all clients who required it. Agencies may define the term somewhat differently, but basically, the staff on a health-care agency unit is divided into districts. Each team is responsible for the care of the clients in its district, and each team has a designated leader who organizes the work for the rest of the nursing team. Composition of the team depends on agency policy and scheduling but is generally composed of other nurses, L.P.N.s, and nursing assistants. The team members usually do most of the hands-on care, with the leader supervising. This enables fewer professional nurses to be responsible for larger numbers of clients.

Unique features of the concept of team nursing included direct supervision of all clients and team members by a professional nurse; team conferences for planning and problem solving; continuity of care through individualized care plans; and on-site in-service training for team members.

The Korean War

The outbreak of the Korean War on June 25, 1950, once again placed demands on nurses. At the beginning of this conflict, there were only about 5000 nurses in the Army and Navy Nurse Corps and another 6000 on reserve. The Air Force Nurse Corps was just beginning, celebrating its first anniversary in July, 1950. It was faced with mobilizing a large number of nurses to assist in air evacuation of battle casualties from the war zone.

Korea served as a test for the MASH units. These units were equipped with over 100 highly trained individuals including at least 15 physicians, 16 nurses, and 120 support persons. These units were located from 8 to 20 miles from the front lines; because of prompt medical care, many deaths from battle wounds were prevented. The mortality rate from war wounds in Korea was half the corresponding rate from World War II.

Another factor contributing to the reduced casualty death rate was the air evacuation of the severely wounded to the hospitals. Flight nurses and medics provided patient care in the planes used for patient transport. These flight nurses assumed some battlefield risks of soldiers, including the possibility of air attacks, ground fire, and sabotage from North Korean wounded who were treated in the MASH units and transported to hospitals.

When the war was finally ended in July, 1953, medical science had advanced through the development of the ability to give highly skilled and technical medical care on or near the battlefront. Nurses had been a part of this effort and made many contributions to it.

The Vietnam War

American involvement in Southeast Asia occurred during the Truman era, when in 1950 President Truman sent a 35-person military advisory team to assist the French in their battle against the North Vietnamese. Following the defeat of a French garrison at Dien Bien Phu in 1954, France and North Vietnam agreed to partition Vietnam, contingent on free reunification elections. The South Vietnamese government refused, indicating that free elections would not be possible in the North. The following year, President Eisenhower offered South Vietnam economic aid and assistance in training the Army. By 1960, the North had formed the National Liberation Front of South Vietnam (Viet Cong) and terrorism in the South increased. During the next few years, the number of American "military advisors" in South Vietnam continued to increase from 2000 in 1961 to over

15,000 by the end of 1963. American nurses arrived in Vietnam in 1962. Of these 300 military nurses, 200 were Army nurses assigned to the Eighth Field Hospital at Nha Trang, 37 were Air Force flight nurses, 39 were Navy, of whom 29 were aboard a hospital ship. The number of female Army nurses reached a peak of 900 in 1964. A congressional bill authorized the appointment of male nurses to the Army, Navy, and Air Force Nurse Corps and was approved by the president in 1966. By the end of 1967, 1032 men had joined the Army Nurse Corps making up 22 percent of the Army's nurse population.

This war was different from previous wars in that no traditional front lines could be defined. This was due to the guerrilla tactics used by the Viet Cong. The American strategy included dividing the country into different zones, each one patrolled from a central camp. Hospitals therefore were more permanent than the MASH units used in Korea and the temporary field hospitals of World War II. Also, since it was difficult to secure roads in Vietnam, hospitals could not use ground evacuation of wounded. It became necessary to use helicopters. Despite such problems, medical care supplied to the wounded was rapid and complete. About 98 percent of those who were hospitalized for wounds, injuries, or diseases recovered, while about 90 percent of these returned to duty. The death rate of Vietnam was about 1.5 percent for those Americans who were hospitalized following injury.

Nurses have, to one degree or another, always been at the battlefront during times of war. Despite enemy attacks, nurses at the front have always risked their lives in caring for the ill and wounded.

NURSING EDUCATION

In the 1700s and early 1800s, most nurses in America were associated with religious communities. Catholic nursing orders, such as the Ursuline Sisters, based in France, trained their own nurses and established themselves in various settlements throughout the New World. In addition to these nursing sisters, other women who provided services to the sick were either family members or hired servants. Guided by practical experience and home remedies, they varied greatly in their abilities and skill. The term "nurse" was applied to anyone hired to care for ill people.[80]

The first organized attempt to train nurses in the United States began in 1839 in Philadelphia.[81] A Philadelphia physician, Dr. Joseph Warrington, organized a number of elementary classes for nurses that included medical lectures and practice on mannequins.[82] In 1862, a training program was organized for nurses at the Women's Hospital of Philadelphia.[83] This six-month program was required of all nurses who were hired to work at the hospital, and although no diploma was awarded, the graduates were recognized as trained nurses.[84] In 1873, Linda Richards was recognized as the first nurse to graduate from a training program in the United States. She attended a year-long program at the New England Hospital for Women and Children in Boston.[85]

The Civil War (1861–1865) acted as a catalyst in bringing the need for more highly skilled nurses to the attention of society. In 1873, three important schools of nursing were founded: Bellevue Hospital School of Nursing (New York City), Massachusetts General Hospital School of Nursing (Boston), and the Connecticut Training School in New Haven. All were based on the Nightingale model established for nurses in England.[86]

Hospital Diploma Schools

The Nightingale model was a hospital-based apprenticeship program that provided instruction in scientific principles and practical experience for skills mastery. Lectures were generally given by the hospital medical staff, and there was a contractual agreement between the school and the hospital to ensure teaching facilities.[87,88]

The three early American schools differed from the English model principally in terms of financial backing. The American schools had some independent backing but not the larger endowments afforded to schools in the English system. As a direct consequence of this, the American schools became more dependent on their associated hospital institutions. To offset costs associated with the presence of student nurses, the hospitals required a certain amount

of ward work in exchange for room, board, and instruction. As client care improved with the addition of student nurses, hospitals began to enjoy a better reputation and greater financial rewards. Nursing, too, became more respectable as a working opportunity for women, and many were attracted to the field. Hospital schools of nursing flourished, and by 1890, there were 15 schools; by 1900, over 400.

Compared to conditions during most of the 1800s, these turn-of-the-century diploma schools represented a grat deal of change for the status of nursing and certainly for the status of hospitals. The education components of these schools, however, were not given a high priority, and formal instruction was often lacking or nonexistent. There is considerable documentation supporting the view that hospital diploma schools existed primarily for the benefit of the hospital enterprise and not for the education of nurses.[89] Mastery of ward procedures was the emphasis, and it was not unusual for students to staff all areas of the hospital including kitchens, laundries, and supply departments.[90]

Nursing leaders recognized early in the twentieth century that this system of nursing education was inadequate to prepare nurses for professional nursing practice.[91] A number of nurse leaders such as Isabel Hampton Robb, Mary Adelaide Nutting, and Annie Goodrich all worked to enlighten both nurses and the public about the need for educational reform. Professional organizations and nursing school alumni groups were formed; many of these became active in calling for changes in nurse training programs and furthering the ideas of licensure and accreditation.

The various landmark studies described earlier dealt largely with issues of nursing education. The Goldmark Report, for example, noted that the majority of nursing schools failed to provide an education equivalent to that in other professions and that a primary reason for this lack was insufficient funds allocated for education by hospitals.[92,93]

Additional studies recommended major changes in nursing education, but there was very little support for implementing any of them. Hospitals were very protective of their nursing schools and were reluctant to support changes that would give them less control. For prospective students, hospital diploma schools offered an attractive arrangement financially. Most students or their families did not have the means to pay for an education. The general public continued to be pleased with the tremendous strides in the quality of hospital care and were not particularly involved with, aware of, or concerned about the status of nursing education. Also, society's attitude toward the role of women and higher education for women was a factor in the inertia.

The diploma model for nursing education continued to predominate for over 60 years. During this time there were educational improvements, and by early 1940, nursing school standards were being enforced by state boards of nurse examiners. Some schools had associations with universities or colleges, and the average length of the programs had increased from one to three years.

The mid-twentieth century diploma nursing school curriculum was typically 36 months in length and prepared nurses for roles in hospitals and similar inpatient settings. Graduates were skilled in carrying out tasks associated with bedside care and assisting physicians with procedures and other aspects of medical care. Nursing courses followed a disease-oriented framework (the medical model) and many programs offered introductory courses in the social as well as biological sciences. Students continued to rotate clinically through most departments in the hospital, and some schools offered introductory experiences in public health and psychiatric nursing outside the hospital setting. Clinical rotations typically included evening, night, and weekend hours. Students commonly lived in a nurse residence or dormitory within the hospital and were required to meet a number of personal as well as educational qualifications.

Collegiate Education in Nursing

The movement of nursing education from hospitals to colleges and universities took a long time. During the period when diploma schools were flourishing, a few early collegiate programs did become established. In 1909, the University of Minnesota established what is considered the first nursing program to be administered wholly within a university setting.[94,95] The Yale School of Nursing was established in 1923 and is considered the first autonomous collegiate school of nursing in the United States. The movement grew slowly, but by 1940 there were 76 baccalaureate nursing programs in the United States.[96] Almost all of these programs were specialized for public health nursing or for administration, teaching, and supervision in hospitals and schools of nursing.[97]

In the period following World War II, colleges and universities began to expand, and significant gains were made in establishing collegiate nursing programs.[98] The success of the Cadet Nurse Corps, established to meet the nursing needs of the military during the war, also helped associate nursing with higher education. Nurses trained within this program spent their first nine months in a university setting learning the basic sciences and fundamentals of nursing.[99] After the war, many of these nurse veterans took advantage of the G.I. Bill of Rights and continued their education.

At this time, baccalaureate programs in nursing varied significantly in curriculum, content, and quality of faculty. In 1948, the Brown Report called for the stratification of nursing and nursing education into practical and professional, the latter taking place firmly within the collegiate setting. The report further recommended upgrading all present programs and faculty, mandatory inclusion of psychiatric nursing preparation in baccalaureate programs, public financing of nursing education, and instituting a system of accreditation of nursing schools.[100–102]

The recommendations set forth in the Brown Report had far-reaching effects in promoting baccalaureate education for nursing. Efforts to accredit nursing schools were accelerated, and the task of identifying appropriate and acceptable curriculum content was begun.

During the 1950s, two distinct types of baccalaureate nursing programs developed. The first was called the basic degree program and was designed for students who had no previous education in nursing. The second type was usually called a general nursing program and was designed for diploma graduates or nurses who had been trained in other kinds of programs.[103] By 1957 these latter programs had been discontinued, and diploma graduates were admitted to regular college programs with advanced standing.[104] Curricula began to emphasize more liberal arts.

The year 1965 was a landmark in the history of nursing education. The ANA, after several years of study and research, took a firm public stand on collegiate education for nursing. In an official position paper published in December of 1965, the ANA Committee on Education recommended that the baccalaureate degree be the minimal educational preparation for professional nurses.[105] A distinction was made between professional nursing practice and technical nursing practice. Professional nursing practice was described as theory oriented rather than technique oriented and involved coordination of illness prevention and health maintenance as well as aspects of caring and curing.[106] This type of practice was further described as having a responsibility to supervise, teach, and direct all those who give nursing care.[107] Technical nursing practice was described as centering around specific nursing measures and medically delegated techniques, which were carried out with a high degree of competency and skill. The minimum preparation recommended for technical nursing practice was the associate degree.

Although the issue of collegiate versus diploma education had always been controversial, the ANA paper intensified feelings and heightened conflicts of opinion. Prior to this, the issue had been merely a topic to consider for most nurses. With such a strong statement from the major professional nursing organization, diploma nurses in particular felt threatened and confused. Hospital administrators and many nurse administrators were angry. Instead of fostering collaboration and cooperative planning among nurses, the position paper "became an issue that, to this day, has caused polarization between nurse educators and nursing service administrators and a divisive force in the profession as a whole."[108]

Despite the stormy controversy and resentment generated by the position paper, it has proven to have profound effects in its proposal to end an age-old conflict. Since 1965, diploma schools have steadily declined and college and university programs have taken their place.

The Lysaught Report. In 1968, the National Commission for the Study of Nursing and Nursing Education (NCSNNE) was founded. Fully supported by the ANA and the National League for Nursing, this commission launched a comprehensive study to analyze how nursing and nursing education could be improved to meet the health care needs of society.[109] The results of this study, commonly known as the Lysaught Report, was published in 1970 as *An Abstract for Action.* Dr. Jerome P. Lysaught was project director of the study. The Lysaught Report identified three major problems in nursing education: a shortage of qualified faculty, inadequate and outmoded facilities, and a lack of funds and financing for schools of nursing.[110] Final recommendations included increasing research efforts regarding nursing practice and nursing education, improving the educational environment based on findings from this research, and clarifying professional roles.

The Lysaught Report was a credible study, and the majority of nursing organizations, allied health professions, and other public interest groups supported and applauded the recommendations. The commission was funded for three more years for the purpose of attempting to initiate some of the recommendations. In light of a history of commissioned studies and the landmark studies resulting in little followup action, it was clear to nursing leaders that bona fide changes were not only necessary, but were crucial for both nursing and society. A second Lysaught Report, *From Abstract into Action,* published in 1973, detailed a number of positive accomplishments, among them the establishment of statewide master planning committees in nine target states to promote nursing education within the mainstream of general education.[111]

In the meantime, and despite the upsurge of two-year associate degree nursing (A.D.N.) programs, bachelor of science nursing (B.S.N.) programs have made significant gains in the periods following the ANA Position Paper and the Lysaught Reports. In 1982 there were 393 B.S.N. programs in the United States.[112] These programs are fully collegiate in the sense that the university or college administration is responsible for creating the major in nursing, overseeing the planning for course selection and faculty appointment, and assigning credit. Educational standards and policies are consistent with other academic programs offered by the institution.

B.S.N. programs are generally four years in length and include courses in the biological, physical, and social sciences, the humanities, and nursing practice.

The general aim of these programs is to prepare nurses as general health-care providers and for potential leadership positions in nursing. Graduates are prepared to give nursing care to people of all ages and in all types of settings. Emphasis is placed on health promotion and illness prevention in addition to the clinical nursing care of people who are ill.

Associate Degree Nursing Programs. One of the effects of the 1965 position paper was the proliferation of associate degree nursing programs. The idea for these technically oriented nursing curricula was born in the early 1950s, when small community-based junior colleges began to flourish. Mildred Montag proposed the first plan in her doctoral thesis, *Education of Nursing Technicians,* published in 1951. A pilot research study was undertaken in 1952 by Teacher's College, Columbia University, and included seven junior colleges and six hospitals.[113] The study results were released in 1957 and demonstrated that nurses could be educated totally within an academic setting, be technically and competently trained as bedside nurses, and successfully pass the state board licensing examination for registered nurses.

The number of A.D.N. programs expanded rapidly, and by 1985 there were 776 accredited schools.[114] The early A.D.N. curriculum was characterized by a ratio of one general education course to one nursing theory course. More recently the ratio is closer to one general education course to two nursing courses. Some programs require one or two summer sessions, in addition. Associate degree programs now are in the majority. Chapter 2 provides a comparative view of the three types of nursing programs in 1982.

A.D.N. programs clearly have filled the need to train more bedside nurses and have been a strong motivating force in moving nursing education out of the hospital and into the college.

Graduate Education. Graduate education for nurses has existed since 1899, when Columbia University Teachers College established a program for nursing leaders.[115] Most of the early programs that followed were highly specialized and generally not consistent. Some were nearly all clinical, and others just the opposite.[116]

In the 1950s a number of attempts were made to organize graduate education. The National League for Nursing sponsored several conferences for the purpose of formulating guidelines for organization, administration, curriculum, and testing in masters education in nursing. In 1955, the master's degree was termed the "second professional degree for nurses," and the National League for Nursing identified specialization and research as its primary focus.[117]

Graduate education on both the master's and doctoral levels has received increasing attention since the 1960s. Programs are available in nearly all areas of the United States for nurses who want to pursue additional education in teaching, administration, research, and specialized practice. Today, programs that lead to a master's degree in nursing provide students with an opportunity to[118]:

- Acquire advanced knowledge from the sciences and humanities to support advanced nursing practice and role development
- Expand their knowledge of nursing theory as a basis for advanced nursing practice
- Develop expertise in a specialized area of clinical nursing practice
- Acquire the knowledge and skills related to a specific functional role in nursing, e.g., teaching, administration, management
- Acquire competence in conducting research
- Plan and initiate change in the health-care system and in the practice and delivery of health care
- Further develop and implement leadership strategies for the betterment of health care
- Actively engage in collaborative relationships with others for the purpose of improving health care
- Acquire a foundation for doctoral study

Doctoral programs were slow to develop, as they depended on the efforts of nurses who were prepared at the doctoral level in other disciplines. The first doctoral program in nursing was established at Teachers College, Columbia University, in 1920, and until 1961 there were only three such programs in the United States.[119] At present, there are 44 programs that lead to the doctoral degree. These programs offer one of three types of degrees: the Doctor of Nursing Science (D.N.Sc.), the Doctor of Education (Ed.D.), and the Doctor of Philosophy (Ph.D.).[120]

Doctoral work is highly specialized, focusing on research and the development of scientific theory in nursing. Many faculties of nursing now require the doctoral degree, and there is increasing recognition that doctoral preparation is necessary for the attainment of true professional status.

Reform in nursing education continues into the 1980s. Although the idea of collegiate education has rooted itself firmly as the emerging entry level to practice, much needs to be done. Having more than one type of basic preparatory program, for example, is confusing to both nurses and the public. In addition, service-oriented programs (diploma schools) tend to increase the cost of health care and penalize graduates in terms of educational mobility.

Many influences in today's society point nursing toward a clear and unified approach to education. Various professional, political, and socioeconomic trends, as well as new advances in the health-care system, are forcing the related issues of quality care and competence in nursing. As the result of these influences, the issue of nursing education will, it is hoped, be placed on a more defined and unified path, one that is acceptable and accessible to both nursing and the needs of society.

SUMMARY

The history of nursing goes far back into early civilization, although most accounts begin with Florence Nightingale's work in the 1800s. Nightingale is known as the founder of modern nursing; through her ideas and efforts the practice of nursing was organized. She laid the groundwork for nursing as a theory-based profession with its own body of knowledge.

It is important for contemporary nurses to understand the influences of Nightingale and the many nurse leaders who followed her. These early nurse leaders gave a richness to the profession that has helped to shape the practice of nursing today.

Over the years, various organizations and groups have undertaken studies on the state of nursing in America. Several of these studies have been characterized as landmark studies.

Study Questions

1. List several ways in which history affected the development of nursing in America.

2. What were Florence Nightingale's contributions to nursing?

3. What are some factors that have helped nursing evolve toward professional status?

4. How did the status of women affect nursing?

References

1. Deborah M. Jensen, *History and Trends of Professional Nursing*, 4th ed. (St. Louis: C.V. Mosby Co., 1959).
2. M. Louise Fitzpatrick, *Prologue to Professionalism* (Bowie, MD: R.J. Brady Co., 1983), 2.
3. A.C. Kaviratna, transl., *Charaka-Samhita*, n.d., 102–103.
4. Ibid, 103.
5. K.K.C. Bhishagratna, transl., *The Sushruta Samhita.* (Calcutta: J.N. Base, 1907), 305–307.
6. R.H. Shyrock, *The History of Nursing: An Interpretation of the Social and Medical Factors Involved* (Philadelphia: W.B. Saunders Co., 1959), 26.
7. T.E. Christy, *Historical Perspectives on Accountability*, in J.A. Williamson (ed.), *Current Perspectives in Nursing Education* (St. Louis: C.V. Mosby Co., 1976), 3.
8. Patricia Donahue, *Nursing: The Finest Art* (St. Louis: C.V. Mosby Co., 1985), 141.
9. M. Adelaide Nutting and Lavinia L. Dock, *A History of Nursing*, vol. II (New York: G.P. Putnam's Sons, 1937).
10. J. Howard, *An Account of the Principle Lazarettos in Europe.* (London: Johnson, Dilly, & Cadel, 1791).

11. Jensen, *History and Trends*, 91.
12. Isabel M. Stewart and Anne L. Austin, *A History of Nursing: From Ancient Times, A World View*, 5th ed (New York: G.P. Putnam's Sons, 1962), 101.
13. Sr. Charles Marie Frank, *Foundations of Nursing* (Philadelphia: W.B. Saunders Co., 1959), 98–99.
14. Annie Matheson, *Forence Nightingale* (London: T. Nelson & Sons, 1913), 137.
15. Cecil Woodham-Smith, *Florence Nightingale, 1820–1910* (New York: McGraw-Hill Book Co., 1951), 66.
16. Ibid., 63.
17. F.T. Smith, "Florence Nightingale: Early Feminist," *Am J Nurs, 81* (May 1981):1021–24.
18. Stewart and Austin, *History of Nursing*, 101.
19. J.A. Dolon, *History of Nursing*, 12th ed. (Philadelphia: W.B. Saunders Co., 1968), 215–16.
20. Florence Nightingale, *Notes on Nursing, What It Is and What It Is Not* (New York: Appleton & Co., 1860), 65.
21. Bonnie Bullough and Vern Bullough. *The Emergence of Modern Nursing* (New York: Macmillan Co., 1969).
22. Philip A. Kalisch and Beatrice J. Kalisch, *The Advances of American Nursing*, 2nd ed. (Boston: Little, Brown, & Co., 1986), 18.
23. Ibid., 24.
24. Jensen. *History and Trends*, 183.
25. Kalisch and Kalisch, *The Advances of American Nursing*, 62.
26. Lois R. Wiggins, "The Nurse's Cap, Symbol of a Proud Profession," *J Prac Nurs* 23 (January 1973):22–23.
27. Kalisch and Kalisch, *The Advances of American Nursing*, 141.
28. Agnes G. Deans and Anne L. Austin, *The History of the Farrand Training School for Nurses* (Detroit: Alumnae Association of the Farrand Training School for Nurses, 1936), 58.
29. G.J. Griffin and H.J. Griffin, *History and Trends of Professional Nursing*, 7th ed (St. Louis: C.V. Mosby Co., 1975) p. 87.
30. E. Ware, *Transcript of Interview* by C. Schofield (Baltimore: Johns Hopkins Archives, 1939).
31. Teresa E. Christy, "Nurses in American History: The Fateful Decade, 1890–1900," *Am J Nurs* 75 (July 1975):1163–65.
32. Fitzpatrick, *Prologue to Professionalism*, 223.
33. Teresa E. Christy, "Portrait of a Leader: Isabel Hampton Robb," *Nurs Outlook* 17 (March 1969):26–29.
34. Jensen, *History and Trends*, 106.
35. Lillian D. Wald, *The House on Henry Street* (New York: Henry Hall & Co., 1938), 4–8.
36. Teresa E. Christy, "Portrait of a Leader: Lavinia Lloyd Dock," *Nurs Outlook* 17 (June 1969):72–75.
37. Lavinia L. Dock, *Textbook on Materia Medica for Nurses* (New York: G.P. Putnam's Sons, 1890).
38. Mary M. Roberts, "Lavinia Lloyd Dock—Nurse, Feminist, Internationalist," *Am J Nurs* 56 (February 1956):176–79.
39. Helen L. Bundge, "Research is Every Professional Nurses' Business," *Nurs Res* 7 (1958):816.
40. Louise C. Smith, *Helen L. Bundge* (Madison, Wisconsin: School of Nursing, University of Wisconsin, 1979), 1–4.
41. Lois R. Wiggins, "Lydia Hall's Place in the Development of Theory in Nursing," *Image* 12 (February 1980):10–12.
42. "Progress in Nursing Education," Editorial, *Am J Nurs* 19 (1919):220–22.
43. Report of the Committee on Nursing Education, Editorial, *Am J Nurs* 22 (1922):878–80.
44. Lucie Y. Kelly, *Dimensions of Professional Nursing*, 4th ed. (New York: Macmillan Co., 1981).
45. Josephine Goldmark, *Nursing and Nursing Education in the United States, Report of the Committee for the Study of Nursing*. (New York: Macmillan Co., 1923).
46. Ibid.
47. Committee on the Grading of Nursing Schools, *Nurses, Patients, and Pocketbooks* (New York: Committee on Grading of Nursing Schools, 1928), 17.
48. Fitzpatrick, *Prologue to Professionalism*, 224.
49. Committee on the Grading of Nursing Schools, *Nurses, Patients, and Pocketbooks*, 20.
50. "Nurses, Patients, and Pocketbooks," *Am J Nurs* 28 (July 1928):674–76.
51. M.A. Burgess, "The First Grading," *Am J Nurs* 29 (1929):429–34.
52. Ibid., 429–32.
53. Fitzpatrick, *Prologue to Professionalism*, 228.
54. Esther Lucille Brown, *Nursing for the Future* (New York: Russell Sage Foundation, 1948), 2.
55. Ibid., 1–2.
56. Sr. Charles Marie Frank, *The Historical Development of Nursing* (Philadelphia: W.B. Saunders Co., 1953), 339–47.
57. Fitzpatrick, *Prologue of Professionalism*, 236.
58. *Planning for Nursing Needs and Resources* (Bethesda, Maryland, Division of Nursing, U.S.

Department of Health, Education, and Welfare, Bureau of Health Manpower Education).

59. Ibid.
60. Fitzpatrick, *Prologue to Professionalism,* 44–45.
61. Griffin and Griffin, *History and Trends,* 166–69.
62. Annie W. Goodrich, "The Contribution of the Army School of Nursing" in the *National League of Nursing Education,* Annual Report, 1919, and *Proceedings of the 25th Convention* (Baltimore: Wilkins & Wilkins, 1919), 146–56.
63. Bullough and Bullough, *The Emergence of Modern Nursing,* 169.
64. Griffin and Griffin, *History and Trends,* 168.
65. Fitzpatrick, *Prologue to Professionalism,* 28.
66. M. Louise Fitzpatrick, "Nursing and the Great Depression," *Am J Nurs* 75 (December 1975):2188–90.
67. Bullough and Bullough, *The Emergence of Modern Nursing,* 189.
68. Philip A. Kalisch and Beatrice J. Kalisch, "From Training to Education: The Impact of Federal Aid on Schools of Nursing in the United States During the 1940s," Final Report of NIH, U.S. Public Health Research Grant, N.U. 00443 (Ann Arbor: University of Michigan, 1974).
69. Beatrice J. Kalisch and Philip A. Kalisch, "The Cadet Nurse Corps—in World War II," *Am J Nurs* 76 (February 1976):240–42.
70. Ibid.
71. Beatrice J. Kalisch and Philip A. Kalisch, "Slaves, Servants or Saints," (An Analysis of the System of Nurse Training in The United States, 1873–1948), *Nurs Forum* 14 (1973):222–63.
72. Ibid., 242.
73. "The Nurses' Contribution to American Victory Facts and Figures from Pearl Harbor" *Am J Nurs* 45 (September 1945):683–86.
74. A.R. Clarke, "Thirty-seven Months as a Prisoner of War," *Am J Nurs* 45 (May 1945): 342–45.
75. Bullough and Bullough, *The Emergence of Modern Nursing,* 190.
76. E.A. Aynes, *From Nightingale to Eagle: An Army Nurse's History,* (Englewood Cliffs, NJ: Prentice-Hall, 1973).
77. J.O. Flikke, *Nurses in Action* (Philadelphia: J.B. Lippincott, 1943).
78. Bonnie Bullough, "The Lasting Impact of World War II on Nursing," *Am J Nurs* 76 (January 1976):116–20.
79. Kalisch and Kalisch, *The Advances of American Nursing,* 192–94.
80. Fitzpatrick, *Prologue to Professionalism,* 58.
81. Deborah M. Jensen, *A History of Nursing* (St. Louis: C.V. Mosby Co., 1943), 155.
82. Ibid., 155.
83. Fitzpatrick, *Prologue to Professionalism,* 61, 62.
84. Ibid.
85. Ibid.
86. Bonnie Bullough and Vern Bullough, "Educational Problems In a Women's Profession," *J Nurs Educ* 20 (September 1981):6–17.
87. Ibid.
88. Joann Ashley, *Hospitals, Paternalism, and the Role of the Nurse* (New York: Teachers College Press, Columbia University, 1977), 8, 9.
89. Ibid.
90. Fitzpatrick, *Prologue to Professionalism.*
91. "American Nurses' Association's First Position on Education for Nursing," *Am J Nurs* 65 (December 1965):109
92. Fitzpatrick, *Prologue to Professionalism,* 216–22.
93. Ibid.
94. Lillian DeYoung, *Dynamics of Nursing* (St. Louis: C.V. Mosby Co., 1981), 92.
95. Fitzpatrick, *Prologue to Professionalism,* 71.
96. Bullough and Bullough, "Educational Problems," 6–17.
97. DeYoung, *Dynamics of Nursing,* 95.
98. Bullough and Bullough "Educational Problems," 6.
99. Fitzpatrick, *Prologue to Professionalism,* 74.
100. Ibid., 236.
101. Ibid., 235–39.
102. Brown, *Nursing for the Future.*
103. DeYoung, *Dynamics of Nursing,* 89.
104. *Mosby's Comprehensive Review of Nursing,* 10th ed. (St. Louis: C.V. Mosby Co., 1981), 486.
105. "ANA Position Paper," *Am J Nurs* 1965, 107.
106. Ibid., 107.
107. Ibid., 108.
108. Fitzpatrick, *Prologue to Professionalism,* 246.
109. Jerome P. Lysaught, *An Abstract for Action,* Report of National Commission for the Study of Nursing and Nursing Education (New York: McGraw-Hill Book Co., 1970).
110. Ibid.
111. Fitzpatrick, *Prologue to Professionalism,* 254.
112. AACN, Washington D.C. Oct 1987, personal communication.
113. Fitzpatrick, *Prologue to Professionalism,* 92–94.
114. National League for Nursing Statistics, 1982.
115. Stewart and Austin, *A History of Nursing,* 205.
116. Janie H. Brown, "Masters Education in Nursing 1945–1969," in *Historical Studies in Nurs-*

ing by M. Louise Fitzpatrick (New York: Teachers College Press, 1977), 112.

117. Ibid., 111.

118. National League for Nursing, *Characteristics of Graduate Education in Nursing Leading to a Masters Degree* (New York: National League for Nursing, 1978).

119. Fitzpatrick, *Prologue to Professionalism*, 83.

120. AACN, Washington D.C. Oct 1987, personal communication.

Annotated Bibliography

Baer, E.D. 1985. Nursing's divided house—an historical view. *Nurs Res,* 34(1):32–38. Historical analysis of data was used in this study to examine the nature and scope of the divisions in nursing in America in the last third of the nineteenth century. The author presents the story of nursing's reform origins, the post-Civil War social context, and explains changes relevant to women during this time of social turbulence.

Berges, F., and Berges C. 1986. A visit to Scutari. *Am J Nurs* 86(7):811–13. The authors of this article give an account of their visit to the quarters where Florence Nightingale lived during the Crimean war. They also provide a historical account of the lives of men who were wounded in the Crimean War.

Carnegie, M.E. 1986. *The Path We Tread. Blacks in Nursing, 1954–1984.* Philadelphia: Lippincott. The author of this book presents the reader with the contributions of black nurses, both past and present, and their influence on the development of professional nursing.

Curtis, D.E. 1985. The Way It Was. *Am J Nurs* 85(10):1253–54. The author of this article gives a first-hand account of nursing during World War II.

Donahue, M.P. 1985. *Nursing: The Finest Art.* St. Louis: C.V. Mosby. This coffee-table-sized book is designed to be a classic nursing book. It contains an illustrated history of nursing and is unique in its reliance on art to present that history.

Fitzpatrick, M.L. 1983. *Prologue to Professionalism.* Norwalk, Conn.: Appleton-Century-Crofts. This book was designed to provide the reader with a historical background of nursing in order to understand the profession today. Included are such topics as: nursing education, professional organizations, nursing practice, and accreditation in nursing. Simulated nursing care plans are included, depicting nursing care during various stages of nursing development.

Flanagan, L., comp. 1986. *One Strong Voice.* Kansas City, Mo.: American Nurses' Association. This book was prepared by the ANA to review the impact the role of nursing has had on health care from the time of the Revolution to 1976.

Kalisch, P.A., and Kalisch B.J. 1986. *The Advance of Modern Nursing.* 2nd ed. Boston: Little, Brown. This excellent text provides a comprehensive analysis of the transition of nursing into a profession. It includes hundreds of photographs and drawings concerning health care and nursing from ancient times to the present.

Nightingale, F. 1859, 1984. *Notes on Nursing.* London: Harrison & Sons (facsimile reproduced by Lippincott). This classic book was designed for women, who were responsible for children and households to tell them how to nurse. Its focus is on hygiene. This 76-page book is very interesting and highly readable, especially for those interested in Nightingale and the history of nursing.

Nutting M.A., and Dock L.L. 1912. *A History of Nursing.* New York: Putnam's. This classic four-volume collection contains a description of the evolution of nursing from prehistory to the early twentieth century. It includes interesting drawings and photographs.

Reverby, S. 1987. The caring dilemma: Womanhood and nursing in historical perspective. *Nurs Res* 36(1):5–11. This excellent article gives a broad overview of the concept of caring and considers the impact of Nightingale and the changes in the profession of nursing.

Richards, L.A.J. 1911. *Reminiscences of Linda Richards, America's First Trained Nurse.* Boston: Whitcomb & Barrows. In this short book, the experiences of a nurse in the 1800s are described, and a fascinating picture of the role of the nurse during this early period of American nursing is given.

The Way We Nursed. 1985. *Am J Nurs* 85(10):1119–34. This article written for the 85th Anniversary of *AJN* offers excerpts from the first half of this century. This article is interesting and fun to read.

Woodham-Smith, C. 1951, 1983. *Florence Nightingale.* New York: McGraw-Hill. (reprinted New York: Atheneum). This thorough biography is one of the most complete on Nightingale.

Chapter 2

Contemporary Nursing

Phyllis B. Heffron

Chapter Outline

- Objectives
- Glossary
- Introduction
- Health and Illness
- Definitions of Nursing
- Trends in Nursing Education
  Entry into Practice
  Nursing School Enrollments
  Graduate Education, Master's Level
  Graduate Education, Doctoral Level
- Nursing Roles
  Episodic Nursing Roles
  Distributive Nursing Roles
  The Expanded Role in Nursing
  International Nursing
- Contemporary Issues in Nursing
  Nurse Shortages
  Reality Shock
  Burnout Syndrome
  Computer Technology and Nursing
- Summary
- Study Questions
- References
- Annotated Bibliography

Objectives

At the completion of this chapter the reader will be able to:

▶ Differentiate health and illness as viewed by the medical model and the holistic health model

▶ Compare and contrast three stated definitions of nursing
▶ Identify and describe the different types of nursing programs
▶ Compare and contrast episodic nursing roles with distributive nursing roles
▶ Discuss the meaning of the expanded role in nursing
▶ Discuss international nursing roles
▶ Discuss solutions for the problem of reality shock
▶ Identify relevant issues on the question of nurse shortages
▶ Identify the stages of burnout in an employment situation
▶ Identify four ways in which computers can assist nursing practice.
▶ Discuss the status of graduate-level nursing programs in relation to purpose, focus of content, and enrollment trends

Glossary

Burnout. A stress-induced syndrome affecting experienced nurses characterized by general job frustration, fatigue, depression, irritability, and other physical symptoms.

Dependent Nursing Actions. Actions that nurses carry out as a result of written or verbal orders of others on the health-care team.

Distributive Health Care. Care directed toward health maintenance and illness prevention; usually takes place in an outpatient facility, the home, or community setting.

Episodic Care. Care directed toward a cure that usually takes place in a hospital or other inpatient setting.

Expanded Role. Nursing practice characterized by an ability to assume greater autonomous responsibility and perform nursing skills beyond the level of preparation offered in basic nursing education programs.

Health. A dynamic state of being that moves back and forth on a continuum.

Health-Illness Continuum. A hypothetical, graduated scale intended to measure an individual's total health status, as he or she perceives it.

Illness. A state of being in which an optimal health state, for a variety of reasons, is not being maintained.

Independent Nursing Actions. Those actions performed by nurses based primarily on professional knowledge and judgments.

Independent Nursing Practice. Practice by a registered nurse that takes place in a setting other than traditional institutions or organized health-care systems and/or is carried out by self-employed nurses.

Interdependent Nursing Actions. Those actions that nurses perform in collaboration with others on the health-care team.

Medical Model. A framework of health care based on pathophysiological states, disease classification, and physical diagnosis.

Nurse Practitioner. A registered nurse who has completed a nurse practitioner program (master's or certificate level) beyond basic nursing school; these nurses are qualified to function in an expanded role and have greater decision-making skills in assessment and treatment of health problems.

Nursing Information System. A collection of computerized programs that contain nursing and selected client and medical data. The system may or may not be a part of a larger medical information system used to record, review, monitor, and analyze these data.

Primary Care. Health care that takes place at the time of the client's initial contact with the health-care system or health provider. It usually takes place in an office or clinic setting, but may take place on admission to a hospital.

Primary Nursing. A method of nursing-care delivery whereby one nurse is assigned to coordinate and administer nursing care to an individual client from the time of admission to discharge.

Reality Shock. The experiences and feelings a newly graduated nurse or a nurse returning to the workforce after an extended leave often faces because of differences between expectations of the employer and preparedness of the nurse. Reality shock is partially a result of the quick transition from classroom to workplace.

Wellness. Ever-changing growth toward fulfilling an individual's potential, considering individual needs, abilities, and disabilities.

INTRODUCTION

The concept of contemporary nursing is highly dynamic in character, reflecting the social, political, and health-care climate of the time. Nursing is a complex system with various educational philosophies and levels of meaning. On a primary level it is a professional occupation that provides a unique and vital service to society. It is a scientific discipline that studies and produces information about human beings and their environment, human health, and adaptation. On another level, nursing is a skilled practice that requires intelligence, imagination, logic, and creativity. In addition, it involves a spiritual level, one that embodies warmth and caring, empathy, personal ethics, and the give and take of human sharing.

It is the combination of all these levels, along with history, educational processes, and professional roles that provide nurses with perspectives from which to view and understand the concept of nursing today.

This chapter seeks to explore the concept of present-day nursing through discussion of health and illness, professional definitions, educational requirements, and current roles. Current trends and issues within the nursing community are also discussed.

HEALTH AND ILLNESS

To think about the concept of nursing and what it means to deliver nursing and health care, the basic terms of health and illness, and wellness, need to be understood. These terms describe *subjectively* a person's general state of being and are all relative according to a wide range of variables. Health and illness mean different things to different people but both are a reflection of an individual's physical, physiological, psychological, sociological, and spiritual state at any given time.

Health traditionally has been viewed in terms of the absence of disease, pain, illness, or injury. This framework of thought, commonly referred to as the **medical model,** is based on an organized and precise classification of signs, symptoms, syndromes, and specifically named diseases that represent some type of physiological or psychological pathology. This model has dominated western medical and nursing schools for many years. Hospitals commonly use a medical classification system for assigning clients to rooms. Courses are taught on immunology, cardiology, and ophthalmology. Many health insurance companies require clients to be assigned an official medical or injury code before they can be reimbursed for health care.

In 1971, the World Health Organization (WHO) adopted a new definition of health in its official constitution. The WHO definition was comprehensive, and specifically stated that "health is a state of complete physical, mental, and social well being and not merely the absence of disease or infirmity."[1] During this time period, American consumers were becoming more interested in having a voice in health care, and there was an increasing awareness regarding the effects of social and psychological stress on the body. The holistic health movement, which started in the 1960s, coined the term "high-level wellness"—a concept that expanded and offered a whole new way of approaching health and health care.[2]

According to the holistic health model, **health** is seen as a dynamic state of being that, for each individual, moves back and forth on a continuum. Figure 2–1 illustrates this hypothetical and graduated scale, commonly called the **health-illness continuum.** This scale is intended to measure the total health picture as the individual perceives it—not solely as a judgment by the health-care provider. **Wellness** is defined as ever changing growth toward fulfilling an individual's potential, considering individual needs, abilities, and disabilities.[3] A key assumption in holistic health is that the perception of health is an individual decision, promoting self-responsibility and self-control. Health and **illness** are not mutually exclusive, as defined within this model. A person with a disease process, such as cancer, may place him- or herself at different places along the wellness continuum at different times—including optimal health if the person feels he or she is functioning to his or her highest potential relative to the condition.

The holistic view of health has gained a great deal of popularity among health-care professionals, particularly nurses. In addition to the symptoms and signs of illness, people who assess wellness look at a wide variety of health behaviors. Health behaviors are activities a person does to understand his or her health state, maintain an optimal state of health, prevent illness and injury, and reach maximum physical and mental potential. Behaviors such as eating habits, exercise, attention to signs of illness, following treatment advice, and avoiding known health hazards, such as smoking, are all examples. The ability to relax, emotional maturity, productivity, and self-expression are other

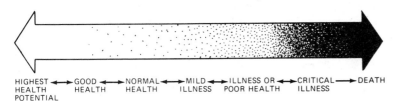

HIGHEST ←→ GOOD ←→ NORMAL ←→ MILD ←→ ILLNESS OR ←→ CRITICAL →DEATH
HEALTH   HEALTH   HEALTH   ILLNESS POOR HEALTH   ILLNESS
POTENTIAL

Figure 2–1. The health-illness continuum.

examples that reflect one's total health picture.

Nurses give health care in a variety of settings; some emphasize a medical orientation to health, such as acute-care facilities, and others emphasize a more holistic approach, such as primary-care clinics, preventive health centers, and specialized agencies like birthing centers and hospices. Many health-care institutions and agencies are a combination of both models of care, and it is often the individual practitioner who sets the tone and assists the client in gaining a realistic understanding of what "health" means in his or her circumstances.

DEFINITIONS OF NURSING

Nursing has been defined in many ways and by many people since its earliest days. There are as many definitions of nursing as there are nursing leaders and state legislatures that license nurses.[4] Others that define nursing include schools of nursing, health-care institutions, and professional organizations.

There was a time when nurses functioned primarily as physician's helpers. At the present time, independent and theory-based practice are emerging characteristics of nursing. Table 2–1 presents a number of selected definitions of nursing in chronological order that reflect some of these changes and provide insight into how people define nursing.

Narrow and Buschle state that the content of a definition of nursing should meet the following criteria[5]:

- Description of its uniqueness
- Consistency with current practices and laws
- Reflection of a philosophy or set of beliefs

Throughout this textbook, the reader will learn about nursing relative to many specific concepts. Each concept contributes ideas that help to define nursing as it is viewed today and will shed light on one or more of the above criteria.

In 1980 the American Nurses' Association (ANA) issued a public statement on the nursing profession that affirmed nursing's social responsibility and delineated the nature and scope of nursing practice. The following definition of nursing was asserted: *Nursing is the diagnosis*

and treatment of human responses to actual or potential health problems.[6] This definition is one that maintains the orientation of nurses to the provision of care that promotes well-being in the people served and, at the same time, reflects the influence of nursing theory.

TRENDS IN NURSING EDUCATION

Chapter One has provided information regarding the historical aspects of nursing education. As American society and the health-care system continue to experience rapid change, the concepts of health-care delivery and roles of health-care providers change also. Inherent in these changes are attempts to modify and restructure the educational systems that prepare health-care professionals. Nursing education, particularly in the area of entry-level program criteria, is no exception, and nursing leaders are currently laying the groundwork for a number of critical changes that could profoundly affect the nursing profession into the next century.

Entry into Practice

Nursing education in the United States continues to comprise three levels of education programs that lead to licensure as a registered nurse. These three levels, two-year (associate degree), three-year (diploma), and four-year (baccalaureate degree), are all well-established programs with their own respective histories, philosophies, curricular designs, and expected practice outcomes for graduates. Table 2–2 gives a current overview of these three programs. The existence of multiple programs, the product of longstanding disagreements on how to best prepare registered nurses, has been a critical issue confronting the profession for many years. Confusion has resulted, particularly regarding the real differences between the three types of graduates and how their abilities and potential employment roles should be categorized. Prospective students are confused as to which program they should choose, employers of nurses are either not sure which type to hire for what job or they make little distinction, and consumers often have no knowledge about the different levels of preparation.

Currently, the impact of this confusion has

TABLE 2–1. SELECTED DEFINITIONS OF NURSING

Source	Definition
Florence Nightingale 1860	Nursing is a noncurative practice in which the patient is put in the best condition possible for nature to act.
Isabel Hampton Robb 1893	The hands of the nurse are the physician's hands lengthened out to minister to the sick. Her watchful presence at the bedside is a trained vigilance supplementing and perfecting his watchful care; her knowledge of his patient's condition an essential element in the diagnosis of disease; her management of the patient, the practical side of medical science. If she fails to appreciate her duties, the physician fails in the same degree to bring aid to his patient.
Education Committee for Curriculum Guide 1917	"Health" nursing is just as fundamental as "sick" nursing and the prevention of disease at least as important a function of the nurse as the care and treatment of the sick. . . . The nurse is essentially a teacher and an agent of health.
Committee on Curriculum of the National League for Nursing Education 1937	The word "nursing" can also be interpreted broadly to mean health conservation in its widest senses, including the care of normal children and adults; the nursing or nurture of the mind and spirit as well as the body; health education as ministration to the sick; the care of the patient's environment, social as well as physical; and health service to families and communities as well as to individuals.
Sister Olivia M. Gowan 1944	Nursing in its broadest sense may be defined as an art and a science which involves the whole patient—body, mind, and spirit; promotes his spiritual, mental, and physical health by teaching and by example; stresses health education and health preservation as well as ministration to the sick; involves the care of the patient's environment—social and spiritual as well as physical; and gives health service to the family and community as well as to the individual.
Frances Reiter 1961	. . . the nature of nursing . . . a disciplined art, an eclectic science and a personal service to patients that has long-term human value and social worth.
Virginia Henderson 1966	The unique function of the nurse is to assist the individual, sick or well, in the performance of those activities contributing to health or its recovery (or to peaceful death) that he would perform unaided if he had the necessary strength, will or knowledge, and to do this in such a way as to help him gain independence as rapidly as possible.
American Nurses' Association Committee for the Study of Credentialing in Nursing 1979	Nursing is defined as a health nurturing discipline: a field of study which encompasses the total occupation of nurturing the health of human beings, sick or well, through assistance with the activities that the human being cannot do or does not have the knowledge to do for himself, or assisting a dying patient to a peaceful death.
Dorothea Orem 1980	Nursing has as its special concern the individual's need for self-care action and the provision and management of it on a continuous basis in order to sustain life and health, recover from disease or injury, and cope with their effects.

Gertrude Torres, "Florence Nightingale" in Nursing Theories (Englewood Cliffs: Prentice Hall, 1980), 29.

Isabel A. Hampton, et al., "Educational Standards for Nurses" in Nursing of the Sick, 1893, Lucille Petry, cons. ed. (New York: McGraw-Hill Book Co., 1949), 2,3.

The Education Committee of the National League for Nursing Education, Standard Curriculum for Nursing Schools (New York: National League for Nursing Education, 1919).

Committee on Curriculum of the National League for Nursing Education, A Curriculum Guide for Schools of Nursing (New York: National League for Nursing Education, 1937).

Sister Olivia M. Gowan. Unpublished papers (The Catholic University of America, School of Nursing, 1944).

Frances Reiter, Improvement of Nursing Practice (New York: American Nurses' Association, 1961).

Virginia Henderson, The Nature of Nursing (New York: Macmillan Co., 1966).

Committee for the Study of Credentialing in Nursing, A New Approach, Staff Working Papers, vol. 2 (Kansas City, Mo.: The American Nurses' Association, 1979).

Dorothea E. Orem, Nursing: Concepts of Practice, 2nd ed. (New York: McGraw-Hill Book Co., 1980).

TABLE 2–2. COMPARATIVE OVERVIEW OF TYPES OF NURSING PROGRAMS

	Diploma	Associate Degree	Baccalaureate Degree
Setting	Hospital/medical center	Community or junior college	College or university
Approximate length of program	3 yr	2 yr	4 yr
Number of schools in 1984	273	777	427
Number of graduates in 1984	12,200	44,394	23,718
Curriculum content (approximate %)	67% nursing courses 33% cognate courses	50% nursing courses 50% cognate courses	30% nursing courses 40% cognate courses 30% liberal arts and other general education courses
General qualities	Students may take room and board at the hospital Clinical experience is introduced early in program and the total time is longer Graduates are prepared as generalists and competency is high at time of graduation Cost of education is relatively low for students	Students usually commute and often are employed part-time during studies Students are highly diversified in age, background, and cultural heritage Students prepared as generalists with emphasis on acute-care settings Graduates have strong technical skills and clinical competency is achieved early	Students commute or live on campus and are exposed to a variety of programs Emphasis is a combination of general and professional education Emphasis in curriculum on leadership roles and independent practice Graduates are prepared for a variety of roles in all settings
Focus of care	Individuals with common, well-defined health needs with predictable outcomes	Individuals with common, well-defined health needs with predictable and unpredictable outcomes	Individuals and social groups with health needs related to illness and wellness
Examples of minimum competencies of new graduates	Develops nursing care plans using the nursing data base and incorporating principles of organization and management	Develops nursing care plans through utilization of the nursing data base in consultation with other nursing personnel	Develops nursing care plans using data bases in structured and unstructured settings for both well and ill individuals and social groups in collaboration with members of the health team
	Performs independent nursing measures according to the needs demonstrated by individuals and families	Performs nursing care by implementing nursing care plans according to a priority of needs and established nursing protocols	Implements nursing care according to current health status and health potential of individuals or social groups based on nursing theory and research

P.A. Kalisch and B.J. Kalisch, The Advance of American Nursing 2nd ed. (Boston: Little, Brown, 1986), 704–709.

National League for Nursing Council of Baccalaureate and Higher Degree Programs, Baccalaureate Education in Nursing 1985–1986, NLN Publication #15–1311 (New York: National League for Nursing, 1985).

National League for Nursing Council of Associate Degree Programs, Associate Degree Education for Nursing—1985, NLN Publication #23–1309 (New York: National League for Nursing, 1985).

National League for Nursing Council of Diploma Programs, Education for Nursing: The Diploma Way, NLN Publication #16–1314 (New York: National League for Nursing, 1985).

Riffle, K.L., et al., "Entry into practice: The continuing debate," in Current Issues in Nursing, 2nd ed., J.C. McCloskey and H.K. Grace, eds. (Boston: Blackwell Scientific Pub., 1985), 197–218.

National League for Nursing Task Force on Competencies of Graduates of Nursing Programs, Working Paper, NLN Publication #14–1787, (New York: National League for Nursing, 1979).

P. Rosenfeld, "Nursing education: Statistics you can use," Nurs & Health Care (June 1986):327–330.

reached an all time high as the entire health-care field undergoes dramatic economic, orga-nizational, technological, and ethical changes. At the heart of the nursing education issue is the establishment of an entry-into-practice man-date that would lessen this confusion, be more cost-effective for all, and give clarity to standard educational qualifications for beginning prac-titioners. In order to appreciate the current sta-tus of the entry into practice issue, it is impor-tant to keep in mind how the nursing profession has dealth with this issue in the past 20 years. The following list of past and recent events pro-vides a brief review.

1965   ANA issued a position paper, which rec-ommended that the baccalaureate de-gree be the minimum educational preparation for professional nursing practice.[7]

1978   ANA called for two labels of nursing personnel and urged work groups to define the competencies inherent in the two categories.[8]

1982   The National League for Nursing (NLN) took the position that the bac-calaureate degree represents prepa-ration for *professional* nursing prac-tice and that other levels represent preparation for *technical* nursing practice.[9]

1984   ANA established goals for states to im-plement the baccalaureate degree for licensure of professional nursing, and endorsed the title of Registered Nurse (R.N.) for professional nurses and the title of Associate Nurse (A.N.) for technical practice.[10]

1985   NLN Board of Directors issued a state-ment that indicated that, in addition to its support for professional and tech-nical (associate) levels of nursing prac-tice, the NLN should endeavor to work with the ANA to define scopes of prac-tice for the two levels.[11]

1986   The North Dakota Board of Nursing took action to standardize educational requirements for two levels of nursing practice by revising rules that govern education programs.[12]

1986   Maine became the first state to adopt legislation calling for standardized educational requirements for two lev-els of nursing practice.[13]

The joining together of the NLN and ANA to work toward resolving the entry-into-prac-tice issue represents significant progress in this continuing dilemma. There appears to be a growing consensus that there should be two cat-egories of nursing practice, that these two cat-egories (professional and technical, or associate) be clearly differentiated, and that accreditation and titling mechanisms be established separately for both.

Coming to agreement on two levels of nurs-ing practice will not be an easy task. Titling and separate licensing procedures will be especially controversial in coming to grips with the en-try-into-practice question. There is general agreement that registered nurse (R.N.) should continue to be the title of the professional nurse, but there is not yet consensus on what the title of the technical nurse should be.[14] However, with the two major nursing organizations work-ing together on these issues as the profession moves into the 1990s, there is new hope that nursing will be able to unify and meet the chang-ing needs of society.

Nursing School Enrollments

Enrollment statistics from the nation's nursing schools have been carefully tracked over time by the National League for Nursing and various other professional and government organiza-tions. These statistics provide ongoing insight into the current state of the profession as well as provide educators, policy makers, and em-ployers with direction for the future. In recent times, 1977–1978 was the peak academic year for total nursing graduates with 77,874 grad-uates. Nursing enrollments have held fairly steady until 1984 when there was a plunge in all types of nursing programs, both in public and private colleges and schools. Table 2–3 gives a summary of enrollment figures since 1975.

The nationwide slump in enrollments is a cause for concern among educators and major nurse employers and is attributed to a number of factors. Overall there are fewer students

TABLE 2–3. SUMMARY TABLE OF ENROLLMENT TRENDS IN NURSING EDUCATION SINCE 1975

Year	Enrollments		
	Diploma	AD[a]	BSN[b]
1975	60,213	89,492	100,680
1976	56,091	92,404	101,046
1977	52,858	92,387	102,494
1978	48,059	92,961	101,239
1979	43,651	93,485	100,444
1980	41,048	95,626	98,190
1981	41,009	101,365	96,099
1982	42,348	106,732	96,429
1983	42,007	111,095	101,621
1984	37,256	104,968	95,008
1985	30,179	90,756	76,232
1986	22,641	90,671	66,654

[a]Associate degree.
[b]Bachelor of Science Nursing.
Nursing Fact Book, 1985 National League for Nursing Nursing Student Census with Policy Implications 1985, (New York: National League for Nursing, 1986).

available for colleges and universities than there were ten years ago. Children of the "baby boom" generation have not yet reached the college-age entry level and the birthrate was remarkably low in the 1960s.[15,16] Students are more selective in their career choices, and women are increasingly choosing once male-dominated fields such as law, engineering, architecture, and medicine. Nursing has also tended to project a negative image in regard to employment conditions of long hours, low pay, and irregular work schedules.

Educational assistance, particularly Federal aid for nursing education, has steadily declined, with sharp reductions in 1982 and further cuts predicted for the future.[17] Another factor linked to low enrollments by some nursing leaders is that prospective nursing students may have decided against a nursing major because of widespread reports several years ago of an excess of nursing personnel, i.e., empty hospital beds and reductions in hospital staffs.[18]

As of the fall of 1987, there is an apparant widespread shortage of registered nurses. This fact highlights the very real and growing concern over decreasing enrollments and mandates that educators, health policy makers, and consumers alike work together toward solutions that will reverse this trend.

Graduate Education, Master's Level

Master's level nursing education provides for the continuing formal education of professional nurses and prepares individuals who can assume increased accountability and leadership in administration and specialized areas of clinical practice. There has been significant growth in the number of master's level programs in the past 20 years, with a 68 percent increase between 1975 and 1984 alone.[19] Along with this and the emergence of nurse practitioners and other nurse specialists with advanced degrees, the scope of nursing services has been vastly expanded. Master's nursing programs are available in increasingly diverse specialty areas and recent data indicate that 81 percent of master's students are preparing for advanced clinical placement; the remaining percentages show 7 percent preparing for teaching and the rest preparing for administration.[20] Table 2–4 gives an overview of master's nursing programs currently accredited by the NLN.

Graduate Education, Doctoral Level

Doctoral programs in nursing have increased dramatically in the past decade, and enrollments have grown over 200 percent. In 1975 there were 12 doctoral nursing programs and 74 graduations. In 1984 there were 31 doctoral level programs and 183 nurses received doctorates, a 32 percent increase over 1983.[21] In 1984 the American Association of Colleges of Nursing and the Division of Nursing, Department of Health and Human Services, sponsored a conference entitled "Doctoral Programs in Nursing: Consensus for Quality." Out of this conference came a significant amount of information on the nature of the nursing doctorate, current issues in doctoral education, and recommendations for quality assurance in doctoral programs in nursing. The following comments, assertions, and conclusions selected from the proceedings of this conference give much insight into the state of doctoral education in nursing today.[22]

- The purpose of doctoral education in nursing is the development of nursing knowledge
- The nurse leaders and researchers who will make the most important differences in the organization and quality of future health care

TABLE 2–4. MASTER'S LEVEL NURSING PROGRAMS: SELECTED AREAS OF STUDY AVAILABLE[a]

Community Health Nursing	Pediatric Nurse Practitioner
Medical/Surgical Nursing	Adult Health Nurse Practitioner
Child Health Nursing	Family Nurse Practitioner
Maternal-Infant Nursing	Primary Care Nurse Practitioner
Adult Health Nursing	Gerontological Nurse Practitioner
Geriatric/Gerontological Nursing	Occupational Health Nurse Practitioner
Psychiatric/Mental Health Nursing	Women's Health Nurse Practitioner
Community Mental Health Nursing	International/Cross-Cultural Nursing
Cardiovascular Nursing	Renal Nursing
Rehabilitation Nursing	Diabetes Nursing
Critical Care Nursing	High-Risk Perinatal Nursing
Occupational Health Nursing	Correctional Health Nursing
Oncology Nursing	Neurological Nursing
School Health Nursing	Rural Health Nursing
Nursing Administration	Chronic Disabilities Nursing
Nurse Anesthesia	Burn/Emergency/Trauma Nursing
Nurse Midwifery	

[a]This list is not an all-inclusive list but represents a cross-section of current NLN accredited programs.
National League for Nursing. Master's Education in Nursing: Route to Opportunities in Contemporary Nursing. Council of Baccalaureate and Higher Degree programs, 1985–1986.

delivery will come from our doctoral programs in nursing

- The doctor of philosophy (Ph.D.) program has a primary emphasis on research and creative scholarship
- The professional doctorate (D.N.S. or D.N.Sc.) emphasizes advanced clinical practice with the integration of research to improve nursing care
- There is a need to further clarify and foster the development of the two degree programs, i.e., that prepare both research and clinical doctors of nursing
- There is a need to identify a basic set of criteria for establishing and maintaining quality doctoral nursing programs; different criteria should be specified for the Ph.D. and the D.N.Sc.

NURSING ROLES

Episodic Nursing Roles

The image of the nurse in white in the hospital setting, providing care and ministering to the sick, is a worldwide concept. Traditionally, nurses have been prepared in acute-care settings such as hospitals. This type of **episodic care** emphasizes the role of the nurse in the delivery of curative and restorative health services to persons with chronic diseases or acute conditions. Episodic practice has become associated with the cure aspect of nursing.

In the episodic or acute-care setting, the role of the nurse is to assess, plan, implement, and evaluate client care. When clients are not able to meet their own needs, nurses assist them. See Table 2–5 for examples of typical nursing actions. As they carry out professional nursing activities, nurses perform many functions that require them to fulfill their professional role in independent, interdependent, and dependent ways. **Independent nursing actions** are those that are performed by nurses based primarily on their assessments, judgments, and knowledge. Nurses carry out these actions without specific orders from health-care professionals. Examples of some of these actions include bathing, dressing, mouth care, hair care, supportive care assessment, formulating nursing diagnoses, care planning and charting, and assisting clients to meet other needs. As primary nurses and nurse practitioners, nurses carry out many of their nursing actions in an independent manner.

Interdependent nursing actions are those that nurses perform in collaboration with others on the health-care team, such as physicians,

TABLE 2–5. EXAMPLES OF NURSING ACTIONS

Assessment

Uses scientific rationale in collection of client data

Contributes to the client data base using resources (client, family, health records, others on the health team)

Identifies changes in client's health state as they occur

Documents client progress

Assesses health state of clients, families, or groups

Assesses self-care needs of clients

Identifies areas where change of behavior is needed

Formulates nursing diagnoses

Planning

Develops individual plan for clients

Prioritizes needs based on assessment

Incorporates client, family, and others in the plan

Validates plan with clients

Establishes goals using outcome criteria

Uses research findings and information from the literature

Communicates the plan in writing and verbally

Implementation

Carries out individualized plans

Maintains client's health state or contributes to a higher state of wellness

Performs technical procedures as necessary

Maintains life support in emergency situations

Uses leadership skills and teaching skills

Serves as a role model for health practices

Collaborates with others to promote health

Accepts responsibility and is accountable for the implementation of the plan

Evaluation

Uses goals and outcome criteria to evaluate the plan

Includes clients and families in the evaluative process

Reassesses

Identifies alternative means of meeting client needs

Evaluates new literature and research findings

Includes other health team members in the evaluation

---

therapists, and nutritionists. Generally, client care decisions are made by this group of professionals, who meet to discuss a client's problems and needs, set goals, and establish priorities. Increasingly, clients and their families are being asked to participate in the problem-solving discussions. Frequently, nurses work interdependently in team nursing or in providing long-term care.

Dependent nursing actions are those actions nurses carry out following the orders of others on the health team. These usually are written by physicians but can be written by physical or occupational therapists, for example. Because the nurse is not prescribing but is carrying out the prescription, the nurse is functioning in a dependent role. However, this does not relieve nurses of accountability and professional responsibility. When acting dependently nurses must:

- Have written orders
- Understand the orders
- Establish their correctness
- Question unclear or erroneous orders
- Perform the prescribed task appropriately
- Assess the outcomes
- Evaluate the outcomes

In recent years, the traditional role of the nurse at the bedside has been expanded in scope. Nurses can choose a wide range of areas and specialized roles in the episodic setting. Intensive and coronary care units, kidney dialysis units, and specialized oncology services are specific examples of clinical areas that provide such roles.

The increase in science and technology has required nurses and health-care providers to develop expertise in using new machinery and new techniques to gain an understanding of client responses to them. Table 2–6 lists some of the specialty areas that nurses can select to work and become expert in.

Many of these new roles require additional training or education. Specialty groups have formed, and many have their own journals and training or education. Specialty groups have formed, and many have their own journals and organizations. Nurses interested in any of these areas can write to those journals or organizations for further information. Although most of these new roles are still at the bedside, some are in areas such as administration, education, or research. A discussion of selected roles in the episodic setting follows.

Primary nursing is care coordinated and administered by one nurse from the time of a client's admission to the time of discharge. Primary nurses are responsible for the care of their clients 24 hours a day during their hospital stay. They develop the plan of care for each of their primary clients, and the plan is followed

TABLE 2-6. SELECTED EPISODIC NURSING ROLES AND PRACTICE AREAS

Administration
Director of nursing
Supervisor of nursing
Head nurse
Assistant head nurse
Clinical coordinator
Charge nurse

Education
Director of continuing education
Continuing education instructor
Client education instructor

Research
Principal Investigator
Research Coordinator
Research Assistant

Practice Areas
Psychiatric nursing
Medical-surgical nursing
Intensive care units
Cardiac or coronary care units
Neonatology
Pediatrics
Rehabilitation nursing
Geriatrics
Dialysis units
Nurse anesthsetist
Operating room
Recovery room
Emergency room
Maternity nursing
    Labor and delivery
    Postpartum
    Nursery
Infection control (nurse epidemiologist)
Enterostomal therapists
Oncology
Orthopedics
Thanotology nurse specialist
Client advocate
Clinical specialist (within any specialty or subspecialty practice area)

by other nurses and other nursing service personnel when the primary nurse is off duty. Proponents of this particular role feel that primary nurses have more autonomy and more responsibility and accountability for holistic client care. There is generally no additional education needed for a general duty primary nurse. Additional training, education, or practice may be required in intensive care or other highly technical areas.

Clinical specialists are leadership positions for nurses who are experts in a specialized area of nursing, for example, gerontology, pediatrics, or medical nursing. Clinical specialists usually have a master's degree in their specialty areas, and their functions may vary from institution to institution. A range of functions generally includes such things as providing direct client care, teaching clients and families, teaching staff new methods of care, and conducting research and consulting with other health-care personnel.

One of the specialty areas that attracts nurses is anesthesia administration. These individuals are called *nurse anesthetists*. Nurse anesthetists are registered nurses who have completed a course of instruction in anesthesia after nursing school. This course of instruction may be a certificate or a master's degree program. They visit a client prior to surgery to assess preoperative medications and anesthesia needs and discuss anesthesia procedures with clients. The duties of nurse anesthetists are similar to physician anesthesiologists, but the nurses are supervised and supported by physicians. During the surgery they administer the anesthesia and assess the client's reponses to drugs and gases being administered, blood loss, etc. After surgery, they accompany clients to the recovery room and evaluate their status and progress.

Enterostomal therapy is another specialty area. Enterostomal nurses teach and assist clients who have had surgery for colostomies, ileostomies, or urinary diversions. Their primary role is to teach clients how to care for themselves and help them adjust to their altered body image. Additional training is available for this, usually provided through a hospital or other health-care-facility-sponsored program.

Geriatric nurse specialists provide comprehensive care to older clients in hospitals, nursing homes, and clinics. Some nurses who practice in this area have advanced certificates or degrees in the care of the elderly.

Infection control nurses (or nurse epidemiologists) monitor the hospital or nursing home environment for infection. They assess infections that have been incubating at the time of a client's admission (community-associated) and those that develop after admission. They assess, report, prevent, and control infections in the acute-care setting. A good working knowledge of asepsis and of microbiology are essential for nurses entering this area.

Oncology nurse specialists work with cancer clients and their families. They provide physical care and emotional support, and some are skilled in administering various types of chemotherapy.

Hospice nurses care for clients who are dying in a hospice. A hospice is a specialized health-care facility for the terminally ill. The hospice concept is a relatively new idea in the United States but has been successfully implemented in some areas of the country. These nurses provide physical care and emotional support for dying clients and their families and assist in coordinating home and hospital care.

Another new area for nursing is thanatology (the study of death). A nurse *thanotologist* is one who helps to meet the physical and psychological needs of the dying client and his family. In addition to this, they teach other staff members how to cope more effectively with death and dying and improve their ability to assist clients through this time.

As the diversity in the episodic care field of nursing continues to expand, the job possibilities will be almost endless. Nurses in the future will be able to choose from an even wider variety of specialities to meet their personal and professional goals.

Distributive Nursing Roles

Nurses who work outside of the hospital setting usually are engaged in some facet of **distributive health care** as opposed to episodic health care. Distributive health care, in turn, is linked to the *care* aspect of health as opposed to the cure. One of the distinguishing features of distributive care is that it is continuous and does not operate within definitive beginnings and endings, such as admission and discharge from a hospital, or declarations of sick and well. In distributive care, the emphasis is on health, and total health needs are planned and assessed in terms of the individual's life span. Activities include such things as risk assessment for potential adverse health states and the promotion of healthful living habits. Episodic illnesses and injuries occur intermittently during the life span and, in one sense, the care provided (episodic care) can be viewed within the larger framework of distributive care. In actuality, people often have both care and cure needs at the same time. Despite this overlap, the terminology is helpful in explaining career choices and categorizing nursing roles in a logical fashion.

Distributive nursing practice is carried out within the framework of the nursing process, and there is emphasis on health maintenance and disease prevention. Health teaching, counseling, and care of the sick at home and in outpatient facilities are major components. A large portion of distributive nursing care services takes place within the realm of community health nursing. (The reader is referred to the chapters on Community Concepts and Family Systems Concepts for a discussion of many of these nursing roles.) Table 2–7 presents an overview of selected distributive nursing roles, including a number of community-based and additional roles not covered in other chapters.

The Expanded Role in Nursing

The trend in the past two decades has been for nurses to take a more active part in patient care, increase their autonomy on the health team, and become more specialized. The **expanded role** is one of the outcomes of this trend. The expanded role generally refers to nursing practice that employs skills and expertise beyond a nurse's basic educational training program.

A nurse practicing in an expanded role usually has attended a specialized program that leads to a certificate qualifying her as a **nurse practitioner.** Nurse practitioner programs generally are specialized according to age of client (e.g., pediatric, adult, geriatric) or according to a clinical specialty, such as community or family health, college health, or oncology nursing. Major components of these programs are advanced training in health assessment and the delivery of primary care. **Primary care** refers to the care that takes place during the client's initial contact with the health-care system or health provider.

Nurse practitioners are able to skillfully elicit a health history and critically evaluate the findings, conduct a physical examination, and evaluate a client's development, maturation, coping ability, emotional well-being, and any presenting complaints. Nurse practitioners are

TABLE 2–7. OVERVIEW OF SELECTED DISTRIBUTIVE NURSING ROLES

Roles and Settings	Characteristics
Community health nurse generalist	Also called public health nurse generalist Most often employed by city or county health departments BSN^a preparation usually required Provides general health care to individuals, families, and target populations Functions as health educator, health counselor, coordinator of services, and giver of direct care within home or clinic setting
Community health nurse specialist	Also called public health nurse specialist Master's degree in nursing preferred Responsibilities may include supervision of other nurses, responsibilities for planning and evaluating health and nursing services in the community, and conducting research
Visiting nurse	Also called home health nurse May be employed by visiting nurse associations, home health-care agencies, public health departments, or be self-employed as a private duty nurse Gives direct care to clients in the home setting, often providing continuous care for chronic disease states and rehabilitation All levels of nursing preparation are in this role; complex families should preferably be cared for by nurses with minimal BSN preparation
Occupational health nurse	Sometimes referred to as employee health nurse or industrial nurse Delivers primary care and preventive health services to individuals in the work setting Educational preparation relative to scope of responsibility; may be prepared as nurse practitioner Experience and expertise in specialized areas of health counseling, such as alcoholism, stress management, and family living may be required
Certified nurse midwife	Registered nurse who has completed a program in nurse midwifery accredited by the American College of Nurse Midwives; some of these programs lead to a master's degree as well as a certificate in nurse midwifery (CNM) A CNM functions as a highly trained specialist in providing prenatal care to women with uncomplicated pregnancies, obstetric care during labor and delivery, and postpartum maternal and infant care; depending on the setting, care may be episodic or continuous throughout the childbearing years Employment may be in group health organizations, private medical offices, hospitals, health departments, or private practice
School nurse	May be employed directly by boards of education, by local health departments, or by private schools Scope of responsibility varies greatly but includes emergency care and referral, health screening and testing, counseling, age-specific health education, and assisting in the management of health-related programs and school policies Educational requirements vary from state to state; special certification is required in some jurisdictions
College health nurse	Employed by a college or university health service or health office Delivers primary care to students, faculty, and staff employees; may provide infirmary inpatient care Educational background varies according to scope of responsibility; may be prepared as nurse practitioner A large portion of care for this age group centers around general health counseling, mental health counseling, and health education
Ambulatory care settings Clinic nurse Office nurse	Settings may include outpatient departments of hospitals, doctors' offices, neighborhood primary care clinics, specialized clinics such as family planning and child health clinics, or other group health organizations *(continued)*

TABLE 2–7. (Continued)

Roles and Settings	Characteristics
Outpatient nurse	Functions and responsibilities vary tremendously and may be broad or specialized; the delivery of primary care (both episodic and distributive) is usually a major component; the degree of health education and health maintenance activities delivered concurrently are determined by the philosophy of the agency and individual health-care provider Registered nurses in these settings may be prepared as nurse practitioners, particularly in pediatrics and in other clinics that perform large numbers of routine physical examinations
Nursing of specialized populations	There are a variety of roles and employment opportunities for nurses in specialized institutions and settings, where care may range from acute episodic to long-term distributive, or a combination of both. Examples include: Nursing in correctional institutions, e.g., prisons Camp nursing Nursing in homes for the mentally retarded or handicapped Public buildings or businesses, e.g., department stores, museums, zoos Recreational enterprises, e.g., circuses, rodeos, fairgrounds, sports events

*a*BSN = Bachelor of science in nursing.

guided, through theory and experience, to discriminate between normal and abnormal findings and between normal variations of development and abnormal deviations. This role clearly includes a number of tasks that heretofore have been the sole province of the physician, particularly those that relate to medical diagnosis and the prescription of therapeutic measures. A critical skill of the nurse practitioner is to use sound judgment in deciding which clients can be cared for by the nurse and which should be referred to physicians or others on the health-care team.

Nurse practitioners work in a variety of employment settings including physicians' offices, ambulatory care clinics, nursing homes, and community health settings. In addition to taking health histories and performing physical examinations, they may collect specimens, order laboratory tests and x-rays, make house calls, and prescribe medications.

Since 1971, 30 states have revised their nurse practice acts to accommodate the expanded role for R.N.s; a number have revised their definitions of nursing to include more autonomous functions within the area of diagnosis and treatment.[23] Only three states at present allow nurse practitioners to prescribe drugs;

Idaho law, for example, allows nurses to prescribe from a limited formulary that includes antibiotics, contraceptives, antihistamines, decongestants, and topical ointments.[24] Certified nurse practitioners are perhaps the largest group who practice in expanded roles. As of yet, there are no legal determinations as to who can be called "nurse practitioner," although the American Nurses' Association has designed an accreditation process for programs that prepare nurses for this expanded role. The National Board of Pediatric Nurse Practitioners and Associates has initiated efforts to certify practitioners by examination. A growing number of nurse practitioner programs are part of B.S.N. or advanced degree programs; e.g., a program may lead to an M.S.N. *and* a nurse practitioner certificate. It is important to be aware that not all nurses who practice in an expanded role are certified practitioners. Increasingly, nurses are acquiring skills through on-the-job training and continuing education.

Independent nursing practice (private practice) is becoming a viable role option for increasing numbers of nurses with advanced training, such as nurse practitioners, certified clinical nurse specialists, and nurse midwives. Nurses who are self-employed or work in settings other than traditional institutions or organized health-care systems fit into this category. Independent nurse specialists are meeting important needs in community mental health centers, home health care, health maintenance organizations, and corporate health settings. A major problem facing these nurses continues to be reimbursement for services through private insurance carriers and government subsidized programs such as Medicaid. Many states do allow nurses to be covered for these services, but the degree of coverage varies and may be limited to certain clinical specialties. Outmoded legislation and lack of public awareness of nurses' changing roles account for much of this problem, as well as competition in the health-care provider marketplace.[25]

International Nursing

Nurses who practice their profession outside of their home country can be considered *international nurses*. In most instances this will involve adjusting to a culture different from one's own and delivering nursing care to individuals with different ideas about health and illness, different customs and beliefs, and different ways of relating to others.

Transcultural nursing requires a body of knowledge related to delivering culturally sensitive nursing care. It requires sensitivity to nursing behaviors, practices, values, and beliefs of people from all cultures. Nurses have been working internationally for many years, but the concept of transcultural nursing has emerged only recently as a separate field of study. It is important to note that transcultural nursing is applicable to both international nurses and nurses caring for culturally different people in any setting. (The reader is referred to Chapter 13 for further discussion.)

There are numerous opportunities for registered nurses to work abroad in community health nursing, primary care, acute care, teaching, and general health-care administration. Prospective employers include foreign governments and business enterprises, religious missions, universities (both foreign and domestic), U.S. military organizations, U.S. government agencies, and various other national and international organizations. Table 2–8 lists some of the recognized health organizations and agencies that provide opportunities for the practice of international nursing and sources of information on nursing opportunities overseas.

CONTEMPORARY ISSUES IN NURSING

Within the framework of revolutionary changes in health care and the society as a whole, a number of professional nursing and nursing-related issues have emerged. One of the most current of these issues, the entry-into-practice debate, has already been discussed. Some of the other issues, such as nursing shortages, have been raised intermittently over the years and periodically reappear as circumstances change. Other issues are related to shifts in economic policies or new scientific and technological developments and their effects on all health-care workers. The following section will highlight some of the dominant issues and current trends that are at the forefront of the nursing profession today.

Nurse Shortages*

A shortage or surplus of nurses is a lack of balance between the number of nursing jobs or positions and the number of qualified nurses available to fill them. From a historic standpoint, a shortage of nurses is characteristic of the profession. The only time in history that an oversupply of nurses existed was during the great economic depression of 1929.

Varying perceptions of the need and demand for nurses, how the supply is estimated and projected, what constitutes a shortage and its causes prevents definitive answers to the questions about shortages. The late 1970s and early 1980s were a period of depressed economic conditions and less demand for health services. By mid-1986, however, there were cries of nursing shortages across the country and the

---

*The section on Nursing Shortages was prepared by Helen V. Foerst.

TABLE 2–8. SOURCE LIST OF INTERNATIONAL NURSING OPPORTUNITIES

Project Hope
c/o Hope Center
Millwood, Virginia 22646
Tel: 703–837–2100

Project HOPE (Health Opportunity for People Everywhere) is an American private voluntary organization that functions to improve health conditions throughout the world. Emphasis is on education and the development of existing health-care systems.

World Health Organization (WHO)
Avenue Appia
CH–1211 Geneva 27
Switzerland

WHO is the official health agency of the United Nations, and its general purpose is to foster the attainment of the highest possible level of health by all peoples. Functions include quarantine and epidemic intelligence, international standardization services, such as statistics, biologicals, and drugs; direct services to governments in surveying their health problems and strengthening their health services; educational and research assistance related to health matters.

Pan American Health Organization (PAHO)
525 23rd Street, NW
Washington, D.C. 20037

PAHO is an intergovernmental public health organization and a specialized agency of the Organization of American States (OAS). It is also the American regional agency for WHO. The purpose of PAHO is to combat disease, lengthen life, and promote the physical and mental health of the peoples of the Americas. It receives and disseminates epidemiologic information, furnishes technical assistance, finances fellowships, promotes cooperation in medical research, and provides professional education in Latin America.

U.S. Agency for International Development
(USAID)
320 21st Street, NW
Washington, D.C. 20037

An agency of the U.S. government that provides a wide range of technical and educational assistance to foreign governments. Included in this range are the building, staffing, and maintenance of medical facilities, water and sanitation projects, and family-planning programs.

The U.S. Peace Corps
806 Connecticut Avenue, NW
Washington, D.C. 20525

The Peace Corps is an agency of the U.S. government that coordinates volunteer services and programs. Peace Corps volunteers work in many parts of the world and provide assistance to host governments in economic and social development including nutrition, nursing education, nursing and hospital administration, and public health nursing.

International Council of Nurses
BOX 42
CH–1211 Geneva 20
Switzerland

Nurses can write to this organization for their publication, *Nursing Abroad,* which provides a description of the services offered by ICN member associations in arranging salaried employment or study abroad.

International Voluntary Services, Inc. (IVS)
1717 Massachusetts Avenue, NW
Washington, D.C. 20036

IVS recruits skilled volunteers to work in developing countries in the broad area of rural development, which includes health.

Intercristo
P.O. Box 9323
Seattle, Washington 98109
Tel: 800–426–0507

An information center on worldwide Christian service. Information on nursing opportunities available on request.

Option
P.O. box 81122
San Diego, California 92138

This agency provides information on volunteer and salaried employment in areas of need, both domestic and international. They publish a monthly newsletter and yearly catalog describing available opportunities.

Technical Assistance Information Clearinghouse
200 Park Avenue South
New York, New York 10003

A publication list is available that includes a directory of U.S. organizations in development assistance abroad and reports of development projects by country.

Adapted from VeNeta Masson "International Nursing: What Is It and Who Does It?" Am J Nurs (July 1979) 1245.
Curriculum papers, Undergraduate Program, The Catholic University of America, School of Nursing, Washington, D.C., 1980.

debate was underway again. In order to understand and evaluate this situation, the question of a shortage must be examined in terms of societal conditions, expectations, and values.

The registered nurse resources of the country, the nurses educated and available for nursing positions, are related to a number of major factors. The number of students who enter and graduate from nursing schools and then remain actively engaged in nursing is the primary indicator of the nurse supply. A large number of nurses who maintain a current license practice part-time or do not practice at all. Inactive or part-time employment is related to marital status, sex, age, and family responsibilities. Low pay for available positions, poor working conditions, and few opportunities for career advancement also cause nurses to leave employment or change jobs.

In addition to the number of nurses available for practice, another factor in the adequacy of the nurse supply is the demand for nursing services in the different health-care settings. As health-care facilities expand, new treatments are developed and new types of care are made available to clients; therefore, more nurses are required. New hospital beds, specialized nursing services, such as intensive care units, kidney dialysis units, and ambulatory care centers, contribute to the demand for nurses.

These characteristics of the nurse supply give rise to the question of a shortage or surplus of nurses. Those who believe there is a surplus of nurses point out that registered nurse resources have grown tremendously and are not fully used. A large number of nurses (about 24 percent) who maintain a current license do not practice.[26] In addition, 53 percent of employed nurses work part-time.[27] On the other hand, the number of vacant positions for nurses in the health-care agencies and the difficulties in recruiting and filling the positions are highlighted. It is said that nursing staffs are used to their fullest productivity and work considerable overtime. To counter understaffing, health-care agencies have to resort to hiring temporary staff from supplemental agencies.

This is only part of the debate. The way the adequacy of the nurse supply is judged is another issue. The nurse supply is the number of registered nurses who are employed or are available for employment. Basic to determining the adequacy of the nurse supply are the concepts of demand and need. *Demand* defines requirements primarily on the basis of economic factors. Demand is assessed by determining how many dollars are available from employers to pay salaries. It is measured by the number of budgeted nursing positions required for the nursing services the population will use and that can be paid for. *Vacancies,* a measure of shortage, are the number of budgeted positions that are not filled. *Need,* on the other hand, defines requirements by considering the standards of good care and the number of nurses that can be expected to be available as determined by health professionals. Need is assessed by applying criteria considered to produce optimum levels of nursing care or service to the health-care needs of the population to be served. Assessments of the nurse supply are interpreted differently depending on need and demand concepts, predictions of the number of nurses in training, and the proportion of trained nurses that practice. It has been proposed that looking at the adequacy of the nurse supply based on the aggregate numbers of nurses itself leads to perception of a surplus. Relying on the annual output of the nursing educational system to augment the supply also contributes to a false perception of the balance between supply and demand for nurses. Over the years, the solution to the nurse shortage has been to educate and graduate more nurses, ignoring the fact that a certain proportion of these nurses will be inactive, work part-time, or drop out of the profession. Some believe that the shortage of nurses is not a function of the number of nurses but of poor use of them. They suggest that in the hospital, for example, nurses are frequently expected to assume the responsibilities of other departments. Nurses act as pharmacists, aides, housekeepers, secretaries, and messengers. If they were free to practice nursing, the shortage would be reduced. The solution lies in better management and improved use of nurses. In this same regard, another interpretation is that the supply of nurses will never reach demand, unless appropriate responses are made to shortages. Attention needs to be focused on the health-care delivery system, the roles and responsibilities of nurses, improved working conditions, career development, and ways to retain nurses in the work force.

Nursing has accumulated a large body of knowledge about its practitioners and has developed and refined methods for determining the number of nurses available and needed for nursing practice. The first counts of the number of registered nurses were made in the states that had laws requiring registration. (New Jersey passed its registration law in 1903.)[28] Even today, the chief source of data on the nurse supply is the number of nurses licensed by the state nurse licensing boards.

Since the beginning of the century, the number of registered nurses has grown in increasing proportion to the population. These relationships are shown in Table 2–9. The national average of the number of nurses per 100,000 population climbed from 55 in 1910 to 520 in 1980, an increase of 465 nurses per 100,000 population. The number of nurses per 100,000 is not uniform among regions of the country, however.

The Northeast tends to have the largest number of nurses per 100,000 population and the South the least number. The growing proportion of nurses to the population is assumed to reflect the increased demand for nurses. But the adequacy of the supply must be addressed in terms of the different areas of the country,

the structure of the health services, the needs and demands for services in the area, and their availability. The characteristics of nurses in the area and their work force participation must be analyzed to determine the significance of their numbers versus need or demand.

The 1963 report of the Consultant Group appointed by the Surgeon General of the United States Public Health Service highlighted national nursing shortages both quantitatively and qualitatively. The Consultant Group set goals for the number of nurses required through 1980, including the numbers prepared for particular health-care settings, fields of nursing practice, and areas of responsibility. In response, the Nurse Training Act of 1964 was enacted by Congress. Through this and extended legislation, the Federal government has supported a broad range of programs designed to increase the quantity and quality of the nurse supply. The Nurse Training Act has provided student aid for basic and postgraduate training and education, funds for construction of nursing schools, institutional aid for operating schools, and grants for improvement of nursing education programs.

With the Nurse Training Act of 1979, Congress authorized a study to determine if there still was a shortage of nurses and a need for continued Federal financial assistance to nursing

TABLE 2–9. NURSE: POPULATION RATIOS BY REGION 1910–1980

| Year | Number of Nurses in United States | Nurses per 100,000 Population | | | | |
		United States	North-east	North central	South	West
1910	50,476	55	75	47	34	104
1920	103,879	98	133	87	60	166
1930	214,292	175	239	159	104	262
1940	284,159	216	304	193	134	299
1950	374,584	249	321	233	174	318
1960	525,374	293	349	270	245	340
1970	750,000	368	491	367	281	355
1980	1,272,851	520	620	547	423	529

1910–1950: US Department of Health, Education and Welfare, Public Health Service, Health Manpower Chart Book PHS Pub. No. 511 (Washington, D.C.: U.S. Government Printing Office, 1957), 51.
1960: US Department of Health, Education and Welfare, Public Health Service, Health Resources Administration. Source Books: Nursing Personnel. DHEW Pub. No. (HRA) 75–43 (Washington, D.C.: US Government Printing Office, 1974), 13.
1970 & 1980: Division of Health Professions Analysis, Bureau of Health Professions: Supply and Characteristics of Selected Health Personnel. DHHS Pub. No. (HRA) 81–20 (Hyattsville, Md.: Health Resources Administration, June 1981), 115.

education. The report of a study committee on nursing and nursing education conducted by the Institute of Medicine (IOM), National Academy of Sciences, was issued in January, 1983.[29]

It concluded that there was an adequate general supply of nurses through 1990 and no substantial Federal support and activities were needed to increase the overall number.

Nursing shortages did exist in certain geographic areas and practice settings, such as inner cities and rural areas. This was seen as a distribution problem. A shortage was seen in the number of nurses with advanced training in administration, teaching, research, and clinical nursing specialities. As the IOM study was published, newspaper and journal articles announced that 37 percent of California hospitals were not hiring registered nurses; 51 percent were reducing weekly work hours; and 17 percent closed client care units. Unemployment, a decline in client admissions, and decrease in client census were cited as reasons.[30] The IOM study analyses of projected supply of registered nurses did take into account the fact that projections were made at a time of economic recession, when there was great concern for cost containment. Changes in demand for health services and nurses would affect changes in output of nurses. Other factors also would influence the supply of nurses, such as the cost of educating them.

It can be concluded that determining the supply and requirements for nurses is not a straightforward definitive process. Both quantitative and qualitative assessments of need and demand involve some subjective judgment and are influenced by personal and professional views of the health-care system and nursing.

The supply of nurses and its adequacy for meeting health-care needs will require continuous monitoring to detect changing situations. A periodic critical assessment will need to focus on the supply as well as trends in the demand for nurses. The many factors that influence whether there is a shortage or a surplus and their implications will need to be evaluated. A response to the periodic assessments and efforts to keep the supply in balance with needs will continue to be a challenge to the nursing profession.

There are many popular reasons for the perceived shortage of nurses, even though the supply is increasing. The staff of the Institute of Medicine study on nursing examined some of these assertions in relation to data on the nurse supply.[31]

- Fewer nurses are employed in nursing. The proportion of the total registered nurse populations actually employed in nursing has increased from 59.3 percent in 1949 to 76.6 percent in 1980.
- Nurses are leaving nursing to work in other fields.
- Nurses are leaving active employment to pursue further education.

As this edition goes to press, there appears to be a frank shortage of nurses, especially in critical care, in many geographic areas across the country. A rising acuity level within acute-care facilities, rebounding census, the move to primary care (resulting in a decrease in ancillary staff), growth in alternative health-care facilities, and sagging school enrollments are some of the reasons cited for this trend.[32]

Reality Shock

Reality shock is an important issue facing beginning nurses and nurses returning to the workforce after being away. Kramer explains **reality shock** as the feelings inexperienced nurses have when they discover themselves in job situations for which they thought they were prepared, only to find that they are not.[33] For example, many students have their clinical experience two to three days per week, during an academic year. They are giving care to only three or four clients at a time, and the clinical experience is structured as a learning experience. Students are closely monitored and assisted by their instructors, and have no ancillary responsibilities on the nursing unit.

According to Kramer, many problems arise from the fact that nurses are educated to believe in professional values but are hired by bureaucratic organizations.[34] Student nurses are taught to provide individualized attention to clients, autonomy in the decision-making process, and independence in nursing behavior. Yet many nurses, particularly those in acute episodic settings, are employed by institutions that are organized around the performance of tasks and are based on examples from industry where products and profitable outcomes are the objectives.[35] When new nurses arrive at their jobs, they are expected by the health-care agency and by themselves to be compentent. The criteria for competency in the work setting is usually far from the type of competency expected in the nursing school experience. In addition to giving direct care to clients, employed nurses are expected to take on their share of the work load in relation to the number of staff on duty, to manage their work load in terms of priorities, and to assist in the supervision of less professional personnel. When they cannot live up to these expectations, they are disappointed and experience feelings ranging from shock and depression to recovery and resolution. Consequently, some nurses do not adapt well and may even drop out of the profession.

To help nurses remain in nursing and lessen their chances of suffering from reality shock, several things need to be done. First of all, student nurses need to be aware that reality shock may occur. Nursing educators can present the reality of staff nursing to students as well as the ideal. Students should be fully aware, for example, that nursing is largely a 24-hours-a-day, 7-days-a-week profession. This is true in all episodic settings and in some distributive settings. Although scheduling and shift rotation expectations vary, nurses are expected to work evening or night shifts, as well as holidays and weekends. New graduates need to be oriented to their assigned shifts and have adequate time to prepare for shift rotation.

Administrators need to be aware that the agency expectations for new graduates need to be flexible and individualized, and an adjustment period should be part of the orientation plan. Nursing administrators, supervisors, and head nurses also need to identify those nurses experiencing reality shock and assist them in resolving it.

Nurses who reach the resolution stage will find strength in the fact that they experienced reality shock and have coped successfully and will continually be challenged by the complex problems that are part of the real world of nursing.

Burnout Syndrome

Burnout is a term used to describe a stress-related syndrome that experienced nurses may develop. Psychologists have found the burnout syndrome to be a common state among nurses, doctors, social workers, teachers, and other professionals who are so busy helping others that they neglect their own needs. In many instances, they do not even recognize their own needs. Some factors that contribute to nursing burnout include: heavy work loads; low pay; long and diverse hours; lack of autonomy; inability to deliver holistic, individualized client care; the inability to assist all clients in positive adaptation; and the continual experience of loss when clients die. Burnout rate is particularly high in intensive care units, burn units, and oncology units, where many people are critically or terminally ill. Although burnout can occur in any setting, it appears to be most concentrated in acute-care settings, such as hospitals.

Donna Diers summarized the work of nurses in the following way:

> Nurses deal with the most basic human needs: feeding, heartbreak, warmth, elimination, suffering, loneliness, birth, and death. Our hands get dirty, our uniforms stained, and our psyches eroded by daily contact with human beings in need—people crying, immobilized, angry, frightened, depressed, and only occasionally joyful. We live with the outrage of the diagnosis made or missed, the crisis of faith in a higher being or a physician; the knowledge of decline, disability, permanent change, death and the consciousness of our own mortality. We must be graceful over vomitus . . . , dignified as we change the dressing, . . . (or) give out bad news. With our hands and eyes we touch the lives of others and are admitted to the privacy of their inner space without even asking.[36]

With this type of responsibility, it is understandable why nurses cannot always cope with the stress of nursing. Experiencing this kind of stress response can give rise to burnout symptoms: fatigue, insomnia, depression, irritability, headaches, stomach distress, susceptibility to contagious illnesses, dread of going to work, dehumanization, and exhaustion.

To combat burnout and increase job satisfaction, many agencies try to increase the nurse:client ratio, enabling nurses to provide more holistic care. This increases satisfaction because nurses have more responsibility for a smaller group of clients, are able to give more comprehensive care, and are therefore more likely to stay.

In some agencies, staff members meet with a counselor to discuss their feelings on a more formal basis. Also, many staff nurses serve as their own support group encouraging other nurses to express their feelings. Sometimes just sharing feelings, frustrations, and problems with other sympathetic nurses is helpful. Because of the symptoms of the burnout syndrome, many nurses are not aware that it is common. Once they are able to talk about their feelings, they are able to generate a plan for change.

Another method of combating the burnout syndrome is rotation out of the high-stress area for a time. For example, a staff nurse in the intensive care nursery would rotate through the normal nursery every other month, to minimize the stress. It is important for nurses to be aware that burnout exists so that they can recognize the symptoms in themselves and others, and take appropriate action to alleviate it.

Individual nurses, too, can take steps to combat burnout. The first and most important step for nurses to take is to realize that there is a problem. Once the syndrome has been assessed, several other steps can be taken. Establishing a daily "decompression time" has been found to be helpful. This involves some sort of relaxing activity. Jogging, walking, swimming, shopping, and going for a drive are examples of how decompression time can be spent.

Other nurses have found exploring their employment options can be a means of reducing burnout. Lateral job transfers or a completely new job are ways of doing this.

Most professional nurses experience some degree of burnout at some time in their career.

Awareness of the symptoms and taking action to reverse the syndrome is the most important means of coping with it successfully.

Computer Technology and Nursing

As science and technology continue to advance, the information generated can be overwhelming. As a result, we are in what some have called an information revolution. In order to organize, store, and retrieve this information effectively, many agencies are turning to computers for support. New roles subsequently have been created for nurses and other health-care providers.

As hospitals and community health agencies begin to computerize their services, departments such as nursing are finding many new ways to improve client care. Computers can be of great advantage to nurses, and some of the ways they are currently being used to assist nursing practice include:

- Classification of clients for workload determination and variable staffing in hospitals
- General nurse scheduling in hospitals
- Budgeting and other fiscal analysis for nursing service departments
- Documentation of client care data in all phases of the nursing process, including computer-generated nursing diagnoses
- Client monitoring applications, such as direct recording of vital signs, stress tolerance levels, and other physiological processes
- Client data analysis to monitor trends in clients' nursing care needs and to assist in research efforts
- Provision of communication interface between departments within a health-care institution, e.g., laboratory, x-ray, social services, dietary services, pharmacy
- Management of supplies; inventory assistance, ordering, crediting
- Assistance with client education and professional nursing education
- Maintenance of reference data for quick access by nurses on the job; e.g., adverse effects of drugs, emergency protocols, community referral listings

The computer eases decision making and communications, and results in the reduction of errors and better use of professional time and effort.

Computers are still a relatively new phenomenon in the health-care system, but the number of institutions and agencies that employ them is rapidly increasing. There are a number of emerging nursing roles in the field of automated data processing and medical and nursing information systems within the health-care agencies.

To understand the role of the nurse, several terms need to be introduced and defined. *Automated data processing* (ADP) refers to the operation of identifying pieces of information, converting them into machine-readable formats, and storing them in a coherent way in a computer, for people and organizations to use. An *automated system* is a defined collection of computerized information that is programmed in a precise way to accomplish specified goals. Automated systems may exist for use solely within one organization, such as hospital personnel system, or may be intended for use by the public at large, such as a bibliographic system in a library. *Hospital information systems* (HIS), often referred to as *medical information systems* (MIS), use computer systems to process information needed to deliver client care within hospitals or other health-care institutions.

Nursing information systems provide computer access to nursing information and selected client information and enable nurses to record, monitor, analyze, and review these data. There are many specific and potential uses of nursing information systems as listed previously in this section. Nursing information systems can be autonomous and exist as single systems within themselves, or they can be integrated as a subsystem to the HIS or MIS in an institution. The latter is more common and provides more flexibility and resource data for delivering client care. Health-related automated systems are moving from institutions into ambulatory care settings such as community health nursing agencies. One of the major contributions of the computer to community health nursing is its ability to rank nursing care needs of clients.

Specific job descriptions for nurses who work with computer technology and nursing information systems are not yet standardized and are specific to the health-care institution. The U.S. Department of Health Services and the National Institutes of Health (NIH) have sponsored an annual computer technology and nursing conference since 1981.[37] At the third national conference, an integrated computer model for nursing was presented.

Much of the current literature, along with findings from the first national computers in nursing conference, echoes a recurring theme regarding nursing roles and nursing involvement in computer technology: nurses must become committed to and have a stake in the development of computerized nursing systems, and they must establish standards for the data content of these systems and develop a taxonomy of terms representing the nursing process. This is one mandate for assuring the survival of nursing functions and allowing nurses to control their own practice. The future for nurses and the computer undoubtedly will expand rapidly in the next few years. Nurses need to become increasingly familiar with computer technology, understand the roles of computer professionals such as programmers and systems analysts, become involved in the acquisition of computer hardware and in software development, and work diligently to clarify and produce a standardized nursing data base.

SUMMARY

The concept of nursing is multidimensional. It is a professional discipline that provides health and illness care to individuals, families, and groups within society. Nursing has been defined variously by nursing leaders, health-care agencies, and nursing organizations. From these definitions and an understanding of the concepts of health and illness, the nurse develops her or his own philosophy and definition of nursing.

Health, illness, and wellness are all relative terms that describe a person's state of being. They are viewed on a continuum and are relative to an individual's age, cultural orientation, personal philosophy, and society. Nurses carry out activities that promote and maintain health, prevent illness, and assist ill and injured persons in returning to their potential health states.

Currently there are three major educational programs that prepare nurses for the R.N. license; the two-year associate degree program; the three-year diploma school; and the four-year baccalaureate degree program. Graduate programs leading to the master's and doctoral degrees have expanded in number since the 1950s, and research efforts in nursing have increased accordingly.

Contemporary nursing is characterized by diverse opportunities in clinical practice, administration, education, and research. Episodic care roles are available in hospitals and other acute-care inpatient facilities. Distributive care roles that emphasize continuous health-promotion and illness-prevention activities take place in the community and ambulatory care agencies. The expanded role includes nurse practitioners, nurse midwives, and other nurses prepared to deliver primary care or highly specialized health and nursing services.

A number of dilemmas in modern nursing have emerged along with the advancements. Nurses in acute-care settings are subject to the burnout syndrome, for example, and newly employed nurses often experience reality shock. Related to both of these is a chronic nurse shortage problem, a problem that is both complex and dynamic.

The application of computer technology to nursing is one of the exciting trends in modern nursing and promises to enhance working conditions for nurses, provide more research opportunities, and improve nursing and health care in general.

The challenges that face the contemporary nurse are numerous. Nurses are highly educated, and there is an increased interest in research, the development of nursing theory, and the use of professional management techniques. Nurses are gaining more autonomy and exercising more control over their practice.

The setting for nursing practice used to be primarily episodic, and now, in common with the health-care system in general, there is a trend toward ambulatory care and a greater demand for preventive services. The needs of society are changing, technology is expanding, and competition among health-care providers is high. There will always be a need for nursing services. Perhaps the greatest challenge throughout the history of nursing has been the attainment of professional status. Today nursing can look at itself with great pride; its professionalism is at an all-time high, and nurses are actively engaged in furthering and maintaining excellence in practice. For the nursing profession, the future is now.

Study Questions

1. Interview a friend or family member in terms of his or her current health status. How does he or she define health and illness? How does he or she make a decision about seeking professional health care? What does he or she perceive as an ideal for high-level wellness?

2. If you were asked to give an opinion on how the nursing entry-into-practice issue should be settled, what would it consist of? How do you think each of the three current types of nursing graduates would feel about your solution?

3. What is episodic nursing practice? List several episodic nursing roles.

4. What is distributive nursing practice? List several of these roles.

5. Describe the way you feel around final exams. How does this resemble burnout?

6. Describe your first day in clinical practice. Did your instructor expect more of you than you felt you could deliver?

7. Interview a nurse who is actively engaged in using a computer in nursing practice. Describe the role the computer plays.

References

1. World Health Organization, *Constitution: World Health Organization* (Geneva: World Health Organization, 1971).

2. Halbert L. Dunn, *High Level Wellness* (Washington, D.C.: Mt. Vernon Publishing Co. 1961).
3. Patricia Flynn, *Holistic Health* (Bowie, Md.: Robert J. Brady Co., 1981), 12.
4. Committee for the Study of Credentialing in Nursing, *A New Approach*. Staff Working Papers, vol. 2 (Kansas City, Mo.: The American Nurses' Association, 1979), 388–91.
5. Barbara W. Narrow and Kay Brown Buschle, *Fundamentals of Nursing Practice* (New York: John Wiley & Sons, 1982), 29.
6. American Nurses' Association, *Nursing: A Social Policy Statement* (Kansas City, Mo.: The American Nurses' Association, 1980), 9.
7. American Nurses' Association Committee on Education, "ANA's First Position on Education for Nursing," *Am J Nurs,* 65 (December 1965):106–11.
8. American Nurses' Association House of Delegates, "Resolutions," *The American Nurse* 10:8, (September 15, 1978):9.
9. National League for Nursing Board of Directors, *1982 Position Statement on Nursing Roles— Scope and Preparation* (New York: National League for Nursing, 1982).
10. American Nurses' Association National Task Force on Nursing Education for Nursing Practice, *Education for Nursing Practice in the Context of the 1980s* (Kansas City, Mo.: American Nurses' Association, 1983).
11. National League for Nursing press release, "News from NLN," (New York: National League for Nursing, November 1985).
12. *The American Nurse* 18(May 1986):1.
13. Ibid.
14. Gail Hood, "At issue: titling and licensure," *Am J Nurs* 85(May 1985):592–94.
15. Lila L. Anastas, *The Washington Post,* April 28, 1985.
16. Paul Woody, "Nursing in the eighties," *The Virginia Commonwealth University Magazine* 15(Fall 1986).
17. Kathleen Michels, "Balanced budget law slashes health programs," *The American Nurse* 18(April 1986):1.
18. Lawrence Feinberg, "Area nursing schools seek cure for decreasing enrollment," *The Washington Post,* August 11, 1986.
19. Peri Rosenfeld, "Nursing education: Statistics you can use," *Nurs & Health Care* (June 1986): 327–29.
20. Ibid.
21. Ibid., 329.
22. JoAnn S. Jamann, ed., "Proceedings of doctoral programs in nursing: Consensus for quality," *J Professional Nurs* 1(March/April 1985):90–121.
23. Bonnie Bullough, "Nurse practice acts," *Nursing 77* (February 1977).
24. Dianne Hales, "A different kind of doctoring," *America's Health* 4(Summer, 1982).
25. Eunice R. Cole, "Nurses are doing more but some insurers won't pay." *The Washington Post,* (Washington, D.C., June 18, 1986):6.
26. Eugene Levine, "The Registered Nurse Supply and Nurse Shortage," *Study of Nursing and Nursing Education Background Paper* (Washington, D.C.: Institute of Medicine, National Academy of Sciences, January 1983).
27. Linda H. Aiken and Robert J. Blendon, "The National Nurse Shortage" *National Journal* (May 23, 1981), 948–53.
28. Sara Erickson, "Spotlight on History," *N J Nurse,* (January/February 1983):9.
29. Division of Health Care Service, Institute of Medicine, *Nursing and Nursing Education: Public Policies and Private Actions* (Washington, D.C.: National Academy Press, 1983), 76.
30. "Layoffs loom as state and federal cutbacks hit California hospitals," *Am J Nurs* 83(February 1983):196.
31. Margaret D. West, "The Projected Supply of Registered Nurses 1990. Discussion and Methodology," *Study of Nursing and Nursing Education Background Paper* (Washington, D.C.: Institute of Medicine, National Academy of Sciences, January 1983), 19, 20.
32. "News," *Am J Nurs* 86(July 1986):851–60.
33. Marlene Kramer, *Reality Shock, Why Nurses Leave Nursing* (St. Louis: C.V. Mosby Co., 1974), viii.
34. Ibid.
35. Patricia T. Haase, "Pathways to practice—part I," *Am J Nurs* 76 (May 1976):806–9.
36. D. Diers and D.L. Evans. "Excellence in nursing," *Image* 12 (February 1980):27–30.
37. Proceedings for the *First National Conference; Computer Technology in Nursing*. NIH, U.S. Department of Health, Education, and Welfare, June, 1981.

Annotated Bibliography

Dailey, A.L. 1985. The burnout test. *Am J Nurs* 85(3):270–72. This article is written by a clinical psychologist with experience in burnout counseling with nurses. It presents a guide to nurses who wish to identify their risk potential for burnout and offers a comprehensive and structured plan for coping with and overcoming burnout.

Lancaster, J. 1986. 1986 and beyond: Nursing's future. *J Nurs Admin* 16(3):31–37. This journal article gives an excellent overview of the status of the nursing profession as it moves into the 1990s. Trends affecting health care and nursing are discussed as well as future directions in nursing. Recommendations are offered regarding effective dealing with nursing's image, educating nurses, attaining public accountability and professional autonomy, and increasing political skills and research activity.

McCloskey, J.C. and Grace, H.K., eds. 1985. *Current Issues in Nursing,* 2nd ed. Boston: Blackwell Scientific, 1985. This book provides a forum in which knowledgeable nursing leaders debate some of the most important issues facing today's nursing profession. There are 12 sections, each of which provides a number of viewpoints pro and con the issue at hand. Examples of issues include role conflict, educational preparation of nurses, quality assurance, changing practice, and ethics.

A Nursing 78 Handbook. 1978. *A Guide to Nursing Specialties.* Part I (A to M), *Nursing 78* 8(10):57–64; Part II (N to Z), 8(11):49–56. These two articles list many nursing specialties and the level of nursing education necessary for those specialties. Also listed are selected educational programs, professional organizations, and specialty journals.

Chapter 3

Theory, Concept, and Process

Janet-Beth McCann Flynn
Phyllis B. Heffron

Chapter Outline

- Objectives
- Glossary
- Introduction
- Philosophy
- Theory
- Concepts
- Frameworks and Models
- Process
- Summary
- Study Questions
- References
- Annotated Bibliography

Objectives

At the completion of this chapter the reader will be able to:

▶ Define the terms theory, concept, and process
▶ Compare and contrast the terms theory, concept, and process
▶ Describe a framework
▶ Discuss why models are needed in nursing

Glossary

Concepts. General, intangible, and symbolic ways of referring to reality.

Framework. An organizational structure for ordering concepts to provide an integrated perspective of a profession, field, or the world.

Model. A paradigm describing a consensually adopted mode of practice in a scientific or professional field.

Philosophy. A set of beliefs that are acquired and interpreted throughout a lifetime of experiences with reality.

Process. The act of continuously moving along in order to meet a predetermined goal or set of goals.

Theory. Systematically related set of statements or concepts that describe, explain, and predict the real world.

INTRODUCTION

The quest for knowledge is a never-ending process, but the acquisition of facts alone is not enough to facilitate adaptation. Facts need a unifying theme to pull them together into a larger system of viewing life and to give them meaning. This is why we have large bodies of knowledge such as philosophies, theories, and concepts.

Philosophies, theories, and concepts organize facts into a structured framework for viewing reality. Once these have been organized and defined, a mechanism must be defined to put the organized frameworks into action. This action phase is called **process.**

Nurses need to understand philosophies, theories, concepts and processes because nursing is a discipline based on using and integrating bodies of knowledge to be able to assess what is needed or to deliver health care.

This chapter describes the terms philosophy, theory, concept and process.

PHILOSOPHY

A philosopher is one who loves wisdom. **Philosophy** is the study of wisdom, of fundamental knowledge, and of the process by which we construct our outlook on life. It is also the study of how people acquire beliefs.[1] The basic beliefs and values that give meaning to one's experiences come from a lifetime of learning through interpersonal contact, religion, education, and the environment.

These beliefs and values determine the manner by which persons relate to each other, the way they work with each other and the way nurses care for clients.[2] A person's philosophy, whether or not that person is able to recognize and articulate it as such, is a set of beliefs and values that direct behavior and attitudes. It can be thought of as a multifaceted lens through which we observe, comprehend, and evaluate the seemingly random events that go on around us—a lens through which we see things as good, evil, healthful, sick, socially or professionally appropriate, irresponsible, and so forth.

Philosophy is a belief about life, human beings, values, and ideals. Each of us has a philosophy of life, but most of us are not fully aware of it. Our philosophy is our overall outlook on life. It is like an umbrella composed of all the concepts we believe in (Fig. 3–1). Individuals use their philosophy of life to orient themselves to the world around them. Nurses, as they work with clients, families, and groups, come into contact with some of the most profound issues that affect human life, such as suicide, child abuse, abortion, and euthanasia. Studying philosophy helps individuals to reflect on personal belief systems and provides a framework for examining one's own value system (Fig. 3–2). "An awareness and understanding

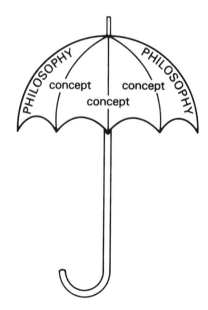

Figure 3–1. Philosophy umbrella.

of one's own philosophy and values and a deliberate expression of one's own beliefs about man are fundamental to the performance of quality nursing."[3]

THEORY

Riehl and Roy define a **theory** as a "scientifically acceptable general principle which governs practice or is proposed to explain observed facts."[4] Yura and Walsh write that a "theory is a systematically related set of statements that describes, explains, and predicts parts of the empirical or real world."[5]

Theory orders abstracted and conceptualized observations and propositions to specify relationships among concepts. It is an attempt to present as clear, rounded, and systematic a picture of the subject as possible. Theory represents the present understanding and thinking surrounding the focus of the theory.

A theory is a proposed structuring of reality, not reality itself, and is used to guide, explain, and predict reality.[6,7] Theories can be verbalized and communicated to others. They are structures for passing on knowledge. Examples

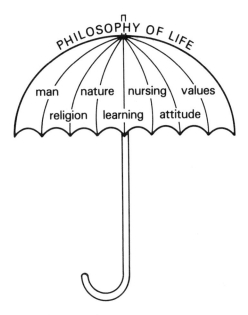

Figure 3–2. Philosophy-of-life umbrella.

The nursing profession needs theories to organize and integrate what is known about humans, health, illness, and nursing. These theories can provide a structured systematic way of examining and directing nursing practice. Theories are the primary force in elevating nursing from a skill-oriented job into a profession. Over the past 20 years, many nursing theorists (see Chapter 4) have struggled to define the nature of nursing and identify its professional purpose through the development of theoretical frameworks.

According to Ellis, the purposes of developing theories of nursing are to facilitate the differentiation between fact and pseudofact and to structure the conveying of facts from other professions.[12] Nursing theory provides the framework to integrate knowledge from the biological and psychological aspects of humankind.

Ellis provides another reason for nurses to be concerned with theory and theory development. She writes that theory directs practice, and through practice, observations can be made that provide the opportunity for theory evaluation.[13]

Theories generally are arrived at by two major processes.* One process is that of *deductive reasoning.* Deductive reasoning is the method of looking initially at the general or universal idea and then moving to the specific or particular. In *inductive reasoning,* the other major process, the direction is reversed. First, the specific or particular action is identified, and then conclusions are drawn about general or universal ideas.

For example, it is observed that people who smoke cigarettes have a higher incidence of lung cancer than those who do not smoke. Is this deductive or inductive reasoning? In what direction does the flow of information take place? Does the process move from the general to the specific or vice versa? In the case of smoking, the process is from the particular (people who smoke) to the general (lung cancer). Therefore, this example demonstrates the inductive method. An example of the deductive method would be to consider that resistance to infection

of well-known theories include Albert Einstein's theory of relativity, Issac Newton's theory of gravitation, and Sigmund Freud's psychoanalytic theory.

Generally speaking, a theory is a "set of beliefs for which there is some, but not completely supporting, evidence."[8] It is a set of untested ideas that results from speculations about reality.[9] Theories are testable and therefore refutable and alterable.[10] Theory guides research through the generation of expected or predicted outcomes (hypothesis) of interventions. A theory is therefore supported or not supported by the empirical data that is obtained through the research it generates. When theories are proven, they become laws. Physical scientific theories are easier to prove than human-based theories. Disciplines, such as chemistry and physics, have more laws than social sciences, such as sociology, psychology, and nursing.

Theories have many purposes. They provide a systematic way of viewing reality. They guide research and provide a framework for evaluation. In addition to guiding practice and identifying research problems, theory provides a basis for evaluating and selecting proposed innovative methods or practices.[11]

---

*Major portion of discussion on reasoning from unpublished manuscript by Dr. MaryAnn Schroeder.

is best in healthy people. Therefore, it can be deduced that people who are chronically ill with a kidney disease probably would be more likely to catch colds than people who are generally healthy.

Some nursing theorists use the deductive method and others use the inductive method. According to Dickoff and James, the determination of what kind of nursing theory is needed for professional practice is dependent upon professional purpose.[14] They write that a professional person, as opposed to a technician, is one who shapes reality rather than one who experiences reality. Nursing theory must therefore be based upon an action orientation and have a purpose.[15]

Dickoff and James suggest that theories evolve through a series of stages or levels, and during development, each higher level presupposes the existence of theories at a lower level.[16] The first level of theory development is the factor-isolating stage, in which relevant facets or concepts of the theories are identified and named. The second level of theory development is observing and noting the relationship between the concepts that were named in stage one. In the third level, concepts are related to each other in such a way that predictions about outcomes can be made. Finally, after the predictive theory is defined, the highest level of theory development is reached. This is called the situation-producing theory, and its purpose is to produce situations in which predicted outcomes are obtained.

According to Riehl and Roy, nursing has not "yet reached the point of clear development on all four levels of theory," but nurses are able to use the elements of situation-producing theory to provide the elements for nursing practice.[17]

Theories rarely occur in isolation but rather, usually reflect the time and culture in which they are conceived. In other words, theories are products of the milieu in which they happen. Two concepts that express these environmental or evolutionary aspects of the climate in which theories arise are the German words *Zeitgeist* and *Weltanschauung.** Zeitgeist describes the general moral and intellectual state of a culture. It denotes the trends of taste characteristic of a given era. Zeitgeist means "the spirit of the times"—the fashion. Weltanschauung is the prevailing philosophy of life, the "world view," or manner of looking at the universe. For example, theories generated in an era of unrest and upheaval, such as in wartime, might reflect concepts regarding anxiety and attempts by individuals to make themselves more comfortable. Theories may support the philosophy of the time or refute it. But it is the rare theory that appears indifferent to the intellectual or philosophical climate of the era.

CONCEPTS

Concepts are the building blocks of theories. They are more fundamental than theories. They are general thoughts or ideas that are intangible and can be thought of as a symbolic or abstract way of referring to reality.[18–20] Concepts are words that describe objects, properties, events, and relationships among them.[21]

Concepts are more than just words or labels. They are significant symbols, words that have been given special meanings in the course of human interactions.[22] Therefore a concept is both a word and an idea with special meaning attached to that word.[23]

A concept is a clear-cut verbal and logical operation in which one uses a series of logically selected ideas to arrive at a decision or conclusion. A concept serves as a process of classification, of placing a number of items into a category.[24] This is achieved by focusing on one or more essential features of an item and disregarding all other individualistic peculiarities. A concept represents an attribute shared by a group of items or ideas. A concept is a stereotype, i.e., a bird has given features and ways of behavior that are associated only with birds; for example, they have feathers, wings, and most can fly.

By using concepts, individuals can anticipate the future, can plan actions to achieve pleasant happenings and avoid unpleasant ones. Concepts serve to tie past experiences with the present and allow for some prediction of the future. For example, preparing a care plan for

*This discussion from unpublished manuscript by Dr. MaryAnn Schroeder.

a postoperative client who is at present in the operating room. A person who has the necessary knowledge can anticipate the needs and plan interventions on the predicted events in the course of postoperative recovery.

Concepts indicate the subject matter of theory and are defined by the specific theory.[25] Conceptual meanings are understood only within the theory of which they are a part.[26] Examples of concepts from nursing theories include self-care, adaptation, interaction, and interdependence. Each theory must define its own concepts, as these vary from theory to theory. Concepts are the tools with which professionals perform their work.

Concepts develop as a part of a theory and are refined as the knowledge base of the theory expands. Refinement of concepts is an ongoing process that, according to Hardy, involves not only sharpening of theoretical and operational definitions, but also modifying existing theory. Concepts are refined by relating the theoretical world to the real world, by organizing many concrete items into a smaller number of classes, and by relating diverse concepts within a more general system of concepts.[27]

Concepts are necessary in nursing in order to relate theory to practice. Horgan, in 1967, researched selected nursing periodicals from 1950 to 1965 and found that, between 1960 and 1965, 18 concepts appeared.[28] Horgan defined a concept of nursing as an expression of ideas that summarize the theorists' view of elements and components of nursing and the nursing process. As time passes and nurses become more sophisticated, more concepts will be defined. Since this particular study was completed, the literature has been rich with concepts and theories. Many of the major nursing theories have been formalized during this time as well. If nursing is to continue to develop as a health-care profession, identification of concepts and research to support them is essential.

FRAMEWORKS AND MODELS

Frameworks are ways of organizing concepts into a broader view of a situation. Conceptual frameworks consist of sets of networks of concepts and attempt to provide an integrated perspective of the world. Conceptual frameworks are not theories. They are broad pretheoretical bases from which theories are derived.[29] Conceptual frameworks are the bases that allow decision making and problem solving. They serve to integrate and synthesize knowledge from one or more fields.

In nursing, conceptual frameworks are used as a means of describing what is present in experience and beliefs. As such, they guide and direct nursing care.

A **model** is a guideline and a standard for practice that is built on a theory.[30] A model is an exemplar or paradigm describing a consensually adopted mode of practice in a scientific or professional field. It includes a science or profession's laws, theories, methods, instruments, and applications.

The nursing literature states that a model is a delineation of the nature of humans, the state of health, the environment, and services provided by nurses. A model is viewed as a systematic set of implicit and explicit ideas that nurses use to direct their activities in the clinical setting. Nursing models, to be complete, must contain several critical elements. These include: the nursing process, a goal, a rationale, a statement of professional role, a client description, and a care setting.

PROCESS

Process is the action phase of a conceptual framework or theory. It is the act of moving forward to meet a goal. The very term "process" indicates continuous movement through a succession of stages until the goal or the outcome has been accomplished. According to Bevis, process is also a change that uses feedback as one proceeds toward the objective.[31] The feedback into the process is due to the data being collected from the environment. How this data analysis is carried out relates to the theoretical or conceptual framework and its definition.

Yura and Walsh write that the perception of a process as an action suggests a power behind the action or someone who strives to complete the action.[32] Therefore there is control over the action and a systematic movement toward completion. Conscious attention and effort must be exerted to complete the process and meet the predetermined goal. The action of moving, or the process, must be based on a needs assessment. Without a goal to direct the process, it would become disorganized and perhaps useless.[33]

Since nursing is action directed and goal oriented, it has a process, a systematic way of providing assistance to clients. It is based upon assessment of clients' needs, making plans with the clients to meet these needs, carrying out the plan, and evaluating its success. Without this systematic process, nursing would lack clarity and be potentially ineffective.

SUMMARY

People need a structure to be able to organize the hundreds of thousands of facts accumulated during life. Philosophies, theories, and concepts serve this purpose. They are frameworks for viewing and making sense of reality.

Nurses need philosophies, theories, and concepts because nursing is a field of diverse facts that need to be related to specific nursing actions. Through theory development, nursing is advancing professionally. Through application, theory becomes reality.

Process is the action phase of a conceptual framework or theory. The nursing process is the action phase in applying nursing concepts in practice. It is an organized framework for systematic problem solving and is goal-directed. Without a systematic and comprehensive theory, process cannot be effective.

Study Questions

1. What is a theory?

2. How do concepts relate to theory?

3. Describe a framework and compare it to concepts.

4. What is a model?

5. What is a process?

6. How does a theory or framework relate to a process?

7. Why do nurses need theories and concepts?

References

1. Van Cleve Morris and Young Pai, *Philosophy and the American School,* 2nd ed. (Boston: Houghton Mifflin Co., 1976), 4.
2. Helen Yura and Mary Walsh, *The Nursing Process,* 3rd ed. (New York: Appleton-Century-Crofts, 1978), 16.
3. Ibid.
4. Joan P. Riehl and Sr. Callista Roy, *Conceptual Models for Nursing Practice* (New York: Appleton-Century-Crofts, 1974), 3.
5. Yura and Walsh, *The Nursing Process,* 16.
6. J. Dickoff and P. James, "A Theory of theories: A position paper," *Nurs Res* 17 (1968):197–203.
7. Riehl and Roy, *Conceptual Models for Nursing Practice,* 3.
8. Morris and Pai, *Philosophy and the American School,* 4.
9. Dorothea E. Orem (ed.), *Concept Formulation in Nursing: Process and Product* (Boston: Little, Brown, & Co., 1979), 55.
10. Margaret Newman, *Theory Development in Nursing* (Philadelphia: F.A. Davis Co., 1979), 6.
11. C.H. Patterson, *Foundations for a Theory of Induction and Educational Psychology* (New York: Harper & Row, 1977), 4.
12. R. Ellis, "Characteristics of significant theorists," *Nurs Res* 17 (1968):217–22.
13. Ibid.
14. J. Dickoff and P. James, "A theory of theories," 197–203.
15. Ibid.
16. Ibid.
17. Riehl and Roy, *Conceptual Models for Nursing Practice,* 5.
18. G. Sartori, *Social Science Concepts: A Systematic Analysis* (Beverly Hills, Calif.: Sage Publications, 1984).
19. Yura and Walsh, *Nursing Process,* 18.
20. A. Jacox, "Theory construction in nursing: an overview," *Nurs Res* 23 (1974):4–13.
21. Ibid., 5.
22. G. Mead, *Mind, Self and Society* (Chicago: University of Chicago Press, 1934).
23. Ibid., 5.
24. M.E. Hardy, "Theories: Components, develop-

ment, evaluation," *Nurs Res* 23 (1974):100–106.

25. A.N. Burscher, "Nursing diagnosis. Where does the conceptual framework fit?" in M.E. Hurley (ed.), *Classification of Nursing Diagnosis* (St. Louis: C.V. Mosby Co., 1986), 76.
26. Mead, *Mind, Self and Society.*
27. Hardy, "Theories: Components, development, evaluation," 100–106.
28. M.V. Horgan, *Concepts about Nursing in Selected Nursing Literature from 1950–1965.* (Master's thesis, The Catholic University of America, School of Nursing, Washington, D.C., 1967).
29. J. Faucett, *Analyses and Evaluation of Concept Models in Nursing* (Philadelphia: F.A. Davis Co., 1984).
30. F. Abadellah and E. Levine, *Better Patient Care through Research* (NY: Macmillan Co, 1965).
31. E.O. Bevis, *Curriculum Building in Nursing—A Process* (St. Louis: C.V. Mosby Co., 1973), 9.
32. Yura and Walsh, *The Nursing Process,* 19.
33. Ibid.

Annotated Bibliography

Ellis, R. 1968. Characteristics of significant theories. *Nurs Res* 17(3):217–22. This classic article reviews the key components of theories.

Hardy, M.E. 1974. Theories: Components, development, evaluation. *Nurs Res* 23(2):100–197. This article discusses basic terms, selection, and evaluation of nursing theories.

Jacox, A. 1974. Theory construction in nursing: An overview. *Nurs Res* 23(1):4–13. This article reviews how scientific knowledge is developed and organized into theories.

Jones, P.S. 1978. An adaptation model for nursing practice. *Am J Nurs* 78(11):1900–1905. This article discusses the conceptual framework of adaptation. It provides an excellent, brief review of the relevant literature and suggests a tool for assessment.

Newman, M.A. 1979. *Theory Development in Nursing.* Philadelphia: F. A. Davis. This brief and excellent book discusses how theories are developed.

Riehl, J.P., Roy, C. 1974. *Conceptual Models for Nursing Practice.* New York: Appleton-Century-Crofts. This text is a collection of contributed chapters that discuss several of the major nursing theories.

Chapter 4

Theorists in Nursing

Edna M. Fordyce

Chapter Outline

- Objectives
- Glossary
- Introduction
- Selected Nursing Theorists
  Virginia Henderson
  Hildegard E. Peplau
  Ida J. Orlando
  Ernestine Wiedenbach
  Dorothy E. Johnson
  Imogene M. King
  Dorothea E. Orem
  Martha E. Rogers
  Joyce Travelbee
  Sister Callista Roy
  Josephine G. Paterson and Loretta T. Zderad
  Myra E. Levine
  Betty M. Neuman
  Other Theorists
- Summary
- Study Questions
- References
- Annotated Bibliography

Objectives

At the completion of this chapter the reader will be able to:

- Define the terms in the glossary
- Name some of the prominent nursing theorists
- Identify the major premise of the perspective of nursing as presented by one or more of the prominent nurse theorists
- State the definition of nursing presented by each of the prominent nurse theorists
- State the view of nursing process as described by one or more of the prominent nurse theorists
- Identify the dominant influences that have persuaded the nurse theorist to view nursing from the particular perspective advocated by her

Glossary

Automatic Nursing Action. Orlando's term for activities or tasks carried out by nurses that have been based on reasons other than the client's immediate needs.

Behavioral System. Johnson identified this as a combination of all the patterned, repetitive, and purposeful ways of behaving that characterize each person's life.

Complementarity. Rogers's principle relating the interaction between the human and environmental energy fields as continuous, mutual, and simultaneous.

Contextual Stimuli. Roy's description of those occurrences as substances in individuals or their environment other than those most immediate to them, that influence client's adaptation; this term is used relative to focal stimuli.

Deliberative Nursing Action. Orlando's term for activities or tasks carried out by the nurse that have been based on an analysis that ascertains or meets the client's immediate needs

Focal Stimuli. Roy's description of those occurrences or substances in individuals or their environment that most immediately influence client adaptation.

Health-deviation Self-care. Orem's category of client care activities that are necessitated because of illness, injury, or disease.

Helicy. Rogers's human development principle describing the nature as well as the direction of the human and environmental energy fields and their interaction.

Nursology. The study of humanistic nursing practice as defined by Patterson and Zderad.

Residual Stimuli. Roy's terminology for influences of adaptation in humankind, such as an individual's beliefs, attitudes, or traits.

Resonancy. Rogers's principle describing the human and environmental energy fields according to the pattern and organization of shorter and longer wave patterns.

Self-care. The central theme of Orem's nursing theory that refers to those activities that individuals personally initiate and perform on their own behalf for the purpose of their health and well-being.

Universal Self-care. Orem's definition of those activities individuals do in everyday life to meet their basic human needs.

INTRODUCTION

The purpose of this chapter is to identify leading nursing theorists and their conceptual models of nursing. A study of nursing literature provides indications of the maturation of nursing. During the last several years the profession of nursing has progressed from developing definitions of nursing and nursing practice to endeavoring to identify the theoretical dimensions of what constitutes nursing. The growing collection of publications by nurse-authors within a relatively few years indicates the emergence of many theories of nursing.

The development of definitions of nursing was essential, particularly for determining the legal boundaries of nursing for the nurse prac-

tice acts of the various states. Another significant historical trend in the development of nursing theory was the identification and definition of conceps that provided a framework for nursing practice and nursing education. Concepts have been referred to as the building blocks of a body of knowledge. Webster's New Collegiate Dictionary defines a concept as an abstract or generic idea generalized from particular instances.

In discussing theory construction in nursing, Jacox defines concepts as "abstract representations of reality."[1] Concepts are symbolic descriptions, and when several are combined in a meaningful way, a theory is developed. Concepts might be characterized as the workhorses that, when harnessed together in a systematized way, become theory. Theory enables the performance of a task or set of tasks. For example, theory guides the practice of nursing.

Theory provides first, the framework for the analysis of one set of facts in relation to another, and second, a belief, policy, or procedure proposed or followed as the basis of action. Another perspective commonly accepted in describing theory is the grouping of related concepts to describe, explain, or predict some part of reality. When defining theory, Jacox stated, "it is a systematically related set of statements or propositions."[2] Thus, theory in nursing would include a description of nursing, explain nursing practice, and predict the influence of this practice.

One nurse author of contemporary times, Dorothy Johnson, has emphasized the importance of developing a theoretical base for the practice of nursing, if professional stature is our concern. She stated, "if nursing is indeed an emerging profession, nurses must be able to identify clearly and develop continually the theoretical body of knowledge upon which practice must rest."[3] In describing the characteristics of a profession, she noted that "a profession's service to society is an intellectual one, and a sound, scientific basis for that service is indispensable."[4] Another nurse author, Myra Levine, advised that a theory of nursing must recognize the importance of unique detail of care for a single client within an empiric framework that successfully describes the requirements of all clients.[5]

From the early days of nursing, leaders in the profession have sought to identify and describe the functions of nursing as well as its significant components and dimensions. Modern nursing's founder, Florence Nightingale, a nurse theorist and scientist in her own right, described the knowledge she considered basic to nursing care.[6] Her perspective emphasized fresh air and sanitation. The environment in which the patient was cared for was of paramount concern to her.

In recent times, there have emerged a number of authors espousing specific theoretical perspectives on the practice of nursing. Several of these authors have been selected for discussion in the remainder of this chapter. Each author has contributed to the continuing pursuit of the theoretical base for nursing.

The sequence for the discussion of these nursing theorist-authors was made on the basis of the publication years of each person's writings.

SELECTED NURSING THEORISTS

Virginia Henderson

Virginia Henderson is a writer of international influence whose contributions to nursing have been numerous. She believes her greatest contribution to nursing was the preparation of the *Nursing Studies Index*. Dr. Henderson wishes to be remembered as a practitioner,[7] and indeed, her writings focus on the practice of nursing.

In presenting her view of nursing, Henderson proposed a definition of nursing (see Chapter 2) that still has impact upon nursing today. This definition was previously cited, sometimes with minor variations, in other publications.[8–11] The same central theme is present in the definition wherever cited: that of assisting the client with activities that ordinarily are performed without assistance, and to help the individual regain his or her performance capability as soon as possible. Dr. Henderson viewed

the primary function of the nurse as that of "helping the patient with his daily pattern of living. . . ."[12] This helping function was associated with particular activities or the provision of certain conditions that she described as encompassing basic nursing care, and through which the nurse was seen as a substitute for what the client lacked in physical strength, will, or knowledge.[13, 14] Dr. Henderson delineated the following activities and conditions[15,16]:

- Breathe normally
- Eat and drink adequately
- Eliminate body wastes
- Move and maintain desirable postures
- Sleep and rest
- Select suitable clothes—dress and undress
- Maintain body temperature within normal range by adjusting clothing and modifying the environment
- Keep the body clean and well groomed and protect the integument
- Avoid dangers in the environment and avoid injuring others
- Communicate with others in expressing emotions, needs, fears, or opinions
- Worship according to one's faith
- Work in such a way that there is a sense of accomplishment
- Play or participate in various forms of recreation
- Learn, discover, or satisfy the curiosity that leads to normal development and health and use the available health facilities

Henderson contended that "the nurse is the authority on basic nursing care."[17] Furthermore, Henderson believed that this list of activities and conditions could be used to evaluate nursing, principally by measuring the success attained in helping clients acquire independence in the performance of these functions.[18]

Writing in 1955,[19] Henderson emphasized the significance of providing and promoting activities that would be life-enhancing according to the individual needs of each client. She further noted the numerous ways that the client's daily life was disrupted in respect to these ordinary activities through the hospital experience. She also stated her consequent concerns about "every nursing routine or restriction that is in conflict with the individual's fundamental need for shelter, food, communication with others and the company he loves; for opportunity to win approval, to dominate and be dominated, to learn, to work, to worship, and to play."[20] Henderson was one of the first authors to include responsibilities of the nurse for those who would not recover from injury or illness in her definition of nursing.

Henderson's writings represent her own personal memoirs, and she recounts the many influences that have shaped her perspective of nursing. The view of nursing that she holds is practice-centered. Virginia Henderson's first work in the nursing literature was her authorship of the revision of Bertha Harmer's *Textbook of the Principles and Practice of Nursing,* which was published in 1939.[21] In subsequent writings, a major hallmark of Henderson's perspective of nursing can be found in her definition of nursing and the 14 activities or conditions that constitute, in her opinion, basic nursing care.

Hildegard E. Peplau

Hildegard Peplau wrote a textbook, *Interpersonal Relations in Nursing,* that has made a continuing contribution during the years since its publication.[22] The ideas of prominent psychiatrists (particularly Harry Stack Sullivan) and psychologists of that time were translated and presented in terms understandable to nurses. Dr. Peplau espoused the view that nursing was an interpersonal relationship between a person who needed help and a person who, because of special preparation, could provide the help needed. Psychodynamic nursing was described by Peplau as recognizing, clarifying, and building an understanding of what happens when nurses relate to clients helpfully.

The major themes present in the 1952 publication were the interpersonal relationship with clients and the nurse's self-understanding and developing maturity. Peplau viewed nursing as an interpersonal process. She observed that every nurse–client relationship is an interper-

TABLE 4–1. PEPLAU'S FOUR MAJOR LIFE TASKS

Learning to count on others
Learning to delay satisfactions
Identifying oneself
Developing skills in participation or problem solving

sonal one, where the difficulties of everyday living arise and recur. A significant feature of Dr. Peplau's perspective of nursing was the emphasis on the nurse's own personality growth and maturation, which influenced the kind of nursing care that was given.

Peplau discussed the psychological tasks encountered in the process of learning to live with people. Four major life tasks are emphasized by Peplau (Table 4–1). Each of these developmental tasks of life that the client struggles with indicate the tasks demanded of the nurse in helping the client complete the unfinished psychological tasks of childhood. These problems of everyday life were the concern of the nurse as she endeavored to help clients meet and encounter the various tasks of life. The nurse, according to Dr. Peplau, performed various tasks in facilitating the personal growth of the client. The phases of the nurse–client relationship were identified and described as constituting psychodynamic nursing. Peplau identified four interlocking phases of the nurse–client relationship (Table 4–2). Each phase is characterized by overlapping roles or functions of the nurse and defines the nurse's roles and tasks. The various roles associated with the performance of nursing included that of stranger, re-

TABLE 4–2. THE FOUR PHASES OF THE PSYCHODYNAMIC NURSE–CLIENT RELATIONSHIP

Orientation phase
Identification phase
Exploitation phase
Resolution phase

source person, teacher, surrogate parent, sibling, counselor, technical expert, and others. She also suggested that nurses had a responsibility for the environment of the client.

In addition, Peplau discussed psychobiological experiences (human needs) and factors that interfere with the achievement of discussed goals, such as frustration and subsequent aggression, opposing developmental goals and resultant conflict, and unexplained discomforts—anxiety, guilt, and doubt.

Peplau suggested that observation, communication, and recording are methods for studying nursing as an interpersonal process. She maintained that nursing can be a therapeutic, maturing, educative force in society.

Peplau asserted that her views were a partial theory for the practice of nursing as an interpersonal process. She suggested that nursing was in a unique position for identifying and studying the recurring human problems of everyday living and for studying the skills used by people during these struggles.

She stated that self-understanding and personal maturity determined one's performance in interpersonal relations in nursing situations and thus nursing education had a responsibility to promote personality development and maturation of nursing students.

Ida J. Orlando

During the mid-1950s, Ida Orlando undertook a study of what nursing is, which entailed the examination of numerous nursing situations to determine the outcome of the nursing care provided. Based on her findings she described the process the nurse went through to influence a change in the client's behavior. From this personal study of verbatim nursing notes, she contended that the "purpose of nursing is to supply the help a patient requires in order for his needs to be met."[23] This purpose is achieved as the nurse initiates the process of finding and meeting the immediate needs of clients for help.

The focus of the perspective of nursing, as presented by Orlando, is the process the nurse undertakes to accomplish the purpose of nursing. In contrast to other descriptions of nursing processes presented in nursing literature, Orlando described this process taking place within the nurse.[24, 25] Orlando identified three elements present in a nursing situation[26] (Table 4–3). Whenever the nurse observes the behavior of the client, observation occurs through the nurse's perceptions. These perceptions trigger associated thoughts and feelings in the nurse; in other words, the nurse's reaction to the behavior of the client. Orlando advised that the nursing action(s) is the sharing of these perceptions and the related thoughts and feelings with the client, to determine if this is what the client is experiencing. This action is known as validation. When this process is followed, the purpose can be achieved.

Orlando identified nursing principles that were to guide the nurse in practice, and these principles represented the theory of effective nursing practice that could be taught to nursing students. Orlando identified four practices that she considered basic to nursing (Table 4–4).[27] Orlando stated the principles that guided these practices as:

> Any observation shared and explored with the patient is immediately useful in ascertaining and meeting his need or finding out that he is not in need at that time.[28]

TABLE 4–3. ORLANDO'S BASIC ELEMENTS PRESENT IN NURSING SITUATIONS

The behavior of the patient
The reaction of the nurse
The nursing action designed for the patient's benefit

TABLE 4–4. ORLANDO'S FOUR BASIC PRACTICES IN NURSING

Observing
Reporting
Recording
Carrying out actions for or with the patient

The presenting behavior of the patient, regardless of the form in which it appears, may represent a plea for help.[29]

The nurse does not assume that any aspect of her reaction to the patient is correct, helpful or appropriate until she checks the validity of it in exploration with the patient.[30]

These principles guide nurses in their observing, reporting, recording, and responding through nursing action.

Orlando identified two types of nursing actions. **Deliberative nursing actions** are those that, when decided on, ascertain or meet the client's immediate need. These actions constitute the disciplined nursing response. Any other kinds are **automatic nursing actions** that have been decided upon for reasons other than the client's immediate needs and, consequently, are ineffective.[31]

Orlando stated three requirements for the disciplined nursing process. The process must be included in one's thoughts, must ask a question about the thought, and must consider how the nurse states the thought (i.e., the nurse must claim ownership of the thought).[32]

A major contribution of Orlando's perspective of nursing practice has been her emphasis on the validation of the nurse's perceptions, thoughts, and feelings with the patient. Her description of the nursing process is unique and, historically, was one of the first to be presented in the nursing literature. The writings of Orlando also represent a belief about nursing based on the findings of her personal study of nursing, as documented through verbatim nursing notes. This represents an early example of nursing research on nursing practice to determine the theoretical aspects of nursing.

Ernestine Wiedenbach

After many years of experience in nursing, Ernestine Wiedenbach described clinical nursing as comprising four interlocking components that she identified as philosophy, purpose, practice, and art.[33] Her perspective of nursing is embodied in the descriptions she presents of each of these components.

While a faculty member of Yale University School of Nursing, Ernestine Wiedenbach was associated with Ida Orlando, Patricia James, and James Dickoff. The influence of these colleagues is observable in Wiedenbach's writings.

Wiedenbach described clinical nursing as a helping art.[34] It was a deliberate blending of thoughts, feelings, and overt actions, practiced in relation to an individual who is in need of help. It is triggered by a behavioral stimulus from the individual, is rooted in an explicit philosophy, and is directed toward fulfillment of a specific purpose.[35]

The foundation of the practice of nursing, according to Wiedenbach, is the philosophy that the individual nurse has about nursing and the individual client. The nurse's philosophy is the unique attitude toward life and reality incorporated in one's beliefs and conduct and is exhibited in the way nursing is practiced.[36] Wiedenbach presented three concepts basic to a philosophy of nursing. She suggested these concepts as guiding the choices and decisions of practices. According to Wiedenbach, the nurse's philosophy should include the concepts of[37]:

- Reverence for the gift of life
- Respect for the dignity, worth, autonomy, and individuality of each human being
- Resolution to act dynamically in relation to one's beliefs

As a basis for understanding the philosophy of nursing upon which her publication was predicated, Wiedenbach presented four assumptions about human nature that emphasized a respect for individuals.[38]

Intricately intertwined with the nurse's philosophy is the purpose or goal of nursing. The purpose, or the "why" of nursing, according to Wiedenbach, is "to meet the need the individual is experiencing as a need-for-help."[39] Wiedenbach noted that how the client perceived this need was contingent on the situation and how this was experienced concurrent with the nurse's contact with the client. She also observed that meaningful help from the nurse was used by the client "in enhancing or extending his capability."[40]

The practice of nursing is the "what" that is done to attain the purpose of nursing. The focus for the practice of clinical nursing is the client who is in need of help. Wiedenbach delineated the interrelated and interdependent knowledge, judgment, and skills that are essential attributes of the nurse for effective nursing practice. In addition, Wiedenbach cited four distinct components of practice to be used in meeting the client's needs. Three components are "directly related to the patient's care" and are[41]:

- Identification of the patient's experienced need-for-help
- Ministration of help needed
- Validation that the help provided was indeed the help needed

The fourth component is an indirect part of patient care, though an important aspect, and involves the coordination of "resources for help and of help provided."[42]

The art of helping clients includes the identification, ministration, and validation components of practice through the application of nursing knowledge and skill to fulfill the purpose of nursing. This art, or the "how" of clinical nursing, is a helping process and is action individualized for the patient.[43] Three principles of helping are presented by Wiedenbach as integral to the art of nursing. The principle of inconsistency-consistency alerts the nurse to heed any inconsistencies observed in the situation. The principle of purposeful perseverance requires the use of nursing judgment as to how long to persevere as well as resourcefulness in communication skills. The principle of self-extension enables the nurse to recognize her or his own limitations and enlist whatever help is indicated by the situation, including the participation of the client.[44]

Wiedenbach described the essence of clinical nursing as deliberative action that "holds the key to consistency in obtaining results the nurse seeks to obtain through what she does in giving nursing care to her patients."[45] Wiedenbach has succinctly described the "way, why, what, and how" of clinical nursing in the interlocking components of the philosophy, purpose, practice, and art of nursing.

TABLE 4–5. JOHNSON'S SEVEN BEHAVIORAL SYSTEMS

Attachment/affiliative
Dependency behavior
Ingestive
Eliminative
Sexual
Aggressive
Achievement

Dorothy E. Johnson

Dorothy E. Johnson has developed a **behavioral system** model for nursing that focuses on "efficient and effective behavioral functioning in the patient to prevent illness, and during and following illness."[46] Johnson stated that "all the patterned, repetitive, and purposeful ways of behaving that characterize each man's life are considered to comprise his behavioral system."[47]

Johnson identified seven behavioral systems (Table 4–5) associated with the human. The first, the attachment or affiliative subsystem, is the most critical and is one of the first to develop. The other six subsystems develop simultaneously or subsequently as part of the total behavioral system. Each subsystem has specialized tasks to be accomplished for the system as a whole.

Each of the subsystems has a structure as well as a function. Johnson has described four structural elements present in each subsystem. The behavior of the person is an observable element. Although not observable, the other three elements—drive, set, and goal—are each essential.

Nursing, according to Johnson, is "an external regulatory force which acts to preserve the organization and integration of the patient's behavior at an optimal level under those conditions in which the behavior constitutes a threat to physical or social health, or in which illness is found."[48]

For development and maintenance, the subsystems and the system as a whole require protection, nurture, and stimulation. As the external regulator of the environment, the nurse becomes the source of these functional requirements to meet the client's basic needs. Consequently, nursing intervention, in accordance with the Johnson model, entails four specific modes of intervention (note the association with the sustenance imperatives). The nurse restricts, defends, inhibits, or facilitates.

In discussing the Johnson model, Grubb describes a four-stage nursing process: a two-level assessment, diagnosis, interventions, and evaluation.[49]

Johnson's model is a systems model. Johnson believes that the human person functions according to the laws that govern all systems. The system of humans like other systems, seeks the maintenance of balance and a steady state, and generally there is enough flexibility in the system to attain this. However, there may be times when, because of a physical illness or a crisis situation, the system balance is disturbed enough that some external assistance may be required. Nursing may be the force that supplies this assistance through the external regulation of the environment.

Johnson believes that nursing is a service complementary to medicine and other health professions but that it also "makes its own distinctive contribution to the health and well-being of people."[50]

Professor Johnson has advanced nursing's progress toward a theoretical perspective through her own behavioral systems model as well as through her academic service and personal challenge to the profession.[51-54] She has influenced further interpretation of her model and the development of new models.

Imogene M. King

Imogene King has developed a view of nursing that incorporates both a general systems theory perspective and the process of human interactions. Dr. King identified aspects of nursing that have endured over time.[55] Then she set out to determine if these aspects continued to constitute the practice of nursing.[56] She also discussed changes in society and nursing.[57] The outcome of King's personal study of nursing has been the development of a conceptual framework that has subsequently emerged into a theory for goal attainment.[58]

King identified nursing as:

> a process of human interactions between nurse and client whereby each perceives the other and the situation; and through communication, they set goals, explore means, and agree on means to achieve goals.[59]

The process of nursing, described by King, is that of human interaction that includes action, reaction, interaction, transaction, and feedback (Table 4–6).[60] Consistent with this viewpoint, King affirmed that the focus of nursing is the care of human beings.[61]

King clearly stated the place of concepts in the formulation of her theory of nursing, as embodied in the process of human interaction, by identifying and describing the essential concepts upon which the theory was founded. The concepts she specified as central to human interaction were: "interaction, perception, communication, transaction, self, role, stress, growth and development, and time and space."[62]

King differentiated three levels of function for nursing that she later referred to as the domain of nursing.[63] These levels of interacting systems represented the care of individuals (personal systems) and groups (interpersonal systems) within society (social systems). The important concepts for each of the three levels are fully discussed in King's publications. King viewed these concepts as the content of nursing.[64] Readers of this chapter are encouraged to pursue study of these references. The three levels of nursing function, the concepts that constitute a knowledge base for each level, and the implications of the concepts for nursing constitute a noteworthy portion of King's theoretical perspective of nursing. The levels of function and the associated concepts related to each level are presented in the following way:

TABLE 4–6. KING'S PROCESS OF NURSING

Action
Reaction
Interaction
Transaction
Feedback

- *Personal Systems (Individuals):* Perception, self, growth and development, body image, space and time.[65]
- *Interpersonal Systems (Groups):* Human interactions, communication, transactions, role, and stress.
- *Social Systems (Society):* Organization, authority, power, status, and decision making.

The concept of health is an integral aspect of King's view of nursing. She succinctly described the goal of nursing as helping "individuals and groups attain, maintain, and restore health."[66]

To faciliate the application of her goal attainment theory, King developed a goal-oriented nursing record based on the problem-oriented medical record.

In developing her systems approach to describing nursing, King systematically clarified the specific concepts basic to her theory. A notable aspect of King's contribution to theory development in nursing is her own research designed to test the ideas set forth as a theory for nursing. Her description of the process of nursing as a human interaction, the levels of nursing functions, and the related concepts central to nursing practice reflect the scholarly dedication that is a hallmark of this author.

Dorothea E. Orem

Dorothea Orem's formalization of concepts based on the premise of self-care have become a focal point in the development of curricula for numerous schools of nursing. Although her first major publication on concepts of nursing practice did not appear until 1971, a definition of nursing and a perspective of nursing were initially published in 1959.[67] The writings of Dorothea Orem reflect some striking similarities to the view of nursing presented by Virginia Henderson. The diagrams depicting the themes in Henderson's and Orem's concept of nursing, prepared by the Nursing Development Conference Group, are a good source for the study of these comparisons.[68]

The central focus of Orem's perspective of nursing is the emphasis on each individual's **self-care** agency. Self-care, as defined by Orem, "is

the practice of activities that individuals personally initiate and perform on their own behalf in maintaining life, health, and well-being."[69]

Orem differentiates three types of self-care: **universal self care;** developmental self-care; and **health-deviation self-care.**[70]

Universal self-care is synonymous with those everyday life experiences that are designated as activities of daily living or basic human needs. Orem categorized the components of universal self-care (Table 4–7).[71]

Developmental self-care is associated with physical and mental growth and development processes during the life cycle and events that effect that development.

Health-deviation self-care includes all the variations in care necessary because of illness, injury, or disease experienced by individuals.[72]

Orem viewed nursing as a human service concerned with "the individual's need for self-care action and the provision and management of it on a continuous basis in order to sustain life and health, recover from disease or injury, and cope with their effects."[73]

Orem advocated the design of nursing systems that would incorporate the various activities indicated by the extent of deviation in self-care experienced by the potential patient or client and the situation. When the client is unable to perform self-care actions, a *wholly compensatory* nursing system is indicated. The *partly compensatory* nursing system would be designated when both the nurse and client perform the self-care. The third nursing system, a *supportive-educative* (or developmental) system, is used when the client can learn the required self-care measure(s) with the guidance and support of the nurse. The client's needs for

TABLE 4–7. OREM'S COMPONENTS OF UNIVERSAL SELF-CARE

Maintenance of sufficient intake of air, water, food
Care associated with elimination process and excrements
Balance between activity and rest
Balance between solitude and social interaction
Prevention of hazards to life functioning and well-being
Human desire to be normal

meeting self-care requisites determine the design of the nursing system and the subsequent variation in role(s) for the nurse and the client.[74]

According to Orem, nursing practice encompasses social, interpersonal, and technological dimensions. The technological aspect of nursing practice as described by Orem, includes a three-step nursing process. Orem's view of the nursing process is presented as[75]:

Step 1   A determination of whether nursing care is needed
Step 2   The designing of the nursing care system and planning of nursing care according to that system
Step 3   The provision of the indicated nursing actions

Orem stated that nursing situations had characteristics of helping situations. Orem identified methods of assisting or helping used by the nurse.[76] The five general methods she suggested were viewed as applicable to a variety of situations:

• Acting for or doing for another
• Guiding another
• Supporting another (physically or psychologically)
• Providing an environment that promotes personal development
• Teaching another

Each of these methods of helping is used in conjunction with a specified nursing system according to the appropriate role of nurse and client.[77]

Dorothea Orem has contributed a unique perspective of nursing using the framework of self-care. She has provided nursing with a new vocabulary to describe the components of nursing practice.

Martha E. Rogers

Martha Rogers has advocated "a science of unitary man" as the focus of her theoretical viewpoint of nursing. She perceives nursing as the science that "seeks to study the nature and direction of unitary human development integral with the environment, and to evolve the descriptive, explanatory, and predictive principles basic to knowledgeable practice in nursing."[78] People are at the center of nursing's purpose, according to Rogers, and the science of nursing is directed toward describing the life process in humans as well as explaining and predicting the nature and direction of human development.

Rogers identified "four building blocks" as essential elements in the development of her conceptual system of nursing. The first of these four, *energy fields,* views both the human and the environment as energy fields. The second building block, *openness,* is predicated on a belief in a universe of open systems. *Pattern and organization* are identifying characteristics of the energy field that is undergoing continuous change. Both the human and environmental fields are considered unique and are characterized by the concept of *four-dimensionality* (see Table 4–8).[79]

An evolutionary picture of the individual's development as a unidirectional progression through life was emphasized by Rogers. Rogers suggested that the Slinky walking spring toy demonstrates the rhythmic nature of life progressing through time and space.[80] Simultaneous with this life progression is the continuous interaction of the human energy field with the energy field of the environment.[81]

To describe the nature and direction of the development of unitary man, Rogers has stated and defined three principles[82]:

• The principle of **helicy,** which describes the nature as well as the direction of both the human and the environmental fields and their interaction
• The principle of **resonancy,** which describes the human and environmental fields accord-

TABLE 4–8. ROGERS'S FOUR BUILDING BLOCKS

Energy fields
Openness
Pattern and organization
Four-dimensionality

ing to the pattern and organization of shorter and longer patterns

- The principle of **complementarity**, which relates the interaction between the human and environmental fields as continuous, mutual, and simultaneous

The development of the science of nursing, with a specified body of knowledge, is a critical need, if the goals of nursing are to be accomplished. According to Rogers, "nursing aims to assist people in achieving their maximum health potential."[83] The goals of nursing include the maintenance and promotion of health and the prevention of disease through nursing diagnosis, intervention, and rehabilitation. Rogers contends that her theory, the science of unitary man, has implications for nursing practice in such areas as the aging process, hypertension, and hyperactivity.[84]

Rogers recognizes the constant exchange of energy between the human and environmental fields as integral to the life process.[85] Consequently, Rogers summarized the professional practice of nursing as seeking

to promote symphonic interaction between man and environment, to strengthen the coherence and integrity of the human field, and to direct and redirect patterning of the human and environmental fields for realization of maximum health potential.[86]

The science of nursing proposed by Dr. Rogers "aims to provide a growing body of theoretical knowledge whereby nursing practice can achieve new levels of meaningful service to man."[87] The body of knowledge constitutes the science of nursing, which makes possible the application of knowledge that is the art of nursing practice.[88]

The science of nursing proposed by Rogers is one of the most complex of the theories of nursing. Nonetheless, the serious student of nursing will endeavor to master the dimensions of this conceptual framework, which has been adopted as the basis for some nursing curricula and the practice of nursing.

Joyce Travelbee

The interpersonal relationship between the patient and the nurse (the human-to-human relationship) and the existential dimension of life are the distinguishing features of Joyce Travelbee's beliefs about nursing. Travelbee observed that the purpose of nursing was achieved through the establishment of the nurse–client relationship.[89]

Victor Frankl and Karl Jaspers, noted existential writers, were major influences in Travelbee's perspective of nursing. Joyce Travelbee was a student of Ida J. Orlando, and her influence is evident in Travelbee's emphasis on the disciplined intellectual approach to nursing.

The definition of nursing presented by Travelbee succinctly summarizes the premise on which her approach was formulated. Travelbee described nursing in the following way:

Nursing is an interpersonal process whereby the professional nurse practitioner assists an individual or family to prevent, or cope with, the experience of illness and suffering and, if necessary, assists the individual or family to find meaning in these experiences.[90]

From this definition, Travelbee derived her statement regarding the purpose of nursing.[91] Travelbee describes this interpersonal process between two human beings, one the client and the other the nurse, as experienced in four phases culminating in the human-to-human relationship.[92]

Nursing is viewed by Travelbee as a process, an experience, or a happening "between a nurse, an individual, or group of individuals in need of the assistance the nurse can offer."[93] This process is undertaken to meet needs and necessitates observation, validation of inferences, decision making, and planning of nursing action, as well as evaluation of the extent to which the needs have been met.

Establishment of the human-to-human relationship is preceded by four phases of experience. The initial phase, the original encounter, occurs when the nurse meets the ill person for the first time. The impressions or inferences that develop at this time are significant because they determine the nurse's subsequent behavior toward that person. The task of the nurse in this phase is to recognize the uniqueness of the client. When this is done, the second phase, emerging identities, is initiated. A bond between the nurse and client is established during this phase. The identities of each are seen as distinctly separate, and each appreciates the uniqueness of the other. The nursing task of this phase includes becoming aware of one's perception of the other person (the client) and distinguishing the similarities and differences between oneself and the client. Then empathy, the third phase, can occur. Empathy is described as an intellectual and emotional comprehension of another person to such an extent that the behavior of that person can be predicted. One's perceptions of the other person's thoughts and feelings are accurate when empathy is present.[94] Empathy is followed by the fourth phase, sympathy. Sympathy is characterized by an urgent desire to respond through action to alleviate the distress perceived in the other person.[95] The task of the nurse in this phase is to provide helpful nursing action.

The outcome of these four phases is experienced as *rapport* and the establishment of the *human-to-human* relationship. Rapport, in Travelbee's view, is synonymous with relatedness and is expressed in how two persons perceive each other and behave toward one another. Travelbee further described rapport as "a cluster of interrelated thoughts and feelings . . . communicated by one human being to another."[96]

Readers are urged to note the unique definitions and descriptions of empathy, sympathy, and rapport presented by Travelbee, and to refer to her publications for a more complete discussion of these crucial experiences.

Several major concepts are basic to the view of nursing emphasized by Travelbee and are foundations of her perspective of nursing: the human being, client, nurse, illness, suffering, hope, communication, and therapeutic use of self.

The nurse–client relationship is a central point in Travelbee's distinctive view of nursing. It is this relationship that enables the nurse to accomplish the purpose of nursing. Travelbee observed that nursing was in danger of losing its caring functions. She suggested that every activity performed by the nurse could be used as a vehicle through which caring could be expressed. This concern was impressively expressed in her own words. "To care for, and in the caring for, to care about is the very heart of nursing."[97]

Sister Callista Roy

Sister Callista Roy describes an approach to nursing based on findings in the study of adaptation. The Roy Adaptation Model was first developed in 1964, when Roy was a graduate student of Dorothy E. Johnson, and the first formulation of this model was developed in association with that experience. Roy stated that her model was both a systems model and an interactionist model.[98]

Roy was persuaded that adaptation could provide a conceptual framework for nursing. Consequently, she adopted the perspective of the psychologist, Dr. Harry Helson, as the theoretical base for her framework.

The view of the person and the adaptation process held are explicitly stated in eight assumptions. A basic premise of the model is the view of the human person as a bio-psycho-social being along a continuum of health–illness. Because of various stimuli that surround the person, some kind of adaptation constantly is required.

Based on this framework, Roy subsequently stated that the function of nursing "is to support and promote patient adaptation."[99] Thus, the practice of nursing based on this model endeavors to facilitate adaptation through whatever activities are indicated.

Roy observed that, both in health and illness, four particular ways of adapting are characteristic of a person. These modes of adaptation were identified by Roy as physiological needs, self-concept, role function, and interdependence relationships.[100]

Derived from her study of Helson, Roy proposed that the individual's adaptation level is influenced by three types of stimuli: focal, contextual, and residual. The stimuli influencing adaptation that are most immediate to the person are referred to as **focal stimuli. Contextual stimuli** include all stimuli influencing the person other than that most immediate to him or her. Though not as readily identifiable as focal or contextual stimuli, **residual stimuli,** which include an individual's beliefs, attitudes, or traits, also influence either adaptive or maladaptive behavior in life situations.[101] The nurse becomes concerned with these stimuli both in making assessments and during nursing intervention.

The goal of nursing, as stated by Roy, is "to promote man's adaptation in each of the adaptive modes in situations of health and illness."[102] Roy maintained that a nursing process, using problem solving as its basis, represents a scientific approach to the service that nursing could provide for society. The nursing process that Roy developed for her model entails six specific steps.

Assessment is undertaken at two levels. Initially the nurse acquires information about the individual's behavior in each of the adaptive modes and seeks to determine whether the behavior is adaptive or maladaptive. Subsequently, the second level of assessment is initiated as the nurse undertakes the identification of the various stimuli (focal, contextual, residual) that are influencing the patient's behavior. Data from these first two steps then are used to formulate a statement regarding the client's adaptive or maladaptive behaviors for the third step, problem identification. This activity is synonymous with making a nursing diagnosis. Roy is actively involved with the ambitious efforts of the National Conference Group endeavoring to establish a diagnostic classification system for nursing. When the problem has been clearly identified, the nurse is ready to embark upon step four, goal setting. Nursing intervention, step five, focuses on adaptation problems through the manipulation of stimuli as the nurse seeks to promote the patient's adaptation. The final step, evaluation, is focused on determining the effectiveness of the nursing interventions undertaken.

The basis of the Roy model is adaptation. The approach described by Roy is explicitly stated in the eight assumptions central to her model and also form the framework for it. The Roy Adaptation Model has become one of the most popular theoretical approaches to nursing during the relatively short time since its inception.

Josephine G. Paterson and Loretta T. Zderad

The publication, *Humanistic Nursing,* coauthored by Paterson and Zderad, describes the nursing situation that can be existentially experienced. The authors state that "nursing is a responsible searching, transactional relationship whose meaningfulness demands conceptualization founded on a nurse's existential awareness of self and of other."[103]

Paterson and Zderad emphasized that nursing is "an experience lived between human beings."[104]

They observed that the nurse experiences peak life events with other human beings. Peak life events include: birth, death, separation, and various other crises. It is through these experiences that the nurse can come to know self and others as these experiences are reflected on. These experiences must then be described. In presenting this humanistic nursing practice theory, Paterson and Zderad view nursing "as the ability to struggle with other men through peak experiences related to health and suffering in which the participants in the nursing situation are and become in accordance with their human potential."[105]

The essence of these human-lived experiences must be described by nurses. Nursing situations warrant description, and only nurses can describe them. As nurses describe these human phenomena of nursing situations, ultimately nursing theory and science will be developed. This endeavor also will affect the nursing situation and the nurse's knowledge of the human capacity for beingness.

Nursology (a term invented by Paterson and Zderad) is the study of humanistic nursing practice. Paterson and Zderad have proposed a methodology that they describe as occurring in four phases. The first phase entails the preparation of the nurse for the "task of knowing," which necessitates an openness to the situations that will be encountered. Knowing the client 'intuitively' and how he or she views the world is the focus of the second phase. This phase requires the nurse to be a part of what is studied. In the third phase, the nurse reflects on the experience and seeks to record as many aspects of the experience as possible. The final and fourth phase allows for greater understanding of the phenomena under study when the nurse takes "an intuitive leap" as the specific ideas and views of many situations are applied to other situations.

The approach to nursing presented by Paterson and Zderad is predicated on the nurse's involvement with the client and the experience between them as it is lived in the nursing situation. Paterson and Zderad have called this the "active presence" of the nurse. They recognize that in the actual nursing situation, the nurse may not be able to be "wholly present" to every client to the same degree. However, they encourage nurses to strive toward this difficult goal.

Paterson and Zderad have proposed that nurses consciously and deliberately approach nursing as an existential experience. They view nursing as a lived experience that must be described. Descriptions of these experiences between nurses and clients in the real world must be shared in order to develop a humanistic nursing theory.[106] An understanding of existential terminology and literature is helpful in appreciating the scholarly perspective of nursing set forth by Paterson and Zderad.

Myra E. Levine

Myra E. Levine describes a perspective of nursing that focuses on nursing's responsibility for maintaining or restoring wholeness for clients. She sees nursing as a keeping-together function. The individual client is the central focus for nursing practice. According to Levine, nursing is concerned with the unity and integrity of the individual client. To achieve the nursing purpose, Levine identified four principles of conservation that are the framework for conserving the wholeness of the client.[107]

These principles identify the major areas of care and concern of the nurse. The first principle is the *conservation of the individual client's energy*. Nursing intervention uses this principle when the nurse is attentive to the energy resources of the client compared to the energy expenditure associated with his or her response to a situation. Energy depletion is influenced by many factors, for example, the client's general condition and the demands made upon the individual because of the client's illness.

Conservation of structural integrity, the second principle, is predicated on the awareness that structural changes alter function, and pathophysiological processes all threaten structural integrity. Consequently, the nurse incorporates knowledge of bodily structure and function in the application of this principle. A variety of nursing measures can be instituted in daily care to conserve structure and the associated functions. Positioning, care of the client's skin, and personal hygiene are aspects of daily care that can facilitate conservation of the client's structural integrity.

The third principle, *conservation of personal integrity*, encompasses concerns for the individual's self-identity and self-respect.[108] Nursing intervention conserves personal integrity when the patient is accepted, valued, and respected as he is. Consideration for the rights and privileges of each client for privacy; participation in care, and regard for confidentiality are evidence of this principle.

The fourth principle is *conservation of social integrity*. The social integrity of the client is conserved when nursing care facilitates the individual's continuing contacts and relationships with family and other important associations that are meaningful to him or her as a member of society.[109]

According to Levine, nursing is a human interaction. Nursing intervention is therapeutic and supportive. Therapeutic intervention entails influencing the individual's adaptation favorably or toward renewed social well-being. Intervention is supportive when the course of adaptation cannot be altered, or the status quo is maintained. Nursing intervention, according to Levine, "must be designed so that it fosters successful adaptation."[110]

Nursing intervention is a conservation of wholeness for the individual client. The conservation principles embody the major areas of care in which nursing can fulfill this conservation function. Levine has succinctly summarized her perspective of nursing in describing the task of nursing as recognizing the value and wondrous variety of all humankind while offering ministrations that conserve the unique and special integrity of every person.[111]

Betty M. Neuman

Betty Neuman conceptualized a model of health care that she proposed could be used by various disciplines of health-care providers, including nurses. The Neuman perspective of health care focuses on the individual and that individual's environment, with particular emphasis on the relationship to stress. Though the model is referred to as a "total person approach to patient problems," it is recommended for use with families and groups, as well as with individuals.[112] The purpose of the model is to provide a framework for health-care givers to assist in attaining and maintaining a maximum level of wellness through purposeful interventions.[113]

Nine assumptions are presented by Neuman as basic to the development of her model. These assumptions identify beliefs about the individual and characteristic responses to stress that humans develop during their lifetime. The relationship of primary, secondary, and tertiary prevention are noted and defined in the context of this model.[114]

The individual is viewed by Neuman as an open system and is represented in the model diagram by a series of concentric circles. The basic structure of the individual is envisioned as the core. This core is bounded by lines of resistance, a normal line of defense, and a flexible line of defense, which represents the individual's response to stressors that impact upon the individual throughout life.[115]

Intervention by the health-care provider may be instituted at whatever level indicated in respect to primary, secondary, and tertiary prevention levels. The identification of the stressors and the subsequent impact upon the physiological, psychological, sociocultural, and developmental influences as variables affecting the individual determine the timing and locations of interventions.

The application of this model by the nurse (or care givers of whatever discipline) can be facilitated through use of the assessment-intervention tool developed by Neuman. The tool is an interview guide to obtain data essential to determining and providing appropriate care. Neuman emphasized the importance of incorporating the individual client's perception of his or her condition in developing the goals for care.[116]

Neuman has endeavored to describe a framework for health care that includes many possible dimensions. It is recommended for the care of individuals, families and groups by care givers in any health-care setting. Stress and the individual's response to stressors is the basic phenomenon emphasized.

Other Theorists

The work of several other theorists, including Evelyn Adam, Helen C. Erickson, Joyce J. Fitzpatrick, Madeleine Leininger, Margaret Newman, Rosemarie Rizzo Parse, Joan Riehl Sisca, Mary Ann P. Swain, Evelyn M. Tomlin, and Jean Watson have significantly contributed to the expanding literature describing the theoretical dimension of nursing. Their noteworthy perspectives on nursing are presented in a recent publication by Ann Marriner, *Nursing Theorists and Their Work*.[117] Readers are urged to consult this excellent reference for further study of theorists discussed in this chapter as well as these additional authors and their writings.

SUMMARY

The perspective on nursing held by selected nurse authors was briefly presented in this chapter. Each of these authors has contributed to the building of a theoretical foundation for the practice of nursing.

Historical evidence of efforts to state a theoretical premise for the practice of nursing can be found in the writings of Florence Nightingale. During the past three decades, the writings of a growing number of nurses reflect their attempts to enlarge the scientific dimensions of nursing care and state a perspective that is commensurate with those recognized as distinguishing a professional discipline. Several of these authors were selected for presentation in this chapter as representative nursing theorists with whom nurses should be familiar.

In viewing these authors from a historical standpoint, it is evident that personal, cultural, environmental, and theoretical forces influence the focus maintained by each of these nurse theorists.

Though there are notable differences between these authors, there are also some similarities. One common factor is the inclusion of the needs of the client as an important component in determining the role of the nurse as well as the focus of nursing practice. The interpersonal relationship between the nurse and the client is noted as of central importance by many of the authors. The variations observed in the point of view of each author are expressed in the components of nursing practice that are emphasized as well as the conceptual frameworks on which the ideas are centered.

A chart, Comparison of Selected Nurse Authors and their Theories, highlighting the basic premises of authors appears at the end of this chapter. It is hoped that this comparison of authors according to a specific list of variables will aid in the understanding of the noteworthy contributions of those selected for discussion.

Study Questions

1. Name three nursing author-theorists.

2. For each of the individuals named in question 1, identify and briefly state

   A. the definition of nursing given by the author

   B. the view of the nursing process described by the author

3. Describe the perspective of nursing held by each nurse author discussed in this chapter.

4. State the historic progression of the development of nursing theory.

5. Discuss the factors that have been influential for each nurse author identified in this chapter.

References

1. A. Jacox, "Theory construction in nursing: An overview," *Nurs Res* 23 (1974):4–13.
2. Ibid., 8.
3. Dorothy E. Johnson, "The development of theory: A requisite for nursing as a primary health profession," *Nurs Res* 23 (1974):372.
4. Ibid.
5. M.E. Levine, "Adaptation and assessment: A rationale for nursing intervention," *Am J Nurs* 66 (1966):2451–54.
6. Florence Nightingale, *Notes on Nursing: What It Is, and What It is Not* (New York: D. Appleton Co., 1879).
7. G. Safier, *Contemporary American Leaders in Nursing* (New York: McGraw-Hill Book Co., 1977).
8. Virginia Henderson, *The Nature of Nursing* (New York: Macmillan Co., 1966), 15.
9. Bertha Harmer and Virginia Henderson, *Textbook of the Principles and Practice of Nursing*, 5th ed. (New York: Macmillan Co., 1955).
10. V. Henderson, "The nature of nursing," *Am J Nurs* 64 (1964):63.
11. Virginia Henderson and Gladys Nite, *The Principles and Practice of Nursing*, 6th ed. (New York: Macmillan Co., 1978), 34.
12. Harmer and Henderson, *Principles*, 5.
13. Ibid.
14. Henderson, *The Nature of Nursing*, 16.
15. Henderson, "The nature of nursing," 65.
16. Henderson, *The Nature of Nursing*, 16–17.
17. Ibid., 16.
18. Henderson. "The nature of nursing," 66.
19. Harmer and Henderson. *Principles*, 6.
20. Henderson, "The nature of nursing," 65.
21. Bertha Harmer and Virginia Henderson. *Textbook of the Principles and Practice of Nursing*, 4th ed. (New York: Macmillan Co., 1939).
22. Hildegard E. Peplau, *Interpersonal Relations in Nursing* (New York: G.P. Putnam's Sons, 1952).

23. Ida J. Orlando, *Dynamic Nurse-Patient Relationships* (New York: G.P. Putnam's Sons, 1961), 8.
24. Ibid.
25. Ida J. Orlando Pelletier. "The Dynamic Nurse-Patient Relationship." Talk presented at Walter Reed Army Medical Center, Department of Nursing, Washington, D.C., October 1980.
26. Orlando. *Nurse-Patient Relationships*, 36.
27. Ibid., 31.
28. Ibid., 35–36.
29. Ibid., 40.
30. Ibid., 56.
31. Ibid., 60.
32. Orlando-Pelletier. "The Dynamic Nurse-Patient Relationship."
33. Ernestine Wiedenbach, *Clinical Nursing: A Helping Art* (New York: Springer Publishing Co., 1964), 12.
34. Ibid., 2.
35. Ibid., 11.
36. Ibid., 13.
37. Ibid., 16.
38. Ibid., 17.
39. Ibid., 15.
40. Ibid.
41. Ibid., 31.
42. Ibid.
43. Ibid., 36.
44. Ibid., 49–52.
45. Ibid., 107.
46. D.E. Johnson, "The behavioral system model for nursing," in Joan P. Riehl and Sr. Callista Roy, *Conceptual Models for Nursing Practice,* 2nd ed. (New York: Appleton-Century-Crofts, 1980), 207.
47. Ibid., 209.
48. Ibid., 214.
49. J. Grubb, "An interpretation of the Johnson behavioral system model for nursing practice," in Joan Riehl and Sr. Callista Roy, *Conceptual Models for Nursing Practice,* 2nd ed. (New York: Appleton-Century-Crofts, 1980), 238–247.
50. D.E. Johnson, "Behavioral system model." 207.
51. D.E. Johnson, "A philosophy of nursing," *Nurs Outlook* 7 (1959).
52. D.E. Johnson, "The significance of nursing care," *Am J Nurs* 61 (1961).
53. D.E. Johnson, "Tonight's action will determine tomorrow's nursing." *Nurs Outlook* 13 (1965).
54. D.E. Johnson, "Development of theory: A requisite." *Nurs Res* 23 (1974):372.
55. Imogene M. King, *Toward a Theory for Nursing* (New York: John Wiley & Sons, 1971). *x,* 119.
56. Imogene M. King, *A Theory for Nursing*: Systems, Concepts & Process (New York: John Wiley & Sons, 1981), 150.
57. King, *Toward a Theory for Nursing*, 107–118.
58. King, *A Theory for Nursing*, 144.
59. Ibid.
60. King, *A Theory for Nursing*, 145.
61. Ibid., 10, 13.
62. Ibid., 145.
63. King, *A Theory for Nursing*, 13.
64. Ibid., 142.
65. Ibid.
66. Ibid., 13.
67. Nursing Development Conference Group, *Concept Formalization in Nursing*, 2nd ed., Dorothea E. Orem, ed. (Boston: Little, Brown & Co., 1979), 69–70.
68. Ibid., 89–90.
69. Dorothea E. Orem, *Nursing: Concepts of Practice* (New York: McGraw-Hill Book Co., 1971), 13.
70. Dorothea E. Orem, *Nursing: Concepts of Practice*, 3rd ed. (New York: McGraw-Hill Book Co., 1985), 90.
71. Ibid.
72. Ibid., 90.
73. Ibid., 54.
74. Dorothea E. Orem, *Nursing: Concepts of Practice*, 2nd ed., 94–104; 3rd ed., 152–157 (New York: McGraw-Hill Book Co., 1980, 1985).
75. Ibid., 1980, pp. 200–203.
76. Ibid., 95.
77. Ibid., 94–95. 1985, p 138.
78. M.E. Rogers, "Nursing: A science of unitary man," in Joan Riehl and Sr. Callista Roy, *Conceptual Models for Nursing Practice,* 2nd ed. (New York: Appleton-Century-Crofts, 1980), 329.
79. Ibid., 330.
80. Ibid., 330–32.
81. Martha E. Rogers, *An Introduction to the Theoretical Basis of Nursing* (Philadelphia: F.A. Davis Co., 1970), 90–92.
82. Rogers. "Nursing: A science," 330.
83. Rogers, *Theoretical Basis of Nursing*, 86.
84. Rogers, "Nursing: A science," 336.
85. Rogers, *Theoretical Basis of Nursing*, 92.
86. Ibid., 122.
87. Ibid., 88.
88. Ibid., 121.
89. Joyce Travelbee, *Interpersonal Aspects of*

Nursing (Philadelphia: F.A. Davis Co., 1966), 121.

90. Ibid., 5–6.
91. Ibid., 13.
92. Joyce Travelbee, *Interpersonal Aspects of Nursing,* 2nd ed. (Philadelphia: F.A. Davis Co., 1971), 123.
93. Ibid., 8.
94. J. Travelbee, "What's wrong with sympathy?" *Am J Nurs* 64 (1964):68.
95. Ibid., 68–69.
96. J. Travelbee. *Interpersonal Aspects of Nursing,* 2nd ed., 150.
97. J. Travelbee. *Interpersonal Aspects of Nursing,* 2.
98. Sr. Callista Roy, "Adaptation: A conceptual framework for nursing" *Nurs Outlook* 18 (1970):42–45.
99. Joan Riehl and Sr. Callista Roy, *Conceptual Models for Nursing Practice,* 2nd ed. (New York: Appleton-Century-Crofts, 1980), 179.
100. Sr. Callista Roy, *Introduction to Nursing: An Adaptation Model* (Englewood Cliffs, N.J., Prentice-Hall, 1976), 30–33.
101. Ibid., 18.
102. Riehl and Roy, *Conceptual Models for Nursing Practice,* 2nd ed., 182.
103. Josephine G. Paterson and Loretta T. Zderad, *Humanistic Nursing* (New York: John Wiley & Sons, 1976), 3–7.
104. Ibid., 3.
105. Ibid., 7.
106. Ibid., 76–83.
107. M.E. Levine, "Holistic nursing," *Nurs Clin North Am* (1971):258.
108. M.E. Levine, "The four conservation principles of nursing," *Nurs Forum* 6 (1967):50–54.
109. Myra E. Levine, *Introduction to Clinical Nursing,* 2nd ed. (Philadelphia: F.A. Davis Co., 1973).
110. Myra E. Levine, "Adaptation and assessment: A rationale for nursing intervention," *Am J Nurs* 66 (1966):2452.
111. Ibid.
112. B. Neuman, "The Betty Neuman health-care systems model: A total person approach to patient problems," in Joan Riehl and Sr. Callista Roy, *Conceptual Models for Nursing Practice,* 2nd ed. (New York: Appleton-Century-Crofts, 1980), 119.
113. Ibid.
114. Ibid., 119, 121.
115. Ibid., 120.
116. Ibid., 127.

117. Ann Marriner, *Nursing Theorists and Their Work* (St. Louis: C.V. Mosby Co., 1986).

Annotated Bibliography

Henderson, V. 1966. *The Nature of Nursing.* New York: Macmillan. Dr. Henderson presents her professional memoirs in this reference. Not only has she included her view of nursing, but she identifies the individuals and experiences that have been most influential in her professional life and have contributed to the perspective of nursing she holds. Her views on nursing practice, nursing education, and nursing research also are presented.

Johnson, D.E. 1980. The behavioral system model for nursing. In *Conceptual Models for Nursing Practice,* 2nd ed., ed. J. Riehl and C. Roy. New York: Appleton-Century-Crofts. Dr. Johnson presents a concise summary of her view of nursing in this chapter. She includes descriptions of the components of her model with a documented explanation of each of the behavioral subsystems she identified as comprising the human behavioral system.

King, I.M. 1981. *A Theory for Nursing.* New York: Wiley. An update of Dr. King's perspective of nursing, with findings from her personal research, is presented. The concepts she has identified as basic to her theory are thoroughly discussed, with substantial documentation of related literature included. The progression of Dr. King's view of nursing is evident when this reference is compared with her previous publications.

Levine, M.E. 1973. *Introduction to Clinical Nursing,* 2nd ed. Philadelphia: F.A. Davis. This reference was written for the beginning nursing student. Levine's view of nursing is presented within a conceptual framework and emphasizes a client-centered approach. The holistic approach of nursing held by this author is explained, including the application of conservation principles that she has identified and described in this and previous publications.

Neuman, B. 1980. The Betty Neuman health-care systems model. In *Conceptual Models for Nursing Practice,* 2nd ed., ed. J. Riehl and C. Roy. New York: Appleton-Century-Crofts. Betty Neuman described and illustrated her model for nursing incorporating a total-person approach. The assessment-intervention tool associated with the model is presented and explained. The diagram of the model (first published in *Nursing Research* in

1972) provides the reader with an excellent road map of the components of the model.

Orem, D.E. 1985. *Nursing Concepts of Practice,* 3rd ed. New York: McGraw-Hill. This third edition expands the self-care conceptual view of nursing developed by Orem and described in the first (1971) and second (1980) editions. This reference, like its forerunners, includes a comprehensive guide to this author's perspective on nursing.

Orlando, I.J. 1961. *Dynamic Nurse–Patient Relationships.* New York: Putnam's. A vanguard view of nursing and the nursing process. This author's description of the nursing process was one of the first publications to use this terminology and explain its place in nursing practice. This publication is a classic of nursing theory development literature. It is noteworthy to observe that the research findings of this author were obtained in the practice setting and influenced the view of nursing that she developed.

Paterson, J.G. and L.T. Zderad. 1976. *Humanistic Nursing.* New York: Wiley. A scholarly perspective on nursing as an existential experience lived between a nurse and other human beings. The process of developing a humanistic nursing theory is described by the authors.

Peplau, H.E. 1952. *Interpersonal Relations in Nursing.* New York: Putnam's. A classic in psychiatric nursing. Dr. Peplau translated the ideas of prominent psychiatrists, especially Harry Stack Sullivan, M.D., and psychologists of that period into understandable language for nurses. Her application of this knowledge base for nursing practice included identifying phases in the nurse–patient relationship and the roles, functions, and tasks of the nurse in facilitating the personal growth of the patient.

Rogers, M.E. 1970. *An Introduction to the Theoretical Basis of Nursing.* Philadelphia: F.A. Davis. Dr. Rogers's theoretical view of nursing science and unitary man is presented in this reference. Though the text may appear to be complex to readers just beginning study of nurse theorists, it is a comprehensive description of the view of nursing advocated by this influential nurse author.

Roy, Sr.C. 1976. *Introduction to Nursing: An Adaptation Model.* Englewood Cliffs, N.J.: Prentice-Hall. Roy's adaptation model is presented by its author and her nursing colleagues in this reference. The application of the model is demonstrated throughout the publication. Both beginning nursing students and experienced nurses will find material helpful to their practice in this publication.

Travelbee, J. 1959. *Intervention in Psychiatric Nursing: Processes in the One-to-One Relationship.* Philadelphia: F.A. Davis. This classic book presents Travelbee's beliefs about interpersonal relationships between patients and nurses. It uses an existential framework based on the writings of Frankl and Jaspers. Travelbee's application of this knowledge to nursing culminated with her description of nursing as a human-to-human relationship.

Wiedenbach, E. 1964. *Clinical Nursing: A Helping Art.* New York: Springer. The components of nursing and their application to practice are emphasized in this historic reference. Wiedenbach was one of the first nurse authors to develop a theoretical framework for nursing practice incorporating the personal philosophy of the nurse as an important element. In this reference she presents three concepts she considers basic to a philosophy of nursing.

A COMPARISON OF SELECTED NURSE-AUTHORS AND THEIR THEORIES

	Central Theme	View of the Human Person	Key Terminology	Definition/View of Nursing
V. Henderson 1939, 1955, 1964–1966	Unique and independent function of the nurse	Personhood—mind and body are inseparable	The Nurse is primary rehabilitation agent Patient-centered care Independent role and function of nurse	"The unique function of the nurse is to assist the individual, sick or well. In the performance of those activities contributing to health or its recovery (or to peaceful death) that he would perform unaided if he had the necessary strength, will or knowledge. And to do this in such a way as to help him gain independence as rapidly as possible." (1964, 63) Viewed the nurse as the authority on nursing care Aim of nursing to promote normalcy and independence Nurse is a substitute for what the patient lacks
H. Peplau 1952	Nurse–patient relationship in nursing or interpersonal relations in nursing and the personal growth and development of the nurse	Each person is an individual with the potential for growth, whose personality is developed by the interaction of cultural forces and biological constitutions	Psychodynamic nursing	"Nursing is a significant therapeutic, interpersonal process. It functions cooperatively with other human processes that make health possible for individuals in communities. . . . Nursing is an educative instrument, a maturing force, that aims to promote forward movement of personality in the direction of creative, constructive, personal, and community living." (1952, 16) Nursing is psychodynamic, an applied science, a function Nursing is an interpersonal process Nursing is a human relationship between a patient and a nurse who is able to respond to the need for help Assist patients to meet human problems of everyday life Tasks and performances of the nurse–patient relationship

View of Nursing Process	Other	Applicability of Theory/Model	Major Origin(s) of Thought or Influences on Author/Theorist
Individualized care planning with continual analysis to meet the patient's needs	Informational nurse leader Set trend in nursing research—influenced by her wise foresight Presents personal memoirs and historical perspective	Cites implications for practice, research and education based on her concept of nursing	F. Nightingale, Annie Goodrich Need Theory (Thorndike) Rehabilitation experts, Yale nursing colleagues
The phases of nurse–patient relationship: four interlocking phases—orientation, identification, exploitation, resolution Nursing process is educative and therapeutic	The kind of person the nurse becomes makes a difference to the patient and nursing care given Multiple roles of nurse(s) are identified as occur in phases of the nurse–patient relationship	Views of practice, research and education are presented	Harry Stack Sullivan Erich Fromm Staff of Chestnut Lodge and Wm. Alanson White Institute of Psychiatry

(continued)

A COMPARISON OF SELECTED NURSE-AUTHORS AND THEIR THEORIES (Continued)

	Central Theme	View of the Human Person	Key Terminology	Definition/View of Nursing
I. Orlando (Pelletier) 1961, 1980	The dynamic, interpersonal nurse–patient relationship: Identification of principles to guide nursing practice and a theory of effective nursing practice for nursing students		Nursing activities as deliberative or automatic	The purpose of nursing is to supply the help a patient requires in order for his needs to be met (1961, 8) To find and meet the patients immediate needs for help directly or indirectly (the nurse's responsibility) is the practice of professional nursing
E. Wiedenbach 1963, 1964, 1968, 1970	The nurse, elements of practice and process which determines its philosophy, purpose, practice, art of nursing	Four assumptions about human nature are described (1964, 17)	Rational, reactionary or deliberative nursing action	Nursing is a service, a helping art—a goal-directed activity The purpose for clinical nursing is "to facilitate the efforts of the individual to overcome the obstacles which currently interfere with his ability to respond capably to demands made of him by his condition, environment, situation and time." (1964, 14–15) "To meet the need the individual is experiencing as a need-for-help." (1964, 15) Clinical nursing has four interlocking components: Philosophy, Purpose, Practice, Art Why: Purpose Way: Philosophy What: Practice How: Art Nursing action is deliberative action
D. Johnson 1959, 1961, 1980	Behavioral systems and subsystems of Man	Person—bio-psycho-social being Human organism is a complex set of behavioral subsystems and boundaries. Further assumptions see (Riehl and Roy, 1980, 208)	Components of each subsystem: goal, action, set, choice. The nurse is an external regulator of the environment Sustenal imperatives	Nursing is a science and an art Nursing care—a direct service to people "The achievement and maintenance of a stable state is nursing's distinctive contribution to patient welfare and the specific purpose of nursing care." (1961, 64) Activities of nursing are centered on human needs Nursing Action—supply of sustenal imperatives: Nurturance, protection, stimulation

View of Nursing Process	Other	Applicability of Theory/Model	Major Origin(s) of Thought or Influences on Author/Theorist
Process occurs within the nurse Nursing process is tool to do what nurse is to do, the process the nurse follows to get an outcome Nurses' perceptions of the patient's behavior, reaction of the nurse, nursing action (say and do)	Observe, state perceptions and associated thoughts/feelings (validation with patient is essential), then do disciplined nursing response: deliberative nursing process is presented	Focus is on practice Research: publications are findings of her personal study, other possibilities Education: content of instruction	Personal findings from study of verbatim nursing notes
The helping process identification of help needed Ministration of help Validation that help was given Coordination of resources for help and of help provided	Emphasis on philosophy of the individual nurse Principles of helping are identified Presents a tool for analyzing nursing incidents	Focus is on practice Suggests types of research States view of Education	V. Henderson I. Orlando Needs Theory Dickoff and James
Nursing Process as four essential stages: Asessment—1st and 2nd level Diagnosis Intervention—four modes: restrict, defend, inhibit, facilitate Evaluation	Seven behavioral subsystems constitute a behavioral system	Education: the foundation in the science of nursing Research: must provide the base for nursing Practice: is the focus of concern for use and source of knowledge	General Systems Theory Needs Theory

(continued)

A COMPARISON OF SELECTED NURSE-AUTHORS AND THEIR THEORIES (Continued)

	Central Theme	View of the Human Person	Key Terminology	Definition/View of Nursing
I. King 1968, 1971, 1973, 1981	Conceptual nursing framework for a theory for nursing; a theory of goal attainment. Interrelationships of concepts and the process of human interactions	Persons are open systems (1981, 20) Specific assumptions about human beings are identified (1981, 143)	Major concepts are interaction, perception, communication, transaction, self, role, stress, growth and development, time and space. (1981, 145)	"Nursing is a process of human interactions between nurse and client whereby each perceives the other and the situation, and through communication, they set goals, explore means, and agree on means to achieve goals." (1981, 144) "The goal of nursing is to help individuals and groups attain, maintain, and restore health." (1981, 13) ". . . help individuals die with dignity." The focus of nursing is on human beings The domain of nursing: Personal, Interpersonal and Social systems Identifies factors in nursing that have persisted through time (1971)
D. Orem 1971, 1980	Self-care: Universal and health deviations	Person is unique Man is an integrated whole	Self-care agency Self-care deficit Self-care requirements and demands	Nursing: a helping service, human service Technology and art "A creative effort of one human being to help another human being." (1971, 69) "Nursing is a personal, family and community service within the health field. Its dimension of concern for human life and well-being is shared with other health services. Nursing differs from these services because of the nature of its contributed effort. Provisions for making nursing available in a social group should consider both its shared and its unique dimension." (1971, 41) Goal of nursing: the health and well-being of the individual Focus of nursing: helping the individual to achieve health results

View of Nursing Process	Other	Applicability of Theory/Model	Major Origin(s) of Thought or Influences on Author/Theorist
Human process, an interpersonal process, a process of action, reaction, interaction, transaction between individuals and groups in social systems. Illustrated by interlocking circles, a methodology for study of nursing process (1973, 515)	Presents a goal-oriented nursing record Concepts of framework are presented according to the three interacting systems: Personal–interpersonal–social	Theory derived from her personal research Views her framework as practice Education: concepts as basis of learning the practice of nursing	V. Henderson H. Peplau, I. Orlando General Systems Theory Numerous sources associated with the identified concepts
Nursing an interpersonal process Deliberative action Step one: Nursing diagnosis Initial determination of need for care Step two: Designing and planning a system of nursing Step three: Actions of nurse A cycle of assisting, checking, adjusting and readjusting activities	Design of nursing systems Partly compensatory–Wholly compensatory Supportive–educative (developmental) systems Development of new language about nursing Man's need for self-care is emphasized.	A basis for practice education: Used as curriculum model Suggests research possibilities	V. Henderson General System Theory

(continued)

A COMPARISON OF SELECTED NURSE-AUTHORS AND THEIR THEORIES (Continued)

	Central Theme	View of the Human Person	Key Terminology	Definition/View of Nursing
M. Rogers 1970, 1980	Unitary Man and his life processes Nursing science	Synergistic Man: Four dimensional, negentropic, unified whole Conceptual boundaries of an energy field	Helicy and Resonancy (nature and direction of change)	Nursing a science and an art "Professional practice in nursing seeks to promote symphonic interaction between man and environment, to strengthen the adherence and integrity of the human field, and to direct and redirect patterning of the human and environmental fields for realization of maximum health potential." (1970, 122) Homeodynamics are Principles of Nursing Science Patterning and Organization define field People at center of nursing purpose Responsibility to Society
J. Travelbee 1963, 1964, 1966, 1969	Interpersonal relationship, nature and uniqueness of professional nursing practice	Uniqueness of Man	Coping, meaning, caring, empathy, sympathy	"Nursing is an interpersonal process whereby the professional nurse practitioner assists an individual or family to prevent, cope with, the experience of illness and suffering and, if necessary, assists the individual or family to find meaning in these experiences." (1966, 5–6) Functions of nursing are derived from the definitions and purpose of nursing Views nurse as supporter, sustainer and change agent
Sr. Callista Roy 1970, 1971, 1973, 1974 1975, 1976, 1980	Adaptation and eight assumptions about Man	Bio-psycho-social being Eight assumptions about man, also see (1974, 136–138; 1980, 180–182)	Man has four modes of adaptation: Physiological needs, self concept, role function, interdependence Man has two types of adaptive mechanisms: Cognator, regulator	Nursing is a scientific discipline, is practice oriented "Nursing is concerned with man as a total being at some point along the health–illness continuum." (1970, 43) Goal of nursing: to bring about an adaptive state in the four adaptive modes

View of Nursing Process	Other	Applicability of Theory/Model	Major Origin(s) of Thought or Influences on Author/Theorist
Setting for nursing is life process and human field Nursing diagnosis intervention Evaluation of intervention	Life process and homeodynamics and continuous interaction between man and environment are emphasized A mind extender	Provides a conceptual framework for practice education: used as curriculum base Has been basis for research studies	Physics (Einstein) Systems Theory Field Theory Evolutionary Theory Paranormal Psychology
An Interpersonal Process Phases of a nurse–patient relationship: Original encounter, emerging identities, empathy, sympathy, rapport (1966) Utilization of observation, interpretation, decision making, action, evaluation	Focus on existential aspects of life For the nurse "to care for and to care about."	Basis for practice of nursing Education—model for teaching interpersonal relationships Research—possibilities are inherent	Karl Jaspers V. Frankl Yale Nursing Colleagues (Orlando)
Problem-solving process: Six step Nursing Process Assessment—1st level —2nd level Problem identification Goal setting Intervention Selection of approaches Evaluation	Modification of Johnson Model, based on Helson's Adaptation-Level Theory	Roy suggests her mode offers possibilities for providing "a scientific basis, a body of knowledge for education, and an area of practice." (1970, 44)	Adaptation Theory of Helson Dorothy Johnson

(continued)

A COMPARISON OF SELECTED NURSE-AUTHORS AND THEIR THEORIES (Continued)

	Central Theme	View of the Human Person	Key Terminology	Definition/View of Nursing
Josephine G. Paterson Loretta T. Zderad 1976	Humanistic nursing The existentially experienced nursing situation Individuals: knowing and becoming	Unique, holistic, intellectual ever evolving person	Nursology, reobjectification, active presence, all-at-once, withness, "thing itself" "The between" "The stuff of nursing"	Always an interhuman act, a living human act "an experience lived between human beings" a transactional relationship, an intersubjective transaction
Myra E. Levine 1966, 1967, 1971 1973, 1978	Conservation Holistic nursing	Unity of mind and body A living being who responds to change, continually interacting with his environments and adapting to change Wholeness: Holism	Conservation Wholeness Health Integrity Adaptation Integration	Nursing is a keeping together function—the wholeness of the patient Nursing care is "focused on man and the complexity of his relationships with his environment" (1973, 46) "Nursing intervention is, . . . a conservation of wholeness." (1971, 258) Nursing can fulfill its conservation function in four major areas of care: Conservation of patient energy Conservation of structural integrity Conservation of personal integrity Conservation of social integrity (1967, 47–59)
Betty M. Neuman 1972, 1974, 1980	A Health-care systems model for a total person approach to patient problems	Every individual is unique, with a composite of characteristics within a normal range Man is an open system who interacts with his environment	Stressors Flexible line of defense Formal line of defense Lines of resistance Reconstitution	Nursing is ". . . a unique profession . . . concerned with all the variables affecting an individual's response to stressors." (1980, 121)

View of Nursing Process	Other	Applicability of Theory/Model	Major Origin(s) of Thought or Influences on Author/Theorist
"Stuff of nursing includes all possible responses of man; man needing and man helping A clinical process: An experience lived between human beings An active presence: Personal and/or professional	Methodology for studying nursing: phases of phenomenologic nursology 1. Experiencing 2. Reflecting 3. Describing	Developed and used in clinical situation Education: Focus of a course Humanistic Nursing taught by the authors Research: Presents possibilities to be explored	Buber Marcel de Chardin Numerous other scholarly works
Not specifically defined Patient-centered nursing care plans "The substance of nursing science" (1967, 47) is the identifying of specific patterns of adaptation of each individual patient and accurately responding	Precise use of vocabulary and origin of words defined and described Focus of concern on the individual Therapeutic and Supportive intervention defined	Practice centered 1973 text was prepared for an introductory nursing course Many possibilities for research are inherent in this nursing approach	Paul Tillich Walter Cannon Rene Dubos Hans Selye Others
An assessment/intervention tool provides for obtaining: Biographical data of the client Stressors as perceived by the client Stressors as perceived by the care givers Identifying of intra-, inter-, and extra-personal factors (Model diagram) Statement of the problem Summary of goals Intervention plan	Man and his environment is the basic phenomenon An individual's reaction to stress and factors that begin reconstitution Utilizes primary, secondary, and tertiary prevention levels	Developed and utilized as a conceptual model for a graduate nursing course Presents a framework for health care providers including nursing and other disciplines Many research possibilities	Gestalt Theory Field theories Hans Selye

Chapter 5

Systems Theory and Adaptation

Phyllis B. Heffron

Chapter Outline

- Objectives
- Glossary
- Introduction
- General Systems Theory
    Overview and Significance
    Definition of a System
    The Hierarchy of Systems
    Boundaries
    Input, Output, and Throughput
    Open and Closed Systems
    Steady State or Dynamic Equilibrium
    Feedback
    Equifinality
    Energy, Entropy, and Negentropy
- Adaptation Theory
    Definition of Adaptation
    Biological Adaptation
    Physiological Adaptation
    Stress and Adaptation
    Psychosocial Adaptation
    Anthropological Adaptation
- Nursing Implications
    The Adaptive Nature of Humans
    Nursing as an Adaptive System
    Health Care and Holism
    Nursing Education
- Summary
- Study Questions
- References
- Annotated Bibliography

Objectives

At the completion of this chapter the reader will be able to:

- Define each term in the glossary
- Discuss, using examples, the meaning of the phrase "the whole is greater than the sum of its parts"
- Describe the relationships between feedback, steady state, and equifinality
- Distinguish between homogeneity and ordered differentiation in systems in terms of entropy and negentropy
- Explain the concept of adaptation as it relates to general systems theory
- Identify six system processes that contribute to the adaptation of open systems
- Identify four ways that psychosocial adaptation can be measured
- Explain the importance of social and anthropological adaptation and provide examples of each
- Discuss a general concept of humankind, using general systems terminology and the principles of adaptation
- Explain how a general systems approach can be applied to the concept of health care
- Describe three ways in which the theories of systems and adaptation have had an influence on nursing education

Glossary

Adaptation. A dynamic, ongoing, and life-sustaining process whereby living things continually adjust to environmental changes.

Adaptation Theory. The body of knowledge that describes and predicts concepts and principles about adaptation, its process, relationships, and consequences.

Boundary. A real or imaginary line of demarcation that separates one system from another and from its environment.

Closed System. A system that does not change or allow any input or output exchanges with the environment; also used to describe relatively closed groups.

Dynamic Equilibrium. A state of balance in living systems that is ever-changing because of continual environmental movements and subsequent cyclical processes of input, throughput, and output.

Energy. The capacity for doing work; the product of a force (e.g., thermal, electrical, chemical), that acts on a body.

Entropy. A systems energy state that measures the system's tendency toward disorder.

Equifinality. A systems principle stating that the system tends toward equilibrium and can arrive at a final goal through various methods and from different initial states.

Evolution. The historic and ongoing process of how living things have changed or adapted over the ages, since life began.

Feedback. A systems process, circular in nature, whereby system outputs are monitored and regulate subsequent input decisions.

General Adaptation Syndrome (GAS). A predictable and specific set of reactions that occur generally when the body is confronted by a stressor.

General Systems Theory. A universal theory of wholeness that explains the relationships between wholes and parts and describes the characteristics and processes of systems and their functions.

Holism. Pertaining to the idea of wholeness and interrelatedness of component parts in a whole system.

Holistic Health Care. Health care that takes into consideration the bio-psycho-social and spiritual needs of the client and provides for all dimensions of health—preventive, rehabilitative, and primary care.

Homeodynamics. The continuous exchange of energy between humans and their environment. Used synonymously with steady state.

Humanism. Pertaining to the idea of universally applicable human characteristics, of needs, feelings, and responses that signify the total experience of being a person.

Input. Any form of information, matter, or energy that enters from the environment into the system through its boundary.

Negentropy. A systems energy state that measures the system's tendency toward order.

Open System. A system with an open or semipermeable boundary that allows a free exchange of input and output between the system and its environment

Output. Any energy, information, or matter that is transferred to the environment.

Steady State. A state of balance or internal constancy that signifies that a system is in harmony with its environment.

Stress. An ever-present and dynamic state of reaction that results from systems' interactions with their environments; a non-specific response of the body to any demand made on it.

Stressor. Any factor or agent that is responsible for or intensifies a stress state.

Throughput. A process that occurs at some point between the input and output processes.

INTRODUCTION

The nursing profession has experienced many changes over the past two decades. One of the most exciting and fundamental changes has been in the area of theory building and conceptualization in nursing.

The purpose of this chapter is to introduce the student to two general and universally applicable theories that have been widely studied and used by nurses in the past few years—general systems theory and adaptation theory. These two theories were chosen for use in this textbook to orient the student to the definition and function of theories in general. General systems theory and adaptation theory are both concrete examples that can accomplish this orientation, and they can be explained, illustrated, and understood within the context of many concepts.

The second reason these two theories were chosen is that they are basic to a wide variety of nursing concepts, and they are a part of or form the structural framework of much of the thinking and writing going on in nursing today. They have a great deal to offer, and practicing professionals, as well as nursing students, will benefit from a basic understanding and appreciation of their ideas and principles. Systems theory, in particular, is widely used in textbooks, in professional literature, and in educational programs.

GENERAL SYSTEMS THEORY

Overview and Significance

Our modern world is so complex that it cannot be comprehended as a single phenomenon or entity. As a result, people tend to fragment it into understandable, manageable pieces. This fragmentation can be seen in science, which is broken down into elements such as chemistry, physics, microbiology, and sociology. In governments there is the division of states, regions, counties, and townships. In the human body there are organ systems, organs, tissues, cells, and genes.

General systems theory explains the breaking of whole things into parts and gaining knowledge about how the parts work together in "systems." It explains the relationships between wholes and parts, describes pertinent concepts about them, and makes predictions about how these "parts of wholes" will function, behave, and react. The terms *general systems theory* and *systems theory* will be used interchangeably in this text.

The basic concepts and ideas of general systems theory were explicitly proposed in the 1950s by scientists from a wide variety of disciplines. Ludwig von Bertalanffy emerged as one of the primary theorists and went on to develop and introduce systems theory as a universal theory, applicable to many fields of study. The theoretical framework gives us generalizations about systems from which concepts, principles, and models can be transformed to work for a particular discipline. Psychology, biology, education, and computer science are all examples of fields that use systems theory and its applications.

Definition of a System

Bertalanffy defines a system as a set of interacting elements.[1] These interacting elements, or components, may or may not serve a different function, but ultimately they all serve a common purpose—to contribute to the overall goal of the system. In general systems theory, this is one of the most fundamental properties of a system. Families provide us with an excellent example of how this works. Given that the typical components of a family are the mother, father, and children, we can say this family system is a set of interacting components. Each member has a unique role and function that contributes to the overall functioning of the system (e.g., keeping members safe, fed, clothed, loved, socialized).

Likewise, a mechanical system, such as a bicycle, also has related components that interact. The wheels, pedals, bearings, and brakes all function separately but ultimately serve to provide a vehicular system.

From these examples we also can understand another part of the definition of a system. In systems the whole is always greater than the sum of its parts. In other words, each part standing by itself has a certain meaning or value that is enhanced or altered, i.e., it becomes "greater," when it is in interaction with the other system elements. In systems, elements work together in such a way that a change in one element may affect the meaning or use of other elements, as well as of the total system. For example,* consider a man with one leg: the

---

*Example from unpublished Master's thesis, Michael H. Heffron.

only way he can propel himself is by hopping on that one leg. Next, consider a man with two legs: if the two legs are seen simply as a collection of single legs, then the best we can expect that man to do is to hop twice as fast as the man with one leg. But if he uses his two legs together as a system, he can run—an activity unique to the system, not simply the sum of individual characteristics. The earlier example of the bicycle as a mechanical system also illustrates this point.

The Hierarchy of Systems

Systems are hierarchical in nature and are composed of interrelated subsystems. Each subsystem is made up of lower subsystems, until some lowest-level subsystem is reached, or at the other end, some highest-level suprasystem. In most living systems, the bottom line for the elementary, or the top line for the suprasystem is somewhat arbitrarily drawn. Atoms, for example, are elementary subsystems in many systems, but to the nuclear physicist, they are complex systems. Figure 5–1 illustrates a broad and common systems hierarchy.

The assignment of systems, therefore, as subsystems or suprasystems, is relative to the focus of study. For example, nursing might be considered a _subsystem_, within the realm of a health-care system, but a _system_ in the realm of a hospital setting.

Boundaries

In systems theory, **boundaries** are real or imaginary lines of demarcation that separate one system from another or a system from its environment. These boundaries help provide a sense of order to the overall concept of a system. Examples of boundaries are skin around a body system or a brick wall around a prison system. Boundaries serve as a point of exchange between what goes into and what goes out of the system.

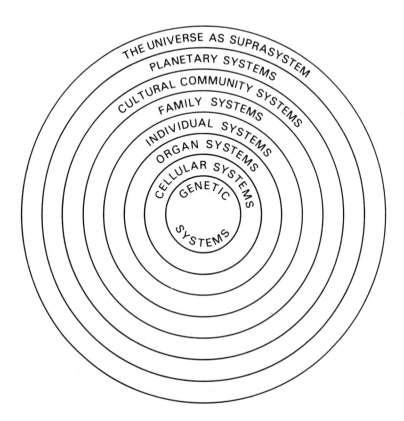

Figure 5–1. A common systems hierarchy.

Input, Output, and Throughput

Input and **output** are processes by which a system is able to communicate and react with its environment (i.e., with what is outside but interactive with a system). Input can be defined as any form of information, energy, or material that enters into the system through its boundary. Output is any energy, information, or matter that is transferred to the environment.

Throughput is a process that occurs at some point between the input and output processes. It enables the input to be transformed in such a way that it can be used readily by the system. When food is put into the human system by way of the mouth, for example, it immediately is subjected to a transformation process as the teeth mechanically grind it and the enzyme ptyalin chemically alters it. Without this and the subsequent processes of throughput, such as internal digestion and metabolism, the initial input could not be made into useful forms of energy for system survival. The throughput process is often referred to as transformation and occurs in manners and degrees of complexity that are highly specific to each organism or system.

Open and Closed Systems

One of the most important concepts advanced in general systems theory is the distinction between open and closed systems. An **open system** is one in which there is freedom and space for the movement of energy, matter, and information into and out of the system—through the system boundary. The boundaries in open systems often are described as *semipermeable*, because they are necessarily equipped to be selective about the movement of input and output. This crucial process of selectivity is discussed further in the sections of this chapter on feedback and equilibrium.

The input and output process in open systems might involve nutrients and wastes, in an animal or plant system, or pieces of information, in a library system. A business system may be described as an open system with the exchange of goods and services the input and output. Likewise, the exchange of feelings, verbally or through body language, in a group system would help classify it as an open system.

All living systems are by nature open sys-

tems; their very survival depends on a continuous exchange of energy, and they are constantly in a state of change. Open systems may vary in their degree of openness, both from system to system and within the same system. Hibernating bears, for example, breathe in oxygen and give off carbon dioxide, but there is little other interaction with the environment until spring. Amoebas and other one-celled animals are highly open systems at all times.

Closed systems are theoretically just the opposite of open systems. A closed system would experience no input from the environment and give no output. It would not change under any circumstances. If openness and closedness were on a continuum, such as in Figure 5–2, all systems would be somewhere in between. In reality, no totally closed system has ever been known to exist. The term *closed system* is used in scientific literature, however, and it is important to keep in mind that it may or may not be in accordance with the definition found in general systems theory. The social sciences, in particular, often make reference to families, particular groups, or societies, as being closed systems. What they mean is that the system in question is *relatively* closed to outside influence or exchange. This might be said about a club or religious group, for example, that only admits members who meet some narrow criterion or that isolates itself from general society.

Steady State or Dynamic Equilibrium

Open systems have to maintain a special balance within themselves to survive. This special balance is referred to as the system's **steady state** or **dynamic equilibrium.** In the human body sys-

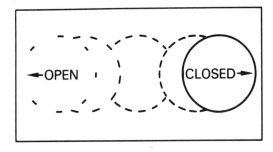

Figure 5–2. An illustrated continuum of open and closed systems.

tem, for example, we can find many instances of this, Maintenance of body temperature, the normal salinity and pH of body fluids, or the proper amount of sugar in the blood and urine are all examples of how the healthy body is in a physiological balance. Psychologically, one also must adapt and maintain a steadiness and balance in one's emotional life. Too much expression of anger, for example, may lead to violent, survival-threatening behavior and alienation from others, whereas too little expression of anger may lead to gastric ulcers, headaches, or other somatic problems.

The concept of steady state does not imply elementary steadiness as one might think of an unmoving hand or an unchanging course at sea. On the contrary, the steady state in systems theory is always associated with the continual input-throughput-output cycle and, while balanced, it is never static. *Homeostasis* is another term that is often used synonymously with steady state, and it too may be misleading in this regard. Stasis clearly implies a stationary or stagnant state, in contradiction to the dynamic nature of the steady state in open systems. Used specifically within the physiological context from which it originates, homeostasis is a time-honored and acceptable term. It seems to lose some of its appropriateness, however, as it is adapted for use in describing the whole of human interactions with the environment in a broad and extended way. **Homeodynamics** is yet another term used in describing the human dynamic state of balance. Homeodynamics is defined as the continuous exchange between humans and their environment of energy that characterizes life itself—its growing, changing, and learning.[2] Whichever terminology is used, and you will see all of these terms used in this text as well as in the general literature, the principle is the same: In open systems there is a life-sustaining balance at all levels that is maintained through the continual input and output exchange process within the environment.

Feedback

The maintenance of the steady state is highly dependent on a mechanism called **feedback**. Feedback is a system's self-regulatory process whereby system outputs are monitored and the result is used to control subsequent input. It is not unlike the feedback mechanism that occurs in the communicaton process where there is interaction between the sender and the receiver; or in perception theory, whereby input messages are encoded, processed, and decoded with the help of feedback to promote adaptation and a system steady state.[3]

Examples of the feedback mechanism can be found within community, family, and group systems as well as in individuals. Persons interacting with their various community systems receive feedback via rules, regulations, and laws. For example, a driver in a great hurry may drive through a stoplight, be stopped by a policeman, and be given a traffic ticket. The act of getting the ticket is the feedback, which probably causes the driver to modify input behavior when reentering the transportation system.

Children within a family system receive feedback from parents regarding their behavior. The harmony and steady state of the family depends greatly on how this feedback is used.

Equifinality

Open systems tend toward a dynamic equilibrium that allows them to maintain their functions and survive. An important principle of systems theory, which is also a characteristic of the steady state, is the principle of equifinality.

Equifinality is a goal-seeking process in which the system strives to reach a particular final state or goal, regardless of the means. A classic example is in the growth and morphogenesis of organisms, particularly the case of identical mammalian twins occurring from one ovum. The goal is the fully formed organism, which can be reached in either of two ways—from a single egg or from half of a divided egg.[4]

The chapters on Family Systems Concepts and Group Concepts provide illustrations of equifinality and how groups of people tend to be goal seeking, reach their goals in different ways, and have the potential for changing from their original states. In addition, individual behavior also reflects an equifinality. Coping mechanisms, for example, that help us to adapt and reduce stress, are highly varied and used by individuals in differing combinations and degrees. One person may seek out the company of a listening friend to reduce stress or anxiety (maintain a steady state), whereas another person may have a glass of wine, meditate, or take a walk. A third person may use a combination of these. The process is goal seeking, and the same goal can be reached through different methods.

Energy, Entropy, and Negentropy

Energy, as a concept in general systems theory, may be looked at from several viewpoints. A basic dictionary definition of **energy** is the capacity to do work. Traditionally, energy is further defined in terms of its source, e.g., the sun or the wind. It also can be talked about in terms of its method of action, what it looks like, what kind of qualitative effect it has, and how much is needed by whom or what. In systems theory, we look in addition and very specifically at the maintenance of adequate amounts of energy and its distribution and movement.

We have noted that open systems are constantly in a dynamic state as the processes of input, throughput, and output are recurring. As these processes continue, the differentiated features of individual components in the systems may tend to lose their distinctiveness, their individuality, and to blend together with the other system components into a homogeneous entity. Contrary to what may be our first intuitive feeling about this process, this tendency toward homogeneity is a tendency toward disorder, that is, a breakdown of organized distinctions. This tendency is called **entropy**. It can be defined as a measure of the tendency toward disorder in a system. Conversely, negative entropy, or **negentropy**, occurs when the system is tending toward order and increasing organization. Negentropy is defined as a measure of a system's tendency toward order.

To understand these concepts more clearly, it is important to recognize what order and disorder really mean in terms of living systems and how systems are affected by entropy and negentropy. Increasing organization, as defined within the context of a system, is an ordered differentiation of system elements, as opposed to homogeneity. Thus, entropy may be understood as dissipation of energy or a diversion of that energy required to maintain the differentiation of system components. If allowed to predominate, it will cause a system to run down and fail to accomplish meaningful goals. Ne-

gentropy, on the other hand, allows the system to differentiate or distinguish its energy flow and provide for order and purpose. Input energy is transformed uniquely and carefully, according to a more specific plan, and there is differentiation or increased organization as system goals are attained.

Yura and Walsh provide an illustration of what these concepts mean as they discuss the use of entropy as measurement of an individual's health state. Health state is equated with the steady state or systems goal, i.e., the goal of a healthy living system is to maintain a steady state as negentropy is maximized and the human organism tends toward order.[5] The human organism, in order to seek and maintain health, must expend energy to understand and define what "good" health is in its particular situation, identify a plan for working toward this goal, mobilize the means for reaching it, and then carry it out. All of these steps take organization as the person (system) interacts with the environment and adapts to the goal of steady state or "good" health. Negentropy is maximized when this is the case.

ADAPTATION THEORY

Definition of Adaptation

The concept of adaptation has been around for many years, as we have studied and observed ourselves in relation to the world around us. A basic encyclopedic definition of **adaptation** in a general biological context is the adjustment of living matter to environmental conditions and to other living things. There are many recorded descriptions and references to adaptation, and in almost all contexts it is characterized as a dynamic process that effects change and involves interaction and response. Human adaptation is much more complex than that of other animals and occurs on three levels: internally (the self), socially (with others), and physically (biochemically by nature).[6] Adaptation is thought by many scientists to be perhaps the one attribute that most clearly distinguishes the concept of life from the concept of inanimate matter.[7]

Within a general systems framework, adaptation is a process that must be ongoing to ensure the survival of living, open systems; it is the process that fosters regulatory mechanisms in systems and works toward a homeodynamic goal or steady state. The processes of input, throughput, and output, as well as feedback, negentropy, and equifinality, are the major system processes that are associated with and contribute to the adaptation of open systems.

Because it is used in so many disciplines and is present in all forms and aspects of life, adaptation means many things to many people.[8] Biologists, sociologists, psychologists, and physicians are among the numerous professionals who use adaptation and apply its principles. This interest and recognition are invaluable to the study of human beings and to such fields as nursing because they allow adaptation to be looked at holistically, as a process that affects the whole person, and not just selected parts.

To understand **adaptation theory** in its broadest sense, it is important to understand more about how the various disciplines view it and make its application meaningful. For the purpose of this discussion, we will look briefly at adaptation theory as developed in biology, physiology, and selected areas of nursing, psychology, and the social sciences.

Biological Adaptation

Biology, the study of life, gives us one of the broadest ranges of information and understanding about adaptation theory. Charles Darwin studied the adaptation of many life forms as he was formulating his famous theory of evolution. He observed that most organisms produce far more offspring than can possibly survive. Those that survive do so because they are best adapted to cope with their environment. Among these survivors, some are better adapted than others, and these would leave the greater number of offspring, the principle of natural selection.[9] Natural selection, according to Darwin, is the process that supports **evolution.** Evolution is the historic and ongoing process of change and adaptation of living things since life began. The well-adapted survivors have passed on accumulated changes to their offspring, and for three billion years, living things have been adapting through succeeding generations to their environment and each other.[10]

Biology is ultimately concerned about the

surival of living things. Various animals and plants are adapted for securing their food and for surviving extremes of temperature and water supplies. The cactus, for example, is adapted for survival in hot, dry climates. Animals like fish and birds each show anatomical adaptations that suit them for life in the water or in the air. Camels are not only built to withstand heat and scarcity of water, but they also have a second row of thick eyelashes that gives them protection against sandstorms.

Ecology, which is the study of plants and animals in relation to their total environment, is concerned with both anatomical and physiological adaptation. Human ecology, which is most relevant to nursing, provides us with additional information on physical, cultural, technological, social, and behavioral adaptation.[11] Within human ecology, people are viewed as open systems in constant interaction with their environments. Their responses to various environmental conditions—weather, temperature, air quality, water purity, noise, toxic substances—are all concerns of adaptation that have become profound and threatening issues in present-day society. Such man-made environmental hazards as high-speed automobiles, chemicals, drugs, and nuclear devices unfortunately are teaching us much about maladaptation as well as adaptation.

Physiological Adaptation

Physiology, a branch of biology, involves the functions, maintenance, and reproduction of living organisms. It is concerned basically with cellular function and the internal environment of the body. Adaptation at this level is looked at within the context of maintaining intracellular homeostasis (i.e., preserving the correct fluid composition and temperature for the cells to carry on their functions). As these cellular systems are grouped together into tissue systems, organs, and so forth, the homeodynamic processes are different; as systems' goals change, environmental exchanges become more complex, and there is a need for more intricate mechanisms of adaptation.

Kidney filtration, one of the most common homeostatic mechanisms, provides an excellent example of the complexities of physiological adaptation. Brunner and Suddarth bring out this complexity by describing quantitatively the filtering and excretion processes that go on in a typically healthy person at rest. Within a 24-hour period, a healthy person at rest, will recirculate about 3 L of plasma per minute through the kidney, 170 L of water, 170 g of glucose, and 560 g of sodium will be filtered. Of these amounts, virtually the same exact percentages are either excreted or reabsorbed, according to cellular or other systems requirements for homeostasis.[12] This is not to mention the myriad of other possible inputs to this system such as drugs or excess water, to which healthy kidneys can adapt.

Thus far, adaptation has been defined as a homeodynamic process in which various body systems adjust to their exchanges and interactions with other internal systems and external environmental exchanges.

Stress and Adaptation

Within living systems, **stress** can be defined in numerous ways. It is a difficult term to describe, as a single phenomenon or typologically, such as psychological, physiological, or sociological stress. Furthermore, stress can be viewed as both a cause and an effect.[13] We often say that illness imposes a stressful condition on our bodies and, at the same time, we refer to stress as the cause of the illness. Dr. Hans Selye, a physiologist who studied stress extensively, offers a definition of stress as both an effect and, through his term **stressor**, as a cause. Selye defines stress as the nonspecific response of the body to any demand made on it, and a stressor as any factor or agent that is responsible for or intensifies a stress state.[14] Because stress causes the body to change in some way, the need for adaptation is created. The responses or adaptations that take place can be chemical, structural, or both (Fig. 5–3). Chapter 26 elaborates on stress and adaptation and specifies adaptive and maladaptive mechanisms that may take place.

Psychosocial Adaptation

Psychosocial adaptation involves the way a person adjusts mentally and emotionally as a self-system, as a person relating to others, and to society in general. These relationships include thinking, acting, and feeling, and can be measured, to a very large degree, by the state of a

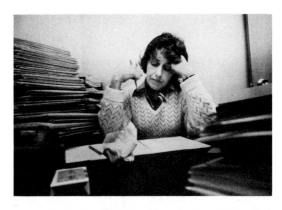

Figure 5–3. The ability to adapt to stressful situations is dependent on interactions from all of a person's subsystems.

person's identity, personal esteem, and level of fulfillment. All of these psychological "states" can be quite complex and never can be totally separated from other kinds of adaptation, such as physiological and biochemical. Also, not as much research has been done in the area of social and psychological adaptation as in physiological homeostasis and there are not as many guidelines as to which variables are important.[15]

At present, more is being studied and written about the application of adaptation principles to psychosocial issues. Selye's theory of the **general adaptation syndrome,** for example, has been applied by a number of nurse authors to the area of psychosocial assessment.[16–18]

In addition, the application of general adaptation concepts is being used to describe and present issues in the study of nursing.[19–22] Social adaptation has been addressed from the viewpoint of medical sociology, as has anthropological and family adaptation.[23–25] The following discussion will outline briefly some of the recent ideas regarding the psychosocial adaptation of human beings.

Sister Callista Roy, a nurse theorist, developed a systems adaptation model for the practice of nursing. The Roy model views the human as a bio-psycho-social being and describes adaptation as occurring in four modes. Three of these, the self-concept mode, the interdependence mode, and the role mode, are concerned with the ways the individual adapts psychosocially. The self-concept mode addresses such areas as esteem, self-concept, and ego integrity. The interdependence mode deals with how a person adapts to others. Changes in relationships, such as death or separation, can disrupt the giving and receiving of affection, social resources, and other need fulfilling activities. The role mode addresses how the individual adapts to the various and changing roles he or she must perform to maintain a homeodynamic balance within self, family, and society. Any change in role, such as a new job or new baby, requires adaptation to bring the system back into balance. Adaptation processes will be geared to changing any lost or maladaptive behaviors related to these changes.[26, 27]

Psychological adaptation is defined by Murray and Zentner in terms of behavioral adequacy and the attainment of appropriate human relationships. Adaptation is achieved through the processing of the conscious self (ego), the unconscious self (id), and the inner self (superego). These are primarily defense mechanisms that allow the person to adjust to and cope with stressful situations. Adaptation, according to these authors, can be evaluated using Selye's general adaptation syndrome.[28]

Lancaster talks about the full range of adaptation behavior within the context of an ecological framework. She defines adaptation as a dynamic, active process by which the individual living system meets its basic needs within a constantly changing environment.[29]

David Mechanic, a prominent medical sociologist, defines social adaptation as a process that requires a person's psychological capacities, skills, and qualities to meet and adjust to the demands of his or her physical and social environments.[30] Take, for example, the social adaptation of people who are hospitalized. The social demands of hospitalization include such things as the relinquishment of privacy, adherence to predetermined eating, bathing, and sleeping schedules, the separation from familiar people, and tolerance of often uncomfortable examinations and treatments (Fig. 5–4). These demands seem relatively beyond the tolerance limits of people accustomed to leading an independent life over which they exert control. For these people, adaptation may be difficult in the hospital setting and may depend on complex coping mechanisms. Yet there are some people

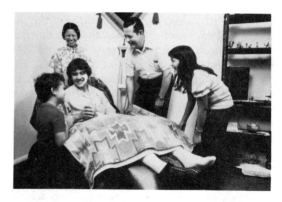

Figure 5–4. People are bio-psycho-social and spiritual beings.

who, because of previous stressful events or other factors may adapt quickly and gratefully to the role of being a dependent client in a hospital. Other factors that affect this kind of social adaptation are the prior experiences the individual has had in adapting to similar situations, how family and friends have adapted, and what one's values are in regard to such issues as privacy and authority. This list of variables appears endless when considering adaptation within this kind of sociocultural framework.

Anthropological Adaptation

Anthropology offers us yet another broad and comprehensive view of adaptation theory. Similar to biological adaptation, anthropological adaptation refers to the capacity of a particular group to tolerate selective forces in its environment and to master environmental problems by developing effective structures, behaviors, and forms of social organization. Humans, in contrast to other living systems, rely more heavily on "learned" ways of adapting rather than on instinctive or inherited methods. Human populations can make complex and extensive changes in a relatively short period of time. As new tools, ideas, and ways of living emerge, cultural adaptation takes place.[31] Culture can be viewed as a determinant of adaptation.[32]

Anthropology loooks at people and adaptation longitudinally as well as comprehensively. Through a time and space perspective, human adaptation is seen in relation to the past, present, and future. As this knowledge is gained and combined with geographical, physical, and sociocultural aspects, a unique and comparative view of the human and adaptation emerges.[33]

NURSING IMPLICATIONS

The ideas and principles within systems theory and adaptation have had considerable influence on nursing and the health professions. In nursing these theories have provided useful frameworks for the definition of major concepts and sound theoretical foundations for education and practice.

The remaining portion of this chapter will focus on how systems and adaptation theory have been applied in the areas of health care, clinical practice, and nursing education.

The Adaptive Nature of Humans

Systems and adaptation theory allow people to be viewed within a dynamic, humanistic, and holistic framework. **Holism** and holistic are terms that reflect the idea of wholeness and the interrelatedness of component parts in a whole system. **Humanism** refers nonjudgmentally to the qualities and essences of being human and to universal human characteristics, such as beliefs, values, and feelings.

Human beings are complex organisms made up of distinct groups and subgroups of related components. The interplay between these human components (i.e., behaviors, feelings, and thoughts), as well as structural and physiological human aspects, involve many unique and complementary relationships that are at the very core of human adaptation. Together, these systems and adaptation provide for a comprehensive view of humankind.

In the nursing profession, the human being is frequently viewed from a holistic and dynamic perspective. In this way, the individual can be looked at within the context of his own individual system, as well as other systems and subsystems in the environment. From this broad, ecological viewpoint, nurses can better understand some of the complexities of human behavior and better meet clients' needs. Clients undergoing planned admissions to the hospital, for example, show highly diverse reactions to seemingly simple procedures such as filling out forms, securing valuables, and going for x-rays. A second look at these reactions, from a systems viewpoint, can provide insight into some of the reasons for them. Attitudes and fears from childhood (psychological subsystem), present economic situations (economic social system or self-social subsystem), and previous community experiences (community systems) are some examples of systems interactions that might influence a person's reactions.

Living systems are goal seeking. They have the potential for growth and development and are allowed flexibility and variance as they pursue their goals. Goals are reached through careful organization and channeling of energy for effective interaction (adaptation) between all the parts. Nursing practice is benefited and enhanced in many settings by looking at people in this way. The community health nurse, for example, looks at goal seeking and growth within the context of a wide variety of human subsystems. Here, clients may be individuals, family groups, or the community at large. All three of these entities are systems within themselves and subsystems of one another that are constantly striving to reach certain goals, all within the context of how they should relate with, depend on, and help each other. Consider an elderly crippled widow who wishes to remain at home, despite her inability to care completely for herself and follow a medication regimen. The community health nurse is able to help this client reach her goal of partial self-care by contacting two family members and another community agency for help. Through mutual planning and health teaching by the nurse, the client feels supported and is able to remain semi-independent during her convalescence.

In another instance, the surgical intensive care nurse must look critically at human physiological goals. In this case, the physiological system will dictate certain priorities of care as homeostasis returns and tissues are repaired, but a look at the psychosocial subsystems will be equally important in promoting the overall return to health. By assessing such things as the will to live, the degree and source of any psychological stress, and family attitudes toward the client's illness, the nurse is acknowledging that mind and body are not separate, but function and respond as a whole unit.

Nursing theorists have given additional evidence of the usefulness of systems and adaptation theory as a way of looking at people. Orem, for example, views the human being as a system with an internal physical, psychological, and social nature that all react to the external elements—the environment.[34] Sister Callista Roy, whose systems adaptation model was mentioned earlier, sees the human being holistically as a bio-psycho-social being who adapts according to various modes or components. These modes of adaptation correlate with the characteristics of each component subsystem of the individual.

Nursing as an Adaptive System

A systems adaptation framework also can help to define and clarify the scope of professional nursing.

The practice of nursing takes place in a variety of settings and in a number of ways. A necessary and major facet of this practice is the *nursing process.* Inspired by several theories, one of which is general systems theory, the nursing process is an organized problem-solving approach by which nurses interact with their clients to promote adaptation. Found in virtually every contemporary nursing book, it is a step-by-step goal-seeking process that is hierarchical in nature and uses a feedback mechanism. The five phases or steps of the nursing process are fully described in Chapter 7. The advancement of this process has benefited nursing in unparalleled ways. It is described as the essence and core of nursing and provides the profession with a positive self-concept, one that functions in an organized and adaptable fashion from a scientific base.[35]

Health Care and Holism

Professional nurses carry out the nursing process interactively and interdependently within a larger system called the health-care system. In American society, the term health-care system identifies a confusing and highly complex network of health and medical components that vary greatly in their goals, meanings, and actual functions. Chapter 6 elaborates on this and provides insights into the subsystems of the health-care system and the relationships among them. In the past few years, the ideas and principles

of general systems theory have helped numerous groups of people think about the plan for a more comprehensive kind of health-care system.

Holistic health and **holistic health care** are terms that became very popular during the 1960s, when many people began to voice dissatisfaction with the existing structures of health care and other American institutions. Holistic health care involves the whole person within his or her environment and reflects the systems concept that the whole is greater than the sum of its parts. It is mandated to consider all the components of health as an open system: health promotion, health education and prevention, health maintenance, and restorative-rehabilitative care. Nurses and other advocates of the holistic approach feel that all of these components are equally important in the process of identifying health needs, planning for care and intervention, and in evaluating the results (Fig. 5–5).

Selye's research and findings on stress and adaptation helped to further thinking on the merits of holistic health care. His book, *The Stress of Life,* increased the interest in stress and stress-related illnesses. Both health professionals and health consumers became more concerned about the totality of stress, about its being the consequence of many interactions with the environment (e.g., chemical, biological, psychological, physical, sociocultural), with potentially damaging effects on the body. This interest and concern has helped evolve a holistic

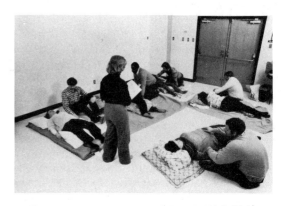

Figure 5–5. Health teaching is a part of holistic health care.

orientation in nursing, as well as foster a more holistic approach in medicine and other health professions.

Nursing Education

In nursing education, models such as systems theory and adaptation have proven to be very important and useful as teaching frameworks within which human beings, nursing, and health care can be explained.

An early example of this can be seen in the writings of Florence Nightingale. Although Nightingale's methods of nursing are not explicitly identified as theoretical and are less well known than her other contributions in nursing education, she used a framework of thought similar to that of adaptation theory. Her philosophy included frequent references to the effects of the environment on the patient and how these effects could hamper or help the healing process. In her nurse's training program, she stressed the importance of fresh air, sunshine, pure water, and a clean, quiet environment. In essence, she said that if these elements are poorly attended to, patients will have to expend too much of their available energy to adapt to the environment rather than to get well.[36, 37]

Although a number of early nursing leaders, such as Nutting and Robb, wrote about nursing as a more humanistic and integral science, the medical model remained the dominant theoretical framework for nursing until fairly recently. In the 1950s and 1960s, conceptual frameworks of intrapersonal theory and human needs theory were advanced. Both of these conceptual frameworks were holistic in nature and embraced basic adaptation principles, although neither general systems theory or adaptation theory were specifically credited.

In the 1970s, nursing leaders and educators began to develop and publish more information on theory development and evaluation. Nursing theories were identified as foundations for nursing education, and many baccalaureate nursing programs adopted a specific theory on which to base their curriculum.

Most curriculums in nursing education contain a mixture of several theoretical approaches, but both general systems theory and adaptation theory have had an influence on schools of nursing and, in some cases, are being used as theoretical frameworks for curriculum guidance.

As was mentioned at the beginning of the section on general systems theory, the basic systems conceptual framework allows for a universality and common basis of understanding among different fields of study. This attribute has tremendous benefits for nursing as well as other service-oriented subsystems of the health-care system. Professionals from many disciplines must develop shared meanings and understandings in order to function interdependently and achieve mutual goals of health care.[38] In addition, nurses, psychologists, physicians, and social workers, for example, can benefit from a shared and interdisciplinary language to span conceptual gaps in knowledge and relate to one another's research more effectively.

Adaptation theory, as the basis for systems integrity and survival, also perpetuates a common basis of understanding across disciplinary boundaries. Together, these theoretical frameworks have been applied and have influenced the nursing profession in numerous ways.

SUMMARY

A system is made up of a set of interdependent and mutually interacting components that have a common goal. The end product or whole system is always greater than the sum of its parts.

Systems are arranged hierarchically in terms of other systems and may be classified as subsystems, systems, or suprasystems. Boundaries are lines of demarcation, visible or invisible, that enclose a system's parts and differentiate it from the environment and other systems.

Systems can be open or closed. Open systems are those that relate freely with the environment and allow for the continual exchange of matter, energy, and information across their boundaries. This input material undergoes varying degrees of transformation inside the system, called throughput, which converts it to usable forms of energy. Any material that leaves the system and is returned to the environment is called output. All living systems are open systems in nature, although the term closed system is sometimes used in the social sciences to refer to isolated or relatively closed groups of people.

Living systems show a remarkable capacity to maintain a constant balance or dynamic equilibrium within themselves. This balanced condition may be referred to as the system's steady state or homeostasis and is necessary for survival of the system. A newer term, homeodynamics, emphasizes the nature of this balance in terms of continual change (i.e., the system is constantly exchanging input, and output remains stable).

Feedback is a self-regulatory process in which a system obtains information from or about its output which is then used to monitor its input. It can be thought of as a circular mechanism and is largely responsible for the maintenance of the steady state.

Living systems exhibit a goal-seeking behavior known as the principle of equifinality. As a result of this property, systems tend toward equilibrium and can arrive at a final state via different routes and from different initial conditions. Equifinality also contributes toward the maintenance of the steady state and is necessary for the growth and integrity of the system.

Energy is a major concept in general systems theory and is described in terms of its type and state of distribution and movement. Entropy is a systems energy state that measures the tendency toward disorder in a system and, if allowed to predominate, will cause the system to degenerate and die. Negentropy is a systems energy state that measures its tendency toward order and increasing organization; negentropy allows a system to differentiate its energy in a purposeful way and progress toward a goal.

Adaptation is the process in which living matter adjusts and makes changes in response to interactions with the environment. It is a dynamic and creative process in humans, described theoretically by a number of disciplines.

In general systems theory, adaptation is an umbrella-term encompassing system processes that lead to the steady state. All open living systems require adaptation for continued functioning and systems survival.

Likewise in the fields of biology and ecology, adaptation connotes the adjustment and survival of living things, to each other and to environmental conditions. Ecology views adaptation holistically, to include all aspects of living organisms.

Psychosocial adaptation refers to that part of human adaptation that involves emotional stability and the quality of interactions with other people and society in general. Adaptive processes within this realm are highly complex because of the great number of variables that are available; the uniqueness of psychological variables within each individual, in combination with all respective characteristics of society, gives rise to this sometimes unpredictable and inconsistent state of affairs.

Anthropological adaptation provides a broad view of human adaptation. The reactions of selected groups of people to all aspects of their environment are studied and looked at in a sociocultural framework over time. Adaptive mechanisms are described comparatively and according to various cultural characteristics.

Many of the basic concepts of professional nursing can be explained and understood within the frameworks of general systems theory and adaptation. The human being can be seen as an open living system made up of interrelated parts that are in constant interaction with the environment. Additionally, the human being is a goal-seeking organism that uses many feedback mechanisms for self-regulation and maintenance of a homeodynamics or a steady state.

Adaptation is necessary for human survival and can be used as a measurement tool in the assessment of health status and planning for nursing care. Health care is described as holistic when it takes into consideration the bio-psychosocial and spiritual needs of people and provides for, or makes referrals for care in all these areas.

In nursing education, systems and adaptation frameworks are used in the teaching-learning process. There is also a trend toward holistic types of course integration in professional curricula. This philosophy reinforces the concepts of the human being as an open system and of nursing as a process that promotes adaptation within a holistically structured health-care system.

Finally, the universality of both of these theories has been a major factor in their capacity to influence nursing. By perpetuating a common basis of understanding across disciplinary boundaries, general systems theory in particular has helped to increase the knowledge base of nursing and foster a holistic approach in the pursuit of professionalism.

Study Questions

1. Describe a family you know in terms of components, boundaries, input, output, feedback, and steady state.

2. Develop a chart showing the hierarchy of systems and subsystems within your school of nursing.

3. List as many examples as you can of behaviors, mechanisms, or factors that have contributed to an increase in your personal negentropy status in the past 48 hours.

4. Describe two homeostatic mechanisms within the human body and list adaptive behaviors and mechanisms for each.

5. Write a short critique of your own health-care needs in the past year. From a systems perspective, were they met in a holistic fashion? Why or why not?

6. Interview two classmates regarding their experience of coming to college for the first time. Compare their various reactions to the processes of social adaptation and methods that helped them cope and adapt.

References

1. Ludwig von Bertalanffy, *General Systems Theory* (New York: Braziller, 1968), 55.
2. Arlyne B. Saperstein and Margaret A. Frazier, *Introduction to Nursing Practice* (Philadelphia: F.A. Davis Co., 1980), 88.
3. Helen Yura and Mary B. Walsh, *The Nursing Process* (New York: Appleton-Century-Crofts, 1973), 65.
4. Bertalanffy, *General Systems Theory*, 40.
5. Yura and Walsh, *The Nursing Process*, 42.
6. Philip K. Bock, *Modern Cultural Anthropology* (New York: Alfred A. Knopf, 1969), 209.
7. René Dubos, *Man Adapting* (New Haven: Yale University Press, 1965), 256.
8. Ibid., 257
9. Theodore W. Torrey, *Morphogenesis of the Vertebrates* (New York: John Wiley & Sons, 1971), 5.
10. Malcolm E. Weiss, *Clues to the Riddle of Life* (New York: Hawthorn Books, 1968), 25, 29.
11. Jeanette Lancaster, *Community Mental Health Nursing, An Ecological Perspective* (St. Louis: C.V. Mosby Co., 1980).
12. Lillian Brunner and Doris Suddarth, *Textbook of Medical-Surgical Nursing* (Philadelphia: J.B. Lippincott Co., 1980), 106–7.
13. Marjorie L. Byrne and Lida F. Thompson, *Key Concepts for the Study and Practice of Nursing* (St. Louis: C.V. Mosby Co., 1972), 42.
14. Hans Selye, *The Stress of Life*, rev. ed. (New York: McGraw-Hill Book Co., 1976).
15. Lancaster, *Community Mental Health Nursing*, 19–20.
16. Ellen M. Feeley, Moira S. Shine, and Sharon B. Sloboda, *Fundamentals of Nursing Care* (New York: D. Van Nostrand Co., 1980), 179–180.
17. Ruth B. Murray and Judith P. Zenter, *Nursing Concepts for Health Promotion*, 2nd ed. (Englewood Cliffs, N.J.: Prentice-Hall, 1979), 44–45, 48.
18. Byrne and Thompson, *Key Concepts*, 44, 45, 48.
19. Jeanine R. Auger, *Behavioral Systems and Nursing* (Englewood Cliffs, N.J.: Prentice-Hall, 1976) 51, 162, 168.
20. Lancaster, *Community Mental Health Nursing*, 52–54.
21. Carolyn C. Clark, *Mental Health Aspects of Community Health Nursing* (New York: McGraw-Hill, 1978), 4–6, 69.
22. Joan P. Riehl and Sr. Callista Roy, *Conceptual Models for Nursing Practice* (New York: Appleton-Century-Crofts, 1974), 135–51.
23. Madeleine M. Leininger, *Nursing and Anthropology: Two Worlds to Blend* (New York: John Wiley & Sons, 1970), 5.
24. Murray and Zentner, *Nursing Concepts for Health Promotion*, 179–180.
25. David Mechanic, *Medical Sociology* (New York: The Free Press, 1968), 2, 57, 68, 179.
26. Riehl and Roy, *Conceptual Models*, 135–38.
27. Baccalaureate Curriculum Subcommittee, The Catholic University of America School of Nursing, *CUA Systems Adaptation Model* (Washington, D.C.: The Catholic University of America, 1978), 16, 19, 22.
28. Murray and Zentner, *Nursing Concepts for Health Promotion*, 170–74.

29. Lancaster, *Community Mental Health Nursing,* 52–54.
30. Mechanic, *Medical Sociology,* 57.
31. Bock, *Modern Cultural Anthropology,* 208, 209.
32. Murray and Zentner, *Nursing Concepts for Health Promotion,* 175.
33. Leininger, *Nursing and Anthropology,* 208, 209.
34. The Nursing Theories Conference Group *Nursing Theories* (Englewood Cliffs, N.J.: Prentice-Hall, 1980), 66.
35. Yura and Walsh, *The Nursing Process,* 1.
36. Julia George, *Nursing Theories the Base for Professional Nursing Practice,* 2nd ed (Englewood Cliffs, N.J.: Prentice Hall, 1985), 33.
37. Frances T. Smith, "Florence Nightingale: Early Feminist," *Am J Nurs* (1981):1023–24.
38. Lillian DeYoung, *Dynamics of Nursing* (St. Louis: C.V. Mosby Co., 1981), 68.

Annotated Bibliography

Auger, J.R. 1976. *Behavioral Systems and Nursing.* Englewood Cliffs, N.J.: Prentice-Hall. This text presents a behavioral systems approach to nursing practice. General systems theory is discussed, as is the structure and function of behavior. An assessment tool and case examples are included.

Hall, J.E., Weaver B.R. 1985. *Distributive Nursing Practice: A Systems Approach to Community Health,* 2nd ed. Philadelphia: Lippincott. This entire text uses a general systems theory approach to community health nursing. Chapters 3 and 4 give clear explanations of general systems concepts and provide examples of how they can be applied to components of nursing practice.

King, I. 1981. *A Theory For Nursing Systems, Concepts, Process.* New York: Wiley. A conceptual framework is presented by linking nursing concepts essential to understanding nursing as a system with health-care systems. There are sections on social systems, personal systems, interpersonal systems, and goal attainment. A good reference for understanding how to use a systems framework in nursing.

Neuman, M. 1984. Looking at the whole. *Am J Nurs* 84:1496–99. This article defines and clarifies the concept of nursing diagnosis within a conceptual framework based on general systems theory. Emphasizes that nursing assessment must embrace holism, i.e., nursing diagnosis results from assessment of the total person's pattern of health. Contains examples.

Chapter 6

The Health-care System

Sr. Rosemary Donley

Chapter Outline

- Objectives
- Glossary
- Definition of the Health-care System
- The Health-care Inputs
    The Client
    Media
    The Public
    Health Professionals
    Technology
    Health-care Centers
    Unions and Professional Associations
    Planners, Regulators, and Accreditors
    Health Insurers
    Legislation
- Health-care Throughputs
    Client Care
    Client–Family Education
    Education of Health Professionals
    Research
    Standards and Regulations
- Health-care Outputs
    Healthy People
    Health Professionals
    Health-care Centers
    Standards of Care and Practice
    Health-care Plans
    Health Laws
    Reimbursement Policies
- Feedback
- Summary
- Study Questions
- References
- Annotated Bibliography

Objectives

After completion of this chapter the reader will be able to:

- Name inputs into the health-care system
- Discuss how inputs affect each other
- Name some processes or throughputs in the health-care system
- Discuss how health throughputs compete with each other for resources
- Name some health outputs
- Discuss the interrelationships among outputs
- Explain how feedback is used to change health-care systems
- Discuss how nursing inputs affect other subsystems within the health-care system

Glossary

Academic Health Center. A complex of a medical school, a university hospital, and one other health school, usually a school of nursing.

Access to Care. Availability and acceptability of services to people.

Accreditors. A group or a professional association that sets criteria, evaluates institutions, and develops a listing of agencies that meet standards.

Case Mix. The diagnosis-specific makeup of a hospital's clients. Case mix directly influences lengths of stay and intensity, cost, and scope of the services provided by a hospital.

Certification. Recognition of special competence or eduction.

Diagnosis-related Groups (DRGs). A system of classifying clients according to type of disease. It was developed by researchers at Yale University and contains 467 mutually exclusive and exhaustive disease categories or groups. Medicare's prospective payment system is based on DRGs.

Health-care Team. The group of health professionals that provides care. Physicians and nurses are members on the team.

Health Maintenance Organization (HMO). Prepaid health plans that encourage outpatient and preventive health services.

High Technology Medicine. The use of machines to diagnose, monitor, treat, and relay information.

Home Health Agency. A public agency or private organization that is primarily engaged in providing skilled nursing services and other therapeutic services in the client's home and that meets certain conditions designed to ensure the health and safety of the individuals furnished these services.

PL. Abbreviation for public law.

Planners. Volunteer or public agencies that design and recommend building and program proposals for health-care institutions.

Prospective Reimbursement. A system of payment in accord with prearranged policies that are negotiated before services are provided.

Regulators. A group responsible for controlling operations or enforcing standards.

Reimbursement Policies. Decisions and agreements that control how health-care professionals and institutions are paid.

Secondary Care Facilities. Institutions that provide routine treatment and inpatient care to moderately and seriously ill people.

Tertiary Care Facilities. Institutions that admit directly or on referral seriously ill people or people who require highly specialized diagnosis and treatment.

DEFINTION OF THE HEALTH-CARE SYSTEM

Health-care systems or health-delivery systems are phrases used to describe the method by which health care is given. This chapter will analyze health-care patterns using the language of systems theory. It is important to understand the concepts in systems theory; the reader is referred to Chapter 5, in which Heffron notes that input, throughput, output, and feedback are words used to order discussions. The health field is a complex system. There are many inputs, multiple throughputs, serial outputs, and elaborate feedback mechanisms.

Figure 6–1 lists the components of the health-care system as they will be presented in this chapter. Some of you may find, as you examine the list that you disagree with this classification system. For example, it may be argued that regulations are "inputs" or that client care is an "output." Both of these are correct. The task of assigning a label as "input" or "throughput" to components of an open system enables us to discuss their inter-relationships. Relationships among parts are significant to goal achievement. In an open system there is a constant exchange of energy, activity, and information. Consequently, the classification system proposed in Figure 6–1 presents one way of understanding how clients, doctors, nurses, institutions, and noninstitutionalized care settings work together to achieve health care.

Each section of the health system operates with different values, goals, and information. Sometimes health systems experience trouble or dysfunction because of these differences. On the other hand, the system usually works to the satisfaction of clients, nurses, and the public. The discussion of the health-care system will begin with a close look at the inputs. Health systems need clients, people trained to help them, and places in which the system can work.

THE HEALTH-CARE INPUTS

The Client
Who are the patients or clients and how do they enter the health system? Although most clients seek health care because they perceive a lack of

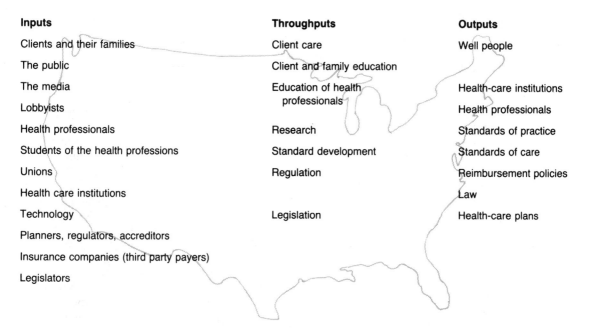

Inputs	Throughputs	Outputs
Clients and their families	Client care	Well people
The public	Client and family education	
The media	Education of health	Health-care institutions
Lobbyists	professionals	Health professionals
Health professionals	Research	Standards of practice
Students of the health professions	Standard development	Standards of care
Unions	Regulation	Reimbursement policies
Health care institutions		Law
Technology	Legislation	Health-care plans
Planners, regulators, accreditors		
Insurance companies (third party payers)		
Legislators		

Figure 6–1. Components of the health-care system.

well-being, there are various states of health. People can be worried well, mildly ill, moderately ill, acutely ill, chronically ill, or dying when they seek health care.[1] Consequently, one of the first actions to occur is diagnosis. Assessment of well-being is so important that a client cannot be admitted to an institution, a noninstitutionalized setting, or treated by a professional without a diagnosis. The answers to the questions: What is wrong? or Why did you come for help? describe the diagnostic process. Physicians classify clients according to disease states (acute gallbladder attack or myocardial infarction), body systems (cardiovascular or neuromuscular), types of treatment (medical or surgical), and degrees of illness (critical or chronic).

Hospital and home-health-care administrators assess the degree of illness of clients to determine needs for special services and to estimate the costs of care. For example, clients in need of surgery are placed in one section of the hospital. The high cost of hospital care requires that clients and their families, doctors, nurses, and administrators work together from the beginning to determine which treatments are most effective and least costly. In the cost-conscious

world of the eighties, assessment includes an evaluation of the client's ability to pay for services and an assessment of which care setting is medically appropriate as well as cost effective.

Nurses use the diagnoses of their medical and administrative colleagues. They also make nursing diagnoses.[2] For example, nurses speak about limited mobility, change in body image, or describe the ability to participate in self-care. In practice, however, nurses are bi- or trilingual in that their work requires that they speak the languages of nursing, medicine, and administration. Because nurses spend more time with clients and their families than other health workers, they often translate between clients and health-care professionals. This role is important because clients and families often are surprised by diagnoses and plans of treatment. Nurses help clients understand how the health-care system works. They help clients express their needs, and they advocate client rights. Advocacy is an important role in a complex system. Some critics of modern health organizations argue that clients are no longer considered to be important influences in health-care decisions. They suggest that professionals or those who pay the health-care bills control what happens to clients, who are not consulted. (See Figs. 6–2A, 6–2B.) To the degree that this description is accurate, the health-care system is ineffective. You may wish to conduct an informal survey of client input in plans of care. Ask your clients how they are consulted about their treatment, its costs or the sites where their care is provided.

The client as input can be examined in two ways. Clients enter health-care systems to receive treatment. Once diagnosed, they "go through the system" and recover. Another view of the client as input looks at the client's input. In this model, clients are defined as partners who contribute actively to the resolution of their illnesses, the improvement of the environment, and reduction in health-care costs.

Media

The media influence the health-care system. The press, radio, and television shows, and popular

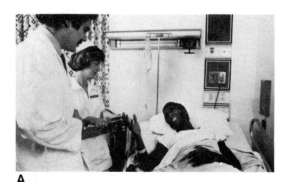

A

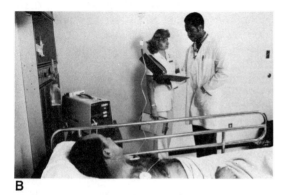

B

Figure 6–2. A. The client as a partner. **B.** The client as an observer.

literature portray a typical day in the life of an ordinary client. Sometimes stories about sophisticated breakthroughs in the treatment of serious illnesses excite the public. Occasionally the media serve as the public's conscience and bring attention to unmet needs. The 1970 articles depicting the shameful treatment of the institutionalized aged shocked and mobilized Americans against scandals in the nursing home industry.[3] The media have played an important role in public education about acquired immune deficiency syndrome (AIDS).

For sociological, psychological, and anthropological perspectives on the roles and lives of clients, families, care givers, and institutions, the interested reader is referred to the works of Talcott Parsons and Erving Goffman. Parsons' classic description of "sick role theory" uses a sociological framework to explain what happens to personal, family, peer, and societal expectations when a person is ill.[4] Goffman's illustrations of "sick people" and their professional care givers add another dimension to the understanding of the complexity of "inputs" in the health-care establishments. In analyzing life careers of mental patients, Goffman examines patients' views of their worlds.[5] In a later text, he describes the behavior of one subset of health professionals, surgeons, and their associates.[6]

On a less serious note, each season brings new hospital television dramas to American living rooms. The medium provides colorful input into the health-care system and reflects public opinion about health care.

The Public

The public contributes to the health-care system by its presence on boards of hospitals, home-health-care agencies, health departments, and planning agencies, and by membership in voluntary, civic, or advocacy health groups. Input from these groups occurs at the levels of planning, program and policy development, and health-care financing. For example **PL 93–641,** the National Planning Act of 1974, and its amendments established public roles in decision making about the allocation of health resources. This Federal law proposed a strategy for the development of local and state planning organizations.[7] It is possible to criticize the complexity of PL 93–641. However, the underlying concept of the importance of citizen participation in the construction or expansion of hospitals cannot be refuted. In addition to working on planning boards, citizens are members of governing boards of hospitals and community agencies. Each year, people concerned with the treatment of disease, like heart disease or cancer, raise millions of dollars to aid research and to provide client services. In addition to raising money for health care, or making decisions about the conduct of hospitals, citizens can change specific health practices. For example, public demand for family-centered care enabled fathers to participate in childbirth classes and to be present during labor and delivery.[8] Employers and major purchasers of health insurance have encouraged cost containment through endorsement of prepaid health plans.

The public exchanges information with the health system. This communication occurs within therapeutic relationships between clients, nurses, and doctors. It takes place at board meetings and in fund-raising activities. Public views about health care also are presented in newspapers, magazines, and television serials. The information that is generated is fed back into the system and influences future actions and decisions.

Health Professionals

Who are the health professionals and what do they do? In the modern health system, nurses, doctors, and dentists are joined by nutritionists, dieticians, pharmacists, social workers, medical and radiologic technicians, physical and occupational therapists, accountants, medical record librarians, managers, and executives. These individuals are called the **health-care team** (Fig. 6–3).

Some health workers perform public services, such as community-oriented nutrition ed-

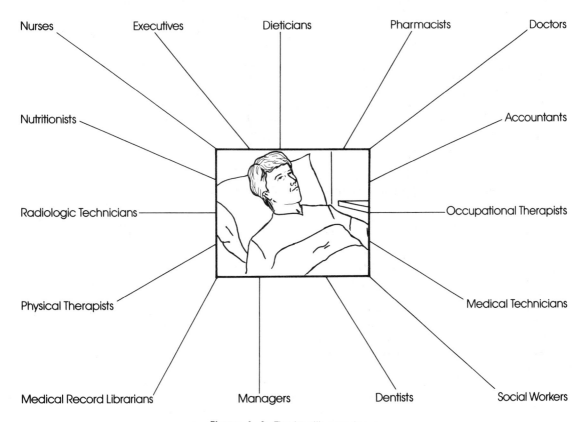

Nurses   Executives   Dieticians   Pharmacists   Doctors

Nutritionists   Accountants

Radiologic Technicians   Occupational Therapists

Physical Therapists   Medical Technicians

Medical Record Librarians   Managers   Dentists   Social Workers

Figure 6–3. The health-care team.

ucation. Others, like physical therapists, work with specialized groups of clients. Others perform their services away from the clinical area (medical record librarians). The complexity of health-care services requires teams of experts. While the traditional hub of health-team activity is the hospital, health teams function in school systems, health departments, industrial health centers, home-health agencies, specialized institutions for handicapped individuals, and in community based emergency or primary care programs.

Health professionals assess, diagnose, triage, treat, refer, care, and cure. They develop or contribute to care plans, record the process and outcome of their work, direct the activities of technicians and assistants, and manage resources.

The input of health professions usually is described by direct-care activities. However, health professionals shape and direct the system of care. Earlier in this chapter the public roles of citizens were described. Health professionals also sit on planning boards, hold positions on voluntary health associations, serve on hospital and home-care boards, and head health departments. They order and manage the health system in addition to providing services. They set standards, develop criteria, and participate in peer and institutional evaluation. Health professionals have multiple inputs into the system.

Because there are so many interesting and different career opportunities in the health field, it is not surprising that health careers attract many students.

Students in the various health-care professions also contribute input to the system. Recruitment and retention of good students is important for the maintenance and development of the system. Recognizing this, Federal and state governments and private foundations have established programs to provide financial assistance. Nursing fortunately has been enriched by program support to schools and financial grants to students. Schools of nursing have used Federal dollars to prepare clinical specialists and nurse practitioners and to develop outreach programs of continuing education for registered nurses. Nurses educated for new forms of practice work in rural settings, community hospitals, home-care centers, health maintenance organi-

zations (HMOs), and medical centers. Advanced education has changed the input that nurses have in health-care delivery and created expanded and independent nursing roles.

Systems theory suggests that a change in one part of the system affects the whole. Rapid developments in the field of nursing have caused some ripples in the system. You are studying nursing during a period of innovation. You can influence and contribute to the professional dialogue. Major disagreements center around the scope and nature of the "nursing input." Questions are raised: Is the nurse an independent provider of health care? Should nurses work under orders and supervision of physicians? Should there be only two levels of education, practice and licensure? You may wish to study how the changing role of nurses has influenced nursing's input into the health-care system.

Recruitment and retention of health professionals is another important input. Historically, Federal investment in the training of health professionals has been based on two premises: health professionals are a national resource, and Federal intervention is needed to resolve the shortage of physicians and nurses.[9,10]

Recent national studies suggest that there is no shortage.[11,12] These studies have been used in a climate of cost containment to reduce Federal investment in professional training and to limit support for graduate medical education under Medicare.[13]

Technology

Perhaps the most striking new force in the health system is the rapid growth in the use of technology. Machines and new drugs have enhanced diagnostic and therapeutic capabilities and improved professional communications. Technology has made diagnostic assessment quicker, safer and easier for clients. For example, computerized axial tomography (CAT) scanners make it possible to visualize the body without intrusion. Dialysis units, blood oxygenators, and respirators enable treatment of end-stage renal disease, serious cardiac insufficiency, and acute or chronic respiratory failure. Drug research has simplified the treatment of hypertension, depression, and some forms of cancer. Computers have enabled the health team to store and retrieve information about client care and health-care costs.

Any input this powerful and pervasive has another side. "The technological tiger" is indicted as a culprit in rising health-care costs.[14] Rationing of high technology is proposed as strategy for reducing costs.[15] Overtreatment or overuse of technology is always possible in a highly technological society. Concern for privacy, consent, or compassion is sometimes ignored as health professionals work their way through computerized monitors, intravenous lines, respirators, and machines that measure oxygenation and cardiac reserve. **High technology medicine** contributes to the complexity of health institutions and determines the **case mix** to a large extent.

Health-care Centers

Lists of health-care centers usually include hospitals, home-care agencies, skilled-care facilities, and ambulatory clinics or centers. However, physicians' offices, health clinics in schools or workplaces, and health departments also offer organized health programs. Health-care centers are classified by:

- Size
- Sponsorship or ownership
- Location
- Type of service
- Level of care
- Cost

Today's health centers are a far cry from medieval monasteries or inns. Some hospitals span city blocks or cluster in sections of cities. "Pill Hill" in Seattle, Washington, is an example of such a health-care complex. In small communities, large hospitals or skilled-care facilities employ most of the residents. To address cost and competition, proprietary and nonprofit hospitals have organized vertically and horizontally.[16] In vertical integrations, one organization owns and controls ambulatory, inpatient, extended- and home-care services. Horizontal integration links health-care centers across a state, region, or country.

Health-care centers develop identities and personalities. Charity Hospital in New Orleans, Louisiana, for example, is intimately associated with the life of the city and with the historical development of the United States. In addition to influencing the lives of clients, their families, friends, and health professionals, health centers affect the standard and cost of health care. For example, technological sophistication of acute-care hospitals and the number of unnecessary hospital beds are cited as factors that have made health care so costly.[17] Because health centers represent a group of interests, their input in the system is more compelling than the influence of small groups of individuals. When efforts are made to change the system, health centers receive most attention. Because the health-care system is an open system, it responds to internal and external pressures. The next section of this chapter examines how groups influence health-care delivery.

Unions and Professional Associations

Earlier in this chapter, health professionals were grouped in teams. Other organized structures of health workers influence particular institutions or the general system. Typically, health-care professionals align themselves with peer groups. These associations provide networks for **certification,** standard development, continuing education, job and salary information, and professional support. Nursing has developed an impressive list of professional organizations. Table 6–1 gives an overview of nursing associations.

Unions are another group active in health fields. In 1974, the Taft–Hartley Act was amended to include workers in nonprofit industries. Since then, labor unions have provided input into hospitals and skilled-care facilities. Some unions follow the industrial model of the American Federation of Labor. Others, like the American Nurses' Association or the American Federation of Teachers, operate along professional norms. Traditional unions and professional associations compete to represent nonprofessional and professional health workers. Health institutions and unions struggle for patterns that meet the needs of workers and management without losing sight of the special mission of the health industry. When the discussions are successful, salaries and working conditions improve. Hospital unions are controversial, although the economic security program has been a major platform of the American Nurses' Association for 40 years.

TABLE 6–1. SELECTED NURSING PROFESSIONAL ASSOCIATIONS

Academy of Nursing	International Association for Enterostomal Therapy
American Academy of Ambulatory Nursing Administration	MARNA—Mid Atlantic Regional Nurses Association
American Association for Nursing History	Midwest Alliance in Nursing
American Association of Colleges of Nursing	National Association of Hispanic Nurses
American Association of Critical Care	National Association of Pediatric Nurse Associates and Practitioners
American Association of Nephrology	National Association of Nurse Recruiters
American Association of Neurosurgical Nurses	National Association of Orthopedic Nurses
American Association of Nurse Anesthetists	National Association of Physicians' Nurses
American Association of Occupational Health Nurses, Inc.	National Association of School Nurses
	National Black Nurses Association
American College of Nurse Midwives	National Center for Nursing Ethics
American Indian/Alaska Native Nurse Association	National Federation for Specialty Organizations
American Nurses' Association	National Intravenous Therapy Association
American Organization of Nurse Executives	National League for Nursing (NLN)
American Society of Ophthalmic RN's	National Male Nurses Association
American Public Health Association Public Health Nursing	National Nurses Society on Substance Abuse
	National Organization of Philippine Nurses
American Society for Nursing Service Administration	North American Nursing Diagnosis Association
American Society of Plastic and Reconstructive Surgical Nurses	Nurses Association of the American College of Obstetrics and Gynecology
American Society of Post Anesthesia Nurses	Nurse Consultants Association
American Urological Association	Nurses House, Inc.
Association of Operating Room Nurses	Nurses Organization of the Veterans Administration
Association of Pediatric Nursing	Oncology Nursing Society
Association of Practitioners in Infection Control	Sigma Theta Tau
Association of Rehabilitation Nurses	Society of Gastrointestinal Assistants
Coalition of Nurse Practitioners	Society of Otorhinolaryngology and Head and Neck Nurses
Commission on Graduates of Foreign Nursing Schools (CGFNS)	Southern Regional Nurses Association
Dermatology Nurses Association	Western Interstate Commission of Higher Education for Nursing
Emergency Department Nurses Association	

Planners, Regulators, and Accreditors

A major direction in health care flows from those who set standards, make plans, or evaluate performance. Some critics of the health system say that **planners** have had no impact on the system. They argue that the health-care industry is unplanned. Usually this point of view is supported by statistics that contrast the number of acute-care beds in a community with the number of nursing-home beds.[18] The methodology for sophisticated, community-based planning developed after the construction of the hospital system. Some reasons for this lie in the history of nonprofit hospitals.

Health-care institutions developed in response to the needs of an immigrant people. Religion, social class, ethnicity, and race stimulated hospital construction more than did medical need. The development and expansion of health institutions were influenced by the same motives that brought them into being. Communities' wish "to have their own hospitals" was encouraged by the Hill–Burton Act, a federally funded program to build hospitals. By the time health planning came to be taught as a subject in schools of hospital administration, health institutions were built. Recent efforts of the Federal government to curb construction and expansion of institutions resulted in a national health planning act.[19] This law mandates public and provider planning for construction, expansions, new programs, and manpower development. While all states have formal health plans, there is not much evidence that state or regional planning has a serious impact on the internal plans and aspirations of institutions.[20] On the other hand, financial constraint, prepaid health insurance, and competitive ambulatory and home-care programs have forced mergers, consolidations, and reduction in bed capacity.

Health-care centers are subject to review by **accreditors** such as state health departments and professional accrediting teams. Institutions are licensed by state health departments. They are accredited by the Joint Commission on the Accreditation of Hospitals (JCAH). Home-care agencies are accredited by the JCAH or the National League for Nursing. These groups apply standards and criteria to health centers. Examples of such criteria might be a fixed ratio of professional nurses to patient populations or a minimum amount of emergency equipment at specific locations in the hospital. Efforts to meet these criteria cause centers to modify procedures or services. Information fed back to institutions after accreditation reviews causes further change. Standards for practitioners or clinical services are set by professional peers. For example, many nurses seek certification through the American Nurses' Association or one of the specialty organizations.

Health Insurers

Americans have a private/public system for paying for health care. Health insurance is a work-related fringe benefit, and private insurers sell health benefits to employers. The major provider of health insurance is Blue Cross, a non-profit health insurance agency. Multipurpose for-profit insurance companies, such as Aetna and Travelers, also offer health insurance. **Health Maintenance Organizations (HMOs)** offer health plans that provide a program of care, rather than illness-related services, for a predetermined price.

In 1965, the Federal government passed two major health insurance bills as amendments to the Social Security Act. Medicare (Title 18) and Medicaid (Title 19) revolutionized the health field. Initially, because of the opposition of organized medicine, Medicare and Medicaid functioned as traditional insurance carriers. In the 1970s, however, the Federal government became the prime financer and standard-setter in the health field. Much has been written since the enactment of Titles 18 and 19 about the input of the Federal government in the health field. Perhaps the major input of Medicare and Medicaid is explained by studying their beneficiaries. Before 1965, employees lost health insurance benefits upon retirement, and the poor were uninsured. Medicare and Medicaid give the aged and the poor access to the health system. Federal money poured into the health-care system since 1965 has caused dramatic increases in health-care costs.

In 1982, Congress passed the Tax Equity and Fiscal Responsibility Act (TEFRA).[21] This first effort in cost containment was quickly followed by the Prospective Payment Act of 1983 (PL 98–21).[22] PL 98–21 changed the way in which the Federal government pays its hospital bills for Medicare recipients. A fixed price has been set, based on the assignment of a patient to a **diagnosis-related group,** the so-called **DRG.** This legislation also changed the pattern of reimbursement from a fee-for-service, retrospective payment plan to a fixed-rate prospective plan.[23] The financial incentives of the flat-rate system encourage physicians and hospitals to delay admission, hasten discharge, and use fewer resources to provide care. The input of health-care financing has had a major impact on the configuration of the health-care system.

Efforts to reduce health-care costs have stimulated new forms of prepaid insurance (HMOs); new programs of care (home care, day surgery, and surgicenters), new professionals (nurse practitioners), and new forms of practice (preferred provider organizations [PPO]).

As has been evident in the discussion of inputs, the health-care system is changing. Major change (expanded roles for nurses, new financing systems) in inputs causes change in the whole system. Today, the health-care system is trying to achieve equilibrium and adjust to new inputs, particularly an innovative system of Medicare payments. You have the opportunity to observe how a complex system uses new information and adjusts its methods and goals.

Legislation

Health legislation can be classified in four ways:

- Legislation to ensure safety
- Legislation to prepare professionals and health workers
- Legislation to establish programs of service
- Legislation to pay for service delivery

Safety Legislation. Nurse and physician practice acts are examples of legislation to ensure safe health care. Federal and state governments also have statutory authority to license health institutions, set the number of beds, establish programs of immunization and disease control, and enforce food and drug safety laws.

Manpower Legislation. Laws that support students through low-interest loans or scholarships are called manpower laws. They help qualified students achieve their career goals. The Health Professions and the Nurse Education Act are examples of comprehensive manpower laws.[24] You may wish to study these laws and note the programs of study that they support. Some sections of the manpower law finance the education of medical or nursing students in exchange for a promise of service in a medically underserved area. Other Federal laws support professional education for military personnel or veterans.[25]

Health Services Legislation. Public health service laws support a wide range of health programs. Until recently, these programs were established by individual titles in the Public Health Service Act.[26] The Budget Reconciliation Act of 1981 altered the role of the Federal government in providing local health services.[27] As a result of this law, 21 Federal programs were combined into four block grants. Programs sent to the states included the Maternal Child Health Grant, the Primary Care Grant, the Health, Prevention and Services Grant, and the Mental Health Block Grant. Federal funding for these programs was reduced.

Health-care Financing Legislation. The most significant health legislation is the set of laws that purchases health care for beneficiaries. Medicare and Medicaid are public health insurance acts.

Medicare is a two-part, Federally administered nationwide health insurance program for the aged and disabled. The payroll-tax-financed hospital insurance (HI) program, or part A, provides protection against the cost of inpatient hospital services, posthospital home-health services, and posthospital skilled-nursing-facility services, with specified deductibles and coinsurance amounts. The supplementary medical insurance (SMI) program, or part B, is a voluntary program that provides protection against the cost of physician and certain other medical services.

Medicaid provides matching funds to states to finance medical care for low-income persons who are in families with dependent children or who are aged, blind, or disabled. Federal financial participation in the medicaid program is based on a matching rate according to a state's per capita income. Although the program is governed by a mixture of Federal and state eligibility requirements, the states are responsible for the administration of their respective medicaid programs.[28] Figure 6–4 provides an overview of the growth of the Medicare and Medicaid programs.

The first section of this chapter has considered inputs into the health-care system. Although each input has been discussed individually, it is apparent that energy and information exchange occurs within the input system. Changes in the nature or degree of any component part affect other inputs. For example, physician or nurse shortage has always triggered Federal legislation to support professional education. Changes in financing influence the delivery of health services. The real test of inputs, however, develops from an examination of the processes or methods within the system.

HEALTH-CARE THROUGHPUTS

Client care, education, research, regulation, standard development, and legislation are processes by which the goals of the health-care system are achieved.

Client Care
Client care is the major throughput in the health-care system. Hospitals and home-care settings are the hubs of client care.

Most hospitals treat adults with medical or surgical illnesses. Community hospitals rival university teaching facilities in their capacity to treat acutely ill people in specialized units. Many health-care observers believe that the line between **secondary** and **tertiary care facilities** is an imaginery one and that the hospital of the

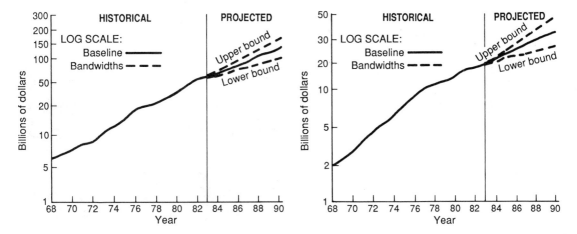

Figure 6–4. Medicare/Medicaid growth care. **A.** Medicare outlays with bandwidths: 1968–1990. **B.** Federal Medicaid outlays with bandwidths: 1968–1990.

future will be a center for tertiary or most complex care. When a client is admitted to the hospital, "throughput" begins. The client, his or her family, and the professionals begin to look for the source of the client's difficulties. The modern medical complex is known by its diagnostic capability. Observation, history, intrusive and nonintrusive examinations of organs, body parts, body fluids, and excretions, are used to identify the cause of the client's discomfort. Once this is accomplished, the client is given the appropriate treatment and is discharged. If, however, the cause of the client's illness is elusive or indefinite, "throughput" continues. When the diagnostic quest is partially or completely unsuccessful, the client and his family experience repeated emotional and physical conflicts. Sometimes, a diagnostic-therapeutic-diagnostic-therapeutic cycle develops. In these cases, one treatment leads to another test to another treatment. The emphasis on diagnosis and cure is so strong that if an illness cannot be treated, the health team often experiences apathy and a sense of failure. Because of the emphasis on cure, few health professionals or institutions possess the resources to manage treatment failures.

One method of examining throughput within a hospital is to trace the therapeutic course of a client. Case studies give new insights into inputs and interactions. Client care has many dimensions. Some common needs for care are summarized below:

- Need for acute care
- Need for maintenance care
- Need for supportive care
- Need for rehabilitative care
- Need for protective care
- Need for hospice care
- Need for health education

Although this section focuses on acute-care hospitals, client care is given in long-term, chronic-care, or psychiatric hospitals, in ambulatory centers, and in the home. Long-term care is underdeveloped and underfinanced. Clients with chronic conditions have not received attention because acute-care modalities emphasize diagnosis and treatment. Recently, several programs have been established to address the needs of the institutionalized aged. In nursing, this program is called the teaching Nursing Home Project. Supported by grants from the Robert Wood Johnson Foundation, this effort is designed to encourage faculty and students to assume clinical decision making in skilled-care facilities.[29]

Since the late 1960s, public and private ambulatory clinics and health maintenance organizations have become centers for client care. *Pri-*

mary care is the term used to describe client care in these centers. Primary care includes:

> a person's first contact in any period of illness with a health care system that leads to a decision about the resolution of the problem and the responsibility for the continuum of care, that is, maintenance of health, evaluation and management of symptoms and appropriate referrals.[30]

This definition highlights the important elements of primary care:

- Coordinated primary care
- Interdisciplinary care
- Comprehensive care
- Preventive care
- Ambulatory care
- Continuous care

An interesting idea about client care in these settings has been promoted by HMOs. The prototypes of HMOs were occupational health units at construction sites. Some industries had found they could provide better, less expensive health coverage for their employees if they combined workplace clinics with general health care programs.[31] The original plan of the HMO supported the use of ambulatory treatment and preventive care for workers and their families. HMOs adopted a new method of paying for health services called **prospective reimbursement.** Individuals and employers contract for certain benefits and pay a flat fee. Membership entitles people to use HMOs for health education, health assessment, immunizations, and treatments. HMOs operate on an old principle: An ounce of prevention is worth a pound of cure. Another source of ambulatory care is the physician in his office.

Studies report that many Americans seek care from their family doctor.[32] However, a physician who practices alone does not seem to be a future-oriented model of client care. Concern with cost containment has stimulated the development of new forms of outpatient care. The storefront clinics of the 1960s have been replaced by surgical centers in office complexes and department stores. Some suburban shopping malls provide a "doc in the box"—a drop-in health service (Figure 6–5) similar to 24-hour banking. Hospitals have opened satellite clinics

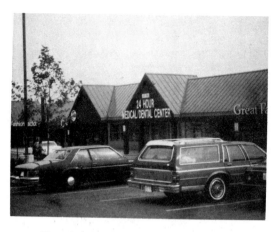

Figure 6–5. The new health-care center.

to reduce costs and ensure a system of client referral. Innovation in ambulatory care is related to reducing costs and to marketing competitive and convenient health care.

Client care is also provided in the home by:

- For-profit home-care agencies
- Voluntary agencies, of which the visiting nurse association is a prototype
- Hospital-based home-care programs
- The Veterans' Administration
- Hospices: care programs for the terminally ill and their families

Each **home health agency** provides client care as a function of its purpose, philosophy, and sponsorship. Hospice home-care programs are designed to help families care for their loved ones at home. The commitment of hospice teams is to support patients and families during dying, death, and bereavement.[33]

Visiting nurse associations operate around a health-education model of care. Visiting nurses in the home aim to teach clients and care givers how to care for themselves. Their plans of care always include health education. Freestanding (usually for-profit) and hospital-based programs also give care at home. Their home-care goals are similar to therapeutic care offered in hospitals. The significant difference in these programs is concern for cost-effective care.

Home care is the most rapidly developing segment in the health-care system. Prospective payment and flat-rate reimbursement under

DRGs have encouraged the discharge of clients who are still receiving active treatments. Home-care agencies have responded to a new client population and have used Medicare, Part B to finance durable medical equipment. Bedrooms now resemble hospital rooms as clients, their families, and home-care nurses maintain such treatment protocols as intravenous therapy and care of surgical incisions. The client's ability to pay and the scope of insurance coverage determine the extent and scope of service in for-profit and hospital-based home-care services.

In summary, client care is given in hospitals, skilled-care facilities, physicians' offices, ambulatory clinics, HMOs, and in the home. These programs are sponsored by Federal, state, and municipal governments, the military and Veterans Administration, private corporations that are proprietary or voluntary in structure, and by individuals.

Client–Family Education

Client–family education is an integral component of client care. Some organizations (HMOs and visiting nurse home-care services) were founded on the belief that health education is basic to client care. Public health agencies and industrial health programs emphasize health education and personal responsibility for health and safety. Nurses and physicians always have included client–family teaching in their care plans. However, within the past 20 years, hospitals have developed formal programs for client, family, and community health education.

Typically, hospitals offer programs in:

- Preparation for childbirth
- Parenting
- Normal and therapeutic nutrition
- Stress reduction
- Weight control
- Living with chronic illnesses (diabetes, arthritis, heart disease, cancer, stroke)
- Preoperative and postoperative instruction
- Discharge planning

Emphasis on health and maintaining a healthy lifestyle have become integral parts of the American culture in the past 2 decades. Many Americans, for example, are conscious of weight control, moderation in the use of alcohol, cessation of smoking, and regular exercise.

Personal responsibility for health makes the work of health professionals easier. Public concern with maintaining healthy minds and bodies gives positive feedback to the health-care system (Fig. 6–6).

Education of Health Professionals

A major responsibility of the health-care system is the education of its health professionals. Historically, health-care agencies have played critical roles in the education of physicians, nurses, and other members of the health team. Today universities and colleges educate most health workers. Table 6–2 shows the movement of professional schools of nursing from hospitals to junior and senior colleges and universities.

There are unresolved questions about the balance between theoretical and practical instruction in the fields of health. In the case of nursing, debates continue between advocates for hospital schools, and associate degree and baccalaureate college-based programs.[34] At stake is the issue of control of the education of nurses. In medicine, the primary care versus specialist training dialogues express a preference for clinical sites. Will young physicians receive clinical training in community hospitals and ambulatory care centers or in tertiary (highly specialized) hospitals operated by schools of medicine? Will young women physicians elect primary care? There are pros and cons to the nursing and medical discussions. Perhaps you and your classmates might stage a debate. Resolved: In the future there will be two levels of entry into practice: professional and technical, with two distinct licenses. The education of health-

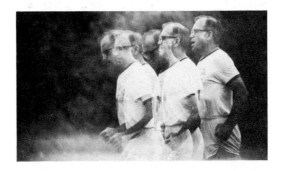

Figure 6–6. Jogging is a national pastime.

care workers is an important throughput. Information learned in discussions about methods of instruction give feedback into the system. This information becomes stimulus for change.

Continuing education for health professionals is a personal, organizational, and public challenge. Professional values and codes address the importance of maintaining and increasing knowledge and skill. The technological and therapeutic advances in biomedical research demand health professionals who like change and value lifelong learning.

Professional associations and employers assist their members by sponsoring continuing education.

It is possible to group continuing education into three categories:

- Orientation
- Maintenance and development
- Professional advancement

Orientation programs present the philosophy and purposes of health-care settings. They acquaint new employees with policies, procedures, and regulations. Some settings have special programs for new graduate nurses. These internship or preceptor programs continue during the first months of employment. Nurses who return to work or change specialties need to be introduced to new techniques and procedures. Orientation programs address the needs of new, returning, and reassigned nurses. A second type of continuing education recognizes that familiar procedures must be reviewed and that new skills must be developed. Hospitals, home-care agencies, and skilled-care facilities present annual programs on disaster training, fire safety, infection control, and cardiopulmonary resuscitation. Programs also introduce new technology, expanded services, or changes in procedure or policy. The expanded and new services offered by home-care agencies require vigorous attention to continuing education. The stimulation and development of stable employees are a challenge to health-care managers. Growth in the health industry is unparalleled. Consequently, vigorous efforts are needed to keep current employees up to date.

The third type of program promotes career advancement. Sometimes courses are conducted within institutions or in colleges or universities. Health-care institutions play significant roles in preservice and continuing education. They also conduct on-the-job training programs for ancillary and technical workers. Today, education is available through correspondence or telecommunication series, as well. The reader is referred to Chapter 11 for further discussion on continuing education.

Research

A final component of health-care delivery is research. Hospitals and ambulatory care centers connected to schools of medicine (**academic health centers**) were the first institutions to conduct research. These major institutions conducted:

- Clinical trials of drugs
- Basic research on disease states
- Development and testing of new treatments and technologies

Research is conducted in all sectors of the health community and by all health professionals. In the field of nursing, there have been significant developments in clinical research.

In 1985 the National Center for Nursing Research was established within the National Institutes of Health to foster funding for research and to increase the number of nurse re-

TABLE 6–2. EDUCATIONAL PATHWAYS FOR NURSING

Program Type	1970		1980		1983	
	Number of Programs	Percent of Change	Number of Programs	Percent of Change	Number of Programs	Percent of Change
Diploma	636	−7.6	311	−6.6	281	−2.4
Associate	437	+13.8	697	+2.8	764	+3.0
Baccalaureate	267	+6.0	377	+3.9	421	+4.7

From the National League for Nursing (NLN), Nursing Data Review 1985, 3.

searchers. The nursing community looks to this center to stimulate fundamental and applied nursing care research, to encourage talented young scientists to select careers in nursing research, and to secure stable funding for nursing research.[35]

Another form of research, health services research, explores the processes and goals of health-care delivery. Health services research is conducted by multidisciplinary teams rather than by single investigators. It addresses practical problems, such as access to care and cost of care.[36]

Hospitals and health centers do informal studies of internal organization, operations, market appeal, and management capabilities. They use data from Medicare and Medicaid reports, Professional Review Organizations, (PRO), records and studies of Health Planning Organizations and Health Systems Agencies (HSA), State Health Planning and Developmental Agencies (SHPDA), and State Health Coordinating Councils (SHCC). This information has helped health agencies compare their institutions to others in the region and the country. Informed hospitals and other health agencies compete to make their programs and services most attractive. National data banks have been developed by the Federal government and large insurance companies.

Interesting changes have occurred in research. Although investigation into the cause of illnesses is still the major research priority, other topics command public attention and public funds. Professionals and health-care agencies use the tools of research to study and improve their practices. The Federal government's Health Care Financing Administration (HCFA) and other insurance companies that pay health-care bills try to find solutions to growing health-care costs.

Standards and Regulations

Regulatory, legislative, and standard-setting agencies influence practice in complex health organizations in the following ways:

- Establishing and enforcing standards of professional practice within states and institutions
- Licensing professionals and institutions
- Specifying types of service to be given by professionals and institutions

- Regulating the growth and expansion of health-care agencies
- Setting fees for reimbursement for professionals and institutions
- Establishing and enforcing safety codes
- Establishing and enforcing conditions of participation for Federal, state and municipal programs
- Establishing and enforcing criteria for the certification of health professionals and the accreditation of health-care institutions

The health-care system has many lawgivers, **regulators,** and standard setters. Table 6–3 lists some agencies with which you should be familiar.

Several presidents have expressed concern with the complexity and cost of regulatory throughput. President Carter directed Federal agencies to simplify regulations. President Reagan proposed deregulation of the health industry. Regulations are mixed blessings. Everyone supported the "straight language" of the Carter administration. However, the application of deregulation in health causes some concern. The popular example given to support deregulation is the airline industry. Deregulation has reduced fares in routes served by competitive airlines. Physicians have a monopoly on medical practice and control reimbursement for health services. They are like those airline companies that hold the only franchise to a desired city. The deregulation of nursing homes proposed by the Department of Health and Human Services provoked public and professional outcries.[37] The deregulation debate offers an example of feed-

---

TABLE 6–3. SELECTED AGENCIES THAT ESTABLISH POLICIES, REGULATE PRACTICE, AND SET STANDARDS

Joint Commission for the Accreditation of Hospitals
State Boards of Nurse Examiners
Health Planning Agencies
State Health Departments
State Legislators
The Congress of the United States
Federal Trade Commission
Specialty Boards of Medicine
American Association of Medical Colleges
National League for Nursing
American Nurses' Association and specialty nurses associations

back in the health system. Those who favor deregulation argue that removal of artificial regulations will free the industry and reduce costs. Those who oppose deregulation say that health care is more a monopoly than a free market and stress the need for regulations to protect the health and safety of captive populations: the institutionalized sick, poor, aged, and retarded. The nature, scope, and extent of regulatory activity is an important issue of the 1980s. Its resolution will impact upon inputs and outputs in the system.

Health-care throughputs are processes by which patients receive care, professionals generate new knowledge and receive training, and health institutions interface with society. The study of throughputs opens windows into the health-care system.

HEALTH-CARE OUTPUTS

Several years ago, the Surgeon General of the United States issued a report entitled *Healthy People*.[38] This study addresses the goals of the health care system and describes personal behavior that leads to health. This American perspective should be read along with the statement of the World Health Organization: *Health for All by the Year 2000*.[39] The report of the World Health Organization balances health-care outcomes in first world countries like the United States with health goals of less developed nations.

The statements of the chief of the United States Public Health Service and the World Health Organization set a broad conceptual base for understanding health-care outcomes.

When health professionals and managers of health institutions discuss health outcomes, they cite:

- Well patients
- Well-managed institutions
- An adequate number of trained health professionals
- Standards of professional practice and care
- Adequate reimbursement for health services
- Evidence of health planning (accessible health services and health-care beds)
- Laws and regulations that ensure public safety

Healthy People

As has been stated many times in this chapter, the major goal of the health system is healthy people. However, when you look within the system for indicators of health, you will uncover indirect measurements. For example, state health departments, hospitals, skilled-care facilities, ambulatory centers, and home-care agencies record:

- Discharge rates by disease
- Infection rates
- Number of falls in institutions
- Number of live births
- Number of deaths per disease category
- Number of suicides
- Number of deaths by accident
- Average life expectancy by sex, race, and ethnic origin
- Number of maternal deaths
- Incidence of certain diseases
- Incidence of communicable disease
- Number of persons receiving workman's compensation or disability insurance

Most of these parameters describe absence of disease rather than signs of health. These data confirm the priority that the identification and treatment of disease (medical model) has in the American health-care system. It seems illogical to define healthy people as people without significant illness or disability. Yet that definition can be best defended in the American health-care system.

Health Professionals

This chapter also records the education of health professionals. The development of an adequate number of trained health professionals is a public goal. Assuring their placement throughout the country remains a national priority. Recent studies report that there are too many physicians and sufficient bedside nurses. They also note that maldistribution of health personnel persists. The geographic maldistribution of physicians and nurses is related to complex social, professional, and economic forces. There are many reasons to practice in urban and suburban areas. There are few incentives associated with rural and inner city practices. The more important question is: Are there enough of the right types of doctors and nurses? In the field of nursing, the Institute of Medicine (the latest group to study the supply of nurses) reports that the 1.33 million nurses in the work force satisfies public need for generalist nursing services. They note, however, a shortage of nurse specialists capable of working in acute-care and long-term environments.[40]

Health-care Centers

It is generally accepted that the United States has a sufficient number of health institutions to meet public need. The problems are **access to care** (overcoming cultural and financial barriers), the balance between acute and long-term care beds, and geographic maldistribution of services. The major concern expressed about institutional care is the cost of inpatient services.[41] Put another way, the United States has developed an enviable system of institutionalized care that is becoming too costly to maintain. We are witnessing efforts to reduce costs by encouraging the use of ambulatory clinics and home care.

Standards of Care and Practice

Mature organizations set standards. These criteria form the basis for evaluation and training. In the field of health, standards are developed by professional associations and the Federal government. You may wish to compare the standards of practice developed by Medicare with those of the American Nurses' Association and specialty organizations like the American Association of Critical Care Nurses and the Association of Operating Room Nurses.

Health-care Plans

Health-care plans are developed by state and local health departments and by the state health planning and development agencies. Mandated by PL 93-641 and amended by PL 96-79, these plans are statements of policy that provide planning frameworks for improving the health status of area residents.

Read a copy of your state's health plan. It will give you a comprehensive view of the health-care system in which you study nursing.

Health Laws

Since President Reagan assumed the presidency, the pattern of health laws has changed. The most complete compilation of current health laws is found in the Budget Reconciliation Act of 1981, which created the block grant program, the Tax Equity and Fiscal Responsibility Act of 1982, and the Prospective Payment Act of 1983 that modified Medicare and Medicaid.

At the state level, you may wish to review medical and nursing practice acts to determine the legality of current practice.

Reimbursement Policies

Given the direction of Medicare and Medicaid, many changes are anticipated in **reimbursement policies**. Competition and cost containment are key concepts in the new schema.

There is also concern about the impact of Gramm–Rudman, the Budget and Emergency Deficit Control Act of 1985, on all sectors of the health-care system.[42] Although Medicaid is exempt from the legislatively mandated sequestration orders and Medicare is somewhat protected, the programs of education, research, and health services have been subjected to reductions.

You have the opportunity to observe the effects of budget cuts and competitive strategies on reimbursement policies.

FEEDBACK

Feedback is the concept that best explains how systems regulate and change themselves. As inputs, throughputs, and outputs are generated, information is gleaned about the system and its functioning. This information is then reintroduced or fed back into the system. Several examples will illustrate how feedback influences contemporary health-care systems.

When major changes in financing health care, introduced by the 1983 amendments to the Social Security Act (PL 98-21), were fed back into the health-care systems, new home health-care agencies were developed to care for clients who were never admitted or were discharged early from acute-care hospitals. Hospitals also adjusted to lowered occupancy rates and a sicker group of clients (an intensified **case mix**) by closing units, reassigning nurses, and substituting registered for licensed practical nurses.

Hospitals have been less successful in adjusting to the costs of providing care to the poor or the uninsured, estimated to be around 35 million. Flat-rate reimbursement makes it difficult to subsidize care for the poor by charging other clients or their insurance companies. Recent policy decisions suggest that health care for the poor is a state, not a Federal responsibility.[43] The Budget Reconciliation Act of 1981, which created block grants, has enhanced the role that states play in programs for the poor. However the states are affected by rising health-care costs, troubled economies, state revenue shortfalls, and the domestic policies of the Reagan administration.

Although the problem of uncompensated care can be analyzed, the health-care system's response has been to deny or ration care or to transfer poor clients from one sector of the health-care system to another—the so-called "dumping" syndrome.[44]

SUMMARY

Inputs, throughputs, outputs, and feedback are described in this chapter using the language and theoretical frameworks of systems theory. Health systems are dynamic, interacting organizations. They exist as units or subsystems (community mental health ambulatory centers), as major systems (mental health centers connected to large academic health centers), and as macro systems (the Hospital Corporation of America).

Every health subsystem provides client care, participates in the education of its staff, and conducts research into its own operations. Major health systems achieve these goals, too. They also act as specialized hospitals to which clients are referred for sophisticated therapy. They educate health professionals and contribute to scientific knowledge. Macro systems offer and influence client care, professional education, and research across a geographic region or throughout the country.

In addition to describing the three classic goals of health-delivery systems, this chapter identifies political, economic, and social influences.

The demands of a highly mobile "third wave society" are played out in its institutions.

Health institutions are not immune to changes in the professions, the economy, and in religious and social values. Because the health-care system is a living, dynamic organism, it also contributes to social change. Public expectations about treatment of illness are a testimony to the successful therapy of health-care institutions. Concerns about the costs of health care indicate that feedback mechanisms have not been successful in regulating rising costs. As students of nursing, you will influence and be affected by health-care systems. As professionals, you will be challenged to advance and alter "the system" so that personalized care, informed education, and humanistic research remains a hallmark of the American health-care system.

Study Questions

1. Name some inputs into the health-care system.

2. Discuss what each "input" contributes to the system.

3. How are clients consulted about their care?

4. What is the most important input that you, a student of nursing, can make in the system?

5. What are some throughputs in the health-care system?

6. Can you prioritize the health throughputs?

7. Can you identify any evidence of feedback in the system?

8. What are some goals of the health-care system?

9. Can you prioritize the goals of the systems?

10. Are goals the same in each institution?

11. Do you think systems theory is a good model to apply to health care? Why or why not?

References

1. M. Terris, Approaches to an epidemiology of health, *Am J Public Health* 65, (1975): 1038–45.
2. M. Gordon, *Nursing Diagnosis* (New York: McGraw-Hill, 1982).
3. M. Medelson, *Tender Loving Greed* (New York: Random House, 1975).
4. T. Parsons, *The Social System* (Glencoe, Ill.: Free Press, 1951).
5. E. Goffman, *Asylums* (New York: Doubleday & Co., 1961).
6. E. Goffman, *Encounters* (Indianapolis: Bobbs-Merrill, 1961).
7. PL 93-641, *The National Health Planning and Resource Development Act of 1974* (Washington, D.C.: U.S. Superintendent of Documents, 1974).
8. M. L. Moore, *Newborn, Family and Nurse* (Philadelphia: W. B. Saunders Co., 1981).
9. Bureau of Health Professions, *Nurse Supply, Distribution and Requirements, Third Report to the Congress. Nurse Training Act of 1975* (Hyattsville, Md.: Bureau of Health Professions, Division of Nursing, 1982).
10. E. Ginzberg, "The future supply of physicians: From pluralism to policy," *Health Aff* 1, (1982):6–19.
11. Graduate Medical Education National Advisory Committee. *Report of the Graduate Medical Education National Advisory Committee to the Secretary* (Washington, D.C.: Department of Health and Human Services, 1981).
12. Institute of Medicine, *Nursing and Nursing Education: Public Policies and Private Actions* (Washington, D.C.: Institute of Medicine, 1983).
13. A. Relman, "Who will pay for medical education in our teaching hospitals? *Science* 226, (1984):20–23.
14. C. Schramm, "The teaching hospital and the future role of state government," *N Engl J Med* 308, (1983):41–45.
15. H.J. Aaron and W.B. Schwartz, *The Painful Prescription* (Washington, D.C.: Brookings Institute, 1983).
16. T. Porter-O'Grady, and S. Finnegan, *Shared Governance for Nursing* (Rockville, Md.: Aspen Systems Corp., 1984).
17. Institute of medicine, *Controlling the Supply of Hospital Beds, No. 2-04602* (Washington, D.C.: Institute of Medicine, 1976).
18. E. Champion, A. Bang, and M. May, "Why acute care hospitals must undertake long-term care." *N Engl J Med* 308, (1983):71–74.
19. PL 93-641 *The National Health Planning and Resources Development Act of 1974.*
20. J. Tierney and W. Walters, "Evolution of health planning," *N Engl J Med* 308, (1983):95–97.
21. PL 97-248, *The Tax Equity and Fiscal Responsibility Act of 1982.* (Washington, D.C.: U.S. Government Printing Office, 1982).
22. PL 98-21, *The Prospective Payment Act of 1983* (Washington, D.C.: U.S. Government Printing Office, 1983).
23. B. Vladeck, "Medicare hospital payment by diagnosis-related groups," *Ann Intern Med* 100, (1984):576–91.
24. K. Smith, U. Reinhardt, and R. Andreano, "Planning a national health manpower policy: A critique and a strategy," In R. M. Scheffler (ed): *Research in Health Economics I* (Greenwich, Conn.: JAI Press, 1979), 1–35.
25. "American medical manpower dilemma: How many doctors and nurses do we need?" *Heatlh Aff* 1, (1982):5.
26. *Compilation of Selected Public Health Service Acts* (Washington, D.C.: U.S. Government Printing Office, 1981).
27. PL 97-35, *The Omnibus Budget Reconciliation Act of 1981* (Washington, D.C.: U.S. Superintendent of Documents, 1981).
28. Special Committee on Aging, United States Senate, *The Proposed Fiscal Year 1983 Budget; What It Means for Older Americans: An Information Paper* (Washington, D.C.: U.S. Government Printing Office, 1982).
29. L. H. Aiken, "Nursing priorities for the 1980s: Hospitals and nursing homes" *Am J Nurs* 81, (1981): 324–30.
30. United States Department of Health, Education and Welfare, *Extending the Scope of Nursing Practice* (Washington, D.C.: U.S. Government Printing Office, 1971).
31. The National Academy of Science, *A Policy Statement: HMOs: Toward a Fair Market Test* (Washington, D.C.: The National Academy of Science, 1974).
32. D. Rogers, L. Aiken, and P. Blendon, *Personal Medical Care: Its Adaptation to the 1980s* (Washington, D.C.: Institute of Medicine, 1980).
33. S. Dobihal, "Hospice: Enabling a patient to die at home," *Am J Nurs* 80, (1980):1448–51.
34. R. Donley and M.J. Flaherty, The entry level into practice: The baccalaureate degree, *Imprint* 33, (1986):45–46.
35. American Nurses' Association, Division of Governmental Affairs, *1986–87 Health Legislation Fact Sheets* (Kansas City, Mo.: American Nurses' Association, 1986).
36. Institute of Medicine, "A Strategy for Evaluating

Health Services," *Contrasts in Health Status, No. 2* (Washington, D.C.: Institute of Medicine, 1973).

37. "Proposed Rules," *Federal Register* (May 27, 1982).

38. The U.S. Surgeon General, *Healthy People, The Surgeon General's Report on Health Promotion and Disease Prevention* (Washington, D.C.: U.S. Government Printing Office, 1979).

39. H. Maher, "Blueprint for health for all," *WHO Chron* 31, (1977):491–98.

40. Institute of Medicine, *Nursing and Nursing Education.*

41. R. Hanft, "The impact of changes in Federal policy on academic health centers," *Health Aff,* (1982):67–82.

42. PL 99-177. The Budget and Emergency Deficit Control Act of 1985. (Washington, D.C.: U.S. Government Printing Office, 1985).

43. States take the lead in indigent care, *The Internists* 27, (February 1986):12–13.

44. U.E. Reinhart, Rationing the nation's health care surplus: An American paradox, *The Internist* 27, (February 1986):11–13.

Annotated Bibliography

These references are examples of government documents or policy papers developed by private or public groups.

American Academy of Nursing. 1984. *Nursing Research and Policy Formation: The Case of Prospective Payment.* Kansas City, Mo.: The American Academy of Nursing. This policy document analyzes the effects of prospective payment on nursing practice and quality care.

Bureau of Health Professions. 1982. *Nurse Supply, Distribution and Requirements, Third Report to the Congress. Nurse Training Act of 1975.* Hyattsville, Md.: Bureau of Health Professions, Division of Nursing. This report to Congress, mandated by public law, represents the work of a division and bureau within the Department of Health and Human Services.

Conference Report to Accompany HR 4961, Tax Equity and Fiscal Responsibility Act of 1982. 1982. Washington, D.C.: Superintendent of Documents. This document is the official report of the agreements reached by senators and members of Congress who conferred on the 1982 tax law.

Special Committee on Aging United States Senate. 1982. *The Proposed Fiscal Year 1983 Budget; What it means for Older Americans: An Information Paper.* Washington, D.C.: U.S. Government Printing Office. This report, prepared by a staff of a Senate committee, examines the Federal budget and analyzes its impact on a specialized population: the aged.

Graduate Medical Education National Advisory Committee. 1981. *Report of the Graduate Medical Education National Advisory Committee to the Secretary.* Washington, D.C.: Department of Health and Human Services. The "GMENAC" report illustrates the work of a specially selected committee that studied medical manpower and filed a report to the Secretary of Health and Human Services. This report was released and became the subject of discussion and debate in the public and professional sector.

Gramm–Rudman sets stage for epic budget battle. 1986. *Am J Nurs* 86:461, 464, 483–84. This article reports the Gramm–Rudman bill and provides insight into ensuing changes in nursing and health care.

Institute of Medicine. 1983. *Nursing and Nursing Education: Public Policies and Private Actions.* Washington, D.C.: Institute of Medicine. This is a final report of a congressionally mandated two-year study of nursing.

The National Academy of Science. 1974. *A Policy Statement: HMOs: Toward a Fair Market Test.* Washington, D.C.: The National Academy of Science. Developed by a think tank of interdisciplinary professionals, this report illustrates private sector influence on public policy.

The Prospective Payment Act of 1983 (PL 98–21) 1983. Washington, D.C.: U.S. Government Printing Office. PL 98–21 illustrates a public law. Available from the local offices of congressmen or senators, it can also be obtained from the Superintendent of Documents in Washington, D.C.

Part II

Nursing as a Process

Nursing has progressed through the years from an intuitive, nurturing type of helping to a structured delivery of health care in which the nurse is legally and ethically accountable for nursing care. This evolution took place as nursing moved into the nineteenth and twentieth centuries. As nurses obtained formal nursing education based on facts, they began to contemplate what nursing was, is, and can be. From this came observations on how nursing care is delivered.

The nursing process has been widely recognized as the framework or core central to all nursing actions. It is the model that allows nurses to provide nursing care in an organized and systematic manner. The expert presentation of the nursing process in this section is highlighted by the introduction of the human needs framework and provides a clear illustration of the relationship of theory to nursing practice. This chapter also includes a care plan divided into the steps of the nursing process: assessment, planning, implementation, and evaluation. The comprehensive care plan also includes examples of nursing diagnoses and patient outcome criteria. Nursing diagnosis and health assessment are addressed separately in this section to provide the reader with more detail in these two important areas.

The nursing process guides the delivery of nursing care, but nurses are also guided by legal and ethical concepts as they provide care. Chapter 10 contains information related to the legal system in the United States and how it has an impact on nursing practice. Accountability, in general, is a key concept for professional nurses today. Chapter 11 addresses this concept in terms of standards of care, quality assurance, the professional literature, accreditation and certification, and continuing education. The final chapter in this section presents an overview of ethics and discusses ethical decision making as it relates to nursing and health care.

Chapter 7

The Nursing Process*

Helen Yura
Mary B. Walsh

Chapter Outline

- Objectives
- Glossary
- Introduction
- Theoretical/Conceptual Frameworks
- Theoretical Bases for Practice
  Human Need Theory
  Perception Theory
- Nursing and Components of Nursing
- Processes in Nursing
- The Nursing Process
  Assessing
  Planning
  Implementing
  Evaluating
- Summary
- Study Questions
- References
- Annotated Bibliography

Objectives

At the completion of this chapter the reader will be able to:

▶ Define the nursing process
▶ Differentiate the nursing process from other processes in nursing
▶ Describe the evolution of the nursing process
▶ Identify the importance and value of using a systematic process in nursing
▶ Describe the value of using a logical framework for performing nursing
▶ Draw resources for nursing from multiple theories that provide a base for nursing practice
▶ Define, describe, and practice nursing through the use of the nursing process
  Assessing: including data collection and data analysis about the client and arrival at conclusions about the client's strengths and limitations (nursing diagnoses)
  Planning: including use of client validation, goal setting, and expected outcomes of care
  Implementing: including carrying out the plan according to client values, client needs, client abilities, available personnel and their level of preparation
  Evaluating: including a review of goals to be achieved and the extent to which client or nurses are able to reach desired outcomes

Glossary

Assessing. The act of reviewing a human situation in order to affirm the wellness state and to diagnose potential client problems; to affirm an illness state; to diagnose the client's obvious problems, determine the potential for problems, and identify the wellness of the ill client.

---

*Adapted from H. Yura and M.B. Walsh, *The Nursing Process*, 4th ed., (East Norwalk, Conn.: Appleton-Century-Crofts, 1983).

Evaluating. The appraisal of changes experienced by the client in relation to goal achievement as a result of actions of the nurse.

Goal. The expected behavioral result of human need fulfillment experienced by a client.

Implementing. The initiation and completion of actions necessary to accomplish the defined goal of optimal fulfillment of human needs.

Nursing Diagnosis. The judgment or conclusion reached by the nurse based on assessment data that indicate the potential for or actual human need fulfillment alteration viewed as an excess, an altered pattern in expression, or a deficit, lack, or limitation for the client as person, family, or community.

Nursing Process. An orderly, systematic manner of determining the client's problems, making plans to solve them, initiating the plan or assigning others to implement it, and evaluating the extent to which the plan was effective in resolving the problem identified.

Outcome Criteria. Specific descriptive behavioral expectations stemming from a specified goal with the level of achievement expected and the time interval for measurement of achievement.

Planning. The determination of a plan of action to assist the client toward the goal of optimal wellness based on the highest level of fulfillment of human needs and to resolve potential and obvious nursing diagnoses.

INTRODUCTION

The nursing process is the core and essence of nursing; it is central to all nursing actions; it is applicable in any setting and within any theoretical conceptual reference. It is flexible and adaptable, adjustable to a number of variables, yet sufficiently structured so as to provide a base from which all systematic nursing actions can proceed. . . .There is a basic theme that underlies the process; it is organized, systematic, and deliberate.[1]

The nursing process was not a familiar term in nursing prior to the middle 1960s. As defined, described, and developed by Yura and Walsh, the nursing process was born in 1967 at the Catholic University of America. The Continuing Education Committee of the School of Nursing defined the nursing process components, and eight sessions of evening classes were planned and presented to nurses in the community. Yura and Walsh were the persons responsible for implementing that significant and historic series.[2] The report of these 1967 proceedings, published by the Catholic University of America Press, is considered to be the first edition of the nursing process text. The fifth edition will be published by Appleton & Lange in 1988, to celebrate the 20th anniversary of the birth of the nursing process. What began as a low rumble in 1967 has now grown to a loud roar in terms of the significance, importance, and impact of using an organized, systematic, and deliberate process when nurses care for clients.

Prior to 1967, a select few nurses used the term nursing process. These included: Hildegard Peplau,[3] Lydia Hall,[4] Dorothy Johnson,[5] Ida Orlando,[6] and Ernestine Wiedenbach.[7] All these authors touched on what was to become a gold mine of knowledge for professional nursing. The mine was there for many years, but now it is being refined qualitatively as professional nurses see the advantage of proceeding deliberately and with intention rather than proceeding intuitively. Identification and deliberate use of a process in nursing has enabled the profession to proceed systematically to produce a data base on which research can proceed to improve practice and to duplicate nursing actions that are qualitatively developed. The nursing process is further enhanced through theoretical frameworks that give breadth and depth to knowledge about people and their needs. The future of nursing with the use of the nursing process is boundless.

Further dimensions to consider when addressing the nursing process include criteria for a profession, a code for professional nurses, standards of nursing practice, and a definition of nursing.

Although many people refer to their occupation as a profession, strictly speaking, an occupation should meet certain criteria to be viewed as a profession. Several sources of criteria are available, for example, A. Flexner[8] and E.H. Schein.[9]

Recently, Gail Stuart[10] summarized suggestions of various authors on professionalism in nursing as follows. Nursing as a profession:

- Has a history
- Has a commitment to the profession
- Has a professional organization (American Nurses' Association)
- Continues to progress
- Provides services for those in need
- Is beginning to identify and establish an autonomous practice

To convince others that nursing is a profession, Stuart suggested that:

- The knowledge base should be expanded to establish nursing science as a recognized body of knowledge
- Nursing research should be expanded
- Autonomy and power should be used to convince others that nurses can identify and implement independent functions of nursing

One criterion of a profession is that a code of ethics is essential. The most recent revision of the Code for Nurses stresses self-determination of the client, the role of the nurse as client advocate, and the need for quality assurance and peer review.[11]

Standards of nursing practice are important criteria that are developed by nurses to guide the evaluation of nursing. The use of standards is a means to ensure that quality care is provided.

The struggle to reach universal agreement about a definition of nursing was evident in the nursing literature for many years. Two early nursing leaders who proposed definitions of nursing that apply across all ages were: Sister Olivia Gowan[12] and Virginia Henderson[13] (see Chapter 2). Their words of wisdom are as appropriate today as they were when they were written.

The most recent definition of nursing is that presented by the American Nurses' Association as part of the Social Policy Statement.[14] In 1980, the Congress for Nursing Practice completed a charge given to them by the American Nurses' Association, namely, to define the nature and scope of nursing practice. The charge was assumed by a seven-member task force who used input from distinguished scholars in nursing and

responses from many groups of nurses to contribute to the report. One outcome of this valiant effort was the use of historical data and current trends to define nursing as follows: "Nursing is the diagnosis and treatment of human responses to actual or potential health problems."[14]

Two directions are evolving for the present development of nursing and the ultimate specification of the science of nursing:

- Identification of the theoretical/conceptual frameworks for functioning
- Use of the nursing process for the performance of nursing

THEORETICAL/CONCEPTUAL FRAMEWORKS

It has been suggested in the philosophy of science literature that philosophers have experienced false starts and held numerous debates among themselves while striving to identify their scientific bases in the development of a philosophy of science. It seems important to get on with the work of identifying frameworks for nursing that are consistent with the underlying philosophies about nursing. It has been suggested that in order to do this[15]:

- The identification of frameworks is important
- Definitions and labels are important
- Knowing when one is using proposed theories or using jargon without committing to the idea of the theory is important

During the 1960s and 1970s, a number of nurse authors developed and reported their ideas about nursing, including definitions of nursing, views about the human person with clear references to beliefs about fellow humans, and perceptions about nursing and the nursing process. Nurse writers of the 1960s who made an impact on the development of a theoretical framework for nursing include: Faye Abdellah,[16] Dorothy Johnson,[17] Myra Levine,[18] Ida Orlando,[19] Joyce Travelbee,[20] and Ernestine Wiedenbach.[21]

In the 1970s, further development of scientific bases for nursing was made by Imogene King,[22] Betty Neuman,[23] Dorothea Orem,[24]

Martha Rogers,[25] Sister Callista Roy,[26] and Josephine Paterson and Loretta Zderad.[27]

Another development that has had a continuing effect on nursing is the embryonic identification of a classification system for nursing diagnoses. Writers who have contributed to this effort are Kristine Gebbie and Mary Ann Lavin,[28] Marjorie Gordon[29] and Phyllis Kritek.[30]

Historically, the terminology of **nursing diagnosis** can be found in the nursing literature over the past 30 years; it has been identified as an integral part of the nursing process since nurses began to organize the practice of nursing in the systematic format of the Nursing Process. It was not until 1973, however, that a separate thrust for the identification of nursing diagnosis was initiated.[31] The movement began with a group meeting of interested clinicians, led by Gebbie and Lavin at St. Louis University. Since then the group has grown in numbers and in achievements. There is now an international association known as the North American Nursing Diagnosis Association (NANDA), with offices at St. Louis University School of Nursing in St. Louis, Missouri. At the first meeting of the newly formed NANDA in 1984, quite substantive issues were addressed over a three-day period.[32] Qualitative papers were presented and productive discussions were held. The activities of this pioneering group to date offer hopeful prospects for the future of the nursing diagnosis movement.

In March, 1986, over 600 nurses met at the Seventh Biennial NANDA Conference in St. Louis. The groups considered the many dimensions involved in defining nursing diagnoses, the discussion including such subjects as conceptual frameworks, acceptable classifications and taxonomy, results of clinical testing of suggested diagnoses, and the etiology and defining characteristics of nursing diagnoses. A total of 72 diagnoses were identified as acceptable at this conference.

Scientifically defining the territory of nursing is a valuable endeavor, especially when it is integrated within the nursing process to enable practitioners to use nursing diagnoses as bases for patient care planning. Many writers, nurses, and theorists are continuing their efforts into the 1980s. Others are joining them by building

on their published ideas, applying theories and concepts to practice, and conducting research to prove the validity, value, and potential of the work accomplished during the 1960s and 1970s.

THEORETICAL BASES FOR PRACTICE

Recent advances in technology have been exciting, stimulating, breathtaking, and potentially overwhelming. It is no longer possible to present all there is to know in one class, one course, one program, or in any one person's educational career, no matter how long. To order available knowledge, it is necessary to establish some means of organizing data. Determining theoretical or conceptual frameworks is one way to organize knowledge.

The multifaceted nature of nursing makes client care in a large variety of settings necessary. The recipient of services (the client) is individual and complex, bringing religious, cultural, economic, educational, sociological, psychological, and physiological dimensions to every encounter. The provider of nursing brings that same variety to each client encounter. To reconcile and consider all these dimensions with reasonable attention, some schema is necessary.

A large variety of theories and concepts that enable the pursuit of quality client care is available to the nurse. Use of a theoretical base can facilitate the use of available knowledge and can maximize the quality of care delivered.

Among the various theories that can guide the use of the nursing process are: general systems theory; communication theory; decision theory; problem-solving theory; human need theory; and perception theory.* General systems and theories that flow from it are discussed in other chapters in this text. In this chapter human need and perception theories are discussed.

---

*A more detailed discussion of all theories that underlie the nursing process can be found in H. Yura and M.B. Walsh, *The Nursing Process,* 4th ed. (E. Norwalk, Conn.: Appleton-Century-Crofts, 1983), Chapter 2, Theoretical Frameworks for the Nursing Process.

Human Need Theory

A human need is viewed as an internal tension resulting in an alteration in some part of the person that is expressed in some type of behavior, usually goal directed, and that continues until satisfaction is achieved.[33] A basic or vital human need is one that must be satisfied to sustain life.

Maslow emphasizes the holism of a person, and states that most needs cannot be isolated, localized, or considered as if they were the only events occurring. Any one desire or need is a need of the whole person.[34] Motivation is stressed as a basis for developing fundamental goals or needs. Rarely is behavior expressive of human motivation except in relation to a situation or to other persons.[35] The character of the person is an important variable here, as is the degree of intensity of the situation. For example, in responding to situations of great intensity, such as extreme joy, sorrow, fear, or threat, one displays the most unified or completely integrated behavior. If the situation becomes overwhelming, however, disintegration may occur.[36]

To understand how needs are fulfilled, they should be grouped or classified.

As can be seen from Figure 7–1, fundamental physical needs described by Maslow[37] are strongly similar to those vital human needs identified by Montagu.[38]

Gratification or fulfillment of needs and deprivation or lack of need fulfillment are important concepts. When vital human needs are satisfied, the next-higher-level needs emerge and seek gratification or fulfillment. In order to understand and relate to human behavior, it is important to understand the level of need on which a person is functioning at a particular time. Gratification has to do with the power or strength of any one of the human needs. Each level of the hierarchy denotes a group of needs that is less strong or less powerful than the preceding level. For example, safety and security needs are stronger than are needs for love and belonging; unless a person feels safe he or she will be unable to exhibit love or to demonstrate a healthy state of belonging to another human or group of humans. In like manner, physical needs, those on the lowest level of the hierarchy, are the most powerful, or the strongest. Unless needs for food and sleep are met, people cannot consider the need for self-esteem. Safety sometimes is completely ignored in an extreme need for food. Therefore, one can conclude that the higher the level of need, the less imperative it is for survival and the longer gratification can be postponed. This need could disappear perma-

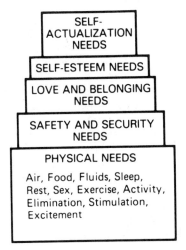

5-Level
Maslow's Hierarchy
of needs

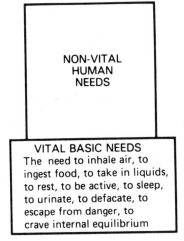

Montagu's 2-Level
Structure
of needs

Figure 7–1. Theoretical views of human needs.

nently, but the pursuit and gratification of higher level needs leads to a healthier person.[39]

Another perspective on human need theory suggests that all humans have a single need in common: a force within each human by which he or she continually seeks to become more adequate in coping with life.[40] For this singular need to be met, there must be a healthy body, because it is the body that is responsible for perceiving the self.[41] According to this theory, the goal is to maintain the perceived self as an independent and distinct self, capable of dealing with present and future events of life. Motivation is inherent in each individual and is an internal force that provides direction, drive, and organization for the functioning of each person. The needs as specified by Montagu and Maslow are perceived as the goals, the achievement of which satisfy the need of the person for adequacy. Development of a person's perceptions contributes to the development of awareness. The need for adequacy is met or there is an effort to meet the need for adequacy based on a person's perception of any one event at any one time. The focus for action becomes the means to achieve its fulfillment.[42]

Perception Theory

What is perceived is determined by each person's unique perceptual field; this field includes more than the direct experience of the senses.[43] A person perceives only what previous experience has made it possible to perceive.[44] Experience suggests that one sees what one wants to see; what one anticipates as a result of experience is so firmly established in one's thinking that one may be "blinded" to the real world.[45]

Limitations in the functioning of the sense organs, the brain, and the nervous system create limitations in perception.[46] For example, severely brain damaged persons try to maintain organization by avoiding situations that would strain their impaired capacities.[47] In certain situations, however, some positive outcomes may be experienced, such as deaf persons development of a high degree of proficiency in the ability to see.

The process of perception is integrated with those of identification, classification, and coding. These processes are dependent on learning, memory, attention, reasoning, and language.

The ability to perceive form, position, and movement of objects in relation to the position and movement of the body is very important in understanding adjustment to normal surroundings.[48] Profound changes in perception can occur when one is exposed to unvarying situations or stimulation over a long period of time.

Inferences that a person makes about the nature of objects and events involve knowledge and expereinces. Information seldom is derived simply from an instantaneous perception that is immediately forgotten. Impressions last for a while, and this provides some continuity in perceptions of the environment and enables persons to remember past experiences.[49]

Accurate perception of the environment is essential to preserve life, however, and individual differences are apparent. Persons may perceive and react to stimulation without being fully aware of their percepts. Motivation and emotion have an affect on arousing, directing, facilitating, or inhibiting the perception of situations and events, but differences in knowledge and acquired skill, of intelligence and ability are of greater importance than motivational influences. For example, witnesses to an accident may give as many and varied reports of the same situation as there are individual witnesses.

The ability to modify immediate perception through reasoning is developed as a person matures; however, experience and learning may have a marked effect on the stage at which it begins to develop.

Persons as perceivers are not always aware of the many aspects of complex situations in the natural environment. Perceptions of form in everyday life may not involve accurate identification of minute detail, although there is the capacity to do this. Generally, there is an overabundance of sensory information, and the observer must select the relevant data to describe objects or events and discard the irrelevant. The observer makes inferences in situations like this.[50] Although observers are prone to make inferences from fragments of data, these inferences are influenced by what one expects to perceive; the expectation is that certain stimuli will appear, and perhaps the observer will identify certain stimuli that would have been missed in other situations.[51]

In addition to peceiving form, objects, languages, space, and movement, a dimension of perception involves people, their emotions, and their actions. People perceive other people in a unique manner. Their faces and behavior are integrated into a special scheme by observers. Perceivers are more aware of the intentions, emotions, and personality characteristics of persons than they are aware of the details of physical characteristics.

Perception plays a crucial role in life; it is a major means by which a person gains information about himself, his needs, and the world.

NURSING AND COMPONENTS OF NURSING

By definition, *nursing* is the diagnosis and treatment of human responses to actual or potential health problems; it is an interpersonal situation in which nurses observe, support, communicate, minister, and teach. Nurses contribute to the maintenance of optimum health and provide care during illness until the client is able to assume responsibility for the fulfillment of his own needs, or when necessary, provides compassionate care and support for the dying person and his or her family.

To be responsible for client care and to be responsive to the indications of client need, the nurse uses interpersonal, intellectual, and technical skills.

The use of *interpersonal skills* requires initial and continuing contacts with clients, their families, and significant others, as well as an understanding approach and astute insight into each individual who is important or significant in the client situation.

Establishing a situation where clients can trust nurses and the health-care team suggests a high degree of interpersonal skill. Especially important is the ability to communicate with clients on their level and about topics in which they are interested. Respect and concern for the perceptions of clients are critical to establishing and maintaining relationships that will permit clients to rely on nurses' skills with the degree of comfort necessary for respite and healing.

The nursing process is an empty structure unless the components of the process are fleshed out with data about the client. A high degree of

intellectual skill development is necessary to recognize the significance of the observations that are made about clients and their situations. Creative approaches to the analysis of the observations are very important, and a rich background of knowledge is critical to the performance of nursing care. Continued development of intellectual skills is inherent in the performance of quality care wherever there is a need for nursing.

Nurses have always been recognized for their *technical skills*. In fact, for many years, the perfection of these skills was the only raison d'etre for nurses. Increased use of technology has made it essential that nurses be able to perform technically; they might need to use sophisticated machinery. Technical skills are important to making the client comfortable. Important in their use, however, is the fact that this is only *one* of the skills for the nurse to perfect.

The challenge for the nurse is to maintain a blend of interpersonal, intellectual, and technical skills—to neglect none of them—to analyze the needs of the client accurately so that priorities can be set and those skills that can best meet the requirements of each situation can be selected. This aspect of nursing continues to be a major feat and presents a formidable challenge to every conscientious nurse.

PROCESSES IN NURSING

Nurses rely on interpersonal, intellectual, and technical skills to carry out client care. As professionals, they are the leaders of those responsible for providing nursing care for clients and are accountable to the client for providing the care needed and for maintaining a level of skill development that will enable performance of client care in a superlative manner. To fulfill the responsibilities incumbent on a leader, the nurse carries out a *leadership process* that involves decision making, relating, influencing, and facilitating. The ultimate goal of leadership is to achieve the goals of the group.

One means by which client care can be accommodated is through the *research process*. By systematically examining the various dimensions of nursing care, nurses can gather information about techniques, skills, levels of performance, rationale for care, intellectual decisions, and other phenomena associated with the ministration of nursing measures. Through such activities, nurses are involved in a process of collecting data, analyzing the data that have been gathered, and arriving at conclusions about the data. Ultimately, nurses identify new knowledge about the situation being examined using the research process. Having proceeded through this systematic activity, nurses have a sound basis on which to make decisions and to determine strategies.

The third process that is central to the activity of nursing is the **nursing process,** about which this chapter is written. This process is not unlike the research process in that it is orderly and systematic. It involves assessment (to identify the client's abilities and limitations), planning (to solve identified problems), initiating the plan or assigning others to implement it, and evaluating the extent to which the plan was effective in resolving the identified problem.

THE NURSING PROCESS

A philosophical base provides the foundation for nursing. Each nurse enters a client situation with a set of beliefs and values that directs her activities throughout the client–nurse encounter. Each client holds a set of values and beliefs that the nurse seeks to understand and with which he or she strives to maintain consistency. In no instance can effective care be planned or carried out unless it is consistent with the client's intentions and wishes. If the client is a family or a community instead of an individual, the determination of values and philosophical principles is equally important and more challenging to define.

Within the philosophical direction of care, determination of a theoretical/conceptual framework is a further component that is an integral part of the nursing process. Just as a building is made of walls that divide the total structure into rooms, so too, the theoretical-conceptual framework for nursing suggests a composite of rooms (concepts) within one structure (theory) where nursing will be performed. Values, beliefs, and philosophies influence the manner in which nursing will be performed and the theorectical-conceptual framework designates the manner by which nursing will be carried out. For example, if the beliefs of Dorothea Orem are followed, the self-care abilities of the client will be recognized and will act as guides for carrying out the nursing process; if Sister Callista Roy's ideas are followed there will be more attention to the client's need for adaptation.

Through the orderly, systematic orientation of the nursing process, the nurse puts herself or himself in close proximity with the client. A "needs orientation" provides the structure and direction needed to plan and carry out the required care. If the nurse can identify client "cues," meticulous analysis of the client data, conscientious **planning, implementing,** and **evaluating** will ensure the nurse's accountability for the optimum level of client care. The cyclical process can be repeated as often as necessary, depending on the complexity of the client's needs and the extent to which it is necessary to refine the nursing diagnoses (Fig. 7–2). Careful and accurate projection of the **goals** to be reached (**outcome criteria**) will help the nurse and the client decide when and how well the needs of the client have been met. These client outcomes should be stated clearly so that the client behaviors are known to the client prior to the nurse–client interaction and in terms that are measurable and observable.

Assessing
Assessing is the act of reviewing a human situation based on a data base. This is done to affirm the wellness state and to diagnose poten-

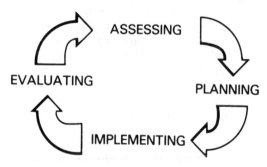

Figure 7–2. The nursing process is cyclical in nature.

tial client problems or to affirm an illness state, diagnosing the client's obvious problems, determining the potential for problems, and identifying the wellness aspects of the ill client. The frameworks provide the structure within which the nurse applies the nursing process and so accomplishes the purpose of nursing, which is the fulfillment of the needs of the identified client.

There are many needs that could be the focus for nurses and clients (Table 7–1). These needs provide the framework for all data gathering, nursing diagnoses, goal designation, specification of nursing strategies, and evaluation of goal achievement. The participation of the nurse in the nursing process, within this framework, requires a high level of intellectual, interpersonal, and technical skills.

TABLE 7–1. SELECTED CLIENT NEEDS

Air
Sleep
Nutrition
Territoriality
To love and be loved
Tenderness
Activity
Structure, law and limits
Confidence
Sexual integrity
Spiritual experience
Protection from excessive fear, anxiety, and stress
Interchange of gases
Adaptation, to manage stress
Safety
Fluids
Elimination
Rest and leisure
Humor
Sensory integrity
Autonomy, choice
Conceptualization, rationality problem solving
Acceptance of self and others
Challenge
Effective perception of reality
Wholesome body image
For self-fulfillment, to be, to become
Value system
Skin integrity
Belonging
Freedom from pain
Personal recognition, esteem, respect
Self-control, self-determination, responsibility
Appreciation, attention
Beauty and esthetic experiences

The assessment phase of the nursing process incorporates all the data-gathering efforts and activities of the nurse, including:

- Taking the nursing history
- Performing the health assessment
- Using data-gathering tools, for example: thermometer, stethoscope, sphygmomanometer, otoscope, cardiac monitor, and tape measure
- Using the techniques of percussion, auscultation, and palpation
- Using all five senses

These activities provide the information needed to make nursing judgments and diagnoses. The purpose of the assessment phase is to identify and obtain data about the client's needs that enable the nurse and the client or his or her family to find potential and obvious problems relating to wellness and illness.

In assessing the level of fulfillment of the needs of the client, nurses consider the influence and interrelationship of factors such as age, sex, education, growth and development, and socioeconomic, cultural, and religious elements.

Nurses assess the educational level of their clients, considering formal and informal education. This includes the use of specialized language related to education or job and special interpretation of terms and phrases used. Nurses assess the socioeconomic status of the client, as well as the client's perception of the status and its implication, and the impact of work on the client's perception of her- or himself. They assess the level of fulfillment or alteration in fulfillment of needs for the client.

More specific data are obtained about the client when the nurse performs a health examination that incorporates physical and psychosocial aspects. A systematic format should be developed and followed by the nurse to assure that the assessment is complete and that no body areas are omitted or forgotten. Additional questions formed from the needs assessment, taken during the nursing history, can be used to obtain more specific data while the physical and psychosocial examinations are in progress. Information and specific inferences about the client's potential and obvious problems related to human need fulfillment are considered.

Data about the client and the client's health status may be gleaned from family members, significant others, neighbors, and teachers, to mention a few. Data about the client and his or her family may be graphed on a genogram, which is a particularly useful tool that provides nurses with a quick visual reference point for the relationship of the client to family members in one or more generations. Such data round out the data provided by the client. Data about living and work environments and about variables that influence the present as well as future health status of the client add to the accuracy of nursing diagnoses and provide information about goal expectations and level of goal achievement.

The time used for data gathering during the assessment phase of the nursing process is time well spent. Not only are data available for nursing diagnoses, but the assessment phase forms the framework for all phases, including goal specification and determination of goal achievement. In other words, the present and immediate health situation for the client is only the first phase of goal-directed actions needed to achieve positive health results. Immediate, intermediate, and long-range expectations are specified. These expectations often extend far beyond the immediate status of the client until he or she is home or back to work. Thus, for hospitalized clients, data gleaned during the assessment phase and subsequent decisions about the data have direct bearing on discharge from the health-care agency and the health follow-up expected after discharge.

It is during the assessment phase that the client begins to participate in the nursing process to ensure the maintenance of the integrity of need fulfillment where there is an alteration. The nursing process offsets the alteration in an expedient, effective, and economic manner. The client participates in all phases of the nursing process as do the family and significant others. If circumstances temporarily limit the client's involvement in his or her own care planning, every effort should be made to involve the family as soon as possible.

During the assessment phase, too, the helping relationship is established between the nurse and the client, beginning with the first nurse–client interaction that determines the client's health status. The initial dialogue with the client should be the beginning of a purposeful inter-

action through all phases of the nursing process. In addition, this beginning interaction initiates the nurse's commitment to the client, a commitment that enhances the holistic view and care of the client.

While the data are being collected, the nurse validates inferences to ensure accuracy in interpretation. When the nurse infers the existence of a problem or assumes a condition or situation from known facts or evidence, she or he confirms or validates the problem, condition, or situation with the client. The client has the opportunity to corroborate or discount the inferences made by the nurse.

The nurse sorts, organizes, categorizes, synthesizes, groups, compares, and analyzes the data obtained about the client. Then the nurse makes judgments ranging from verifying the absence of a problem to verifying a complicated one that the client or family is successfully handling (e.g., from one that requires mechanical or pharmacological aids or the services of other health-team members, to the designation of potential and obvious problems making acute or long-term demands and requiring a multitude of health- and nursing-care services).

The assessment phase concludes with the designation of potential or obvious **nursing diagnoses**. The designation of nursing diagnoses draws heavily on the nurse's intellectual and interpersonal skills and sets the framework for all activities in the remaining process, concluding with evaluation.

Nursing diagnoses can be proposed for each of the needs specified earlier. They can be stated as needs being met excessively, disturbances in the pattern of need fulfillment, or needs being met partially, limitedly, or being totally unmet. The nursing diagnoses can be further specified as acute, chronic, or intermittent, for example, and be qualified with the reason for the alteration in need fulfillment (Table 7–2).

When data to support the nursing diagnosis are evident, the potential or obvious nursing diagnosis is specified and the reason for or cause of the alteration is stated. For example, the alteration may be related to or caused by: personal and situational occurrences; environmental affronts; medical, pharmacological, and nursing therapies (commissions and omissions);

TABLE 7–2. PROPOSED NURSING DIAGNOSES BASED ON NEEDS ASSESSMENT

Human Need	Proposed Nursing Diagnoses
Acceptance of self and others, by others	Overacceptance of self and others, by others Disturbance in pattern of expression of need for acceptance Rejection of self and others, by others
Activity	Excessive activity Disturbance in patterns of expression or fulfillment of the need Insufficient activity
Adaptation, to manage stress	Excessive adaptation Disturbance in pattern of expression or fulfillment of the need to adapt Insufficient adaptation
Air	Excessive aeration Disturbance in pattern of expression or fulfillment of the need Insufficient aeration
Appreciation, attention	Excessive appreciation and attention Disturbance in pattern of expression or fulfillment of the need Lack of appreciation, attention
Autonomy, choice	Excessive autonomy, choice Disturbance in pattern of expression or fulfillment of the need Lack of autonomy, choice
Beauty and esthetic experiences	Preoccupation with beauty and esthetic experiences Disturbance in pattern of expression or fulfillment of the need Lack of beauty and esthetic experiences
Belonging	Excessive belonging Disturbance in pattern of expression or fulfillment of the need Lack of belonging
Challenge	Excessive challenge Disturbance in pattern of expression or fulfillment of the need Lack of challenge
Conceptualization, rationality, problem solving	Preoccupation with conceptualization, rationality, and problem solving Disturbance in pattern of expression or fulfillment of the need Inability to conceptualize, rationalize, and solve problems
Confidence	Overconfidence Disturbance in pattern of expression or fulfillment of the need Lack of confidence

(continued)

TABLE 7–2. (Continued)

Human Need	Proposed Nursing Diagnoses
Elimination (end products of metabolism, toxins, poisons, chemicals, drugs)	Excessive elimination Disturbance in pattern of expression or fulfillment of the need Lack of or diminished elimination
Fluids (intake)	Excessive hydration and electrolytes Disturbance in pattern of expression or fulfillment of the need Depletion of fluids and electrolytes
Freedom from pain	Excessive freedom from pain, lack of appropriate pain signals Disturbance in pattern of expression or fulfillment of the need Inability to experience pain relief
Humor	Excessive or continuous use of humor, hilarity Disturbance in pattern of expression or fulfillment of the need Inability to experience humor
Nutrition (intake)	Excessive nutritional intake Disturbance in pattern of expression or fulfillment of the need Insufficient or lack of nutritional intake
Effective perception of reality	Hypersensitive perception of reality Disturbance in pattern of expression or fulfillment of the need Ineffective, inaccurate perception of reality
Personal recognition, esteem, respect	Over-recognition, respect, excessive esteem Disturbance in pattern of expression or fulfillment of the need Lack of recognition, esteem, respect
Protection from excessive fear	Excessive fear Disturbance in pattern of expression or fulfillment of the need Lack of expression of fear, lack of protection
Rest and leisure	Excessive rest, irresponsible use of leisure Disturbance in pattern of expression or fulfillment of the need Restlessness, lack of rest, or leisure
Safety	Excessive preoccupation with thwarting safety Disturbance in pattern of expression or fulfillment of the need Diminished safety or lack of it
Self-control, self-determination, responsibility	Excessive control, determination, responsibility Disturbance in pattern of expression or fulfillment of the need Diminished or lack of self-control, self-determination, responsibility
Self-fulfillment, to be, become	Independence, preoccupation with becoming Disturbance in pattern of expression or fulfillment of the need

TABLE 7–2. (Continued)

Human Need	Proposed Nursing Diagnoses
Self-fulfillment (cont.)	Lack of fulfillment of self, or feeling of becoming, prolonged dependence
Sensory integrity	Sensory overload Disturbance in pattern of expression or fulfillment of the need Sensory deprivation
Sexual integrity	Preoccupation with sexual dimension Disturbance in pattern of expression or fulfillment of the need Lack of attention to sexual integrity
Skin integrity	Preoccupation with maintenance of skin integrity Disturbance in pattern of expression or fulfillment of the need Diminished or lack of skin integrity
Sleep	Excessive sleep Disturbance in pattern of expression or fulfillment of the need Insufficient or lack of sleep
Spiritual integrity	Preoccupation with or excessive spiritual integrity Disturbance in pattern of expression or fulfillment of the need Ineffective, diminished or lack of spiritual integrity
Structure, law, and limits	Excessive structure, law, and limits Disturbance in pattern of expression or fulfillment of the need Diminished or lack of structure, law, limits
Tenderness	Excessive smothering tenderness Disturbance in pattern of expression or fulfillment of the need Diminished or lack of tenderness
Territoriality	Excessive territorial requirement Disturbance in pattern of expression or fulfillment of the need Diminished or lack of territorial space
To love and be loved	Excessive expression of love and requirement for love and to be loved Disturbance in pattern of expression or fulfillment of the need Diminished or lack of ability to love and be loved
Wholesome body image	Excessive valuation of overall image or of selected body parts Disturbance in pattern of expression or fulfillment of the need Diminished or poor body image
Value system	Excessive or rigid application of value system Disturbance in pattern of expression or fulfillment of the need Diminished or lack of value system

specific pathological states; specific psychopathological states; physiological miscalculations or nonacceptance; congenital alterations (reparable, irreparable); philosophical, ethical, and religious impositions; social and economic affronts; educational affronts; growth and developmental affronts, and others. The nurse has logically specified the client's potential and obvious problems based on data. This information is strategic to planning, particularly for goal specification and goal expectation and for prescribing nursing strategies to prevent or offset disturbances in need fulfillment. In addition, the nurse will support the fulfillment of those human needs currently met fully or reasonably well.

The assessment phase of the nursing process assures that the nurse and client focus on those needs that are reasonably well met by client or family in addition to those in which there is evidence of disturbance in need fulfillment. Using a framework for nursing provides the client with the best assurance that all dimensions for the person (well and ill) will be recognized. Inherent in this protection is evidence that disease will be prevented and wellness promoted by diagnosing potential problems of the client.

When assessment data verify the human needs that are met, those having a potential to be unmet, or those unmet, and the client supports the judgments made, the planning phase of the nursing process begins. Plans are made to maintain the well state if needs of the client are considered to be met, and potential nursing diagnoses are specified or plans are made to offset an illness state if a few or many needs of the client are considered to be unmet. For the ill client, the needs that are reasonably met and those with a potential to be unmet are also the focus for planning.

Planning

Planning is the phase of the nursing process where nursing action plans are determined, to assist the client toward the goal of optional wellness. The purposes of this phase are to:

- Signify the priority of the client's potential and obvious problems
- Specify the behavioral outcomes or goals for the client and the expected time of achievement of these outcomes

- Differeniate client problems and those that could be resolved by nursing intervention from those that could be referred to other members of the health team
- Designate the specific actions or nursing strategies, their frequency, and results
- Write the client's potential and obvious nursing diagnoses, nursing actions and their frequency, and the expected outcomes on the nursing care plan

The planning phase terminates with completion of the nursing care plan, which is the blueprint that provides direction for implementing the plan and provides the framework for evaluation.

In terms of priority setting, the more life-threatening the client problem, the higher the priority. Nurses use their own judgment but also consider the designations of priorities as viewed by the client. Priorities can be conveniently classified as high, medium, and low. As high-priority problems are resolved, fully or in part, a reordering may be needed. Problems in the medium- and low-priority categories may be considered a high priority at some time. For instance, if constipation is a problem it may receive a place quite high on the priority list if it persists. Each client problem should be so ordered that the integrity of the client can be maintained. If there are differences in the designation of priority among the nurse, the client, and other members of the nursing or health team, collection of additional data usually brings about resolution of the differences. The nursing focus is on preserving the well aspects of the sick person while diminishing ill aspects of the person.

If no obvious problems exist or a problem exists potentially, the nurse verifies the client's state of wellness and plans with the client for periodic verification of the state. Information and support services may be provided for the client's use. If, in the interim, symptoms appear or the client feels he or she has a problem, the client is instructed to return to see the nurse immediately. In using the nursing process with the well client, the nurse and client participate in the assessing and planning phases, and the client assumes responsibility in the implementing and evaluating phases.

The expected behavioral results or goals for

the client are specified for each obvious or potential nursing diagnosis. This holds true for a family or community nursing diagnosis, as well as for the individual. For example, if the client's nursing diagnosis is overnutrition caused by excessive eating, the expected behavioral result of intervention would be attainment of a well-balanced nutritional level in accordance with the age, height, target weight, and life-style of the client. The level of human need fulfillment that can be achieved by the client should be realistic considering the reason for the disturbance. A date when the behavioral result is expected should be indicated.

Once determination is made of the time when goal achievement is expected and the specific outcome criteria are defined, the nurse designates possible interventions for each nursing diagnosis. Solutions offered by the client should be considered and incorporated. The possible success of each solution is estimated considering the human variables of age, sex, sociocultural background, level of growth and development, for example, and drawing on scientific principles and sound research results. The best solutions are selected and a judgment is made as to the persons—the nurse, the client, the family, the nursing or team members—who will carry out the action.

The nursing diagnosis and supporting data, the goal descriptions and expectations, the date and time for expected goal achievement, as well as the time interval for measurement of the level of achievement of need fulfillment, and the specific prescribed nursing strategies with frequencies complete the development of the nursing care plan and are the blueprint for action. The format for the nursing care plan should flow from the goals of the nursing care plan and draws heavily on the intellectual skills of the nurse. A sample client situation with a developed nursing care plan follows. Note that the format uses the human need theory framework.

Client Situation: Mrs. Martha Bender

Mrs. Martha Bender, aged 81, has been admitted to the nursing unit of a health-care agency with severe headaches. She is a known hypertensive and has been hospitalized four times in the past two years for control of hypertension. She lives alone and manages a two-story, three-bedroom house, which has been the family home for generations. Mrs. Bender's husband died following a stroke four years ago, and her three children are married with families of their own. Each lives within ten miles of the mother's home. Each of the children has offered Mrs. Bender a home with them, but she refused, stating that she needed to have her own household; she had to be independent and be "her own boss." Close contact has been maintained between Mrs. Bender and her children. In fact, her children planned among themselves the personal and phone contact with their mother as well as the availability of one of the children at all times. Mrs. Bender also stated that if she became unable to care for herself, she would go to a nursing home. Years ago, she and her husband made investigations and tours of nursing homes in the area in case a nursing home experience should be necessary. One nursing home was selected on a contingency basis.

The assessment data obtained by the nurse verified a severe headache mainly in the occipital area that diminishes when Mrs. Bender's head is elevated. The sensation of pain is lessened by the use of cold compresses to the temporal area. This intervention was made by Mrs. Bender prior to admission and has been continued on admission at her request.

She complains of loss of appetite accompanied by a distaste for food. She is unsteady on her feet and stated that she bumped into the bathroom door, causing an area of ecchymosis with an abrasion on her left shoulder and leg. Mrs. Bender appears tired and stated she could barely get around and take care of herself since her headache started two days ago. Her blood pressure was 210/100 on admission; pulse 80, respiration 15. She is 5'1" and weighs 120 pounds. The physician prescribed Lasix (furosemide) 40 mg daily, PO; Inderal (propranolol) 20 mg BID, PO to reduce her blood pressure; a low-salt diet; activity as tolerated; Tylenol (acetaminophen) 650 mg for headache PO q 3 to 4 hours prn, and continuation of cold compresses to head as desired.

Additional data obtained by the nurse through the health assessment of Mrs. Bender includes difficulty focusing her eyes and sensitivity to light. She wears eyeglasses for reading. She has some difficulty hearing, especially noted on the left side. She yawned, looked sleepy, and complained that she slept little for the past two nights. She generally sleeps six hours a night and gets to bed after an 11 P.M. television news report and awakes about 5:30 A.M. She spends the first half hour of bedtime praying and reading the Bible. She generally has been taking a one-hour nap after lunch and bathes in the evening.

Upon completion of the nursing history and health assessment, needs that were reasonably well met were verified and those needs found to be partially or fully unmet or with the potential to be unmet were identified. Nursing diagnoses (potentially, partially, and fully unmet human needs) were determined and shared with Mrs. Bender for validation and accuracy. A nursing care plan with goal determination and achievement was prescribed. The nursing care plan developed for and with Mrs. Bender emerged (Table 7–3).*

Implementing

Implementing is the initiation and completion of actions necessary to accomplish the defined goal of optimal fulfillment of client needs. The implementation phase is directed by the nursing care plan. The persons to be involved in the implementation have been identified on the care plan. Participation in this phase requires nurses to have a high level of intellectual, interpersonal, and technical skill. Decision-making, observation, and communication skills are significant enhancements. These skills are used with the client, nursing-team members, and health-team members.

During this phase, the viability of the nursing care plan is tested. The nurse continues to collect data about the client, the condition, problems, reactions, and feelings. Additional information is gleaned from other health-care personnel, family, neighbors, teachers, and medical or health records. The success of failure of the nursing care plan depends on the nurse's ability to judge the value of new data and his or her creative ability to make adaptations to account

for the uniqueness of the client. For example, the nursing care plan for Mrs. Martha Bender has considerable data along with goal expectations and nursing strategies. New data will emerge as nursing strategies are used and Mrs. Bender responds physically, emotionally, psychologically, and socially to these actions as she proceeds toward the achievement of the goals.

It is strategic that the nurse distinguish and perform the independent nursing functions inherent in the planned actions and those that are interdependent, contributing to the fulfillment of the medical care plan designed by others in the health-care team. The amount of time spent with the client may be short or long but should be goal directed and purposeful.

The nurse may use a specific strategy or action to meet many needs simultaneously. For example, the nurse may plan a caring activity such as a bath, to meet the needs for skin integrity, belonging, and elimination. When the nurse performs a technical action, decision-making skills are used continually to judge when modification is needed in procedural method, in timing of technical action, and in obtaining consultation and assistance from others to ensure safe, effective action.

In each contact with the client, the nurse focuses on the goal of the interaction and continually expands her or his perceptive ability, gathering data about the client that would indicate the correctness of the planned action. Data are sought that indicate the correctness of the planned strategies or that indicate other problems caused by unmet or poorly met human needs. If the nurse is working with other nursing- or health-team members, efforts should be exerted to maintain a client-centered focus. The client should benefit from the actions rather than be overwhelmed.

The implementation phase concludes with the completion and recording of the planned actions. This includes the results of the actions plus the reactions of the client. All data that give direct evidence of goal achievement should be recorded. This evidence designates the status of problem solving and provides information for the direction of continued problem solving. For example, behavioral data about Mrs. Bender should be recorded in relation to each obvious and potential nursing diagnosis and in relation

---

*The authors are grateful to Patricia Frensky Orfini for reviewing this client situation and nursing care plan. Her thoughtful, useful suggestions have been incorporated and have strengthened the presentation.

TABLE 7–3. NURSING CARE PLAN—MRS. MARTHA BENDER—OCTOBER 1

Client Need	Nursing Diagnosis	Goals with Outcome Criteria	Nursing Strategies with Frequencies

Freedom from pain	Experience of pain related to:
	
	Pathological affront of hypertension
	Injury
	Ecchymosis
	Abrasion
		Relief of pain as evidenced by:
		
		Control of pain within 24 hr
		Statements regarding absence of pain 3–4 hr during first 24 hr
		Verbalizing the absence of pain after 48 hr
			1. Assessment for Mrs. Bender: (to be completed in 18 hr)
			  a. Location of headaches
			  b. Circumstances or events that impact upon headache—either diminish or increase it
			  c. Extent of pain relief with acetaminophen; amount of time needed; interval of recurrence
			  d. Character of pain
			  e. Sensation and symptoms accompanying pain
			  f. Areas for pain, numbness, tingling, and discomfort other than head, i.e., extremities, back, abdomen
			  g. Associated symptoms, i.e., weakness, paralysis, etc.
			2. Offer and administer acetaminophen for pain
			  Check level of pain relief
			  Plot the onset of and relief of headaches in conjunction with blood pressure recording, Tylenol (acetaminophen) administration, diuretic action, and look for relationships
			  Do not delay acetaminophen when pain recurs; instruct Mrs. Bender to report onset of headache immediately
			  Look for precipitating events
			  Report failure to obtain pain relief to physician
			  Observe for nausea, vomiting, skin rash
			3. Continue the cold compresses to the occipital area while headache persists
			  a. Facilitate Mrs. Bender's participation by:
			    providing cold compress setup within reach
			    maintaining cold temperature of water-ice solution
			    providing adequate shoulder covering to prevent chills
			    arranging for waterproofing of pillows and head covering
			    supplying additional washcloths to wipe drippings
			  b. Check skin for evidence of irritation, breakdown q 2 hr
			  c. Massage neck and shoulders to promote relaxation and pain relief
			4. Position Mrs. Bender so that her head is elevated at all times to prevent increased intracranial pressure
			  Asses what degree of elevation seems most comfortable and record here

(continued)

TABLE 7–3. (Continued)

Client Need	Nursing Diagnosis	Goals with Outcome Criteria	Nursing Strategies with Frequencies

Freedom from pain (cont.)			5. Administer furosemide as prescribed by physician at 8 A.M.
			  a. Check blood pressure every 2 hr
			  b. Note any headache relief with lowering of blood pressure
			  c. Look for manifestations of drug allergy to furosemide, i.e., skin rash, hives, itching, nausea, vomiting, diarrhea, dizziness, blurred vision
			    If found, discontinue drug administration and notify physician
			  d. Look for side effects of furosemide
			    Orthostatic hypotension
			    Check for decreased Na, decreased K, muscle weakness and cramping, confusion, tingling in extremities
			    Check for sugar in urine
			    Check for confusion, tingling
			6. Administer Inderal (propranolol) 20 mg before breakfast 7:30 A.M. and before dinner 4:45 P.M.
			  Take apical pulse before giving drug
			  Report change in pulse rate rhythm, blood pressure recordings; report pattern to physician
			  Check intake:output ratio; record
			  Check for adverse drug reaction: dry mouth and eyes, nausea, vomiting, confusion, hair loss, skin changes, profound bradycardia, palpitation
			7. Teach Mrs. Bender relaxation exercises, particularly to face, scalp, neck, shoulders
			  15 min p.c. and bedtime (8:30 A.M., 12:30, 5:30, and 10:30 P.M.)
			8. Adjust environment
			  Quiet, pleasant surroundings
			  Ask Mrs. Bender about number of visitors and length of stay she desires
			  Adjust lighting
			  Minimize frightening noises
			9. Gently comb her hair
			  Avoid hairstyles that put traction on scalp
			  Avoid tight head covering or bands
			10. Suggest comfortable, loose-fitting nightgown, robe, and slippers
			11. Observe for signs of TIAs
			  Weakness, numbness
			  Temporary dizziness and unsteadiness
			  Temporary loss of speech; difficulty understanding speech
			  Diplopia
			  Change in personality or emotional state
			  Sudden loss of vision or temporary dimness

TABLE 7-3. (Continued)

Client Need	Nursing Diagnosis	Goals with Outcome Criteria	Nursing Strategies with Frequencies
			12. Solicit assistance of family members in observing for signs and symptoms noted in #11
Fluids (Intake)	Potential loss of fluid volume and Na & K related to: Pharmacological action of furosemide (Lasix) Fluid loss Na loss K loss	Maintenance of adequate fluid volume in three days as evidenced by: Serum K 3.5–5.0 mEq/L Serum Na 132–142 mEq/L Skin, tongue, oral mucosa moist, intact, smooth 5 lb weight loss with stabilized weight after 48 hours	1. Assess fluid intake and output for Mrs. Bender every shift Record quantity of fluids Record type of fluids Encourage citrus juices, milk, apricot nectar, tomato juice, coffee to maintain adequate K Elicit the assistance of Mrs. Bender in recording intake Check color, concentration of urine 2. Observe for signs of hyperkalemia daily Decreased pulse Orthostatic hypotension Muscle weakness and cramping Confusion Tingling sensation in extremities 3. Observe for signs of hypokalemia Weakness Nausea, vomiting Abdominal distention Rapid, irregular pulse Lethargy Confusion 4. Check the status of skin, tongue and oral mucosa for texture, level of dryness or moisture, integrity of tissue. Check for thirst every shift. 5. Check weight daily before breakfast—7 A.M. 6. Assess electrolyte reports daily
Sensory integrity	Diminished sensory integrity related to: Pathological affront of hypertension Aged state Change in sensory input	Enhanced sensory integrity as evidenced by: Improved ability to communicate with staff, using nonverbal techniques, etc. by 48 hr Improved vision and experience of visual comfort within 48 hr Verbalization or improved skin sensation within one week Expression of improved taste within 3 days	1. Complete the assessment of Mrs. Bender within 24 hr Determine if focusing difficulty occurs with near and/or far objects Determine level of light needed to obliterate photosensitivity Determine level and quality of hearing loss 2. Adjust bed position so Mrs. Bender is faced away from window and bright lights Provide Mrs. Bender with dimmer attachment for bed lights Refrain from shining flashlight into eyes of Mrs. Bender during evening and night hours Check that eyeglasses are worn if reading 3. Adjust bed position so that Mrs. Bender's right side is accessible to facilitate hearing Stand in front of client when speaking Speak clearly, slowly and distinctly

(continued)

TABLE 7–3. (Continued)

Client Need	Nursing Diagnosis	Goals with Outcome Criteria	Nursing Strategies with Frequencies
Sensory integrity (cont.)			Verify that Mrs. Bender has received the message Instruct nursing and auxiliary staff on position and method of articulation Refer hearing problem to physician for hearing evaluation, audiometer, value of aid appliance Provide for hearing aid mechanism for telephone if feasible and useful 4. Use touch and nonverbal communication to convey acceptance and valuing 5. Demonstrate to family members the techniques to maximize the limited communication time (hand-holding, caressing, articulation, nonverbal communication) 6. Answer call bell in person—do not rely on intercom system 7. Do not chew gum or cover your mouth when speaking 8. Use nonverbal cues to help convey your meaning, facial expressions, hand gestures, writing, pointing 9. Speak slowly and distinctly—do not shout 10. Keep voice at same volume—avoid dropping off at end of each sentence
Nutrition	Potential for disturbed pattern in intake of food and fluids secondary to: Pathophysiological affront of hypertension Distaste for food	Maintenance of nutritional state as evidenced by: Eats three well-balanced meals with bedtime snack totaling 1500 calories daily Oral fluid intake of no more than 2000 ml daily Verbalizes return to normal energy or activity state within 3 days	1. Assess nutritional status: Ask Mrs. Bender about food preferences Prescribe food selection of high K content, e.g., chicken, fresh fish, milk, sweet potato, bananas, all-bran cereals, beef Weigh daily 2. Check for ability to handle regular meal pattern Order small portions if needed Arrange 4 or 6 meal servings rather than 3 if Mrs. Bender cannot handle usual pattern Suggest a milk food at bedtime to promote sleep 3. Incorporate activity and exercise with meal plan to ensure that she would not be too tired to eat 4. Suggest visit by family members during mealtime, because Mrs. Bender may need to solicit assistance of family member's to facilitate eating 5. Explain to Mrs. Bender and family members the basic levels of low salt diet and the need to maintain adequate intake of K 6. Explore with family members their ability to bring in favorite foods 7. Explain to client and family the relationship between hypertension, sodium, fluid intake, and obesity

TABLE 7–3. (Continued)

Client Need	Nursing Diagnosis	Goals with Outcome Criteria	Nursing Strategies with Frequencies
Elimination	Potential for disturbance in urinary and bowel elimination pattern related to: Pharmacological impact of furosemide (Lasix) diuretic Aged state Loss of appetite	Resumption of usual pattern of bowel elimination within 4 days as evidenced by: Adjustment to current urinary elimination pattern in one week Normal moisture evident for skin, oral mucosa, tongue, and lips within 4 days Verbalizes ability to cope with increased frequency	1. Assess the elimination pattern Note time and character of stool Determine level of strength or difficulty with defecation Determine level and character of voiding Note any discomfort with voiding—urgency, burning 2. Check voiding pattern every shift (daily) to determine effect of diuretic Expect maximum urine volume 2 hours after furosemide (Lasix) then gradually diminishing in 6–8 hr; explain to client Contrast output pattern with blood pressure recording every 2 hr during waking hours Note skin turgor, condition of oral mucosa and tongue Determine impact on body weight Check for edema; determine location and type and extent 3. Assess ambulatory ability within first 12 hr 4. Provide for privacy during voiding and defecation 5. Check for signs of dehydration, and low K 6. Encourage participation in elimination surveillance Note when heaviest voiding occurs Note established pattern of diuretic so that social events and interactions can be planned around elimination schedule 7. Facilitate hand washing and have all toilet articles within easy reach and in appropriate space, to minimize the necessity of bending over to pick up items and increase intracranial pressure 8. Report to physician signs of excessive fluid loss 9. Encourage walk in hall BID (10 A.M.–4 P.M.) 10. Assess diet for roughage: Encourage foods high in fiber
Rest and leisure	Diminished rest and leisure related to: Pathological affront of hypertension with resultant high blood pressure Aged state Pharmacological impact of furosemide diuretic Anxiety	Experience of increased rest and wholesome leisure within a week as evidenced by: Verbalizes return to pre-illness state	1. Assess usual rest and leisure pattern Determine the level of strength Determine the amount of energy available to accomplish activities of daily living Note the response to exertion, e.g., going to bathroom, sitting in a chair, using the bedpan in bed, assisting with bathing, eating, etc. 2. Plan rest period after each meal and a nap in afternoon (preferably after

(continued)

TABLE 7–3. (Continued)

Client Need	Nursing Diagnosis	Goals with Outcome Criteria	Nursing Strategies with Frequencies
Rest and lei- sure (cont.)			heaviest voiding period) Instruct client on relaxation exercises Talk about effective ways to experi- ence quiet time Arrange with staff to respect rest peri- ods and quiet times Post sign on door 3. Determine preference for leisure activ- ities. Arrange with family for small radio and guide to programming Suggest phone visits with friends Visit with family members Visit from clergyman 4. Avoid sitting or lying in one position or for prolonged periods of time.
Sleep	Sleep deprivation secondary to: Pathological state of hypertension with resultant elevated blood pressure Headache Hospitalization	Normal sleep pattern re- sumed as evidenced by: Sleeps 6 hr undisturbed within 24 hr Resumption of afternoon nap and usual sleep pattern in 48 hr	1. Complete assessment of usual sleep pattern within 48 hr (see Chapter 23) Record sleep and wake pattern for 48 hr Inquire about client's perception of sleep Determine presleep rituals 2. Arrange room environment so that it is conducive to sleep Eliminate noise Adjust temperature Arrange night light out of direct range of vision 3. Facilitate undisturbed sleep for at least 4 sleep cycles (about 6 hr, 11:30 P.M.—6 A.M.) during the night Maintain usual time to retire Provide milk snack (contains trypto- phan soporific) Partial bath and soothing back rub at 10 P.M. Give Tylenol for headache if needed Assess comfort or discomfort level Allay fears and anxiety if identified Counsel staff on methods of data col- lection without disturbing client, e.g., taking pulse, observational assess- ment during sleep stage III and IV 4. Plan for afternoon nap Provide opportunity for A.M. nap to in- crease REM sleep time Specify the time usually taken *Please Do Not Disturb* sign on the door Inform staff When facilitating afternoon nap, elim- inate voiding times and too late hours so that night sleep is not jeopardized 5. Record and analyze all sleep-related data.

TABLE 7–3. (Continued)

Client Need	Nursing Diagnosis	Goals with Outcome Criteria	Nursing Strategies with Frequencies
Skin integrity	Disruption in skin integrity due to: Pathological affront of hypertension resultant in faulty circulation Aged state	Achievement of intact skin within 72 to 90 hr as evidenced by: Decrease in size of abrasions No evidence of infection	1. Assess the specific reason for the injury, i.e., TIA, dizziness, poor lighting, poor vision, foreign objects in path, inappropriate footwear, etc. 2. Assess texture, quality of skin, tongue, and oral mucosa 3. Check for edema, redness, drainage, change in size of ecchymotic areas Check for signs of allergy to propranolol, furosemide, i.e., rashes, hives, itching 4. Avoid excessive bathing, use of soaps, alcohol or any drying agents on skin Use emollients to facilitate skin integrity Protect skin over bony prominences Wear soft night clothing to protect against roughness of bed linens Mouth care to prevent dryness and cracking 7, 8:30 A.M., 12:30, 5:30, and 10 P.M. on waking and pc and hs and prn 5. Apply warm soaks to ecchymotic areas TID (10,2,6)—clean abrasions with soap and water BID with morning care and at bedtime 6. Observe fluid intake for adequacy Check excessive output caused by diuretic action
Activity	Diminished activity level related to: Pathological affront of hypertension Aged state Hospitalization	Resumption of preadmission activity regimen within one week as evidenced by: Ability to perform self-care Ability to walk length of corridor Ability to get out of bed unassisted	1. Assess Mrs. Bender's preadmission activity pattern within 24 hours. Use family resources 2. Facilitate activities of daily living (ADL) planned with client Plan so that one major activity occurs at a time, i.e., bathing, feeding 5:30 A.M.—arise; wash face and hands; prayers 7:30 A.M.—vital signs 8 A.M.—breakfast 8:30 A.M.—mouth care, range of motion (ROM), relaxation exercise, leisure activity 9:30 A.M.—walk 10:30 A.M.—nap 12 Noon—lunch, BP 12:30 P.M.—mouth care, relaxation exercise, ROM, BP 2 P.M.—visitors 3 P.M.—nap 4 P.M.—walk activity 5 P.M.—dinner 5:30 P.M.—mouth care, relaxation exercise, ROM, BP 6 P.M.—warm soaks, BP 7 P.M.—visitors 9 P.M.—warm bath, BP, mouth care, relaxation exercise

(continued)

TABLE 7–3. (Continued)

Client Need	Nursing Diagnosis	Goals with Outcome Criteria	Nursing Strategies with Frequencies
Activity (cont.)			Plan a rest period after each activity Include walking short distances in the activity schedule; make certain that substantial slippers are worn for walking Assess ability to walk on own or necessity of one person accompanying within 24 hr Refrain from having Mrs. Bender sit or lie for long periods of time Adjust activity related to trips to bathroom; offer bedpan in between when frequent voiding is experienced (9 A.M.–12 noon) Assess how client bathes (in bed, at sink, etc.) and the portion of the bath she can do 3. Provide for ROM exercises while in bed 3 times a day. Teach leg exercises 4. Diminish or increase level of exercise based on degree of strength, blood pressure, and desire 5. Report to physician any unusual activity or loss of motion, e.g., paralysis, hyperactivity of extremities, momentary loss of consciousness, slurred speech 6. Encourage family members to participate in activities, e.g., ROM, accompany to bathroom, walk in hall
Safety	Potential and actual disturbed pattern in safety related to: Pathological state of hypertension Situational occurrence of hospitalization and living alone Aged state Pharmacological impact of antihypertensive and diuretic	No affronts to safety experienced during hospitalization as evidenced by: No falls Asking for help when tired	1. Assess the major affronts to Mrs. Bender's safety during hospitalization. Determine: Steadiness of gait Hazards that might cause injury, e.g., chairs, equipment in walking pathway, electrical cords Incompatibilities, allergy related to furosemide, e.g., possible problem with alcohol ingestion Access to call light and appliances to maintain position in electrically operated bed 2. Explain the need for bedrails Check security of bedrails Assist with getting out of bed and accompany on all walking activities 3. Protect from viral and bacterial infection Do not assign staff with colds, coughs, etc., to care for Mrs. Bender 4. Allow sufficient time for eating Position during eating to facilitate swallowing Have staff available during mealtime

TABLE 7–3. (Continued)

Client Need	Nursing Diagnosis	Goals with Outcome Criteria	Nursing Strategies with Frequencies
Safety (cont.)			5. Assesss the immediate environment for irritating sounds, unnecessary noise, noxious odors, drafts Intervene to eliminate same, to maintain airy, odor free, comfortable room 6. Refrain from jolting Mrs. Bender Announce yourself; tap her shoulder to get her attention Take care in handling the bed and bedding; prevent bumping against bed especially when headache pain is evident
Autonomy	Potential diminution of autonomy, choice related to: Situational occurrence of hospitalization Pathological affront of hypertension Medical, pharmacological, and nursing therapies Aged state	Resumption of autonomy and choice regarding self and environment as evidenced by: Ability to perform activities of daily living Ability to make sound decisions Ability to solve problems adequately	1. Ask Mrs. Bender how she sees herself participating in her care 2. Seek client's advice on timing of caring activities, menu food selections, timing for visitors, etc. 3. Listen to reminiscences of times when client had full control over herself and situation 4. Talk with family members about ways to maximize client's autonomy while yielding to a dependency state until her blood pressure is stabilized Support family members' efforts to allow autonomy for Mrs. Bender within limits of her state of health and their need to intervene temporarily to conduct her affairs as delegated 5. Facilitate delegation of household affairs to family members while client is hospitalized 6. Keep Mrs. Bender informed of options in medical and nursing care provided Offer choices whenever possible 7. Determine with client and family members how emergency health situations will be handled in the future Assist in establishing surveillance system when client returns to her home.
Self-control, self-determination, responsibility	Potential for diminished opportunity for self-control, self-determination, responsibility for self related to: Hospitalization Pathological affront of hypertension Aged state	Maintenance of control over self, self-determination and responsibility as evidenced by: Continues decision making regarding care and welfare from onset of hospitalization Delegates to significant others those specific areas where intervention is appropriate and desired from onset of hospitalization	1. Involve Mrs. Bender in her care as much as is appropriate and safe Gradually increase involvement as headache subsides and blood pressure is reduced to normal limits 2. Determine how knowledgeable client is about the cause of her headaches and the potential hazard of elevated blood pressure Explore fears related to present and future states of health 3. Compliment Mrs. Bender on her handling of physical crises that resulted in admission to the hospital Review signs and symptoms for which client should be alert, i.e., changes in memory, perception, affect, reason-

(continued)

TABLE 7–3. (Continued)

Client Need	Nursing Diagnosis	Goals with Outcome Criteria	Nursing Strategies with Frequencies
Self-control (cont.)			ing, brief periods of loss of consciousness, any weaknes or numbness, temporary dizziness, unsteadiness, temporary loss of speech, sudden loss of vision or temporary dimness, recurrence of headache, diplopia Review these signs and symptoms with family members and ask them to be alert to change in personality or emotional state Plan with Mrs. Bender and family members how this surveillance will be conducted and what should and can be done in the event of occurrence Teach family members to take blood pressure for Mrs. Bender and themselves Check blood pressure of family members to determine base-line recording, refer family members to physician if elevated readings found after rest and recheck Provide Mrs. Bender and family members with information on community's electronic medical response systems services for elderly, disabled, or all persons in the home 4. Help client to work through the fact that needing care through the intervention of another person need not diminish her control or responsibility for herself or her situation
Self-fulfillment	Potential for diminished self-fulfillment related to: Situational occurrence of hospitalization Pathophysiological state of hypertension Aged state	Experience of enhanced self-fulfillment within one week as evidenced by: Expressions of positive views about her condition: feeling neither overwhelmed nor excessively optimistic States that she is not overly concerned about aspect of dependency brought on by her hospitalization and describes how she expects to resume full control over herself as her situation improves Ability to focus on problems outside herself and can muster energy to get involved in these Expresses a fresh appreciation for the basic things in life	1. Assess client's perception of herself 2. Facilitate fulfillment of usual pattern of activity and contacts with family and friends within the restriction imposed by diminished strength and pain Contract visiting times and length Arrange communication modality if desired: Phone Letter and note writing materials Suggest contacts with neighbor and church groups—particularly those who could be counted on for support

TABLE 7–3. (Continued)

Client Need	Nursing Diagnosis	Goals with Outcome Criteria	Nursing Strategies with Frequencies
Personal recognition, esteem, respect	Potential for diminished amount of personal recognition, esteem, respect secondary to: Hospitalization Situational occurrence of potential stigma of hypertension Aged state	Experiences personal recognition, esteem, and respect as evidenced by: Verbalization of these needs	1. Assess the level and quality of communication (verbal and nonverbal) conveying recognition, respect 2. Work with staff to call Mrs. Bender by name with each contact Maintain client-focused conversation in the environment at all times Listen when Mrs. Bender speaks, noting position, posture and other nonverbal clues 3. Assist Mrs. Bender gently and firmly when assisting her to bathroom, out of or into bed, on short walks 4. Respect need to be slow, need to repeat requests, anecdotes, etc. 5. Ask for clarification to assure meanings are conveyed during conversation 6. Support family members' efforts to show respect and build esteem of client Encourage family members to share these feelings with Mrs. Bender 7. Introduce new or different staff members involved in care 8. Explain all procedures thoroughly giving Mrs. Bender enough time to adjust and prepare herself for these 9. Explore further any communication from Mrs. Bender that indicates self-worth feelings: "I'm too old. . ." "I'm not good to anyone." "I'm always in and out for the same sickness."
Appreciation, attention	Potential for diminished amount of appreciation, attention secondary to: Hospitalization Situational occurrence of potential stigma of hypertension Aged state	Experience of appreciation, wholesome attention from onset of hospitalization as evidenced by: Verbalization of these needs	1. Assess the amount and quality of attention received from staff, family, and friends Spend 10 minutes 3 times a day with client 2. Encourage family members to express to Mrs. Bender their appreciation of her efforts to care for herself Encourage client to allow family members to contribute to her welfare by assisting in caring activities, i.e., mealtimes, brief walks Encourage Mrs. Bender to allow family members to look after her home for her while hospitalized Family members voice desire and willingness to do so Family members report what they have done for their mother 3. Convey progress made in recovery to Mrs. Bender and compliment her efforts to comply with nursing and medical strategies.

(continued)

TABLE 7–3. (Continued)

Client Need	Nursing Diagnosis	Goals with Outcome Criteria	Nursing Strategies with Frequencies
To love and be loved	Potential for diminished ability to be loved and to love related to: Hospitalization Situational occurrence of potential stigma of hypertension Aged state	Experiences love from significant others and conveys love to others as evidenced by: Many visitors, phone calls, and flowers Verbalization	1. Assess the relationship of family members and staff in conveying love to Mrs. Bender within 5–6 days 2. Assess Mrs. Bender's manner and ability of conveying love to family members and staff within 1 wk 3. Point out observations of love shared by family members to client Encourage family members caressing, hand holding, kissing Mrs. Bender if this is their usual pattern Provide privacy for Mrs. Bender and family members while visiting 4. Encourage client to share anecdotes in which she gave or was the recipient of love by family and friends 5. Allow client an opportunity to express her love needs and strategies to meet these Plan 15 min with Mrs. Bender 3 times a day Use touch to convey caring and love for Mrs. Bender Provide assistance to Mrs. Bender for note writing thank you notes to generous family and friends 6. Introduce Mrs. Bender to other clients her age when headaches subside and blood pressure is down to facilitate mutual support system.

ADL = activities of daily living; BID = twice a day; K = potassium; Na = sodium; REM = rapid eye movement; ROM = range of motion; TIA = transient ischemic attacks; TID = three times a day.

to goal expectation. These data provide evidence for formalized evaluation, the final phase of the nursing process.

Evaluating

Evaluation, the fourth phase of the nursing process, is the appraisal of client changes as a result of nurse actions or of the client's behavioral changes as these relate to nurse actions. Evaluating, therefore, audits the behavior of the client, consistent with determined goals.

As the final component in the sequence of the nursing process, evaluation was, for many years, a neglected nursing activity. At first, major attention was given to assessment. There was a preoccupation with tool development to assist in data collection. Some tools were long, involved, and so complex that they were impractical. Other tools were so specific and limited

to such a small population that they were impractical. Until nurses realized they were collecting information about the client that would contribute to a definition of his or her needs or problems, nurses were not goal-directed in the development of assessment instruments. Gradually, the focus for assessment has been clarified and the data gathered about the client's needs, habits, behavior, strengths, and problems are analyzed in a systematic manner, so that a plan of care for the client can be developed and goals for health can be defined.

It is the plan of care and the goals for health that establish the foundation for evaluation. Based upon the identified problems and needs of the client, the nurse sets goals for care. Validation with the client of needs or problems is critical. Client involvement in goal setting is vital, too. Having specified what the thrust of care will be, the nurse implements strategies and then asks: How effective were the strategies? What client changes resulted because of nurse actions?

Just as the preoccupation at one time was on tool development for assessment, at present it appears to be on the development of tools for evaluation. These form the *structure* of evaluation and are important; however, the priority in evaluation must be established. To spend all one's time developing a form for evaluation defeats the purpose of evaluation. Structure is important, and guidelines are essential, but these must be developed and decided on so that the nurse can get on with evaluation.

The *process* of evaluation is an important component, too. Whether evaluation is done via direct observation while care is being given, direct observation of the client after care is given, written reports, taped reports, interviews, or various other means, the rationale for determining a process of evaluation is to provide the best means possible for collecting data on which to evaluate client care. A combination of measures may be used to evaluate care. Incorporating the evaluation component within the care plan format is the most efficient way to accomplish evaluation and the most certain way to ensure its completion. In the care plan for Mrs. Bender, the components for evaluation are integral parts of the care plan (Table 7–3). For example, the nurse plans to provide comfort to Mrs. Bender and identifies when freedom from pain should be achieved; the nurse also records the frequency with which a report of her comfort or discomfort is elicited from Mrs. Bender in order to determine how the client is progressing toward the relief of pain.

When all facets of care have been examined to determine the quality of care rendered, the *outcome* of evaluation is determined, reported, and recorded. Quality of outcomes may vary depending on the *criteria* that were established at the outset of care. A qualitative assessment precisely defines the state of the client when care began. The nurse, in collaboration with the client, when possible, defines how the state of the client should change as a result of nursing care and specifies what should be the length of time necessary to achieve the ultimate goal or final outcome; periodic time checks are built into the evaluation plan to determine the extent

to which, and the rate at which, the planned care is leading to problem resolution. These definitions and specifications of expected client behaviors and physical characteristics are called outcome criteria.

In Mrs. Bender's situation, one goal is to relieve her headache within 48 hours; various nursing strategies are defined with the specified goal to relieve the headache entirely. Periodic checks with Mrs. Bender (every 3 to 4 hours) are made to determine the status of the headache. When the nurse has collected the data about the client and determined the nursing diagnoses and when she or he sets in place a plan of care to include goals, nursing strategies, and time frame for goal achievement, essential components are in place to provide efficient, high-quality client care. If it is determined, through evaluation, that goals are accomplished and client problems are resolved (if Mrs. Bender's headache is gone) the goal of nursing has been accomplished and nursing care may no longer be necessary; the client may be able to manage her care independently. If it is determined through evaluation that some portion of the care plan needs revision, if more data are necessary, if additional problems have developed, or any other alteration has changed the previously stated goals, then the nurse reassesses, replans, and reevaluates while proceeding with client care implementation. The cyclic nature of the nursing process and the continual overlapping of all components of the process become obvious when the nurse deliberately examines nursing actions in the light of client outcomes.

The care plan for Mrs. Bender suggests one way that all components of nursing activity on behalf of the client can be recorded. There are various methods by which client data can be noted for communicating with those persons whose activities are guided by such records. The exact format and specific components of the record can vary from one setting to another, provided the following data about the client are considered:

- What are the needs?
- What are the nursing diagnoses (problems, actual and potential)?
- What are the goals to be achieved?
- When should the goals be achieved?

- What is the time interval for determining progress toward goal achievement?
- What are the nursing strategies?
- What are the outcomes of care (changes in the state of the client)?

Data about the client, the plan of care, and the rate of progress toward goal achievement are critical to any client situation. Communication between health-team members as each works toward client care goals is essential. When there is effective, accurate, and complete communication among those responsible for health care, the care of the client is maximized.

SUMMARY

Within the past two decades, major progress has been made in the identification, development, and use of the nursing process. A number of nurse leaders have written about the science of nursing, and increasing numbers of nurses are using and applying these ideas in the practice of nursing. Guiding these efforts are accepted criteria for a profession, a code for professional nurses, standards of nursing practice, selected definitions of nursing, as well as specification and research about theories and concepts that are viewed as foundations for nursing.

The core and essence of nursing is the nursing process. Although distinct from the leadership and research processes, nurses use both these processes to carry out the nursing process through the use of intellectual, interpersonal, and technical skills. Following the orderly systematic activity of the nursing process enables the nurse to assess client needs; diagnose client problems that are amenable to nursing intervention; and plan, implement, and evaluate the client's care. The deliberate use of this process is the best assurance that the client—individual, family, or community—will receive the nursing care that is needed to maintain wellness or to resolve problems at the appropriate time. The human need framework is a logical framework for the performance of the nursing process and the achievement of the goal of nursing: the maintenance or fulfillment of the human needs of the client.

Study Questions

1. Define nursing.

2. Define the nursing process.

3. Document each cited definition according to the author who proposed the definition.

4. Name and define the elements, phases or steps of the nursing process.

5. Cite the sources for these labels and definitions.

6. Differentiate the nursing process from the nursing research process.

7. Differentiate the nursing process from the nursing leadership process.

8. Explain the recency of nursing process identification.

9. Cite at least three people who have contributed to the development of the nursing process:
   - in the 1960s
   - in the 1970s

10. Specify a theory or concept (or a combination of theories or concepts) that is consistent with your values and beliefs and that you can or do use for providing client care.

11. Explain the way that such a theoretical-conceptual framework enables quality care performance.

12. Cite a specific client situation and illustrate the relationship of the theoretical-conceptual base to the care of that client.

13. Explain the use of assessment in a specific client situation.

14. Present the means by which this client care is planned.

15. Discuss the implementation of this client care.

16. Examine the way by which client care is evaluated.

17. Comment on the value or limitations of using the nursing process in this client situation.

References

1. Helen Yura and Mary B. Walsh, *The Nursing Process: Assessing, Planning, Implementing, Evaluating,* 4th ed. (E. Norwalk, Conn.: Appleton-Century-Crofts, 1983), 1.
2. Helen Yura and Mary B. Walsh, (eds.), *The Nursing Process: Assessing, Planning, Implementing, Evaluating* (Washington, D.C.: The Catholic University of America Press, 1967).
3. Hildegard Peplau, *Interpersonal Relations in Nursing* (New York: G.P. Putnam's Sons, 1952).
4. Lydia E. Hall, "Quality of nursing care," Public Health News (June 1955).
5. D.E. Johnson, "Philosophy of nursing" *Nurs Outlook* 7, (1959):198–200.
6. Ida J. Orlando, *The Dynamic Nurse–Patient Relationship* (New York: G.P. Putnam's Sons, 1961).
7. Ernestine Wiedenbach, *Clinical Nursing: A Helping Art* (New York: Springer Publishing Co., 1964).
8. A. Flexner, *Universities* (New York: Oxford University Press, 1930).
9. E. H. Schein, *Professional Education: Some New Directions,* Carnegie Commission on Higher Education (New York: McGraw-Hill Book Co., 1972).
10. G.W. Stuart, "How professional is nursing?" *Image* 13 (1981):18–33.
11. American Nurses' Association. "Code for nurses," *Am Nurse* 8 (1976):5,8.
12. M. Olivia Gowan, *Report of the Proceedings of the Workshop on Administration of College Programs in Nursing* (Washington, D.C.: The Catholic University of America Press, 1944).
13. Virginia Henderson: *The Nature of Nursing* (New York: Macmillan Co., 1966), 15.
14. American Nurses' Association, *Nursing: A Social Policy Statement* (Kansas City, Mo.: American Nurses' Association, 1980), 9.
15. F. Suppe, "Implications in recent developments in philosophy of science for nursing theory," In *Fifth Biennial Eastern Conference on Nursing Research* (Baltimore, Md.: University of Maryland, 1982).
16. Faye Abdellah and E. Levine, *Better Patient Care Through Nursing Research,* 2nd ed. (New York: Macmillan Co., 1979).
17. D.E. Johnson, "The behavioral system model for nursing," in J.P. Riehl and C. Roy, eds. *Conceptual Models for Nursing Practice,* 2nd ed. (New York: Appleton-Century-Crofts, 1980), 207–16.
18. M.E. Levine: "The four conservation principles of nursing," *Nurs Forum* 6, (1967):45–59.
19. Orlando, *Nurse–Patient Relationship,* 36.
20. Joyce Travelbee: *Interpersonal Aspects of Nursing* (Philadelphia: F.A. Davis Co., 1966).
21. Wiedenbach, *Clinical Nursing: A Helping Art,* 23.
22. Imogene King: *Toward a Theory for Nursing* (New York: John Wiley & Sons, 1971).
23. B.M. Neuman and R.J. Young, A model for teaching total person approach to patient problems, *Nurs Res* 21 (1972).
24. Dorothea E. Orem, *Nursing: Concepts of Practice* (New York: McGraw-Hill Book Co., 1971).
25. Martha E. Rogers, *Nursing Science: Introduction to the Theoretical Basis of Nursing* (Philadelphia: F.A. Davis Co., 1970).
26. Sister Callista Roy, *Introduction to Nursing: An Adaptation Model* (Englewood Cliffs, N.J.: Prentice-Hall, 1976).
27. J.G. Paterson and L.T. Zderad, *Humanistic Nursing* (New York: John Wiley & Sons, 1976).
28. K.M. Gebbie and M.A. Lavin, eds. *Classification of Nursing Diagnoses* (St. Louis: C.V. Mosby Co., 1975).
29. M. Gordon, "Nursing diagnosis and the diagnostic process," *Am J Nurs* 76 (1976):1298–1300.
30. P.B. Kritek, "The generation and classification of nursing diagnoses: Toward a theory of nursing," *Image* 10 (1978):33–40.
31. Gebbie and Lavin, *Classification of Nursing Diagnoses.*
32. M.E. Hurley, ed., *Classification of Nursing Diagnoses,* Proceedings of the Sixth Conference (St. Louis: C.V. Mosby Co., 1986).
33. Ashley Montagu, *The Direction of Human Development* (New York: Hawthorn, 1970).
34. Abraham Maslow, *Motivation and Personality* (New York: Harper & Row, 1970), 29.
35. Ibid., 26, 28.
36. Ibid., 29.
37. Ibid., 36–38.
38. Ashley Montagu, *On Being Human* (New York: Hawthorn, 1966), 49.
39. Maslow, *Motivation and Personality,* 97–100.
40. A. Combs, A.C. Richards, and F. Richards: *Perceptual Psychology: A Humanistic Approach to*

the Study of Persons (New York: Harper & Row, 1976), 57.

41. Ibid., 80.
42. Ibid., 68.
43. Ibid., 86.
44. Ibid., 128.
45. Ibid., 104.
46. Ibid., 67.
47. Ibid., 52.
48. M. Vernon, *Perception Through Experience* (London: Methuen, 1970), 3.
49. Ibid., 4–5.
50. Ibid., 59.
51. Ibid., 99.

Annotated Bibliography

Bower, F.L. 1977. *The Process of Planning Nursing Care: A Model for Nursing Practice,* 2nd ed. St. Louis: C.V. Mosby. This brief book fully describes the importance of a nursing care plan to organize and direct nursing care.

Inzer, F. 1981. "Evaluation Patient Actions," *Nurs Outlook* 29:178–79. This article discusses methods of measuring outcomes of nursing in terms of client behaviors.

Kim, M., and Moritz, D.A. 1982. *Classification of Nursing Diagnoses.* New York: McGraw-Hill. This book presents material presented and developed at the third and fourth National Conferences on the classification of nursing diagnoses in 1976 and 1980. In addition, a development of nursing diagnosis is presented.

Malasanos, L., Barkavskos, V., Moss, M., and Stoltenberg-Allen, K. 1981. *Health Assessment,* 2nd ed. St. Louis: C.V. Mosby. This excellent and comprehensive text fully explains techniques, from history taking through integration of assessment. Special areas focus on pregnant clients, assessment of children, and the aging client.

McLane, A. 1987. *Classification of Nursing Diagnoses: Proceedings of the Seventh Conference.* St. Louis: C.V. Mosby. A presentation of the papers and discussion that guided the deliberation of the seventh conference, at which the classification and taxonomy of nursing diagnoses were considered. This 1986 session was the second international meeting of the North American Nursing Diagnosis Association (NANDA).

Price, M.R. 1980. Nursing Diagnosis: Making a Concept Come Alive. *Am J Nurs* 80(4):668–71. This important article discusses what a nursing diagnosis is, how to develop one, and how to use it.

Rothberg, J.J. 1967. Why Nursing Diagnosis? *Am J Nurs* 67(5):1040–42. In this classic article, the author maintains that nursing diagnosis is essential for nursing practice.

Yura, H., and Walsh, M.B. 1988. *The Nursing Process,* 5th ed. East Norwalk: Appleton & Lange. This book delineates the steps in the nursing process and uses case studies to demonstrate its usefulness. It also discusses the need for a theoretical framework for nursing practice.

Chapter 8

Nursing Diagnosis

Cathie Guzzetta

Chapter Outline

- Objectives
- Glossary
- Introduction
- Nursing Diagnosis and the Nursing Process
    North American Nursing Diagnosis Association
- Nursing Diagnosis Format
    Problem
    Etiology
    Signs and Symptoms
    Different Approaches to P-E-S Format
    Writing the Diagnostic Statement
    Case Study
- Summary
- Study Questions
- References
- Annotated Bibliography

Objectives

After completing this chapter, the reader will be able to:

▸ Differentiate between a nursing and medical diagnosis
▸ Describe how nursing diagnosis fits into the nursing process
▸ Describe the importance of the work of the North American Nursing Diagnosis Association

▸ Discuss the steps involved in the nursing diagnostic process
▸ List the parts included in the diagnostic statement
▸ Discuss two different approaches to the P-E-S format
▸ Discuss how one should begin using nursing diagnoses in clinical practice
▸ Formulate a list of nursing diagnoses from the assessment of a client in clinical practice

Glossary

Critical Defining Characteristics. Those signs and symptoms that must be present and observed in a client for the nursing diagnosis to exist.

Diagnostic Statement. A statement connecting the identified client problem and etiology by the phrase "related to."

Etiology. The probable cause of the problem or factors related to its development.

Nursing Diagnosis. A cluster of signs and symptoms describing an actual or potential health problem that nurses, because of their education and experience, are licensed and able to treat.

Nursing Diagnostic Process. The steps nurses go through to arrive at a nursing diagnosis; involves the Problem-Etiology-Signs-and-Symptoms (P-E-S) format.

Nursing Orders. Specific actions that the nurse performs that are designed to solve the client's problem and achieve the desired outcomes.

Problem. A brief statement of the client's actual or potential health problem.

Signs and Symptoms. The specific client behaviors that lead a nurse to believe the client has a specific problem.

Taxonomy. A classification system based on science and theory that results in established categories.

INTRODUCTION

Nursing diagnosis involves a way of identifying, classifying, and naming client problems. Because nursing diagnosis is a relatively new concept in nursing practice, it is important for the nurse to become familiar with its definition, terminology, steps, and application.

The word *diagnosis* is derived from the Greek word *diagignoskein* meaning "to distinguish." *Diagnosis* is the act of gathering information about what is causing a difficulty, what needs to be corrected, or what is interfering with normal functioning. Although there are many ways to define a "nursing diagnosis," a commonly accepted definition is by Gordon, who states that a nursing diagnosis is a "cluster of signs and symptoms describing an actual or potential health problem (state-of-the-client) which nurses, because of their education and experience, are licensed and able to treat."[1] This step involves translating the data into words that precisely communicate the client's situation. For nursing, this usually is a statement of the impact of a functional deficit on the client's condition.

It is important to distinguish the difference between a medical and a nursing diagnosis. Medical practice is guided by the biomedical model, which traditionally has been involved with the pathophysiology and cure of disease. Thus, medical diagnoses are involved with identifying the cause of disease and treatment is directed toward this cause. In contrast, nursing practice is guided by the holistic model that reflects the inter-relationship of the body-mind-spirit and focuses on maintaining or regaining health.[2] Nursing diagnoses, therefore, are involved with human responses to stressors or other factors that adversely affect optimal health. Treatment is directed toward causes of the response or factors influencing it.[3]

When distinguishing between a nursing and medical diagnosis, it is important to note that nursing diagnoses involve those problems that nurses are licensed and able to treat independently. Therefore, a health problem is not considered a nursing diagnosis if it is treated through modalities that are legally defined by the practice of medicine (e.g., surgery, prescription drugs, radiation). In addition, medical problems treated with standing orders or standing medical protocols are not called nursing diagnoses.

NURSING DIAGNOSIS AND THE NURSING PROCESS

In 1967, at The Catholic University of America, Yura and Walsh identified the phases of the nursing process. These phases included: (1) assessing, (2) planning, (3) implementing, and (4) evaluating.[4] These steps were designed to fulfill the purpose of nursing practice, which is maintaining the client's health or providing quality nursing care to return the client to a state of health. Since 1967, the nursing profession and also the nursing process have undergone many changes and advances. The framework for nursing practice has shifted from the biomedical model to the holistic model of health care. The development of quality assurance programs, nursing audits, prospective payment for health care, and the revision of nurse practice acts have all influenced the nursing process. Thus, in the 1980s, such groups as the American Nurses' Association,[5] the American Heart Association,[6] the American Association of Critical Care Nurses,[7] and the North American Nursing Diagnosis Association[8] have all judged that problem identification or nursing diagnosis is a clear and distinct step in the nursing process. Consistent with such thinking in the 1980s, the American Nurses' Association Congress for Nursing Practice has defined nursing as "the diagnosis and treatment of human responses to actual or potential health problems."[9] This definition of nursing is an exciting one because it establishes and supports the importance of nursing diagnosis in practice.

To understand the concept of nursing diagnosis, it is necessary to discuss how it fits into the expanded steps of the nursing process (Fig. 8–1) (see Chapter 7 on the nursing process). The first step in the nursing process is the *assessment,* which provides the basis for the rest of the nursing process. A systematic biopsychosocial assessment, using a nursing data base, incorporates all body-mind-spirit information related to the client's history, physical examination and results of laboratory data.[10]

Problem identification or nursing diagnosis, the next step in the nursing process, involves a new way of describing actual or potential health problems that are identified in the assessment phase. Nursing diagnoses are summary statements of the health assessment phase and help to designate priorities in dealing with client problems and give direction and purpose to the nursing process. They increase nurses' accountability by providing for more precise record keeping and delineating more specifically the purpose(s) for nursing actions.

After nursing diagnoses are identified, specific and concise *client outcomes* are developed. One or more outcomes are developed for each diagnosis. Client outcomes must be measurable and provide a direct statement of the end the nurse hopes the client will reach. When the client outcomes are clearly stated, the nurse can evaluate whether the outcomes have been achieved.

The next step in the nursing process involves developing the *plan* of care. The plan is guided by the client outcomes and is developed in terms of nursing orders. **Nursing orders** are specific actions that the nurse performs that are designed to solve the client's problem and achieve the desired outcomes. *Implementation* involves carrying out the plan or nursing orders. *Evaluation* is done to determine whether the client outcomes have been achieved (not to determine whether the nursing orders have been completed). Evaluation and reassessment also take place during all phases of the nursing process because of the dynamic nature of human beings and the frequent changes that may occur in health and illness.

North American Nursing Diagnosis Association

Although nurses have always been involved in identifying client problems, there has never been a consistent method developed to standardize and communicate the terminology. The North American Nursing Diagnosis Association (NANDA) has been involved over the past decade in defining, explaining, classifying, and validating nursing diagnoses.[11] They have begun to standardize the terminology regarding client problems encountered by nurses. The results of this work have also provided improved communication and clarification about health problems to all members of the health team.

NURSING DIAGNOSIS FORMAT

NANDA has formalized the **nursing diagnostic process** as consisting of three steps known as the *Problem-Etiology-Signs-and-Symptoms (P-E-S)* format:[12, 13]

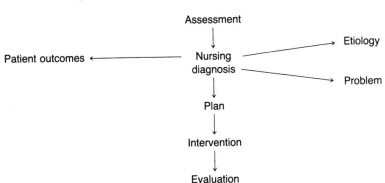

Figure 8–1. The nursing process. (From B. M. Dossey and C. E. Guzzetta, "Person centered caring in the nursing process," In C. E. Guzzetta and B. M. Dossey, eds., Cardiovascular Nursing: Bodymind Tapestry [St. Louis: C. V. Mosby Co., 1984], with permission.)

P = **Problem:** a brief statement about the client's actual or potential health problem (or state-of-the-client)

E = **Etiology:** the probable cause of the problem or factors that may lead to its development

S = **Signs and Symptoms:** the specific client behaviors (also called defining characteristics) observed during the assessment phase that lead the nurse to believe the client has a specific problem

When writing a nursing diagnosis using the P-E-S format, the problem and etiology (the P-E) are connected by the phrase "related to" to form the **diagnostic statement.**[14] If the client's problem is "anxiety" and the probable cause of the problem is the "impending surgery," then the diagnostic statement would be written as "anxiety related to impending surgery." The phrase "related to" rather than "caused by" or "due to" is legally recommended because the causes for most nursing diagnoses have not yet been proven by research.[15] Another example is seen when a client develops redness and a rash behind the ears and on the inside of the wrists with the probable cause being a new perfume. In this case the diagnostic statement would be "impairment of skin integrity related to use of new cosmetic." In summary, the nursing diagnostic process involves three steps known as the P-E-S format, and the nursing diagnostic statement includes the problem and etiology connected by the phrase "related to" (Fig. 8–2).

Problem

The **taxonomy** accepted by NANDA is included in Table 8–1. The problem may be an actual or potential health problem or one for which the client may be at high risk. It is important to state the problem clearly and concisely so that it is easily understood and useful at the bedside. The problem should also be one that nurses are licensed, able, and legally allowed to identify and treat. The problem should reflect what needs to be changed to achieve a state of health and is used to identify client outcomes in the care plan.[16]

It is also important that the nurse refer to the list of accepted nursing diagnoses found on Table 8–1 so that the correct terminology for the problem is consistently written. One of the purposes of the nursing diagnosis movement is to provide a means of consistent terminology so that client problems can be communicated from one nurse to another, from one shift to another, from one hospital to another, and from one area of the country to another. By using consistent terminology, communication will be enhanced, and specific outcome criteria and nursing interventions will be established by research.

It should be noted that the nursing diagnoses listed in Table 8-1 have been accepted by NANDA for clinical research testing and are not necessarily accepted for clinical practice. The process of adopting and approving a specific nursing diagnosis is dynamic and ongoing; much research is still needed to determine if each of the nursing diagnoses actually exists in clinical practice and whether they are useful in describing client problems and in directing nursing interventions at the bedside. The accepted list of nursing diagnoses will continue to be modified, expanded and supported as research is conducted to validate each of the problems.[17]

Table 8–1 represents the nursing diagnoses that have been refined and modified over the years by NANDA during seven National Conferences on Nursing Diagnoses.[18] A specific procedure for accepting each nursing diagnosis has been developed. The name of the diagnosis, together with its definition, defining characteristics, related factors, and substantiating or supportive materials are submitted to NANDA and are reviewed and approved by the Diagnosis Review Committee and the NANDA Board of Directors. After such approval, the diagnostic labels and supportive materials are sent to the NANDA membership for a vote. If the diagnostic label is approved by the membership, it is added to the accepted list.[19]

Because of the method used in developing

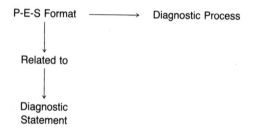

Figure 8–2. Nursing diagnostic process versus the diagnostic statement.

TABLE 8–1. NURSING DIAGNOSES ACCEPTED FOR CLINICAL TESTING (APPROVED APRIL, 1986, BY THE NORTH AMERICAN NURSING DIAGNOSIS ASSOCIATION)

Activity intolerance
Activity intolerance, potential
Adjustment, impaired[a]
Airway clearance, ineffective
Anxiety
Body temperature, potential alteration in[a]
Bowel elimination, alteration in: Constipation
Bowel elimination, alteration in: Diarrhea
Bowel elimination, alteration in: Incontinence
Breathing pattern, ineffective
Cardiac output, alteration in: Decreased
Comfort, alteration in: Pain
Comfort, alteration in: Chronic pain[a]
Communication, impaired: Verbal
Coping, family: Potential for growth
Coping, ineffective family: Compromised
Coping, ineffective family: Disabling
Coping, ineffective individual
Diversional activity, deficit
Family process, alteration in
Fear
Fluid volume alteration in: Excess
Fluid volume deficit, actual
Fluid volume deficit, potential
Gas exchange, impaired
Grieving, anticipatory
Grieving, dysfunctional
Growth and development, altered[a]
Health maintenance, alteration in
Home maintenance management, impaired
Hopelessness[a]
Hyperthermia[a]
Hypothermia[a]
Incontinence, functional[a]
Incontinence, reflex[a]
Incontinence, stress[a]
Incontinence, total[a]
Incontinence, urge[a]
Infection, potential for[a]
Injury, potential for: (poisoning, potential for; suffocation, potential for; trauma, potential for)
Knowledge deficit (specify)
Mobility, impaired physical
Neglect, unilateral[a]
Noncompliance (specify)
Nutrition, alteration in: Less than body requirements
Nutrition, alteration in: More than body requirements
Nutrition, alteration in: Potential for more than body requirements
Oral Mucous membrane, alteration in
Parenting, alteration in: Actual
Parenting, alteration in: Potential
Post trauma response[a]
Powerlessness
Rape trauma syndrome
Self-care deficit: Feeding, bathing/hygiene, dressing/grooming, toileting
Self-concept, disturbance in body image, self-esteem, role performance, personal identity

Sensory-perceptual alteration: Visual, auditory, kinesthetic, gustatory, tactile, olfactory
Sexual dysfunction
Sexuality patterns, altered[a]
Skin integrity, impairment of: Actual
Skin integrity, impairment of: Potential
Sleep pattern disturbance
Social interaction, impaired[a]
Social isolation
Spiritual distress (distress of the human spirit)
Swallowing, impaired[a]
Thermoregulation, ineffective[a]
Thought processes, alteration in
Tissue integrity, impaired[a]
Tissue perfusion, alteration in: Cerebral, cardiopulmonary, renal, gastrointestinal, peripheral
Urinary elimination, alteration in patterns
Urinary retention[a]
Violence, potential for: Self-directed or directed at others

[a]Diagnoses accepted in 1986
From McLane, A.M. (ed.). 1987. Classification of Nursing Diagnoses: Proceedings of the Seventh Conference. St. Louis: C.V. Mosby Co., with permission.

the accepted list, it is well known that many useful nursing diagnoses still need to be added. When reviewing the list, for example, it is apparent that there is need to develop many more diagnoses that are physiologically related. As the list of nursing diagnoses is expanded in the future, it is hoped that it will be developed to include all client problems encountered and dealt with by nurses.[20]

What should nurses do if they identify a client problem that is not on the accepted list of nursing diagnoses? A common error encountered when beginning to use nursing diagnoses is the belief that if a problem is not on the accepted list, then it should not be used. This belief may partially stem from a lack of understanding about how the accepted list of nursing diagnoses was actually developed. Knowing, however, that the list currently is not complete may help to clarify this misunderstanding. Thus, the accepted list in Table 8–1 should be used whenever possible, but there will be times when the nurse identifies a problem not on the list. If the client exhibits observable signs and symptoms that indicate that a new diagnosis exists, the nurse should word the problem concisely and identify the probable cause. For example, if the client exhibits signs and symptoms that indicate "unhealthy denial" (a diagnosis not found on the accepted list), the nurse should identify the probable cause of the denial (e.g., chronic illness) and write the diagnosis on the care plan (e.g., unhealthy denial related to chronic illness). Therefore, the accepted list of problems (nursing diagnoses) should be used when appropriate, but if the diagnosis is not found on the list, nurses should use their education and experience to identify and write the new diagnosis.

Etiology

The etiology is used to identify the actual or probable cause of the health problem. The cause should be stated clearly and concisely and it should be easily understood and useful at the bedside. The etiology helps to identify what is causing or maintaining the problem. When developing the plan of care, the etiology is used to determine what must be changed to achieve a state of health.[21] The probable etiologies for many of the nursing diagnoses have been identified in several publications.[22-24]

Signs and Symptoms

Before the diagnostic statement is written, the nurse must first assess the client's status. The data from the client assessment is analyzed, conclusions are drawn, and nursing diagnoses are formulated. Therefore, even though the nursing diagnostic process involves the P-E-S format, the S part of the format comes first. (Perhaps it should be renamed the S-P-E format.) The signs and symptoms are assessed to identify a specific problem as well as to differentiate among various diagnoses. Signs and symptoms, specific for each nursing diagnosis, have also been called the **critical defining characteristics**. When the critical defining characteristics are observed in a client, the diagnosis is said to exist. Partial listings of signs and symptoms for each nursing diagnosis are available to assist nurses in determining the presence or absence of a particular nursing diagnosis.[25-28] However, for most diagnoses, the list of critical defining characteristics that *must be present* for the diagnosis to exist are still being developed. Nevertheless, after assessing the client's condition and formulating a tentative diagnosis, the nurse should refer to a list of signs and symptoms to determine if these signs and symptoms were actually observed in the client. If the observed signs and symptoms match those in the list, then the nursing diagnosis is confirmed and written on the care plan. However, if the list of signs and symptoms for a particular diagnosis is unclear, incomplete, or not available, then nurses must use their education and experience to determine whether the assessed signs and symptoms actually indicate an actual or potential health problem. If they do, the nursing diagnosis is made.

Different Approaches to P-E-S Format

Several approaches to the P-E-S format have been recommended.[29-34] Nurses learning to use nursing diagnoses may find one or more of these approaches useful. The first approach is recommended for nurses who are beginning to use nursing diagnoses in the clinical setting. It provides written documentation that the client exhibits specific signs and symptoms that support the existence of a specific nursing diagnosis. It also provides the data that can guide the nurse in developing the outcomes and plan (nursing orders) and in evaluating the client outcomes.

The P-E-S format can be documented all in one statement. The diagnostic statement (problem and etiology) is written together with the observed signs and symptoms. The signs and symptoms can appear before, with, or after the diagnostic statement. For example[35,36]:

1. Figure 8–3 illustrates how the signs and symptoms might be listed in a column *before* the nursing diagnosis on the care plan.
2. Signs and symptoms may be written *with* the diagnostic statement: "Knowledge deficit about coronary artery disease related to inadequate health teaching manifested by inability to describe meaning and signs and symptoms of an acute myocardial infarction."
3. Signs and symptoms may be written *after* the diagnostic statement: "Knowledge deficit about coronary artery disease related to inadequate health teaching."
   a. Client asked: "What is a heart attack?"
   b. Client unable to list early warning signs of acute myocardial infarction and unable to describe coronary artery disease risk factors.

Related problems can be written together in the first main clause when they are so closely

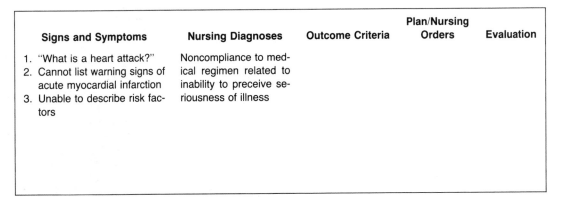

Signs and Symptoms	Nursing Diagnoses	Outcome Criteria	Plan/Nursing Orders	Evaluation
1. "What is a heart attack?" 2. Cannot list warning signs of acute myocardial infarction 3. Unable to describe risk factors	Noncompliance to medical regimen related to inability to preceive seriousness of illness			

FIGURE 8–3. Care plan documenting signs and symptoms with diagnostic statement.

related that their etiology and plan are the same. For example[37,38]: "Anxiety and depression related to impending cardiac valve replacement surgery."

Related etiologies can be written together in the second main clause when they are responsible for causing the same problem. For example[39,40]: "Impairment of skin integrity related to immobility and altered circulation."

Health maintenance patterns identified from health behaviors in the client assessment can be written as nursing diagnoses. Although nursing diagnoses have been developed to identify actual or potential health problems, behaviors that indicate health maintenance patterns should not be excluded from the list of possible nursing diagnoses. In the 1980s, health care is shifting from an illness to a wellness model, and nurses must assume responsibility for assisting and supporting clients in illness prevention and health maintenance. A client who may be at risk for coronary artery disease may be successfully attempting to reduce his risk factors. For example[41–43]: "Maintenance of stress reduction related to client accepting responsibility for reducing risk factors manifested by cessation of smoking and taking daily exercise."

Occasionally, the diagnostic statement may consist of only the first main clause (i.e, the problem). The etiology for some problems may be unidentifiable initially. Additional observation and assessment may be needed before the etiology can be identified and included in the diagnostic statement. An example might be anx-

iety, particularly if the cause is rooted in the unconscious of the client. The diagnostic statement might read "anxiety, etiology unknown." Later, when the etiology has been established, it is then written in the diagnostic statement. When the etiology is omitted from the diagnostic statement, however, the nurse does not know what is maintaining the unhealthy state and the care plan cannot be clearly developed. Thus, this approach should not be routinely used.[44,45]

Writing the Diagnostic Statement

There are several guidelines that should be remembered when writing the diagnostic statement to enhance the descriptiveness, usefulness and specificity of the diagnosis.[46–48] Nurses should occasionally refer to the following guidelines to improve their diagnostic skills after generating the list of nursing diagnoses for a specific client:

- Write the dignosis as a nursing, rather than a medical, diagnosis.
  - Incorrect: Congestive heart failure.
  - Correct: Decreased cardiac output related to mechanical factors (preload, afterload, or inotropic state of the heart).[49,50]
- Write the diagnosis as a problem (or health maintenance pattern) rather than as a client need.
  - Incorrect: Need for maintenance of nutritional intake.

Correct: Alteration in nutritional intake (less than body requirements) related to nausea and vomiting.[51,52]

- Write unrelated problems in separate diagnostic statements. Two or more unrelated problems should not be written in one diagnostic statement even if the etiology of the problems is the same. Unrelated problems are defined as those problems that require separate interventions.

  Incorrect: Anxiety and activity intolerance related to frequent episodes of chest pain.

  Correct: Anxiety related to frequent episodes of chest pain.
  Activity intolerance related to frequent episodes of chest pain.[53,54]

- Check to be sure that the problem is written in the first main clause and the etiology is written in the second clause. Occasionally, the problem and etiology are incorrectly reversed.

  Incorrect: Knowledge deficit about hypertensive medication related to noncompliance with daily medication regimen.

  Correct: Noncompliance with daily medication regimen related to insufficient understanding of illness.[55,56]

- Write the diagnostic statement with sufficient clarity and detail to specifically direct the plan of care.

  Incorrect: Potential vascular complications related to therapy.

  Correct: Potential infective or phlebotic vascular complications related to prolonged intravenous therapy.[57,58]

- Write the diagnostic statement so that the problem and etiology do not say the same thing.

  Incorrect: Self-feeding deficit related to inability to feed self.

  Correct: Self-feeding deficit related to activity intolerance.

- Write the diagnostic statement to avoid legal implications.

  Incorrect: Noncompliance to hypertensive medical regimen related to lack of health teaching (implies negligence of health team and intimates that no teaching was done).

  Correct: Noncompliance to hypertensive medical regimen related to inability to perceive seriousness of illness.

- Write the first main clause to reflect an actual or potential problem rather than an environmental problem. Environmental factors are stated in the second clause.

  Incorrect: Excessive environmental stimuli related to monitoring equipment.

  Correct: Auditory and visual sensory and perceptual overload related to excessive environmental stimuli.[59,60]

- It is also important that the diagnostic statement not be expressed in judgmental terms that might tend to label the client (e.g., labels such as irresponsible or uncooperative). Remember not to formulate a nursing diagnosis that is unrealistic for the client or one that should not or cannot be corrected (e.g., depression related to recent death of spouse). Abbreviations and specialized jargon should be avoided to reduce confusion and improve communication.[61,62] When abbreviations are used, it is common practice to first define them and thereafter to use the abbreviations (e.g., coronary artery bypass graft [CABG] surgery).

Table 8–2 lists guidelines that will be helpful when formulating nursing diagnosis.

Case Study

Mr. S.P., a 50-year-old man, was admitted to the coronary care unit with the chief complaint of chest pain without radiation. The pain began the evening before his admission, lasted for 15 to 20 minutes, and was associated with nausea and shortness of breath. Mr. P. said that he had no previous history of chest pain. He complained also of chills, fatigue, headache, and a poor appetite that he called "flulike" symptoms that began two weeks prior to admission.

TABLE 8-2. HOW TO BEGIN USING NURSING DIAGNOSES

Carry a list of the accepted nursing diagnoses (Table 8-1) for several weeks.

Before formulating nursing diagnoses, perform a complete biopsychosocial assessment on the client early in the shift. Be sure to review the history and physical examination, laboratory data, medical and nursing orders, and the previous 24 to 48 hour nurses' and progress notes.

Following the base-line assessment, analyze and synthesize the data to formulate the tentative nursing diagnosis.

Refer to the published lists of signs and symptoms (if available) to determine whether the observed signs and symptoms actually confirm the existence of the diagnosis.

Refer to the accepted list of nursing diagnoses when formulating and wording the diagnostic statement. Because the accepted list is worded in a new way to standardize terminology and enhance efficiency, it is important to use the correct wording whenever possible.

Write down the diagnostic statement(s) in the client's care plan.

If an identified nursing diagnosis is not on the accepted list, then word the problem clearly, identify the probable cause, and write down the diagnostic statement.

Identify the client outcomes and nursing orders (plan) for each nursing diagnosis.

When giving care, refer to each nursing diagnosis, implement the nursing orders, and evaluate the client outcomes.

Throughout the day, reevaluate and reassess each nursing diagnosis and related plan to determine if it is appropriate or is in need of revision.

Refer to each nursing diagnosis when developing and giving client or health-team conferences.

Use each nursing diagnosis as a guide when doing client charting.

Use each nursing diagnosis as the basis for giving end-of-shift reports.

Mr. P. had rheumatic fever as a child and subsequently developed a mitral regurgitation heart murmur. One and a half months prior to his admission, he had an abscessed tooth extracted. He did not receive prophylactic antibiotic medication before or after the extraction.

Mr. P.'s profile and social history revealed a well developed, 5' 10", 165-pound man who was married, with two teen-age daughters living at home. He was highly anxious during the assessment, talking constantly during the interview and jumping from one topic of conversation to another without any purposeful intent. Mr. P.'s past medical and family history were unremarkable.

Upon examination, Mr. P.'s temperature was 100.4°F orally, apical pulse was 110 beats per minute, respirations were 16 per minute and the blood pressure was 126/80 mm Hg. He was pale, and his skin was warm and dry with good tissue turgor. His temporal and jaw muscles were tensed throughout the examination. Motor and sensory functions and reflexes were normal. Bilateral conjunctival petechiae were noted and a 2-mm Roth spot with a surrounding hemorrhagic zone was seen in the right fundus at 2:00. Mr. P. had poor oral hygiene. The chest was normal in contour and symmetry. Bilateral rhonchi that cleared with coughing were heard. A left ventricular heave was palpated at the fifth left-intercostal space, midclavicular line. The apical pulse was regular, with normal first and second heart sounds. No third or fourth heart sounds or rubs were heard. A grade 3/6 holosystolic murmur was heard at the lower left sternal border with radiation to the left axilla. The client had normal bilateral arterial pulses. No splinter hemorrhages were noted on the distal nail beds. No edema, clubbing, pain, swelling or inflammation of the joints was noted. After a diagnostic workup and positive blood culture studies for *Streptococcus viridans,* the diagnosis of subacute infective endocarditis was made. Mr. P. was treated with a 28-day course of continuous intravenous penicillin. The initial nursing diagnoses written on Mr. P.'s care plan were as follows:

- Anxiety related to illness state and potential lengthy hospitalization.
- Decreased cardiac output related to mitral valve infection.
- Potential hazards of impaired physical mobility related to imposed restricted activities.

Experience of the nurse in the specialty area of cardiovascular nursing led to the following additional nursing diagnoses.

- Potential infective or phlebotic vascular complications related to prolonged intravenous therapy.

• Potential hazard of valve reinfection related to inadequate knowledge about prophylactic endocarditis therapy.[63]

SUMMARY

Nursing diagnosis is the diagnostic phase of the nursing process. The framework for formulating nursing diagnoses has been evolving for over ten years. One group, NANDA, has developed a taxonomy of nursing diagnoses and formulated a series of steps known as the problem-etiology-signs-and-symptoms (P-E-S) format to facilitate the nursing diagnostic process. Other authors and nurse leaders have developed their own interpretations of nursing diagnosis terminology and the nursing diagnostic process.

Nursing diagnoses are formulated from the nursing assessment. According to the P-E-S format, a problem or list of problems is identified from the analysis of signs and symptoms. Problems may be actual or potential but must be amenable to treatment within the educational and legal bounds of professional nursing intervention. The etiology is the identified probable source or cause of the problem. The diagnostic statement can be written once the problem and its etiology have been identified. This statement is simply the problem and the etiology written concisely with the words "related to" in between.

The concept of nursing diagnosis is relatively new, and not all practicing nurses are yet accustomed to formulating diagnoses. Among those nurses and institutions who do use the concept, some have developed their own nursing diagnosis definitions and others use the NANDA terminology or a combination of both. The growing interest in using nursing diagnosis as an essential component of the nursing process is an important step in the advancement of nursing as a profession and a science. It is a positive movement that can further define the domain of nursing care and ensure the highest quality of care for clients.

Study Questions

1. What is the difference between a medical and a nursing diagnosis?

2. Why is the nursing diagnosis movement important in advancing nursing practice?

3. How does a new nursing diagnosis get on the "accepted list of nursing diagnoses"?

4. What are the steps involved in the nursing diagnostic process?

5. What parts are included in the diagnostic statement?

6. What are two acceptable approaches to writing the diagnostic statement?

7. What steps should nurses incorporate when beginning to use nursing diagnoses in the clinical setting?

References

1. M. Gordon, "Nursing diagnosis and diagnostic process," *Am J Nurs* 76, (1976): 1298.
2. C.E. Guzzetta and B.M. Dossey, "A holistic approach to nursing diagnosis," in C.E. Guzzetta and B.M. Dossey, eds., *Cardiovascular Nursing: Bodymind Tapestry* (St. Louis: C. V. Mosby Co., 1984).
3. C.E. Guzzetta and B.M. Dossey, "Nursing diagnosis: Framework-process-problems," *Heart Lung* 12, (May 1983):281.
4. H. Yura and M.B. Walsh, *The Nursing Process: Assessing, Planning, Implementing Evaluating,* 4th ed. (New York: Appleton-Century-Crofts, 1983).
5. American Nurses' Association, Congress for Nursing Practice, *Nursing: A Social Policy Statement* (Kansas City, Mo.: American Nurses' Association, 1980).
6. American Nurses' Association Division on Medical-Surgical Nursing Practice and American Heart Association Council on Cardiovascular Nursing, *Standards of Cardiovascular Nursing Practice* (Kansas City, Mo.: American Nurses' Association, 1981).

7. American Association of Critical Care Nurses, *Standards for Nursing Care of the Critically Ill,* (Reston, Va.: Reston Publishing Co., 1981).

8. M.J. Kim, G.K. McFarland, and A.M. McLane, *Classification of Nursing Diagnoses: Proceedings of the Fifth National Conference* (St. Louis: C.V. Mosby Co., 1984).

9. American Nurses' Association, Congress for Nursing Practice, *Nursing: A Social Policy Statement.*

10. C.V. Kenner, C.E. Guzzetta, and B.M. Dossey, *Critical Care Nursing: Body-Mind-Spirit,* 2nd ed. (Boston: Little, Brown & Co., 1985).

11. M.E. Hurley, (ed.), *Classification of Nursing Diagnoses: Proceedings of the Sixth Conference* (St. Louis: C.V. Mosby Co., 1986).

12. M.J. Kim and D.A. Moritz, *Classification of Nursing Diagnoses: Proceedings from the Third and Fourth National Conferences* (New York: McGraw-Hill Book Co., 1982).

13. Hurley, *Classification of Nursing Diagnoses.*

14. Kim and Moritz, *Classification of Nursing Diagnoses.*

15. M.D. Mundinger, and G. Jauron, "Developing a nursing diagnosis," *Nurs Outlook* 23, (February 1975):94.

16. Kim and Moritz, *Classification of Nursing Diagnoses.*

17. C.E. Guzzetta and B.M. Dossey, *Cardiovascular Nursing: Bodymind Tapestry* (St. Louis: C.V. Mosby Co., 1984).

18. Kim, Mc Farland, and McLane, *Classification of Nursing Diagnoses.*

19. Hurley, *Classification of Nursing Diagnoses.*

20. Guzzetta and Dossey, "Nursing diagnosis: Framework-process-problems."

21. Kim and Moritz, *Classification of Nursing Diagnoses.*

22. M. Gordon, *Manual of Nursing Diagnoses* (New York: McGraw-Hill Book Co., 1982).

23. Kim, McFarland, and McLane, *Classification of Nursing Diagnoses.*

24. M.J. Kim, G.K. McFarland, and A.M. McLane, *Pocket Guide to Nursing Diagnoses* (St. Louis: C.V. Mosby Co., 1984).

25. Gordon, *Manual of Nursing Diagnoses.*

26. Kim, McFarland, and McLane, *Classification of Nursing Diagnoses.*

27. Kim, McFarland, and McLane, *Pocket Guide to Nursing Diagnoses.*

28. N.L Lengel, *Handbook of Nursing Diagnoses* (Bowie, Md.: Robert J. Brady Co., 1982).

29. J. Carlson; C. Craft, and A. McGuire, *Nursing Diagnoses* (Philadelphia: W.B. Saunders Co., 1982).

30. C.J. Gleit, and S. Tatro, "Nursing diagnoses for healthy individuals," *Nurs Health Care* 11, (1981):456.

31. M. Gordon, *Nursing Diagnoses: Process and Application* (New York: McGraw-Hill Book Co., 1982).

32. Guzzetta and Dossey, "Nursing diagnosis: Framework-process-problems."

33. Kim and Moritz, *Classification of Nursing Diagnoses.*

34. Lengel, *Handbook of Nursing Diagnosis.*

35. Guzzetta and Dossey, "Nursing diagnosis: Framework-process-problems."

36. Guzzetta and Dossey, "A holistic approach to nursing diagnosis."

37. Ibid.

38. Guzzetta and Dossey, "Nursing diagnosis: Framework-process-problems."

39. Ibid.

40. Guzzetta and Dossey "A holistic approach to nursing diagnosis."

41. Ibid.

42. Guzzetta and Dossey, "Nursing diagnosis: Framework-process-problems."

43. C.J. Gleit, and S. Tatro, "Nursing Diagnosis," *Nurs Health Care,* 1982.

44. Guzzetta and Dossey, "Nursing diagnosis: Framework-process-problems."

45. Guzzetta and Dossey, "A holistic approach to nursing diagnosis."

46. J. Carlson, C. Craft, and A. McGuire, *Nursing Diagnoses* (Philadelphia: W.B. Saunders Co., 1982).

47. Mundinger and Jauron, "Developing a nursing diagnosis."

48. Price, M.R., "Nursing dignosis: Making a concept come alive," *Am J Nurs* 80 (April 1980):668.

49. Guzzetta and Dossey, "Nursing diagnosis: Framework-process-problems."

50. Guzzetta and Dossey, "A holistic approach to nursing diagnosis."

51. Ibid.

52. Guzzetta and Dossey, "Nursing diagnosis: Framework-process-problems."

53. Ibid.

54. Guzzetta and Dossey, "A holistic approach to nursing diagnosis."

55. Ibid.

56. Guzzetta and Dossey, "Nursing diagnosis: Framework-process-problems."

57. Ibid.

58. Guzzetta and Dossey, "A holistic approach to nursing diagnosis."

59. Ibid.

60. Guzzetta and Dossey, "Nursing diagnosis: Framework-process-problems."

61. Ibid.
62. Guzzetta and Dossey, "A holistic approach to nursing diagnosis."
63. C.E. Guzzetta, "Acute and subacute infective endocarditis," in C.V. Kenner, C.E. Guzzetta, and B.M. Dossey, *Critical Care Nursing: Body-Mind-Spirit,* 2nd ed. (Boston: Little, Brown & Co., 1985).

Annotated Bibliography

Dossey, B.M., and Guzzetta, C.E.: 1981. "Nursing diagnosis." *Nurs '81* 11 (June):34–38. This article discusses how to begin using nursing diagnoses and how to use the diagnostic language effectively. A care plan and a case study illustrate the use of nursing diagnoses, client outcomes, and nursing orders.

Gordon, M. 1982. *Manual of Nursing Diagnosis.* New York: McGraw-Hill. This book provides a quick reference of the nursing diagnoses based on the work of the North American Nursing Diagnosis Association. This pocket guide can serve as a ready reference for nurses in the clinical area.

Gordon, M., Sweeney, M.A., and McKeehank K. 1980. "Nursing diagnosis: Looking at its use in the clinical area." *Am J Nurs* 80(April):672–74. Gordon reports the use of nursing diagnosis in a clinical setting. Recommendations are made for standardizing nursing diagnoses.

Guzzetta, C.E., and Dossey, B.M. 1983. "Nursing diagnosis: Framework-process-problems." *Heart Lung* 12 (May):281–91. The current status of nursing diagnosis is discussed in this article. Problems and solutions to using the nursing diagnostic process are offered. A detailed case study and care plan using nursing diagnoses are included.

Hurley, M.E. (ed.). 1986. *Classification of Nursing Diagnoses: Proceedings of the Sixth Conference.* St. Louis: C.V. Mosby. This book presents an overview of the Sixth National Conference on Nursing Diagnoses, held in April, 1984, in St. Louis. It includes the results of several research studies aimed at validating specific nursing diagnoses.

Kim, M.J., McFarland, G.K., and McLane, A.M. 1984. *Classification of Nursing Diagnoses: Proceedings from the Fifth National Conference.* St. Louis: C.V. Mosby. This book presents an overview of the Fifth National Conference on nursing diagnoses. It also contains an extensive annotated bibliography that familiarizes nurses with the literature describing the signs and symptoms of selected nursing diagnoses.

Kim, M.J., and Moritz, D.A. 1982. *Classification of Nursing Diagnoses: Proceedings from the Third and Fourth National Conferences.* New York: McGraw-Hill. This book presents an overview of the National Nursing Diagnoses Conferences held in 1978 and 1980. The book also contains an extensive annotated bibliography on nursing diagnoses articles.

Porter, E.J. 1986. "Critical analysis of NANDA nursing diagnosis taxonomy I," *Image* 18 (Winter): 136–37. The author of this article analyzes the NANDA nursing diagnoses taxonomy in relation to taxonomy in general and its application to nursing practice.

Chapter 9

Health Assessment

M. Gaie Rubenfeld
Elizabeth A. McFarlane

Chapter Outline

- Objectives
- Glossary
- Introduction
- Health Assessment: A Nursing Perspective
    A Framework for Health Assessment
    The Nurse and Other Health-care Providers
- Human Resources for Health Assessment
    The Nurse
    The Client
    Other Health-care Providers
- Techniques of Data Collection
    Interviewing
    Observation
    Measurement
- Dimensions of Health Assessment:
  Data Collection
    Physiological Dimension
    Psychological Dimension
    Sociocultural Dimension
    Spiritual Dimension
- Special Considerations: Developmental Level
- Summary
- Study Questions
- References
- Annotated Bibliography

Objectives

At the completion of this chapter the reader will be able to:

▶ Define the terms in the glossary
▶ Describe a nursing framework that may be used to guide health assessment
▶ Contrast the roles of the nurse, the client, and other health-care providers in assessing health
▶ Describe the data collection techniques of interviewing, observation, and measurement
▶ Use data collection techniques to assess the client's responses within the physiological, psychological, sociocultural, and spiritual dimensions
▶ Consider the impact of the client's developmental level on responses to actual or potential health problems

Glossary

Aeration. A vital life function of oxygen and carbon dioxide exchange.

Assessment. The collection and analysis of client data or information leading to the derivation of nursing diagnosis.

Body Maintenance. The restoration and regulation of a balance of functions achieved by the body and by the individual on behalf of the body.

Circulation. The transport of nutrients, oxygen, chemicals, and hormones and the removal of waste products and carbon dioxide from body tissues.

Cognitive Ability. A composite of a person's capacity to learn, to remember, and to understand.

Elimination. The output of waste products and indigestible materials from the body.

Emotional Status. The overt and covert feelings a person experiences and expresses in verbal and nonverbal communication.

Health-care Practices. Those activities engaged in primarily for the purpose of attaining or maintaining health.

Interviewing. A technique of data collection; a formal or informal process for the purpose of obtaining verbal information about the client's current or past responses to actual or potential health problems.

Life-style. The usual living circumstances and activities in which a person engages.

Measurement. A technique of data collection; the use of a standard to determine capacity or extent of structures or functions.

Nursing. "The diagnosis and treatment of human responses to actual or potential health problems."*

Nutrition. The intake, assimilation, and use of food for energy, maintenance, and growth of the body.

Observation. A technique of data collection; an identification of the client's physical and behavioral responses by looking or reviewing.

Physiological Dimension. The human dimension reflected in a person's biological response to alterations in the body's structure and functions.

Psychological Dimension. The human dimension reflected in a person's cognitive and emotional responses to the self and the environment.

Rest and Activity. The periods that constitute patterns of repose or rejuvenation of the body and those of movement or exertion.

Sensation. The primary means by which a person receives input from the environment.

---

*American Nurses' Association. *Nursing: A Social Policy Statement.* Kansas City, Mo.: American Nurses' Association, 1980.

Sexuality. A pervasive life-force that includes a person's total feelings, attitudes, behavior, and beliefs that relate to being male or female.

Sociocultural Dimension. The human dimension reflected in a person's noninherited intrapersonal and interpersonal responses to socialization practices learned and transmitted from families and communities.

Spiritual Dimension. The human dimension reflected in a person's personal response to inspirational forces.

Support Networks. Family members and significant persons who provide emotional, physical, or financial support to an individual.

INTRODUCTION

The term health assessment has different meanings to different people. To some, health assessment means an examination of the body's biological systems, to others it may imply health screening for the purpose of detecting a physical impairment, such as hypertension. To the nurse, the term health assessment is more comprehensive—a systematic and continuous collection of data related to a person's health state and the person's response to that health state.

This chapter presents health assessment from a nursing perspective and provides a framework to guide the collection of data. The focus of the nurse when doing a health assessment is contrasted with the focus of other health-care professionals. Ability to apply a framework that ensures a nursing focus and knowledge of the techniques of assessment are skills that are fundamental to a comprehensive health assessment performed by a nurse.

HEALTH ASSESSMENT: A NURSING PERSPECTIVE

A Framework for Health Assessment
The nursing process provides the nurse with direction in the provision of nursing care that will assist a client in attaining, regaining, or maintaining optimal health status. **Assessment,** the first phase of the nursing process, encompasses the collection and analysis of data or informa-

tion leading to the derivation of nursing diagnoses. The assessment phase can be described as the power, or energy source, of the process. If the collection of data does not contribute to the identification of actual or potential problems that are amenable to nursing intervention, the planning, implementation, and evaluation phases of the process cannot be put into operation.

The nurse must be concerned with collecting and analyzing client data that will assist in maintaining a nursing focus in the planning and implementation of client care. A nursing focus evolves from awareness and understanding of the purpose of nursing. This purpose is clearly described in the American Nurses' Association's publication *Nursing: A Social Policy Statement,* in which **nursing** is defined as "the diagnosis and treatment of human responses to actual or potential health problems."[1] This definition directs the nurse to collect information about the client that will assist in identifying the response to actual or potential health problems. A comprehensive health assessment provides data that, on analysis, reflect response patterns related to the client's ability to perform activities contributing to the fulfillment of needs. Patterns of response that indicate that the client is unable to take independent actions to fulfill physiological, psychological, sociocultural, and spiritual needs signal a need for nursing care.

The complex nature of the human being, the intricate relationship among needs, and the way those needs are fulfilled lends complexity to the process of health assessment. When a complex phenomenon such as a human being is being analyzed, examined, or assessed, an attempt is made to identify, isolate, and study the parts of the whole. Yet understanding of the whole, how and why it responds as it does, is dependent on the integration of the parts.

The nature of the human, the integration of physiological, psychological, sociocultural, and spiritual dimensions, implies that responses to a health problem cannot be restricted to one dimension. Thus, when the nurse gathers data to determine a client's responses to real or potential health problems, the assessment cannot be limited to one dimension. Because growth or disruption in one dimension has consequences

for the others, the nurse must expand the focus to include all dimensions. The focus of health assessment is presented in Figure 9–1. The wholeness of the human is represented by the circle. The segmented lines separating each dimension within the circle suggest that the dimensions are not separate entities, but rather integrated facets of the human person.

While acknowledging the wholeness and integration of the person, the dimensions provide the means for the nurse to approach the health assessment of the client in an organized manner. The nurse collects data or information relative to each dimension to determine patterns. Each dimension of the person is reflected in the responses. The nurse assesses these through interviews, observation, and measurement. During the health assessment, the nurse evaluates the client's responses in terms of the impact the health problem has had. It is, therefore, important for the nurse to determine if an actual or potential health problem has changed the manner in which the client usually responds.

Health assessment by the nurse should include the collection of data related to physiological, psychological, sociocultural, and spiritual responses of the client to a health problem.

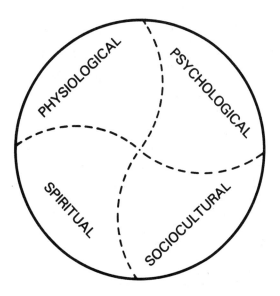

Figure 9–1. The dimensions of the human person.

Analysis of these data will lead to identification of response patterns. If the patterns indicate that the client cannot independently perform activities contributing to the fulfillment of his or her needs, a nursing diagnosis is made, and the planning phase of the nursing process begins.

The four dimensions of human beings are described as follows:

- **Physiological dimension:** Reflected in a person's biological response to alterations in the body's structure and functions
- **Psychological dimension:** Reflected in a person's cognitive and emotional responses to the self and the environment
- **Sociocultural dimension:** Reflected in a person's noninherited intra- and interpersonal responses to socialization practices learned and transmitted from families and communities
- **Spiritual dimension:** Reflected in a person's personal response to inspirational forces

The Nurse and Other Health-care Providers

The focus on the physiological, psychological, sociocultural, and spiritual responses of the client to actual or potential health problems distinguishes the health assessment performed by the nurse from assessments performed by other members of the health team. Although the data collected by the various members of the health team may overlap, each member assesses the client with a different purpose in mind. This purpose defines and gives direction to the assessments made by other health-care providers, such as physicians, nutritionists, dentists, social workers, and psychologists.

Physicians assess health to determine whether or not a pathology exists and how a client is progressing in recovery from that pathology. The focus is primarily on the physiological health of the client. Depending on the area of specialization, a physician may be more concerned with one part of a client's body than with another. Nutritionists are concerned with a person's health as it relates to dietary patterns. Dentists assess a person's health as it relates to the mouth and teeth. Nutritionists and dentists focus on physiological health. Psychologists are concerned with a person's mental status and emotional development and therefore focus on psychological health.

If we use a person with diabetes as an example, the differences in purpose or focus of the various members of the health team become more apparent. A physician diagnoses the pathology, diabetes, by assessing the client's physical health, including blood glucose levels. A nutritionist assesses the client's dietary intake to determine what changes need to be made to decrease the glucose levels. A dentist assesses the person's mouth and teeth to determine the presence of infections or potential infections, knowing that in a diabetic person infections occur frequently and are detrimental to the person's health. A psychologist might assess the person's emotional state as he or she attempts to cope with the chronic illness. The social worker assesses, among other things, the person's financial ability to afford the prescribed treatments and uses that information to assist the client, if necessary, to secure financial assistance.

The nurse is interested in the person's total response to the health problem of diabetes. The nurse assesses the client's physical responses: an indication of a loss or gain in weight; condition of skin, especially at insulin injection sites; condition of feet; and changes in vision. The nurse assesses the client's psychological responses, such as emotional responses to having diabetes or the amount of psychological stress he or she experiences (emotional stress can cause an increase in the body's glucose level). The nurse assesses the client's sociocultural responses: the presence or absence of an effective support system and how the support system influences the client's response to treatment; adherence to social and ethnic dietary patterns that might be inconsistent with a diabetic diet; or language differences that might create misunderstandings about the prescribed treatment. The nurse assesses the client's spiritual responses, the meaning he or she attaches to his or her illness, or religious practices that impinge on receiving health care. Each of these dimensions—physiological, psychological, sociocultural, and spiritual—are reflected in the client's responses to the health problem, diabetes.

HUMAN RESOURCES FOR HEALTH ASSESSMENT

The outcome of the health assessment, its comprehensive nature and quality, is dependent on many factors. The level of the nurse's intellectual, interpersonal, and technical skills affect the breadth and depth of the assessment and therefore the validity of the nursing diagnoses. Sources available for data collection determine the quality of the information found. If the client is conscious and responsive, assessment of the physiological dimension is less complex in terms of searching for information related to health history and usual physiological responses. Availability of family members or other significant persons as sources of information becomes crucial when the client cannot provide the needed data. Other health-care providers and their assessments can provide additional perspectives from which the nurse can supplement or verify information that has been gathered.

The Nurse

The nurse's expertise in doing health assessments is primarily dependent on the level of intellectual, interpersonal, and technical skills. Knowledge and understanding of what constitutes adaptive and maladaptive responses to health problems are essential for decision making about the need for further exploration of the dimensions. The ability and ease with which the nurse can establish supportive relationships with clients, family members, and other health-care providers influences the quality and validity of the data collected as well as the opportunities available for collection and verification of data. The nurse's knowledge of and ability to apply the technical skills used in health assessment determine the nature of the data collected. Effective use of the techniques of observation, interview, and measurement in client assessment is required if the assessment is to be more than the gathering of overt signs and symptoms.

The Client

The client's developmental level, physical condition, and intellectual and emotional status determine the information he or she can provide during the interview and his or her ability to validate the nurse's findings. If able and willing, the client assumes an active role throughout the health assessment, providing information during the interview and cooperating when the nurse uses observation and measurement techniques in assessing quantitative responses. The client will be more willing to assume this role if the nurse is able to ensure physical and emotional comfort during the assessment. If the client is unable to provide information and validate findings, the family and other significant persons become primary sources of information about the client's health history and the impact the health problem has had on the usual manner of responding to needs.

Other Health-care Providers

Although the health assessment is viewed as a complex process for the nurse, the client can experience complexity in terms of the number of health-care professionals who interview, examine, and continually observe him or her. Each health-care institution adopts specific forms that must be completed for each client and retained in the client's record. Much of this information overlaps, and the client is interviewed and examined repeatedly.

The nurse may use the data gathered by other health-care providers if it can be validated. This will eliminate some discomfort the individual experiences from repetitious assessments. Members of the health-care team should seek to identify ways to contribute data that support the focus of other health-care professionals. The physical assessment made by the physician, the dietary assessment made by the nutritionist, and the emotional assessment made by the psychologist provide data and findings that can be essential to the nurse's assessment of the client's responses to health problems. Likewise, the nurse can provide information and findings supportive of health assessments made by other health-care professionals.

Data from the client and family, and the ability to use other health-care professionals as resources add to the breadth and depth of the assessment process and influence the validity of findings. Therefore, the nurse should use all the resources that contribute to a comprehensive health assessment.

TECHNIQUES OF DATA COLLECTION

Interviewing, observation and **measurement** are three techniques used to provide the means to gather information related to the client's physiological, psychological, sociocultural, and spiritual dimensions. Although it is essential to use the three techniques throughout assessment, the types of responses reflected in each dimension determine the extent to which the nurse can use each technique. Physiological responses can best be assessed through measurement, complemented by interviews and observation. Information related to the client's psychological, sociocultural, and spiritual dimensions is collected primarily through interview and observation and may be supplemented by measurement.

Interviewing

Through interviewing, the nurse collects data relevant to the client's general health history, as well as perceptions of his or her present health status. A thorough knowledge of therapeutic communication techniques is necessary to be an effective interviewer. The nurse must maintain an open approach to the client so that the client will feel free to respond fully to the questions asked. Although a set of guidelines to organize questions is helpful, the nurse must take cues from the client and ask additional questions in areas where gaps appear to exist. The most helpful guidelines, therefore, give broad cues for questions. If the client's response to those broad questions indicates a problem area, then the nurse must branch into more specific inquiries and allow the client to relate necessary details. For example, if the client says yes, he or she has discomfort, the nurse must ask where it is, how long it has existed, the nature of the discomfort, and what the client has been doing to alleviate it.

Information acquired during an interview can provide the nurse with adequate data by which a client's responses to an actual or potential health-care problem can be identified or it may provide only clues. In either case, the nurse supplements the interview with other assessment techniques. Observation and measurement could be employed to assist in verifying findings or to gather additional data to follow up clues received during the interview.

The interview can be either formal or informal. When the client enters the health-care system, a formal or structured interview is needed, in which the nurse gathers information that could be essential in determining the client's medical and nursing care. A person's allergies to foods or medicines and usual diet, including sociocultural preferences and religious restrictions, are examples of factors that must be known when planning care. Therefore, factors such as these should be identified early in the client's encounter with the health-care system.

Interviews of a less formal nature are appropriate and necessary for the ongoing, comprehensive assessment that is required throughout the nurse–client relationship. It often takes time for the client to feel comfortable enough to reveal information of a personal nature. Here is an example of a situation in which a less structured interview might occur: A nurse is instructing a client on diet when the client changes the subject and expresses fear about an anticipated diagnostic test. The nurse can use this cue to make further inquiries about the client's feelings toward the health problem and the required tests and therapy.

Another example is the nurse's use of the time when giving a bath to ask the client questions about his skin. Because the skin is observable during that time, questions can be more specific to what is being seen. The client may have a scar on his or her back to which the nurse can refer; in a more formal situation, the client may forget that he had had surgery there for the removal of a mole. That piece of information may be an important determinant of whether the nurse further assesses other moles on the client's body.

These examples also illustrate the importance of questioning the client about past health. Historical questions allow the nurse to see patterns of responses, to identify risk factors caused by cumulative conditions, and to understand the client's previous coping mechanisms, which may be of value or detrimental to the present condition.

Likewise, questions about the client's family health history will give the nurse clues about possible risk factors for illness in the client. If the nurse knows that a client's parents both died at a young age from heart disease, the nurse will know that the client's circulatory status should be given extra consideration during the assessment.

Observation

Observation is the second data collection technique. Primarily, this means the nurse must be alert, seeing the subtle as well as the obvious aspects of the client's behavior. The nurse must observe the client's nonverbal communication while listening to the verbal. This is especially important in collecting data on the client's psychological dimension, which may be difficult for the client to describe in words. Likewise, observing a client's interaction with the family may provide more information than questioning the client about significant relationships. With observation, however, the nurse must guard against jumping to conclusions. Whenever possible, validate nonverbal behaviors with additional questioning.

Accurate observation is often dependent on the setting of the nurse–client encounter. A darkened room may help the nurse assess pupillary reactions, but it will be a disadvantage when looking at a skin lesion. A chilly room may make a client clench teeth and hands, which may be wrongly interpreted by the nurse as a symbol of anger or withdrawal.

There are many tools that aid the nurse in observation. Most essential are the senses of sight and hearing. These senses alone may be used when observing physiological responses, such as rate, rhythm, and depth of respirations, and are essential when observing the client's psychological, sociocultural, and spiritual responses.

Instruments may be used to enhance observations. A flashlight will illuminate a specific area; a tongue depressor may hold the tongue down so that the throat can be seen; a nasal speculum will allow the visualization of the posterior parts of the nose. Likewise, the nurse–client positions will contribute to optimal observations. A nurse must move around to get into the optimal position for observation.

Above all, the nurse must not be afraid to spend time just looking at something. At times, scheduling pressures and demands made by peers or other clients may tempt the nurse to only glance at some aspect of the client that should be studied carefully. Such actions may have grave consequences. Important signs may be overlooked. However, as with other assessment techniques, practice yields precision of observations in less time.

Measurement

Measurement, the third data collection technique, is the most objective and often the most precise method of assessment. Measurement implies that some kind of standard is used to determine the dimensions, capacity, or extent of something. The standards that are used are as varied and complex as the human body that is being measured. Some structures and functions of the body may be precisely measured quite easily; others can only be measured against a general, nonspecific standard. Therefore, standards may be seen as a continuum of precision, one end having exact measurements and the other less differentiated gauges.

Measurement has two components—one is the standard of the measuring device or instrument used, the other is the significance of those measurements against a standard of the body's expected range of responses. Each of these components has a continuum of precision. An instrument such as a ruler, tape measure, sphygmomanometer, caliper, or thermometer gives numeric readings that may be compared to precise numeric ranges of normal. Other instruments are indirect measuring devices that allow the examiner to touch, feel, or hear things that then are compared to less distinct ranges of normal. These instruments do not give the examiner a nominal value, as such, and some judgment is required to make the measurements. Such an instrument may be a percussion hammer, which, when struck against a tendon, may elicit a reflex that then is judged to be absent, weak, strong, or hyperreflexive. Another example is a stethoscope, which can be used to auscultate respiratory sounds that then are compared to a range of normal sounds known by the examiner.

When assessing the client's physiological responses, parts of the examiner's body become the indirect instrument of measurement. Palpation of a client's body allows the examiner to feel with the hands specific organs, muscles, or bones that are not directly measurable with recording devices, such as a tape measure. The amount of mass felt by the hands or fingers is calculated through the examiner's knowledge of sizes within a normal range.

Some precise measuring devices normally are not used as often by nurses as they are by physicians and other health-care professionals. Examples are x-rays or measurements that require invasive techniques, such as surgery, or the extraction of blood or body fluids. Although nurses usually do not initiate such measurements, they do, however, have access to reports of these measurements and should use them whenever they would aid in making nursing diagnoses.

Measurements that guide the nurse in assessing physiological responses are more abundant and precise than those available when measuring psychological, sociocultural, and spiritual responses. Although a variety of inventories, scales, and tests have been developed to measure a client's intelligence, emotional status, and socioeconomic status, these usually are ordered, administered, and interpreted by a psychiatrist or psychologist.

DIMENSIONS OF HEALTH ASSESSMENT: DATA COLLECTION

The nurse must use a framework to organize and guide data collection. Using the dimensions of the human being as a framework, the nurse is assisted in maintaining a nursing focus to diagnose and treat the client's responses to actual or potential health problems. While the holistic nature of the human person is recognized, each dimension and its specific parameters for assessment are addressed separately in this section. This is done in an attempt to provide the reader with an assessment guide that will contribute to the systematic and comprehensive collection of data. These dimensions are interrelated, however, and responses reflective of one dimension may have an impact on other dimensions.

Guidelines for data collection within each dimension and parameters for assessment of data are presented on the following pages. For each parameter, a set of cues for interview, ob-

servation, and measurement are given in table format. Within each dimension, the cues are guidelines for first-level data collection; many additional areas could be assessed, some needing more complicated procedures than appropriate for discussion in this chapter. Numerous texts on assessment can aid the reader in developing additional skills in other data collection techniques. If abnormal or maladaptive responses are found, the nurse should assess further or refer the client to another health-care provider for additional data collection.

The nurse must form questions based on the cues given in the interview guideline tables. Observation cues include nonvalued items that should be noted and some that indicate abnormal responses or changes that should be ruled out. The measurement cues include two parts. The first part of the cue is the item to be measured. The second part (in parentheses) is the tool or method commonly used for that measurement.

Physiological Dimension

The physiological dimension is reflected in a person's biological response to alterations in the body's structure and function. To collect data on the physiological responses of a client, the nurse first must decide what parts of the body are of highest priority in a given situation. Because of the complexity of the physiological dimension, some method of dividing the body into units is necessary. The body's physiological systems—heart, lungs, muscles, and so forth—interrelate; an action of one system affects others. The client's physiological response to a health state is dependent upon the structure and functions of these interrelated body parts. In looking for the responses, the nurse must be aware of the interrelationships.

The following parameters will provide a structure for the nurse's assessment of the physiological dimension: sensation, aeration, circulation, nutrition, elimination, rest and activity, sexuality, and body maintenance. The various anatomical and physiological functions of the body are grouped thus so that all aspects of the body can be assessed. A thorough knowledge of anatomy and physiology is a necessary prerequisite for the nurse who is assessing physiological responses. That knowledge tells the examiner what to look for, what is normal, what is abnormal, and how to describe what is found.

Sensation. **Sensation,** or the use of the senses, is the primary means by which a person receives input from the environment. The skin, eyes, ears, nose, mouth, and their related nerves allow a person to experience physical sensations to which he or she can respond. The skin receives signals about temperature, humidity, touch, pressure, and pain. It also acts as a safety barrier for the rest of the body. Eyes receive visual stimuli, ears receive sound, the nose receives odors, and the mouth distinguishes tastes.

The nervous system and especially the cranial nerves act as a transmitter of these sensations to the brain, which interprets the various signals. A special aspect of sensation is the body's recognition of pain or discomfort. Although this may or may not be directly related to one specific body part, it is included as an important component of the sensation parameter. It is through the sensation of pain or discomfort that alterations in the body's physio-logical responses are often diagnosed. The individual's level of consciousness and respon-siveness is also an important part of sensation.

Collecting information on this parameter is a logical beginning step for the nurse to take in a first-encounter assessment of a client. Guide-lines for assessment of sensation can be found in Table 9–1. Determining the level of con-sciousness, orientation, and the status of the various senses will help the nurse adapt future data collection techniques to that client's re-sponsive abilities. The client's answers to inter-view questions will predict his or her ability to accurately answer questions about other param-eters. These answers, along with the observed and measured responses, tell the nurse the client's level of hearing, sight, smell, taste, and touch, and whether or not he or she is com-fortable enough to tolerate subsequent data col-lection.

Several instruments may aid the observa-tion of certain body parts in this pattern. An ophthalmoscope may be used to see internal eye structures. This instrument can be adapted for

---

TABLE 9–1. GUIDELINES FOR ASSESSMENT OF SENSATION

Interview: Questions and Areas to Discuss

Level of consciousness: Who is the client? Where is the client? What day and time is it?

Pain or discomfort: If so, where? When did it begin? When does it occur? Description of intensity, char-acteristics, treatments tried, and results

Skin: Sensitivity changes, lesions, texture, color, dry-ness, or moisture

Vision: Corrective lenses; changes such as blurring, double vision, halos around lights, spots; changes in lacrimation

Hearing: Loss; ringing in ears

Smell: Changes in ability, nasal discharge, obstruc-tions, bleeding

Taste: Changes in sensation; unusual odors or tastes

Observation:

Level of consciousness: Awake, alert, oriented to sur-roundings

Signs of pain or discomfort: Facial expression, body movement

Skin: Color, vascularity, lesions, signs of scratching or rubbing

Vision: Squinting, excessive blinking, tearing, eye movement (lateral, vertical, and oblique), sym-metry of eyes

External eye structures: conjunctiva moist, nonirri-tated; lid closure full or partial; cornea moist and smooth

Internal eye structures: lens and vitreous clear, retinal structures intact, optic disk defined

Hearing: Hears normal voice tones; leans forward, asking for repetition of words; hearing aid

Outer ear structures: intactness, canal openess (no excessive wax or hair)

Inner ear structures: tympanic membrane intact, canal clear

Smell: Outer nasal structures: nose straight or de-viated, nares flare, discharge

Inner nasal structures: mucosa color, swelling; sep-tum condition; obstructions

Taste: Mouth lesions, breath odor, tongue condition

Measurement:

Skin lesions: Size and character (ruler)

Visual Acuity: Snellen chart

Hearing Acuity: Watch tick, whisper, tuning fork

Smell: Odorous substances

Taste: Application of salt, sugar, lemon, aspirin on parts of tongue

use as an otoscope, which allows the examiner to look into the ear canal; it also can be used as a lighted speculum to look into the nose. A full explanation of the use of these instruments is beyond the scope of this text, but a nurse can learn the mechanics of them and, with practice, will find these are valuable aids to observation of the eyes, nose, and ears.

Instruments of measurement are less complicated and may be readily usable. A simple ruler, preferably calibrated in millimeters and centimeters, allows for measurement. A Snellen chart is a commercially available wall poster commonly used to measure visual acuity. The client reads sets of letters at a distance of 20 feet from the chart, which rates levels of vision numerically. Hearing can be measured simply by holding a ticking watch next to each ear, or by the examiner whispering a phrase behind the client's back to test if it is heard. These are imprecise measurements but are valuable indicators of gross hearing problems. A tuning fork is another simple instrument that, when activated and held against a bone in the skull, can test bone-conducted hearing. It also can be held next to the ear to measure air-conducted hearing.

Smell can be measured by holding a series of distinctively odorous items under each nostril. The client with closed eyes is asked to identify each odor. Taste is similarly measured by swabbing parts of the tongue with substances that are salty, (table salt), sweet (sugar), sour (lemon), or bitter (aspirin).

Aeration. **Aeration** is a vital life function, the exchange of oxygen and carbon dioxide. The mouth, pharynx, nose, and lungs are the primary structures of this parameter. The mouth, pharynx, and nose allow air to pass to and from the lungs, which provide oxygen to the circulatory system and remove carbon dioxide.

Assessment of aeration is a very important function of the nurse. Persons who are immobilized, such as those hospitalized, have a high risk of respiratory dysfunction. Many environmental factors are hazards to respirations, and upper respiratory infections or allergies are very common. Counting respirations per minute always has been part of the assessment trio of "vital signs," that is, the TPR (temperature,

pulse, and respiration). Although the respiratory rate is vital, there are other equally important pieces of data for the nurse to collect.

Many clues to aeration responses can be gained through the simple observations and questions listed in Table 9–2. The measurement techniques are easily learned and applied. Since the lungs are on both sides of the chest cavity, many of the measurements are comparative ones to determine symmetry of functions. *Thoracic expansion* is measured by the examiner's hands being placed posteriorly over the tenth rib area; as the chest expands, the hands should rise equally on both sides. The anterior-posterior diameter of the chest can be estimated visually and compared to the lateral span, or, if indicated, can be measured with a tape measure. *Vocal fremitus* (sound vibration) is felt by the

TABLE 9–2. GUIDELINES FOR ASSESSMENT OF AERATION

Interview:
  Breathing capacity at rest and on exertion
  Allergies
  Air quality in environment
  Coughing: Frequency, type, and productivity
  Frequency of upper respiratory infections (colds)
  Smoking habits

Observation:
  Respirations: Quality and regularity, breathing with mouth or nose
  Color: Nail beds and lips
  Flaring of nostrils
  Condition of nasal mucosa, drainage, swelling
  Condition of mouth, pharynx, especially tonsillar area
  Chest movement: Symmetry, use of accessory muscles

Measurement:
  Respiratory rate: Counted and timed with watch
  Thoracic expansion: Hand measurement during inspiration
  Anterior-posterior diameter: Visual estimation or tape measure
  Symmetry of vocal fremitus: Hands—estimate symmetry
  Symmetry of intensity, pitch, and duration of percussion notes: Fingers, indirect percussion
  Diaphragmatic excursion: Percussion, ruler
  Symmetry and quality of breath sounds: Auscultation with stethoscope

examiner whose hands are placed on the chest while the client vocalizes "99"; these vibrations are compared side to side for symmetry. *Percussion notes* are sounds heard and vibrations felt when the examiner taps over a part of the body. These notes vary in intensity, pitch, or duration depending on the amount of air in the underlying structures. In measuring these notes the examiner can determine where the air-filled lungs end, that is the diaphragm position during inspiration and expiration; these, therefore, determine the *diaphragmatic excursion.* These bilateral notes also are compared and thus measure symmetry of respiratory functions.

Auscultation, or the listening to breath sounds through a stethoscope, allows for further assessment of respiratory functions. By placing the stethoscope on the chest over lung areas, the sounds of air passing into and out of the lungs can be heard, compared for symmetry on both sides, and a qualitative measurement against known ranges of normal can be determined.

Circulation. Circulation is the transport of nutrients, oxygen, chemicals, and hormones and the removal of waste products and carbon dioxide from all body tissues. The heart, blood vessels, and lymph vessels are the primary structures assessed in this parameter.

Because oxygen is a vital substance that is carried throughout the body, circulation responses are linked closely to aeration. If there is an abnormal response in aeration, it is imperative that the nurse collect data on the status of circulation and if circulation is abnormal, it is essential to assess aeration. The pulse and blood pressure are assessed by nurses in almost every client encounter. They are foremost in the measurement category of data collection in this parameter. The usual range of these measurements should also be components of questions put to the client. Questions about the condition of the legs, feet, arms, and hands are also important indicators of the circulatory status of the body.

Most of the observations of circulation are done in conjunction with measurement. Some pulsations in various parts of the body can be seen and should be observed but also should be measured through palpation so that the examiner times and counts their rates. While pulses are being palpated, measurement of their rhythm and quality should be compared to known ranges of normal and compared for bilateral symmetry. There are many locations on the body where pulses may be felt easily. In most instances, when base-line information about a client who has no actual or potential abnormalities in circulation is being collected, a radial pulse is palpated. However, if there is an indication for more precise pulse measurement, all or some of these pulses may be assessed: carotid, temporal, brachial, ulnar, femoral, popliteal, posterior tibial, and dorsalis pedis.

Venous function should be observed over all parts of the body also. Some veins are directly observable; some are not. Any venous area that can be visualized should be checked for discoloration or bulging that might indicate varicosities. The jugular veins are measured for their level of distention or amount of pressure by positioning the patient at certain angles and observing the change in the level of the characteristic pulse wave of the veins. To carry out this measurement, the nurse must study the difference between the carotid pulse and the pulse wave of the jugular vein, because the two can be confused easily.

Auscultation of the heart itself is a valuable data collection technique, allowing for assessment of the sounds and diastolic and systolic phases of the pumping heart. The apical pulse is the most accurate pulse reading, and whenever such precision is indicated, the nurse should listen at the apex of the heart and count the pulse rate there. The nurse should place the stethoscope over the aortic, pulmonic, right ventricular, and apical areas and listen with the bell and diaphragm of the stethoscope so that all ranges of sounds may be heard. With practice and study, the nurse can become more acute in assessing the heart sounds.

Palpation of lymph node areas to determine the size and consistency of these nodes is also an important measurement of circulatory status. Most lymph nodes are in the neck, axilla, and groin, and are not normally palpable. Therefore, if one is palpated, a measurement of its size and consistency is very important. Usually an approximation of size is adequate, but a ruler may be used for more accurate determination.

Finally, any area of the body that appears swollen should be measured. Sometimes, if swelling is unilateral, such as in the extremities, a comparative tape measurement of one side to the other can be made. If it is bilateral, then the pressure of a finger into the swollen area may allow the examiner to approximate "pitting," which usually is recorded on a progressive range of severity from 1+ to 4+. See Table 9–3 for further assessment guidelines.

Nutrition. **Nutrition** is the intake, assimilation, and use of food for energy, maintenance, and growth of the body. The involved body structures are the mouth, teeth, and the abdominal organs. The individual's eating and digestive patterns are critical processes in this parameter.

Assessing nutritional status involves a thorough collection of data regarding: eating patterns; the weight of the person compared to normal ranges for age and height; and the condition of the body structures used for the intake, assimilation, and use of food. Obtaining a thorough picture of a person's eating patterns can be a long and involved process; one of the most accurate records of food intake can be obtained by having a person record the amount and type of food ingested for one week. This process may not be practical, however, so the nurse must find a more expeditious method of getting the data. One way to do this is to ask the person to recall exactly what, when, and how much is eaten in a typical day. The nurse should be aware of inconsistencies in food measurement among people and should suggest standard measurements, such as a cupful, to help the client to identify the perceived amounts.

The instruments for measurement of nutritional patterns are used easily by the nurse. Most health-care facilities have a scale with a height measurement apparatus attached. These two measurements should always be made simultaneously, because a weight without a corresponding height is not very meaningful. Do not assume that the client knows his or her correct weight or height. It is helpful to ask the client, before measurement, his or her perceptions of height and weight. With these data, the nurse gets some idea about the accuracy of the client's perception of size. A measurement of skin-fold thickness through the use of calipers adds another piece of information to the assessment of body size. Although the triceps area is the usual site for such measurement, some persons have an unequal distribution of fat, so it is a good idea to take several readings on various parts of the body and average them.

Measurements of the abdomen are an important part of assessing the structural integrity of the organs involved in digestion. Listening for bowel sounds should be done before the examiner palpates the abdomen. Placing the stethoscope over all four quadrants of the abdomen allows the examiner to determine the degree of activity of the bowels. These are then scaled as inactive, hypoactive, normally active, or hyperactive. Before a judgment of inactive is made, the examiner should listen at least five minutes. Normally, bowel sounds are heard every 5 to 20 seconds.

Other measurements of the abdomen involve techniques of percussion and palpation in all quadrants. Percussion permits the examiner to listen to variations in dullness and tympany.

TABLE 9–3. GUIDELINES FOR ASSESSMENT OF CIRCULATION

Interview:
Chest pain or discomfort

Known alterations in heartbeat

Condition of extremities: Temperature changes, vascularity, swelling, cramping

Tolerance for activity

Usual blood pressure measurements

Observation:
Color of extremities, nail beds, and lips

Pulsations over cardiac area, carotid artery area

Quality of vein areas: Bulging, surrounding coloration, varicosities

Evidence of swelling, especially of the extremities

Measurement:
Blood pressure: Sphygmomanometer and stethoscope

Pulses: Rate, rhythm, quality, symmetry—fingers and watch

Veins: Level of jugular distention—ruler

Heart: Auscultation of rates, rhythm, and quality of heart sounds: stethoscope with bell and diaphragm

Lymph nodes: Palpation with fingertips

Swelling: Tape measure or finger pressure indentation

This allows a fairly accurate determination of borders of organs, such as the liver, the stomach, and the spleen. Borders, when found, can be marked on the abdomen and measured with a tape measure or ruler. Palpating the abdomen also gives the examiner an idea of the size of certain structures and allows for detection of any masses or fluid that normally are not present. Table 9–4 provides an outline for assessment of this parameter.

Elimination. **Elimination** is the output of waste products and indigestible materials from the body. The renal and urinary structures, the rectum, anus, and sweat glands function as eliminative mechanisms. Maintenance of an overall fluid and electrolyte balance is the goal of elimination.

Because the broad goal of elimination is a balance of fluids and electrolytes in the body, the nurse always must compare the output and input of fluids (data from the nutrition parameter). In some situations, especially with some hospitalized clients, precise measurement of fluid output is indicated. These amounts are compared to the client's intake of fluid or fluid-containing substances. Except for perspiration, fluid lost during respiration, and formed stool, most body fluid output can be measured precisely in any calibrated container.

In addition to measurements of the amount of fluid output, questioning the client about elimination patterns will give the examiner baseline information on that person's usual responses. Observations and measurements of the existing elimination, therefore, are more accurate determinants of changes that may be occurring. See Table 9–5.

Other measurements focus on the qualitative state of the body fluids. Urine can be measured for specific gravity and presence of sugar and acetone, or stool for occult blood, without extensive laboratory tests.

Rest and Activity. **Rest and activity** consist of movement or exertion and repose or rejuvenation of the body. The muscular, skeletal, and neurological structures are the primary body parts involved in rest and activity.

Rest and activity are best assessed together, because the balance between the two is crucial

---

TABLE 9–4. GUIDELINES FOR ASSESSMENT OF NUTRITION

Interview:
 Usual weight, changes in weight
 Usual eating patterns, typical day's or week's diet
 Condition of teeth and mouth, dentures, and their effect on chewing and swallowing
 Food tolerance (abdominal disorders affected by eating)

Observation:
 Body size and shape
 Condition of teeth and mouth
 Abdominal shape, symmetry

Measurement:
 Height and weight (scales)
 Triceps skin-fold thickness (calipers)
 Bowel sounds (stethoscope)
 Position and size of abdominal organs and detection of any abnormal fluid or mass (percussion, palpation, examiner's hands, and tape measure)

TABLE 9–5. GUIDELINES FOR ASSESSMENT OF ELIMINATION

Interview:
 Usual bowel patterns, color and consistency of stool, frequency of bowel movements
 Usual urinary patterns, color and odor of urine, frequency of urination
 Usual perspiration patterns, amount, times of increased perspiration
 Use of aids to stimulate bowel or urinary elimination
 Amount, timing, and frequency of flatus

Observation:
 Evidence of perspiration: Appropriateness in relation to environment
 Stool: Color, consistency
 Urine: Color, odor
 Rectal area: Color, intactness
 Unusual drainage such as vomitus, tube drainage: Specific observation depends on type of drainage and expected amounts

Measurement:
 Urine: Amount, specific gravity, sugar and acetone (calibrated container; hydrometer; Uristix, Keto Diastix, or comparable test
 Stool: Amount, occult blood (calibrated container, hemoccult slides)
 Unusual output, such as vomitus, body drainage (calibrated container)
 Intake and output balance (calibrated container)

to well-being. As with other patterns, questions about rest and activity are important in determining the client's usual pattern. This is especially important if the person has an alteration that is affecting some aspect of her or his rest or activity capabilities.

Many clues to the status of a person's rest and activity can be gained through careful observation of movements and facial expressions as the person progresses through the daily activities. Specific measurements of the symmetry of the muscular, skeletal, and neurological functions allow for precise data collection. A logical progression through all joints can determine their range of motion, and any that are in question can be measured with a protractor and compared to normal ranges. Muscle strength should be compared from side to side. The curve of the spine is an important indicator of the symmetrical working ability of the body's bones and muscles. The size of a joint is a critical indicator of its functioning and a valuable clue to detecting abnormalities. See Table 9–6 for additional guidelines for the assessment of rest and activity.

Sexuality. **Sexuality** is the characteristic response of maleness or femaleness of individuals. It includes reproductive functions. The genitalia and breasts are the primary physiological structures of sexuality.

Collecting data in the area of sexuality should be approached in the same manner as data collection in the other physiological parameters. Because of the extremely personal nature of sex, it can be an uncomfortable part of assessment. However, it is the nurse's responsibility to approach it with a degree of comfort that communicates reassurance and openness. Interview questions often set the stage for the degree of comfort felt by the client during the observation and measurement phases. A broad opening question is usually an effective introduction to the subject. Such a question might be, "Are you satisfied with your usual pattern of sexual expression?"

The examiner must be careful to maintain a nonjudgmental approach regardless of the types of sex activity reported by the client. This calls for a study of sexual values and beliefs on

TABLE 9–6. GUIDELINES FOR ASSESSMENT OF REST AND ACTIVITY

Interview:
- Ability to perform activities of daily living
- Usual sleep patterns: Timing, amount, interferences, use of aids
- Usual activity patterns: Job related, home related, specific exercise program; include amount, type, frequency of activity
- Movement of body parts, ability, and limitations
- Relaxation: Type, amount, timing

Observation:
- Alertness; evidence of restlessness, lethargy
- Posture, stance, gait
- Symmetry and coordination of body movements
- Muscle tone

Measurement:
- Hours of sleep, number of interruptions (clock)
- Range of motion of all joints (protractor)
- Muscle strength (examiner resistance over body parts, bilateral comparison)
- Tendon reflexes (reflex hammer)
- Curvature of spine (estimate from observation and palpation with hands)
- Joint size (tape measure if indicated)

the part of the examiner prior to assessing the sexual responses of clients.

Observation and measurement of the genitalia require slightly different techniques for men and women. However, observation and measurement of breasts should be included for both. Breasts should always be palpated to determine the presence of masses, and, if any are felt, an approximation of size and consistency is important.

Because most of the male genital structures are external, the examiner can observe and palpate them without the aid of instruments. The prostate, however, is palpated by the insertion of a finger into the rectum where the prostate can be felt through the rectal wall.

Whereas female external genitalia can be observed easily with no instruments, a speculum is inserted into the vagina to see the internal structures. Palpation of the uterus and ovaries, which are intra-abdominal, is accomplished by the examiner inserting two fingers into the vagina while pushing down on the lower abdomen with the other hand. In this way, the uterus and ovaries can be felt through the vaginal wall and an approximate measurement of these internal structures is obtained.

The Papanicolaou test is a measurement that the nurse may do or assist a physician in doing. This is a measurement of the cells in the discharge of the cervical and vaginal area. The methodology for this test may vary from institution to institution, so the specified method should be learned before doing the test. The examiner collects the discharge and applies it to a slide; a laboratory analyzes the slide and returns a written report to the nurse or physician. Table 9–7 offers guidelines for the assessment of sexuality.

Body Maintenance. **Body maintenance** is the restoration and regulation of a balance of functions achieved by the body itself and by the individual on behalf of his or her body. The endocrine glands, with their hormonal secretions, are a primary regulatory system in the body. The individual person's health maintenance activities, such as preventive immunizations, hygienic activities, and illness treatments are the external balancing functions.

Assessment of body maintenance practices overlaps with the assessment of many other parameters, because it is an indication of how all parts of the body are held intact. Primarily, data are collected through interview questions that focus on the client's perceptions and habits, which are the most important aspects of this pattern.

Special attention is given to the skin and hair because these are critical indicators of the regulating endocrine functions. The thyroid gland is the only endocrine gland easily accessible to examination. Located in the neck, it is not always palpable unless it is enlarged. Its size and consistency should be measured by palpation of the neck area.

Body temperature, easily measured with a thermometer, is an important indicator of the heat regulatory functions of the body. Temperature will usually rise with infective or inflammatory processes.

It is important for the examiner to know what, if any, medications a person is taking, for

TABLE 9–7. GUIDELINES FOR ASSESSMENT OF SEXUALITY

Interview:
Usual pattern of sexual expression—Satisfactory or unsatisfactory
Changes in desire or activity
Use of birth control, type
Changes in breasts
Women: Last menstrual period, number of pregnancies
Men: Changes in testicles, evidence of hernia

Observation:
Signs of gender identification (dress, posture, body language)
Comfort and openness with the subject of sex
Condition of breasts
Women: External vaginal structures—hair distribution, vaginal discharge (color, odor, consistency); internal structures: condition of vaginal walls and cervix
Men: Penis and testicles: hair distribution, color, size, shape, placement of meatus, lesions; femoral regions: scars, lesions, bulging

Measurement:
Any palpable breast lumps: Estimate size, shape, consistency (examiner's fingertips)
Women: Size and shape of cervix and cervical os (estimate by sight using speculum); Papanicolaou test ("Pap smear")—cotton applicator, wooden cervical spatula, glass slide, fixative agent; size, shape, and consistency of uterus and ovaries (estimate through palpation)
Men: Presence of hernia (palpate through inguinal ring); size, shape, consistency of testicles (palpate and estimate); size, shape, consistency of prostate (palpate and estimate)

these may affect many regulatory aspects of the body. A person's preventive health practices, including immunizations, give the nurse an idea of the level of knowledge a person has about her or his health and an indication of the control over health hazards that might exist. A further indication of health hazards is the condition of the client's home, work, and neighborhood settings. Table 9–8 offers guidelines for the assessment of body maintenance.

Psychological Dimension
The psychological dimension is reflected in a person's cognitive and emotional responses to

TABLE 9–8. GUIDELINES FOR ASSESSMENT OF BODY MAINTENANCE

Interview:

Perception of general health status, i.e., level of wellness

Medications: Dosage, frequency, route (include prescribed and over the counter)

Immunization record: Type, date

Frequency and type of preventive health care practices: Dental exams, eye exams, hearing tests, Pap smears, self-breast exams, self-testicular exams

Changes in body temperature, skin condition, hair distribution, energy level

Hygiene practices

Condition of home environment: Water, heating, amount of space, refrigerator, sanitation

Hazards of home, work, or neighborhood: Crime, pests, physical structure, exposure to noise

Observation:

General body appearance

Hygiene

Skin texture, turgor, color, lesions

Condition and distribution of hair

Measurement:

Temperature (thermometer)

Size and consistency of thyroid (palpation and estimation)

the self and the environment. For the purpose of assessment, this description of the psychological dimension directs the nurse to gather data about the client relative to two parameters: cognitive ability and emotional status. Each of these parameters should be assessed separately, as well as in reference to how the client responds to both the potential or actual health-care problem and the treatment and associated therapy that may be required.

The nurse seeks to collect data that will provide information related to the client's cognitive and emotional ability to participate in health care. The nurse seeks to determine if the client can realistically identify strengths and limitations, and how these may impact on the ability and willingness to adhere to recommended therapy. Data-gathering techniques (interview and observation) are used by the nurse to assess this dimension. Measurements of the parameters are made primarily by other health-care providers.

Cognitive Ability. **Cognitive ability** is a composite of a person's capacity to learn, to retain what is learned, and to comprehend or understand. Level of intelligence, past learning experiences, use of the senses, status of the nervous system, and developmental level contribute to a person's cognitive ability.

During interviews the nurse collects demographic data such as the client's age and educational background. These two factors may provide an indication of the client's cognitive abilities as related to achievement in a formal learning environment. Questions should be asked about the client's usual style or pattern of learning. This information will assist in determining the client's cognitive developmental level, the use of sight and hearing in the learning process, and the capacity to learn. The client's capacity to understand may be ascertained through the clarity and appropriateness of verbal responses to the questions asked throughout the interview. If the client does not appear to understand a question, the nurse should reword it and avoid the use of technical terms that may be a source of confusion. Questions related to the health-care problem should be asked so that the client's understanding of the problem and its required treatment and therapy can be assessed.

Information about the client's cognitive ability obtained through interviewing often can be validated or supported through observation. If the client has been taught a health-care procedure that must be carried through, the level of comprehension of what has been described and demonstrated can be assessed by observing performance of the procedure. Observing the client's nonverbal communication, such as a quizzical facial expression, also can provide a clue that the client is having difficulty comprehending information the nurse is giving.

Measurements obtained on the client's visual and hearing acuity, assessed through the physiological parameter of sensation, may provide evidence that indicates that physiological impairment, rather than impairment of cognition, exists. If results of tests assessing level of developmental cognition or intelligence are available to the nurse, they can serve to validate the findings. Table 9–9 provides guidelines for assessing cognitive status.

TABLE 9–9. GUIDELINES FOR ASSESSMENT OF COGNITIVE STATUS

Interview:
  Orientation to person, place, time, situation
  Ability to express self: Verbal communication skills
  Ability to learn: Can the client comprehend information given him or her? Can the client read? What knowledge does the client have of the health-care problem and its required therapy and associated treatment, such as diet, medications, and life-style alterations?

Observation:
  Participation in activities requiring comprehension: Does he or she read? Does she or he engage in conversation with others?
  Performance of self-care activities: If physically able, does the client appear to know how to participate in his or her care? Can he or she perform an activity (e.g., insulin injection) that has been described and demonstrated?

Emotional Status. **Emotional status** is mirrored through the overt and covert feelings a person experiences and expresses in his verbal and nonverbal communication. A person's emotional status influences and is influenced by the effectiveness of the coping strategies he or she uses.

The client's verbal responses that are expressed during the interview and the nonverbal responses as detected through observation are both valuable sources of data in the assessment of the client's emotional status. Questions should be asked that encourage the client to express feelings about the health-care problem and the required treatment. The client's motivation related to the intention to adhere to required therapy or health-care practices can be determined through questions that are non-threatening to the client. Information about past and present methods of coping with problems also should be sought.

In assessing emotional status it is important that, during the interview, the nurse is especially alert to and observant of the client's facial expression, muscular tension, and body movement. For example, a client asked about how a health-care problem will alter life-style may respond, "It's not going to change anything." Yet when the client responds, the nurse notes that the client's facial expression is one of sadness,

his body appears tense, or she is wringing her hands. Certainly the nonverbal cues are in conflict with the verbal response, and more information should be sought. See Table 9–10 for guidelines for assessing emotional status.

Sociocultural Dimension

The sociocultural dimension is reflected in a person's noninherited intrapersonal responses to socialization practices learned and transmitted from families and communities. The responses are influenced by social, political, and economic forces, and are characterized by **life-style, support networks,** and **health-care practices.**

This description of the sociocultural dimension directs the nurse to focus on the three parameters that characterize the client's sociocultural response. These parameters should be assessed in reference to potential or actual health problems and the treatment and associated therapy. The nurse uses interviewing as the primary data collection technique to assess the sociocultural dimension. The relationship of this dimension to the body maintenance parameter of the physiological dimension should be noted.

TABLE 9–10. GUIDELINES FOR ASSESSMENT OF EMOTIONAL STATUS

Interview:
  Mood: Verbal expressions of feelings, particularly in relation to the health-care problem, required treatment and therapy, and alteration of usual life-style
  Coping strategies: How does the client usually cope with problems? How is the client coping now?
  Does he or she perceive this as effective?
  Perception of self: Does he or she perceive self as sick or well?
  Motivation: Does the client perceive him- or herself as capable or incapable of participating in health care? Is the client willing to participate in his or her health care? Is he or she presently adhering to prescribed or recommended therapy?

Observation:
  Mood: Facial expressions (anxious, sad, depressed), muscle tension, body movement (slow, exaggerated)
  Performance of self-care activities: If physically able and knowledgeable, does the client participate in own care?

Life-style. Life-style incorporates the usual living circumstances and activities in which a person engages. It is influenced by employment status, economic status, and routines that become acceptable practices in the person's life.

Demographic data, such as employment status, occupation, and economic status are collected during the client's initial interview upon entering the health-care system. This information provides clues as to the client's ability to afford treatment and associated therapy, (e.g., medications, special diet, required aids—glasses, cane).

The client should be asked about routines, habits, and preferences that could influence health status. For example, if a client's usual daily routine includes drinking large amounts of regular coffee throughout the day and evening, he or she may experience an inadequate sleep pattern caused by difficulty in falling asleep (side effect of caffeine) and nocturia (frequent urination). Gathering information related to the presence of risk factors, such as cigarette smoking, a sedentary life-style, and consistent intake of high-calorie, low-protein foods, is essential. Questions should be asked not only to determine the presence of risk factors, but also to ascertain if and how the client may have tried to overcome them in the past.

Table 9–11 presents guidelines for the assessment of life-styles.

Support Networks. Support networks are made up of family members and significant persons who provide emotional, physical, or financial support to a client. The composition and status of relationships between the client and significant support systems can influence response to treatment and therapy.

During the initial interview, questions can be asked about the client's marital status, family composition, and responsibilities for other persons. Information about friends for whom he or she is responsible and who offer assistance in meeting needs helps to identify actual and potential sources of support on whom he or she can depend (see Table 9–12).

The nurse should seek to gather data that provide clues as to: human and material resources already available to and used by the client; resources available but not used by the

TABLE 9–11. GUIDELINES FOR ASSESSMENT OF LIFE-STYLES

Interview:
   Employment status: Past, present
   Occupation: Does it require physical or cognitive abilities that may be altered by the health problems?
   Economic status: Does the patient have the financial resources to secure the required treatment and associated therapy? Description of residence
   Daily routines: Activity and rest patterns, personal hygiene habits, nutritional pattern, dependence on tobacco, drugs, or alcohol

Observation:
   Type of attire: Appropriate to environment, culturally linked
   Habits: Risk factors

client; and resources that could be available if certain qualifying criteria for use were met. In the first instance, the client's participation in groups such as Mended Hearts, Alcoholics Anonymous, and Weight Watchers gives evidence of health-support networks that are already used. In the second instance, it should be determined whether or not the client is aware of available resources, and if there are specific reasons that influence him or her not to use them. For example, the client may be eligible to use a neighborhood health clinic but has no means to get to and from the clinic. In the final instance, based on the information the client has

TABLE 9–12. GUIDELINES FOR ASSESSMENT OF SUPPORT NETWORKS

Interview:
   Marital status
   Family composition
   Composition of other supportive systems—Their relationship, support to and interaction with the client
   Persons responsible for, dependent upon
   Sources of support: Emotional, physical, financial

Observation:
   Relationships: If hospitalized, does the client have visitors? If so, who and how often?
   If seen in a clinic, is the client accompanied by others?
   If seen in a home, what is the interaction among the persons living there?

given, the nurse may discover that the client is eligible for assistance (e.g., food stamps) but has not made formal application. In this situation, the nurse would use the social worker as a resource for the client.

Health-care Practices. Health-care practices incorporate those activities engaged in primarily for the purpose of attaining or maintaining health. These activities are influenced by the person's beliefs and values about health care, the health-care system, health-care providers, and methods of treatment and therapy.

A person's socialization to accepting and using the health-care system is influenced primarily by family and cultural community. Family and community influence the development of beliefs about and values of health care, adherence to therapy, response to illness, and perception of the health-care system. Values and beliefs will determine willingness to participate in the health-care system.

Questions about how the client usually seeks to resolve health-care problems should be asked. Impressions as to the value of seeking professional care, as well as patterns of adhering to prescribed and recommended therapy, are indicators of potential acceptance of support given by health-care providers. If the client perceives the health-care system only as one that is "out to get my money" or "doesn't care about me," the nurse can deduce that the client may be reluctant to use the system.

The client's usual health-care practices should be explored. Does the client employ nontraditional health care practices? The use of herbs, excessive intake of vitamins, and reliance on psychic healers are examples of practices that could influence the effectiveness of traditional treatments and therapies.

See Table 9–13 for guidelines for assessing health-care practices.

Spiritual Dimension

The spiritual dimension of the human person is reflected by personal response to inspirational forces. It is the inspirational forces that have been and are experienced by a person that contribute to the development of theological, ethical, and spiritual values. Values influence the meaning and purpose ascribed to life and affect

TABLE 9–13. GUIDELINES FOR ASSESSMENT OF HEALTH-CARE PRACTICES

Interview:
Patterns of health care: Usual, present. Does the client use a formal health care system? Does the client use home remedies or nontraditional health care practices?

Illness response: Previous illnesses and hospitalizations, attitude toward hospitalization, meaning attached to role of client, previous history of coping with stress and changes in life-style

Perceptions of health-care system: Beliefs about and attitudes toward: health-care agency, care givers, treatments, and therapies

Observation:
Participation in health-care delivery: Active or passive?

Illness response: Overt or covert?

the manner in which the client responds to actual or potential health-care problems.

A person's religion and spiritual involvement may affirm the inspirational forces he or she experiences and provide a source of inspiration. An organized or formal involvement in religious or spiritual activities can provide a system of support. These activities may be an essential aspect of a person's life and must, therefore, be respected as such.

A person who is a member of a religious group may hold specific beliefs that influence the choice of life-style and health-care practices. An example of this would be a client whose religious or spiritual beliefs require him or her to avoid certain foods or to fast on certain days. A person's view of disease and the acceptance or rejection of prescribed treatments or therapies also may be rooted in spiritual beliefs. The nurse must be aware of these and seek to understand how they affect the client's response to a health-care problem. The reader is referred to Chapter 13 for more discussion on cultural and spiritual dimensions of health care.

In assessing the impact that a person's spiritual dimension has on her or his well-being, it is necessary to consider the way in which a person's spiritual self relates to the physical, psychological, and sociocultural self. Responses assessed in the other dimensions are influenced by the depth and breadth of a person's religious and spiritual beliefs and values. These beliefs

TABLE 9–14. GUIDELINES FOR ASSESSMENT OF SPIRITUAL RESPONSES

Interview:

Religious affiliation: Religion—active or inactive participation, type of participation

Religious or spiritual beliefs influencing

    Health-care practices: Diet, seeking or receiving medical treatment or therapy, rituals or rites

    Perception of illness—a punishment, a test of faith

    Coping strategies

Religious or spiritual values influencing

    Life's purpose and meaning

    Death's purpose and meaning

    Health and its maintenance

    Relationship with God or a higher being, self, and others

Observation:

Religious or spiritual support: Time for personal or group prayer or meditation

Visits from rabbi, minister, priest, or other persons from spiritual support system

Religious or spiritual attitude: Hopeful, trusting, peaceful

and values also provide the parameter for assessing the client's spiritual responses (Table 9–14).

SPECIAL CONSIDERATIONS: DEVELOPMENTAL LEVEL

The client's age and developmental level are important considerations that will influence both the type of data that are likely to be found and the techniques used to obtain data.

The nurse must have a sound knowledge of usual behaviors associated with periods of growth and development. There are many theories that present categories of usual developmental behaviors; these are helpful to the nurse as a broad measurement standard. One such theory is Erik Erikson's, who described eight stages of ego development.[2] While this is a psychological and social orientation, these stages can serve as an organizational scheme for some of the age-specific areas of assessment with which physical changes can be considered.

Infancy is characterized by Erikson as a time of "basic trust versus basic mistrust." It is during this time that a person is totally dependent on others, so the nurse must assess parents

and their reaction and interactions with the infant as well as observe the infant. Naturally, questions must be directed to the parents. During observation and measurement, the accompanying parent assists the nurse by holding the child whenever possible, so that the infant remains secure.

The rate of development in children is very rapid, and there are several instruments designed to test specific levels of development. One such test is the Denver Developmental Screening Test (DDST), which is widely used to evaluate gross and fine motor skills, communication skills, and personal and social behaviors in children from birth to age six years.[3]

The toddler stage is characterized as a period of "autonomy versus shame and doubt." The nurse must carefully assess safety factors in the child's environment as the child begins to walk and explore the increasingly accessible surroundings. It is important to assess developing autonomy during this time when the child is learning to control bodily functions and is beginning to use verbal communication skills.

The preschooler goes through a period of "initiative versus guilt," when the child strives to respond to the expectations of others while testing out initiatives. Information about the child's interactions with other members of the family and with other children are important factors for the nurse to consider. At this age, the nurse can direct questions to the child during some parts of assessment. The child's responses will give the nurse much information about the level of development. It is necessary to determine if the child has a daily routine. Determining the child's level of understanding of dangerous things, like cars on the street or hot stoves, is important to ensure his or her safety.

The school-age years are seen as a period of "industry versus inferiority." In moving outside the home for school, the child begins to develop an identity no longer dependent on the family. Interactions with peers, abilities to "fit in" and be "normal," and school accomplishments are critical indicators of health responses. The nurse can rely more heavily on the child as a source of information during data collection; the child may or may not want parents actively involved during assessment. The nurse must determine the acuteness of the problem and decide the degree to which parents should be involved.

Adolescense, a period of "identity versus role confusion," is a time when a person makes the transition from childhood to adulthood. This developmental stage is sometimes divided into an early, middle, and late period.[4] During these years, depending on the length of schooling, the person plans for and moves into an occupational role. A sex-role identity is very important at this stage, during which puberty matures the body's characteristic male or female functions. When assessing persons in this age group, the nurse must be particularly sensitive to the changes in roles, bodily configuration, and comfort levels of adolescents. While collecting data, the nurse needs to view the client as an adult but allow the person to involve parents in health care if so desired. Adult health habits are formed during this stage. Therefore, the nurse must determine the young person's level of knowledge about physical, psychological, sociocultural, and spiritual responses. Because of adolescents' changing sexual capabilities, there is a need for the nurse to be especially sensitive in assessing sexual responses so that a nonjudgmental, open relationship is established between health-care provider and recipient.

Young adulthood is a time of "intimacy versus isolation." In this period, the person's self-image and ego strength should stabilize, allowing the development of close relationships with others, usually with those of the opposite sex. Choices about having a family are determined, and pregnancy and childbirth are important health issues. Careers or jobs and their related financial rewards are determinants of security and life-styles for these persons. The nurse needs to assess the client for life stressors that may affect health as the young adult copes with a developing family, a beginning career, and contribution to society.

Middle-aged persons are expected to be concerned with "establishing and guiding the next generation."[5] This period is described as a time of "generativity versus stagnation." This is a time of family changes as children (if the person has any) leave and establish their lives separate from parents. While middle-aged adults usually have well-established jobs or carreers, they may become insecure about their age as younger persons enter their work environment. Likewise intimate relationships, while usually well established at this age, may be influenced by aging changes. Menopause is an important body change experienced by women at this time. Chronic illnesses are more frequently seen in this age group. Persons often will be concerned with aged parents and coping with their parents' deaths. These events may be especially stressful as they plan for their own retirement and maturity.

The final developmental stage, later maturity, is a period of "ego identity versus despair." Retirement from a job or career is often a stressful life event, and it is sometimes accompanied by a change in living arrangements and economic status. The nurse must assess the client as well as the environment to determine physical safety hazards, ability to care for him- or herself, relationship with significant others, and ability to cope with inevitable events, such as the death of peers and spouses. An important spiritual concern at this age is the person's beliefs and feelings about death.

In conclusion, the nurse needs to be aware of developmental changes that occur with aging and be able to relate them to effects on health. Developmental stages are presented not as finite time periods, but rather as a continuum of life events. Each individual ages and develops in a unique manner. Consequently the nurse must be careful not to categorize persons on the basis of generalizations. Careful data collection will give objective data concerning each individual client's level of development.

SUMMARY

This chapter presented health assessment from a nursing perspective. A framework based upon the physiological, psychological, sociocultural, and spiritual dimensions of the human person provides a guide for data collection. The nurse's health assessment is contrasted with that of other health-care providers. The roles of the nurse, the client, and other health-care providers are discussed. Interviewing, observation, and measurement are the techniques used by the nurse to establish a comprehensive, objective data base. The techniques are described so as to provide a basic understanding of their use.

For the purpose of guiding the collection of data, each dimension and its assessment parameters are delineated. Developmental stages and their impact on health responses are addressed as important components of health assessment. This first phase of the nursing process is a complex activity. The nurse will add to this foundational level of knowledge through continued practice and the addition of more complex techniques. As the number of client encounters increases, the nurse will sharpen the skills in identifying health assessment priorities for each client. The nurse's job description, health-care setting, and the characteristics of the client population will influence the nature of the data that are needed to determine the client's responses to actual or potential health problems.

Study Questions

1. State how a nursing health assessment differs from a medical health assessment.

2. Describe how the nurse incorporates information from the client and other health-care providers.

3. List tools or instruments that can be used for interviewing, observation, and measurement.

4. Define the parameters for assessment within each dimension of the human being.

5. Choose a stage of development and describe factors that must be considered when assessing a person at that stage.

References

1. American Nurses' Association, *Nursing: A Social Policy Statement* (Kansas City, Mo.: American Nurses' Association, 1980).
2. Gloria J. Block, JoEllen W. Nolan, and Mary K. Dempsey, *Health Assessment for Professional Nursing: A Developmental Approach*, 2nd ed. (E. Norwalk, Conn.: Appleton-Century-Crofts, 1986).
3. W.K. Frankenburg, and J.B. Dodds, *Denver Developmental Screening Test* (Denver, Colo.: University of Colorado Medical Center, 1969).
4. Erik H. Erikson, *Childhood and Society*, 2nd ed. (New York, W.W. Norton & Co., 1963).
5. Ibid, 267.

Annotated Bibliography

Bates, B. 1983. *A Guide to Physical Examination*, 3rd ed. Philadelphia: Lippincott. This frequently used textbook is primarily organized into body systems chapters. It has excellent illustrations to show both the novice and the experienced examiner techniques of examination and the body parts being examined. The text is clear in its directions; examples of abnormal findings are delineated in red. One chapter is devoted to examination of infants and children. Chapters on critical thinking and recording are valuable to show readers what to do with data after examining the patient.

Bellack, J.P., Bamford, P.A. 1984. *Nursing Assessment: A Multidimensional Approach*. Monterey, Calif.: Wadsworth Health Sciences Division. This text includes descriptions of methods used to gather and analyze data during the assessment phase of the nursing process. The chapter on nursing diagnosis, while brief, provides an excellent summary of the formulation of a nursing diagnosis. Frameworks to guide assessment are presented in the sections on developmental, psychosocial, sociocultural, and physiological assessment. In the physiological assessment section, assessment of body systems is incorporated into chapters focusing on functional health patterns: physical integrity, sensory-perceptual-pain, oxygenation, nutrition, fluid and electrolytes and elimination, and activity and sleep. A sample client assessment provides the student with an example that incorporates the collection and analysis of data obtained through a multidimensional assessment.

Block, G.J., Nolan, J.W., and Dempsey, M.K. 1986. *Health Assessment for Professional Nursing: A Developmental Approach*, 2nd ed. E. Norwalk, Conn.: Appleton-Century-Crofts. Outlined according to physiological body systems, this book presents detailed guidelines for health assessment. It integrates content related to differences of age groups within each chapter and gives guidelines for assessing certain life-styles and environmental factors. Numerous photographs and diagrams assist the reader in visualizing assessment techniques and body parts.

Fields, W.L., McGinn-Campball, K.M. 1983. *Introduction to Health Assessment*. Reston, Va.: Reston Publishing Company. This book emphasizes techniques of assessing the healthy individual; thus it is helpful to beginning students. Abnormal findings are presented in separate tables throughout the chapters. Body systems are the major organizational approach for chapters, but chapters on fluid and electrolyte balance, acid-base balance, and integration of health assessment give additional parameters that are valuable to the nurse.

Jones, D.A., Lepley, M.K., and Baker, B.A. 1984. *Health Assessment Across the Life Span*. New York: McGraw-Hill. This book addresses assessment of persons at various developmental phases of life. It is strongly oriented toward a nursing focus on the person's response to developmental changes and on the interaction of the person's body, mind, spirit, and environment. As a precursor to chapters on the various age groups, there is a lengthy introduction on the significance of assessment to nurses and a detailed chapter on the physical examination. Photographs and illustrations are liberally dispersed throughout the book.

LeFrancois, G.R. 1984. *The Lifespan*. Belmont, Calif.: Wadsworth Publishing Co. This text presents information relative to physical, cognitive, social, and moral development of the infant, child, adolescent, and adult. The material included will provide students with information that will enhance their ability to make a comprehensive assessment of clients at various stages of physical development.

Malasanos, L., Barkauskas V., Moss, M., and Stoltenberg-Allen, K. 1986. *Health Assessment*, 3rd ed. St. Louis: C.V. Mosby. This text presents overviews of the interview, the health history, and developmental assessments. Health assessment incorporating a body systems approach is the focus of this text. Sections on health assessment of the pediatric, prenatal, and aging client assist the student in recognizing how the process of health assessment may be tailored to the developmental level of the client. The tables, figures, and pictures enhance the value of the text.

Chapter 10

Legal Aspects

Cynthia E. Northrop

Chapter Outline

- Objectives
- Glossary
- Introduction
- General Legal Concepts
    Sources of Law
    The Court System
- Laws Affecting Nursing Practice
    Torts
    Contracts
    Criminal Law
    Constitutional Law
    Legislation
- Record-keeping Responsibilities
    Access to Records
    Informed Consent
    Common Charting Errors
- Management of Medical Orders
- Accountability for Practice
    Licensure and Nursing Practice Acts
    Clients' Rights and Responsibilities: Best Interests of Clients
    Nurses' Rights and Responsibilities: Best Interests of Nurses
- Summary
- Study Questions
- References
- Annotated Bibliography

Objectives

At the completion of this chapter the reader will be able to:

▶ Discuss sources of law and general legal principles
▶ Compare and contrast negligence and malpractice
▶ Relate to major record-keeping responsibilities and common recording problems
▶ Identify different types of orders and legal implications of each
▶ Describe legal accountability in nursing practice
▶ Discuss the status of mandatory continuing education for today's nurse
▶ Discuss the Code for Nurses
▶ List client rights

Glossary

Agency. Includes every relationship in which one person acts for or represents another by the latter's authority.

Appeal. A complaint to a superior court to reverse or correct an injustic done or an alleged error committed by an inferior court.

Assault. Threat to do bodily harm.

Battery. Committing bodily harm.

Civil Law. Concerned with the legal rights and duties of private persons.

Common Law. Derived from court decisions, judge-made law.

Consent. A voluntary act by which one person agrees to allow someone else to do something.

Constitutional Law. Branch of law dealing with organization and function of government.

Contract. A promissory agreement between two or more persons that create, modify, or destroy a legal relationship. Also, it is a legally enforceable promise between two or more persons to do or not to do something.

Cross-examination. Examination of a witness made, in chief, to test the truth or credibility of the testimony.

Defendant. In a criminal case, the person accused of committing a crime. In a civil suit, the party against whom suit is brought.

Due Process. Certain procedural requirements to assure fairness.

Employer. One who selects the employee, pays a salary or wages, retains the power to dismiss, and can control conduct during working hours.

Expert Witness. One who has special training, experience, skills, and knowledge in a relevant area, and whose opinion testimony is allowed to be considered as evidence; non-expert opinions usually are not admissible as evidence.

Informed Consent. Consent in which the client has received sufficient information concerning the health care proposed, its incumbent risks, and the acceptable alternatives.

Invasion of Privacy. Invasion of the right to be left alone, to live in seclusion without being subjected to unwarranted or undesired publicity.

Jurisdiction. The court has the authority to hear the case.

Law. The sum total of man-made rules and regulations by which society is governed in a formal and legally binding manner.

Lay Witness. One who testifies to what was seen, heard, or otherwise observed.

Legal. Permitted or authorized by law.

Liability. An obligation one has incurred or might incur through any act or failure to act, responsibility for conduct falling below a certain standard that is the causal connection of the plaintiff's injury.

Litigation. A trial in court to determine legal issues and the rights and duties of the parties.

Malpractice. Professional negligence, improper discharge of professional duties, or a failure of a professional to meet standard of care that results in harm to another.

Medical Record. A written official documentary of what has happened to a particular client during a specific period of time.

Plaintiff. The party that brings a civil suit seeking damages or other legal relief.

Police Power. State power to act in order to protect its citizens' health, safety, and welfare.

Policies. Guidelines within which employees of an institution must operate.

Precedent. A previous adjudged decision that serves as authority in a similar case.

Privileged Communication. Statements made to one in a position of trust—usually an attorney, physician, or spouse. Because of the confidential nature of the information, the law protects it from being revealed, even in court. The term is applied in two distinct situations. First, the communications between certain persons (e.g., physician and client), cannot be divulged without consent of the client. Second, in some situations, the law provides an exemption from liability for disclosing information where there is a higher duty to speak, for example, statutory reporting requirements.

Procedures. Mode or proceeding by which a legal right is enforced. A series of steps outlined by the institution to accomplish a specific objective or task.

Proximate Cause. Legal concept of cause and effect; the injury would not have occurred by the particular cause; causal connection.

Reasonable Care. The degree of skill and knowledge customarily used by a competent health practitioner or student of similar education and experience in treating and caring for the sick and injured in the community in which the individual is practicing.

Reasonably Prudent Person Doctrine. Requires a person of ordinary sense to use ordinary care and skill.

Respondeat Superior. "Let the master answer." The employer is responsible for the legal consequences of the acts of the servant or employee while acting within the scope of employment.

Right. Power, privilege, or faculty inherent in one person and incident upon another.

Rules and Regulations. Clear and concise statements mandating or prohibiting certain activity in an institution.

Standard of Care. Those acts performed or omitted that an ordinary prudent person in the defendant's position would have done or not done; a measure by which the defendant's conduct is compared to ascertain negligence.

Standards. Criteria of measuring, and conformity to established practice.

Statutes. Legislative enactments; act of legislature declaring, commanding, or prohibiting something.

Subpoena. A court order requiring one to come to court to give testimony; failure to appear results in punishment by the court.

Suit. Court proceeding where one person seeks damages or other legal remedies from another. The term usually is not used in connection with criminal cases.

Testimony. Oral statement of a witness, given under oath at a trial.

Tort. A legal or civil wrong committed by one person against the person or property of another.

Verdict. The formal declaration of the jury of its findings of fact.

INTRODUCTION

Nursing practice is governed by many legal and ethical concepts. Nurses, because of their health-care-delivery role, are accountable for their professional judgments and behavior. In the past, physicians and agencies assumed much more responsibility for nurses' actions than they do today. This is due partly to the expansion of the nurses' role in the health-care system and the increasing professionalism demonstrated by nurses. If nurses are to be responsible for their acts, then they must be accountable as well. This chapter will discuss general legal concepts and the legal and professional responsibilities of the nurse.

GENERAL LEGAL CONCEPTS

Many concepts from **law** have an impact on nursing practice; therefore, it is important for nurses to know the basics of these concepts. Before this can be accomplished, however, the sources of law and how laws affect nursing practice should be understood.

Sources of Law

There are five major sources of law (Table 10–1). In some situations, each of the five sources may be used by a lawyer representing clients in disputes. In others, only one or two sources may be necessary. For example, if a nurse were wrongly fired from a job at a hospital and then retained an attorney in order to be reinstated or to correct the wrong, the lawyer could examine the facts of the situation and go to several sources of law to prepare the case. Depending on the situation, similar cases might be found in the judicial opinions or judge-written decisions in that particular **jurisdiction.** Federal legislation and regulation on employment practices might also be drawn upon. **Common**

TABLE 10–1. THE SOURCES OF LAW

Constitution: United States, State
Judicial opinions: Federal, State, Administrative
Legislation: Federal, State, Local, City, County
Regulation: Federal, State
Common law principles: Traditions, principle of justice, fairness, autonomy, respect, dignity, precedent

law principles of fairness and justice might be argued by the attorney, depending on how and under what circumstances the nurse was fired. Also, if the nurse were not given notice or reasons for the firing, or not given an opportunity to refute the firing, interpretation of the Federal or state constitution's **due process** clause might assist in proving a violation of constitutional **rights.**

The five sources of law are intertwined. For example, there are judicial opinions that discuss and apply common law principles and interpret the constitution, legislation, or regulation. Courts are bound to follow opinions or previous decisions of their particular jurisdiction. This is the common law principle of **precedent.** Other judicial opinions may be used to persuade the court, but they need not be followed since they did not originate under that court's jurisdiction. Precedent may not be followed if the court can distinguish the facts before them from the previously decided case. In addition, societal views change over time, and this is often reflected in court decisions. The emergent philosophy of an era has an influence on how laws are written. As an era changes, the laws that govern may also change. It is important for nurses to keep up with the status of laws that influence nursing practice. This can be done by reviewing current nursing journals.

The Court System

The Federal court system and individual state court systems are the two main court systems in the United States. The Federal system has three tiers, as do most state systems (Table 10–2). In the lower courts (district and circuit courts), cases are heard for the first time, and evidence is presented. The higher courts are **appeal** courts, where argument is offered to persuade the judges that certain errors may have been made when the case was tried in the lower court. Only under special circumstances is new evidence introduced in the higher courts.

There are other courts that have been established by Congress or state legislatures for selected and limited purposes. For example, disputes dealing with Federal tax issues would be settled in the tax court; custom or patent disputes would be decided in customs and patent courts.

Also established by Congress or state legislatures are administrative law systems that handle certain types of claims. Decisions made in these systems have the force of law and usually may be appealed to a Federal or state court system. For example, if nurses are injured on the job, they may be eligible for workers' compensation. First, a claim would be filed with the state workers' compensation administration. If the claim is denied, the appeal process would have to be exhausted within the administration. Once one exhausted the appeal there, without success, the claim could be filed in the state court system.

LAWS AFFECTING NURSING PRACTICE

Many laws affect nursing practice because the legal system serves to protect the rights of in-

TABLE 10–2. THE U.S. COURT SYSTEM

Federal	State[a]
Supreme Court	Court of Appeals or Supreme Court
U.S. Court of Appeals	Circuit Court
U.S. District Court	District Court

[a]Some states have a four-tier system; most have a three-tier system.

dividuals or groups and determines the responsibilities of individuals in civil and criminal cases (Table 10–3).

Law can be classified in a variety of ways, but the major classifications are criminal law and civil law. Criminal law involves conduct considered harmful or offensive to society. The punishment for committing the crime ranges from a fine to imprisonment. **Civil law** involves legal rights of individuals, primarily disputes between private individuals.

Most legislation involving nursing to date has been civil and not criminal in nature.

Torts

A **tort** is a general term in civil law that describes a legal wrong committed against the person or property of another. The word *tort* comes from the Latin word *tortus* meaning twisted. Disputed, injurious conduct between private individuals is classified as a tort. Civil wrongs usually take one of two forms:

- Simple, direct interference with a person or with property
- Disturbances of intangible interests such as one's reputation

In a civil **suit** involving a tort, only the injured person can begin and maintain the suit. If the decision in the end is to grant a remedy to the injured person, the remedy is money or discontinuance of the disturbance, which is intended to compensate for the injury. The goal of the remedy is to provide the means (funds) so that the injured person can be placed in a similar position to the situation prior to the injury.

Negligence and malpractice are two examples of torts that deal with clinical practice situations. Negligence is an unintended act or failure to act that leads to an injury. Anyone can make a mistake or have an accident that results in injuries to another. Negligence can be defined as carelessness. **Malpractice,** on the other hand, is negligence by a person who is a member of a profession. Individuals are liable for their own negligence. Legal principles of negligence and malpractice that often involve nurses are listed in Table 10–4.

An "ordinary" person (not a member of a profession) is held to an "ordinary" standard,

TABLE 10–3. SELECTED CATEGORIES OF LAWS AFFECTING NURSES

Torts	Negligence and malpractice
	Defamation, libel, and slander
	Assult and battery
	False imprisonment
	Invasion of privacy
Contracts	Nurse and client
	Nurse and agency
	Agency and supplemental staffing agency
	Agency and educational institution
	Nurse and insurance
Criminal	Homicide
	Manslaughter
Constitutional	Due process
	Rights
Legislation	Licensing
	Reporting statutes
	Good Samaritan statutes

meaning that an action will be judged in light of what any other "ordinary" person would have done under the circumstances. The legal doctrine that describes this is called the **Reasonably Prudent Person Doctrine.** The action of a member of a profession is judged by what a similar member of that profession would have done under the circumstances. The "ordinary" person's duty is not the same as that of a member of a profession who, because of increased knowledge and a special relationship, owes a higher duty. Employment in an agency establishes a nurse's duty to carry out services in a

TABLE 10–4. LEGAL PRINCIPLES OF NEGLIGENCE AND MALPRACTICE

Personal liability
Duty and standard of care: Ordinary standard
                                      Professional standard
Breach of duty
Causation, proximate cause
Damage, injury, and remedy
Vicarious liability: Employer
                           Indemnification
Defenses: Contributory negligence
               Comparative negligence
               Immunities and statute of limitation

safe and reasonable manner. In some legal cases, nurses have been held to an ordinary **standard of care**, and in other cases they have been held to a professional standard, known in legal terms as **reasonable care**. Which standard applies varies from situation to situation and state to state. When confronted with a practice dilemma, the safest approach is to decide how a similarly prepared nurse would act under the circumstances in question. Other sources may be used in determining how the nurse should have acted under the same circumstances (Table 10–5).

The breach of the duty owed and the outcome of that breach relate to the rest of the elements of negligence and malpractice. Nurses can make mistakes, such as medication errors, that lead to no injury. For example, no injury might occur if the nurse gave a client a vitamin when one was not ordered by the physician. Nurses have not committed negligence or malpractice if what they did was not the cause of injury. Injuries are usually physical, actual injuries; however, courts and juries grant remedies for psychological injuries, especially if they are in conjunction with physical injuries.

An example of a particular nursing practice situation follows. Examine it in light of the principles discussed thus far and decide whether the nurse who inserted the catheter is negligent.

A client is to have an abdominal hysterectomy. The surgeon orders that a Foley catheter be inserted into the bladder and attached to straight drainage as part of the preoperative preparation for surgery. A nurse mistakenly inserts the Foley into the client's rectum. Never

checking for urinary drainage, the nurse then connects the catheter to the drainage bag and sends the client to surgery.

After the surgery has begun, the surgeon discovers that the client's bladder is full, but sees the drainage bag hanging at the side of the table, and quickly surmises the catheter must not be in the correct location. Still scrubbed, the surgeon reaches under the drapes, grabs the misplaced catheter and pulls it out. In doing so, the catheter flips into the open surgical wound, thoroughly contaminating it with fecal material. Despite precautionary measures taken in the operating room the client suffers a severe infection, pain, extended hospital stay, prolonged recovery period, and develops abdominal adhesions. To recover for injuries sustained, the client sues both the surgeon and the nurse.

The court found only the physician negligent, because placing a catheter in the rectum even though it was the wrong place could not lead to infection, adhesions, and loss of wages. No causal link, or **proximate cause**, between the nurse's mistake and the injuries the client suffered was found to exist.

The following list identifies activities of nurses who have lost legal cases involving allegations of negligence and malpractice.

Some common acts of negligence and malpractice include:

- Failure to count or incorrectly counting the number of sponges or instruments where a duty exists to account for them
- Improper exercise of judgments that bed rails should have been used to safeguard clients
- Lack of supervision of clients at regular and appropriate intervals
- Failure to contact or notify physician of changes in client's condition
- Failure to give emergency treatment to client in hospital
- Failure to recognize adverse signs and symptoms, discontinue treatments, and contact physician
- Lack of judgment in evaluating physician orders
- Failure to administer medications properly (right dose, right route, right client, right drug, right time)
- Failure to apply appropriate principles regarding application of hot and cold

TABLE 10–5. DETERMINING THE APPLICABLE STANDARDS OF NURSING CARE

Specific functions assigned to nurses in written manuals and employer's policy and procedure

Testimony of others that describes the existing usual and reasonable nursing practices under similar circumstances

Education, experience, continuing education

Textbooks, journals, other publications in the field

Standards of professional organizations (e.g., standards of nursing practice, American Nurses' Association)

Standards of accrediting or licensing groups (e.g., Joint Commission on Accreditation of Hospitals)

Policy statements of professional associations (e.g., American Nurses' Association Code for Nurses)

State nursing practice act and regulations

- Failure to assist client with ambulation
- Failure to evaluate client complaints and follow up with physician
- Failure to report to superiors and to physicians changes in client's condition
- Failure to monitor vital signs
- Improper identification of client for surgery
- Failure to take reasonable precautions in regard to client's personal property
- Lack of sterile technique
- Failure to administer anesthetics properly (applies to nurse anesthetist)
- Failure to properly remove a Foley catheter
- Failure to administer correct blood type to a client
- Refusal to admit a client to a hospital floor
- Failure to take a reasonable client history
- Failure to refer a client to a physician for diagnosis and treatment
- Failure to follow proper physician orders and treatments

In cases of vicarious liability, someone else is also held responsible for another's negligent acts. For nurses, that is usually the employer. One type of vicarious liability is **respondeat superior** or "let the master or employer respond." In order for respondeat superior to exist, a negligent act must occur within a relationship of employment and within the scope of duties of that employment. The **employer** shares responsibility with the employee for negligent actions because the employer's responsibilities are to hire reasonable employees and to supervise and evaluate them. A physician who employs a nurse in an office practice has the responsibility as respondeat superior because the physician is the employer.

In determining whom the injured party sues, two main factors are examined: **liability** and ability to compensate for the injury suffered. The fact that nurses are not sued very often relates to both of these factors. Nurses may not be liable or may only be liable to a small degree in a given negligence situation. Nurses, because of societal status and salary, are not viewed as ones with monetary means to compensate for injuries. Therefore, in many situations nursing negligence is the topic of lawsuits not against the negligent nurses but against the hospital or other employer. In situations where the employment or insurance contract allows, a hospital may sue the employee for expenses it incurs in defending the employer. Indemnification allows the employer to recover from the employee the monies spent on litigation or settlement of a claim where the employee is negligent.

In many states, claims of malpractice against physicians and other health-care providers must follow a particular legal process. Each state has unique requirements for beginning a lawsuit where malpractice is the accusation (Fig. 10–1).

The injured person, the **plaintiff,** first seeks the advice of an attorney. Review of the facts and sources of law may determine that the plaintiff has sufficient evidence and legal support to proceed with a lawsuit. The plaintiff's attorney files the necessary papers to describe the claim with an arbitration panel or with a trial court. The initial choice of forum depends on state law and legal procedure. At the same time, the accused person, the **defendant,** is served or sent the same papers that are filed with the panel or court. Usually, at this point the defendant needs to retain a lawyer or, if insured against malpractice, the insurance company needs to be contacted in order to provide legal counsel if that is a provision of the insurance agreement.

In some states nurses may or may not be subject to the rules pertaining to malpractice panels. For example, in some states only claims against physicians and hospitals must go to arbitration first; other state rules or procedure require arbitration for all health-care providers. The arbitration process involves three to five individuals (consumers, lawyers, physicians, or other health providers) and is ideally faster, less formal, and less expensive. The trial court involves a judge, usually 12 jurors, and a longer waiting time before the case is heard. However, several states have abandoned the panel process because their experience with it did not produce the ideal situation.

Documents, primarily **agency** records of the plaintiff's care witnesses, and argument or discussion make up the presentation of the case to the panel or trial court. Both parties may present these items as evidence to either persuade or dissuade the decision makers to favor or reject the plaintiff's claim. Settlement outside

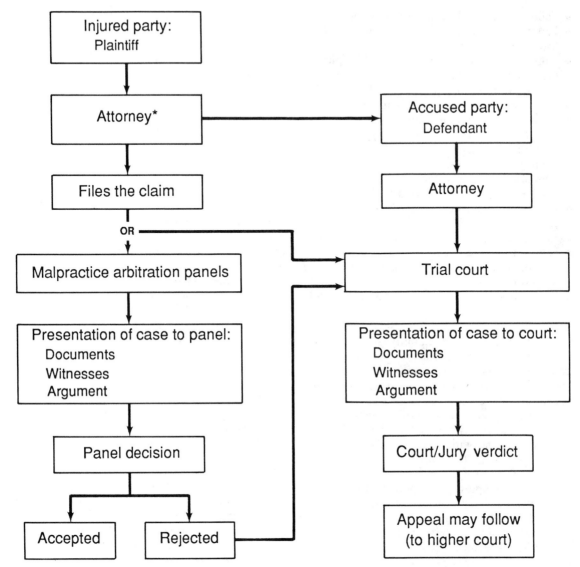

*Settlement may occur at any point until Court/Jury verdict rendered.

Figure 10–1. The civil legal process (varies from state to state). Settlement may occur at any point until court/jury verdict rendered.

the forum may occur at any time before the time when the panel judge or jury renders a decision. Either side may reject the panel's decision and file an appeal in the trial court. If a settlement between the parties occurs prior to a final decision, the question of malpractice is never answered.

An **expert witness,** one who provides an

opinion, often is used by both the plaintiff or defendant in the presentation of the case. This witness usually has no prior connection with the claim and the testimony or consultation with the attorney helps to interpret evidence, clarify questions, or establish what **standards** should be applied to make a decision.

A **lay witness** is one who can say what happened in a particular situation because of participation in or observation of the event. Lay witnesses describe what they saw, smelled, touched, or heard.

Nurses can and have been both lay and expert witnesses in lawsuits that deal with nursing and other situations. A nurse who observed a physician's malpractice may be **subpoenaed** to testify about what was observed. On the other hand, a nurse may be consulted by an attorney to give advice about how much home nursing care would be necessary to rehabilitate an automobile accident victim. While the lay witness can be subpoenaed, the expert witness generally cannot. The expert witness enters into a contractual agreement to consult with and provide assistance to an attorney for a fee. The fee for expert services or consultation should never be contingent on the outcome of the case.

Certain lay witnesses subpoenaed by either party may claim that what they are being asked to reveal in court is a **privileged communication.** The state legislature and legal rules of procedure determine who may claim this privilege not to divulge the information being requested. In most states, physicians, psychiatrists, psychologists, members of the clergy, and husbands and wives are allowed to claim the privilege. In a small number of states, nurses, social workers, and accountants have the privilege. If the legislature does not include nurses under the privileged communication clause, then nurses in that state must testify and reveal confidential information.

The privilege of keeping certain information from a court is not absolute. For example, if a person decides to sue another and needs to present testimony about his or her own mental health, the privilege will be waived because the person to whom the obligation is owed to maintain confidentiality is requesting his or her own psychiatrist to testify. However, the privilege could be claimed if it were the other party's mental health status that is needed in the case and if the other party did not plan to introduce the evidence.

Defamation is a tort involving an action that injures one's reputation in the community. The particular action can be written, called libel, or verbal, called slander. Both of these are defamation. Very few cases exist where a nurse has

been sued for either libel or slander. However, there are a few cases where a nurse has successfully sued other individuals for defamation. Nurses have sued physicians for accusing them of negligence or malpractice in front of family members or fellow workers. Any statement that injures a person's reputation, verbal or written, published or said to someone other than the person who is the subject of the statement, may constitute defamation. The defense to defamation is that the statement is true. The judge or jury must be convinced by the evidence presented that defamation has occurred.

Assault and battery are two torts involving intentional acts. **Assault** is a threat or an attempt to make bodily contact with another person, without the person's **consent.** For example, if a client refused an injection and the nurse then attempted to administer it, this is thought to be assault. If the nurse restrains the client and administers the shot, **battery** has been committed. Battery is the assault carried out.

Every person has the legal right to consent to treatment. Treatments and procedures cannot be carried out without the client's permission. Therefore, obtaining the client's permission before performing nursing care and treatment is an essential part of nursing practice. Without the consent and agreement of the patient, the nurse may commit a battery against the patient.

False imprisonment is a tort that involves intentional placement of someone in an area that has physical barriers. The use of restraints or psychiatric isolation rooms as nursing intervention needs careful scrutiny, because it may constitute the tort of false imprisonment. The only acceptable use of restraints is to protect a client from harm. Restraints should never be used in a punitive manner. Restraints, when necessary, should be used for short time periods and only to safeguard a client through a crisis. Because of recent lawsuits, many health facilities require that restraints be used only after physician review and treatment order. The order for restraint is good for only a short time, after which reevaluation by a physician is required before the order can continue or be renewed.

Invasion of privacy is a tort that involves confidential information that is revealed without permission to someone not entitled to know it. Cases involving this tort in the health care area have been successful. For example, pictures of clients have been taken without their permission and then used in texts for medical education. Permission must be obtained before displaying part of another's body. Another example of invasion of privacy is telling someone who is not part of the health team details of test results or a client diagnosis.

Contracts

Contracts are agreements or obligations into which two or more individuals or agencies enter. They are thought of as promises made between consenting individuals or agencies. Contracts have three elements that, if they exist, the law will enforce in order to protect society's interest in having promises performed. The elements are: offer, acceptance of the offer, and consideration.

Generally speaking, most nurses do not have an employment contract. Most nurses, therefore, are "terminable at will," meaning the employment may end at the will of the nurse or at the employer's will (without cause).

However, employers must abide by their employment **policies.** For example, if there exist policies that state that a nurse's employment cannot be terminated without cause, then termination should be only with cause. In some situations of termination at will, courts have determined that a contract can be implied from employers' actions; in other cases courts will find wrongful discharge if the termination was against public policy. Many possibilities exist; nurses should seek legal advice to determine whether any legal rights have been violated.

Contracts can be made verbally as well as in writing. An employment contract, for example, is usually in writing and sets forth the terms of what the employer and employee will do in order to carry out the employment agreement. Terms of contracts can be negotiated before the offer of a job is finalized. Most often, the act of signing an agreement signals the acceptance of an offer by both parties. The most frequent example of consideration in the employment contract is the exchange of services or work for payment. Both parties gain something

and both give something that, except for the agreement, they would not have given.

Nurses make contracts with their clients daily when negotiating mutual goals. While most are verbal agreements, nurses make promises to clients and vice versa regarding health care. However, most case law discussing contracts and nurses deals with grievance and employment situations and not agreements between nurses and clients in delivering nursing services within an agency. This is not to say, however, that future litigation involving nurses will not focus on this area.

When a nurse contracts with a supplemental staffing agency to be temporarily assigned to another agency, that assignment is based upon a contract between these two agencies. The most important implication for the nurse involved in these contracts is the sorting out of responsibilities of everyone involved. Nurses are personally liable for their own actions; the responsible employer, however, is the supplemental staffing agency and not the agency in which the nurse actually renders the service. Nurses, prior to agreeing to be temporarily assigned, should review all contracts that exist and in particular should note any terms that relate to malpractice, negligence, or insurance.

The relationship between a health-care agency and an educational institution, in which students will use the agency for learning, is also a contractual one. The agency agrees to allow instructors and students into the agency, and the educational institution is thus provided experiences for its students. Most contracts have a term that states that the health-care agency retains responsibility for client care, and the instructor's responsibility is to supervise the students. Should a student make a mistake and be negligent, the contract helps determine who the responsible parties are.

First and foremost, students are responsible for their own actions. If they commit an act of negligence, they will be measured by what a nursing student would have done in a like situation. The instructor and staff of the agency also may be negligent but only if they failed to evaluate or supervise the student. If the instructor knew a student was weak in a particular area and did not take steps to prevent mistakes as a result of the weakness, then the instructor shares liability with the student. Most educational institutions require students and instructors to carry malpractice insurance. In addition, contracts between schools and agencies often require that malpractice insurance be purchased by students and instructors.

Many nurses hold their own malpractice insurance policies. Obtaining this type of insurance involves establishing a contract with an insurance company and paying for the coverage. The two basic questions to ask in determining how much coverage to purchase are: What is the area of practice? What personal assets are at stake? If you are practicing in a high-risk area, such as critical care, anesthesia, or emergency nursing, or if you have substantial personal assets at risk, you will want to obtain higher amounts of coverage.

After these two points are settled, the most important matter to cover with the insurance agent and the contract are the provisions about exclusions, since most insurance for malpractice will cover only that. Therefore, if you are indicted on a criminal charge, legal fees for an attorney will not be covered by your malpractice insurance. Or if you are accused of violating the nurse practice act, your malpractice insurance will not provide legal fees. There are often other exclusions identified in the contract that should be studied carefully.

The other critical point to know about the insurance contract is whether there is a difference in the time it is effective. Some insurance contracts specify that a person will only be covered if the contract is in effect both when the malpractice incident occurred and when the claim of malpractice is made. Other insurance contracts will cover the individual at either of the times mentioned above. Understanding when the contract is effective is important, because the time between an incident of malpractice and when the claim is filed can be a period of several years.

Collective bargaining agreements are yet another example of contractual agreements. Nurses who are subject to such agreements are usually members of a union. Federal and state labor laws have a great impact on collective contracts. The National Labor Relations Board is the primary Federal agency that enforces the National Labor Relations Act.

Criminal Law

A crime is an offense against the public at large. Distinguished from a civil wrong, in which private individuals are the parties involved, a criminal wrong will be prosecuted by the state. The purpose of criminal prosecution is to protect the interests of the public as a whole. The elements of crime and the punishments they carry are usually part of a state's legislation and judicial opinions.

In 1981, Wiley[1] described the experiences of several registered and licensed practical nurses with criminal law. These nurses were employed in intensive care units or medical-surgical units of hospitals, and because the clients they had cared for had died under suspicious circumstances, they were accused of either homicide or murder. The deaths were associated with drugs given by the nurses and their activities involving client life-support mechansims, such as respirators.

While most of the criminal charges were overturned or the nurse was acquitted, the nurses' rub with the criminal justice system led Wiley to make three recommendations:

- Follow hospital (or agency) policies and procedures
- Carry your own malpractice insurance, because a nurse's interest is different from a hospital's
- Retain a lawyer *early*

Constitutional Law

The U.S. Constitution and individual state constitutions set forth the structure and function of the different governments and describe the relationship between government and individual citizens.

One hallmark of **constitutional law** is due process rights. Due process is actually two rights in one. Every citizen is entitled to notice, to the opportunity to be heard, and to have the facts stated as they occurred. For example, if a nurse is accused of violating the state nurse practice act, the government (in this case the state government) must notify the nurse of the charges and set up a time for a hearing. At the hearing, the nurse, through a retained attorney, has an opportunity to hear the charges and to refute them. The evidence presented can be challenged by the nurse, the hearing officer, or nursing board, depending on the state. During the hearing, the nurse has a right to **cross-examine** any **testimony** or other evidence presented.

In the case of a disciplinary action taken by an employer against the nurse, the nurse is entitled to similar due process rights. The nurse is entitled to know why the disciplinary action is being taken and to refute the reason. Because of due process rights, nurses also can examine their own personnel files and insert a statement denying or supporting its contents. In addition, nurses are entitled to know what appeal procedure can be followed in order to challenge decisions made by their supervisors. Federal and state wage and employment laws often determine the answers to employer–nurse disputes. The Civil Rights Act, Age Discrimination Act, Pregnancy Discrimination Act, Fair Wage and Employment Act, Equal Employment Opportunity Commission and other laws exist, which may provide individual protection for nurses.

Legislation

Legislation is law made by various governmentally authorized bodies at the local, state, and federal levels. The legislature is made up of elected officials and is one of three branches of government. Legislation is developed in a formal process that includes bill writing, approval with commitees and houses of the legislature, passage by the entire legislature, and, usually, signing by the president (Federal), governor (state) or mayor (local).

Although legislation has an impact on and shapes nursing practice in general, the area of community health nursing has been particularly influenced by public health laws and regulations. Two examples of legislation, other than licensing laws, that relates to most nurses are reporting **statutes** and the Good Samaritan act.

Reporting statutes are laws that require specified individuals to report to designated authorities events that they have witnessed or suspect to be true. The reporting of suspicions is to be done carefully and in good faith to avoid recklessness and malice. Reporting statutes that affect most nurses are ones that require a nurse to report suspected child abuse or neglect and adult or elder abuse. Although the particular details—to whom and when to report and a

penalty for not reporting—vary among different states, in all states nurses are specifically mentioned as responsible for reporting, along with others.

Good Samaritan acts are state legislation that is intended to encourage people to render emergency first aid or care that may save someone's life at the scene of an accident. The encouragement comes from the fact that if negligence occurs while attempting to save another's life the person who received the negligent care cannot sue the one responsible for the negligence. In some states, nurses are entitled to immunity under Good Samaritan acts whereas in others they are not. The act, however, usually applies only to individuals who do not receive remuneration for what they did; what they did was not gross negligence. Gross negligence is an act that is extremely unreasonable, reckless, or wanton. If a court decides that a nurse acted in a grossly negligent manner, then a lawsuit can be maintained against the nurse. Most states have other legislation that provides immunity from lawsuits for individuals employed by fire departments, rescue squads, or other agencies that deliver emergency medical services.

RECORD-KEEPING RESPONSIBILITIES

Regardless of where nurses work or practice, record-keeping is an important responsibility. Records have many uses in the health-care system.

Records used by nurses in their place of employment can be divided into two categories. Clinical records are all those documents that pertain to the care of a particular client. Administrative records are kept soley for the purpose of administering the agency or facility. The difference between these two major types of records is clearer when one examines selected examples of records used in a health agency.

The client's individual health record is a clinical record. It contains information about the client's stay or contact with every health provider that may be involved in the care. From the time of admission to discharge, details of assessment, plans, interventions, and progress are recorded. These records are called client charts. In most agencies, a client's chart includes the following information.

- The medical and nursing admission information
- A personal data sheet listing name, address, age, marital status, etc.
- Consent or permission sheets (when applicable)
- Medical history
- Nursing history
- Physical examination findings
- Medical progress sheets
- Nursing progress sheets or nurses' notes
- Laboratory finding results sheets
- Procedure finding sheets (e.g., ECG)
- Temperature, pulse, respiration, and blood-pressure flow sheets
- Physician order sheets
- Medicine order sheets
- Discharge planning sheet
- Utilization review sheet

Some agencies that deliver services to families keep family records. These usually contain notes on the family as well as individuals in that family.

Administrative records include documents such as incident reports, valuables lists, or minutes of meetings of different segments of the agency. These records sometimes relate to an individual client but are usually kept separate from the client's clinical record. One purpose, for example, of the incident report is to alert the risk manager, insurance company, or quality assurance director where and what type of mistakes are being made in the institution. Everything that happens to the client is recorded in that clinical record, and an incident report that, when completed, contains similar information to that recorded in the clinical record, is often required by the agency.

Records reflect the quality of care delivered and serve to organize the care given. Clients and health-care providers rely on records' being complete. When clients direct that records be transferred to other agencies or health services, continuity of care can be preserved if records are complete and include a discharge summary. This summary can provide a client's synopsis of the care delivered and the client's reaction to interventions.

Other uses of records include research, data collection, and evaluation of client care. For the agency's purposes, records can be reviewed to examine many aspects of care and organization. Trends in needs and services can be found in records and agencies often plan future services for them. Conducting clinical record reviews within the agency usually does not require the client's permission. Confidentiality, however, must always be maintained. Laws, **rules and regulations** of state and Federal governments, and institutional policies must be followed regarding informed consent and human rights protections when research is involved.

The clinical record is also important in determining financial and economic issues of care. For example, utilization review and peer review use the client's chart to determine length of stay. The diagnoses in the records and documentation of the client's care and needs are factors that determine which diagnosis-related group (DRG) is applicable. The extent of Medicare coverage rests on DRG decisions.

Another major use of the client record is as evidence in a legal dispute. Client records are considered business records of the agency and are admissible as such under rules of evidence. Lawsuits often are won and lost based on what is in the record. Although testimony is also another form of evidence, the written record is seen as more accurate and reliable, since it was written at the time of the incident in question. Because lawsuits sometimes take years to emerge, one's memory (e.g., testimony at trial) is not as reliable as the written record. Because of the reliability of the clinical record, great emphasis is placed on the completeness of the record by individual health-care providers and institutions alike.

Access to Records

A major health-care legal issue is the right of access by clients to their own records. Within the health-care system a range of positions exists. Clients in the military health-care system keep their records with them, for example, whereas in other health care agencies, clients must get a subpoena to obtain access to their records. In the latter situation, the client often has to be anticipating **litigation** or suing the agency in order to get a subpoena from a court.

However, the majority of state legislatures have passed laws requiring agencies to establish reasonable policies and **procedures** so that clients may have access to their own records. A copy of the applicable state law should be part of every agency's policy manual. Policies that have been established often cover when and under what circumstances clients see their records.

In the last 15 years, most agencies have established open and flexible policies so that clients have access to their records more easily than in the past. The only remaining area in which access is still more restrictive is psychiatric records. Some policies allow physicians to object to clients seeing their psychiatric records, in which case, the policy or even the state legislation may provide that the client be provided a summary of the record and an appeal mechanism for challenging the physician's decision to withhold the record.

The legal issue of access to client records has changed dramatically in favor of the client. The law generally recognizes the client's control over the information in the record. The client is the one who holds the right to confidentiality and gives permission for access to the record to those not involved in care in the agency. Permission from the client must be obtained prior to release or transfer of records to others.

Advances in computer technology and access to records is increasingly a concern for both clients and providers. This situation raises legal issues of access, privacy, and confidentiality. Management of **medical records** must involve a mandate to maintain and protect the privacy of clients. The use of computers benefits the delivery of health care but increases the risk of loss of confidentiality. Protection of confidentiality in automated systems includes controls and checks on who can access the data. In addition, code numbers and other methods can be used to guard client privacy.[2]

Informed Consent

Informed consent indicates that clients have had treatments or procedures explained to them and they have given consent based on that information. Informed consent given prior to medical and surgical intervention is an absolute requirement in nonemergency situations. The person conducting the treatment or surgery (usually a physician) is responsible for obtaining the consent, the person who would be committing the tort of battery by touching someone without expressed consent. That person may also be negligent if the consent is not informed.

The nurse's role in informed consent for interventions by the physician is carrying out an agency policy or administrative function. The nurse is accountable for the agency policy. The usual policy requires the nurse to ask the client to sign a form that documents the informed consent given to the physician.

By getting the form signed, the nurse may be the witness to the client's signature. If this is the case, it should be stated on the form: witnessing signature only. If the nurse was present when the physician discussed the treatment or surgery and explained the risks, benefits, and alternatives to a coherent, legally competent individual, then the nurse is witnessing the informed consent and the client's acknowledgment of that fact. In the latter situation the nurse, as a more extensively involved witness, can provide better evidence for the physician should the client later raise the issue of informed consent.

The American Nurses' Association *Code for Nurses*[3] states that obtaining the prior consent of clients to nursing care (not to be confused with medical care where it is the physician's legal responsibility to obtain consent) is an ethical obligation of the nurse. The major elements of informed consent are:

- Consent must be given voluntarily
- Consent must be given by an individual with the capacity and competence to consent
- Consent needs to involve enough information so that the client can be the ultimate decision maker

In emergency situations, health-care providers may intervene to save someone's life without obtaining consent. If the client is a minor, the guardian or parent is the individual legally competent to consent. In many states, minors may consent themselves for selected and specific types of health care. For example, in most states, minors may consent to treatment for mental illness, venereal disease, alcohol and drug addictions, pregnancy, contraception, and abortion. Nurses who have minor patients should obtain a copy of state minor consent laws. In some instances, (e.g., abortion), parental notice may be required.

Common Charting Errors

Despite concerns about the types and uses of records, access to records, and informed consent, major accountability and quality of care of the health provider is reflected in accurate and complete record keeping. Most common failures in recording include failure to:

- Record accurate and complete information
- State objective, factual data
- Document concisely and legibly, in chronological order
- Alter records according to agency policy
- Maintain records in a safe, confidential manner
- Sign with legal name and proper identification
- Observe agency policy on countersigning
- Use accepted abbreviations
- Meet other existing agency policies or bylaws

Most errors are self-explanatory but two are worth further discussion: alterations to records and countersigning. Changes in records become necessary when a mistake has been made in the record. A single line drawn through the mistake with the word "error" printed next to it and the nurses' initials is one appropriate way of correcting the mistake. White-out, cutting and pasting, and obliteration of the mistake is not appropriate. These methods only leave a question in a jury's mind about what the writer is trying to hide. The correct information is placed in the record in chronological order and labeled "late entry."

The effect of countersigning is usually governed by agency policy. Generally, if one countersigns, it is as if what is observed or participated in is being documented equally with the person who actually delivered the care. Countersigning relieves no one of responsibility or accountability for his or her actions. If an agency requires countersigning, its purpose usually is to ensure close supervision and direction for certain types of employees. For example, the nursing supervisor may countersign receipt of physician orders by the staff nurse who has just started the job. The supervisor and staff nurse are equally accountable for the proper processing of those orders.

MANAGEMENT OF MEDICAL ORDERS

One of the many important contributions nurses make to the care of clients is management of medical orders. Receiving, scrutinizing, implementing, and evaluating the effects of medical orders are critical functions of the nurse. It remains one of the dependent functions of the nurse who, according to state law, is dependent on the physician to prescribe medications before they can be given.

Medical orders must come from a licensed physician. In some states, dentists are allowed to **legally** prescribe medications, too. The safest way for nurses to receive medication orders is through written communications by the physician on the doctor's order sheet. Extenuating circumstances occasionally lead nurses to accept verbal orders or telephone orders. If this is the case, orders should come directly from a physician. In the best interest of the clients, nurses, agencies, and physician, once a telephone order has been accepted and written on the doctors' order sheet, the physician should sign for it on his or her next visit to the agency. When nurses are preparing to accept a verbal or telephone order, they may have another registered nurse listen to the order as well and cosign the chart. After taking the order, nurses should read it back to the physician to be certain that it has been written on the chart accurately. The person who takes the order down should sign the physician's name, his or her own name, the date, time, and the letters T.O. or V.O. (to represent telephone or verbal order).

Standing orders are predetermined directions for potential client situations, such as what to do if the client develops a fever. They need to be approved jointly and equally by the physician writing them and the nurse implementing them. Standing orders are to be used in clearly defined, predetermined situations only. Standing orders must be renewed every thirty days. They are more often used in community settings where access to a physician may be limited or distant.

The purpose of standing orders is to provide the nurse with power to act and to expand the usual role into an area of clinical practice. The standing order protects the nurse from charges of practicing medicine without a license. Because of this, nurses should examine their skills, experience, and education in light of the standing order. Nurses should not accept orders they don't feel competent to administer.

The nurse is legally accountable for evaluating physician orders. Nursing judgment must be brought to bear on each order the nurse implements. Appropriate medication, right dose and right route must be observed. Any question about an order should be directed to the originator, and all questions should be answered before any order is implemented.

Because the administration of medications and medical treatments is the area most susceptible to lawsuit, careful scrutiny of orders is essential to eliminating errors and lawsuits involving nurses.

When physician orders involve life-sustaining or resuscitation measures, nurses may be caught between agency policy and physician order. A medical order that, if implemented, would force the nurse to violate agency policy is never an appropriate order. The nurse should notify the supervisor or director of nursing who, in turn, should notify the agency administration. For example, if a hospital policy indicated that no-resuscitation orders must be in writing and the physician refuses to write the order yet expects that no resuscitation will be given, the nurse must follow the agency policy, notify the nursing supervisor, and resuscitate the client. In this situation, the existence of the policy serves to protect the nurse, who, if no resuscitation is given and no written order was recorded, might be liable for negligence or malpractice.

ACCOUNTABILITY FOR PRACTICE

Professional nurses are accountable to many different sources. Nurses relate, report, or account to themselves, others, organizations, and the government. Because nurses must account to such a large variety of sources, sometimes these sources conflict with one another. Nurses also have certain legal duties and responsibilities because of the variety of positions they hold. For example, nurses have a written or verbal contract with their employer; must relate to physician orders to give medications and carry out treatment; must act in their own best interests and in the best interests of their clients; are members of a group of professionals; and are licensed as safe practitioners by the government.

Licensure and Nursing Practice Acts

"Licensure" is a state governmental activity. Each state legislature, through its **police power,** can take steps to protect the public's health, safety, and welfare. Licensure of nurses is designed to ensure that every nurse in that state can function at a minimum level of performance. In this way the state can be sure that when one uses the initials R.N. or L.P.N., the care being received is from someone who is a safe and reasonable practitioner.

State Boards of Nursing. A piece of legislation in each state, the Nurse Practice Act, establishes and identifies certain powers to a board or commission of nursing. This licensing board is part of the executive branch of government. In addition to its power to grant nursing licenses, a board usually has the power to deny or revoke licenses, accredit nursing programs, and write regulations on nursing.

While the act lists many reasons why nurses' licenses may be denied or revoked, the main reasons include:

- Abuse of drugs or alcohol that affects patient care
- Impersonating, by using the initials R.N. or L.P.N. when unlicensed
- Ordinary or gross negligence or unethical conduct
- Conviction of a crime

Through the regulation power, the board may write further detailed rules to govern nursing in that state. Regulations do have the force of law and must go through a formal process that includes public comment before they become effective. The following are selected topics that state nursing regulations cover:

- Examination **procedures**, test development, and fees
- Requirements for renewal of license
- Hearing procedures
- Minimum requirements for approving R.N. or L.P.N. education programs
- Practice of Nurse Midwife
- Practice of Nurse Anesthetist
- Practice of Nurse Practitioner

State boards may require nursing education programs in their state to meet minimum standards written in regulations. In some states, nursing schools must obtain the accreditation or approval of the state board as well as the National League for Nursing, which is a private nursing organization that accredits all schools of nursing. In other instances, schools need to meet government and private group requirements.

Another major aspect of nurse practice acts as a definition of what constitutes nursing practice. See Table 10–6 for examples of state nurse practice acts definitions. Comparison of practice definitions among and across professional groups is essential for understanding what constitutes nursing and where questions of overlap exist. Nursing has independent as well as dependent functions that are delegated to nursing by physicians, such as administering medications.

There are differences in the laws from state to state. Therefore, it is imperative that every nurse obtain and review a copy of the practice act and regulations to which he or she is accountable. These are located in the state code of laws and code of regulation in most public libraries or can be obtained by writing to the state nursing board or commission.

Code of Ethics. The ANA has a committee on ethics that serves as a resource to individual nurses and state nursing associations and whose Council on Practice is charged with implementing the ANA Code (Table 10–7). The Committee has issued *Guidelines for Implementing the Code for Nurses*[4] to be used by state councils when they receive a complaint of unethical conduct by a registered nurse. Other pulications on ethical conduct of nurses are available from professional organizations (see annotated bibliography).

Standards of Practice. Another activity that nursing associations are involved in is the development of standards by which nursing practice can be evaluated. The standards of practice

TABLE 10–6. SELECTED DEFINITION OF REGISTERED NURSING PRACTICE: MARYLAND AND DELAWARE

Maryland	Delaware
Practice registered nursing Health Occupations 7–101 (f)	Practice of professional nursing Chapter 19 Nursing and Schools of Nursing 1902 (6)
Practice registered nursing means the performance of acts requiring substantial specialized knowledge, judgment and skill based on the biological, physiological, behavioral or sociological sciences as the basis for assessment, nursing diagnosis, planning, implementation and evaluation of the practice of nursing in order to: maintain health; prevent illness, or care for or rehabilitate the ill, injured, or infirm.	"Practice of professional nursing" means the performance for compensation of any act in the observation, care and counsel of the ill, injured or infirm, or in the maintenance of health or prevention of illness of others, or in the supervision and teaching of other personnel, or the administration of medications and treatments as prescribed by a licensed physician or dentist requiring substantial specialized judgment and skill and based on knowledge and application of the principles of biological, physical and social science. The foregoing shall not be deemed to include acts of diagnosis or prescription of therapeutic or corrective measures.
For these purposes, practice registered nursing includes: administration; teaching; counseling; supervision, delegation and evaluation of nursing practice; execution of therapeutic regimen, including the administration of medication and treatment; independent nursing functions and delegated medical functions; and performance of additional acts authorized by the board under 7-205.	

TABLE 10–7. AMERICAN NURSES' ASSOCIATION CODE FOR NURSES

The nurse provides services with respect for human dignity and the uniqueness of the client, unrestricted by considerations of social or economic status, personal attributes, or the nature of health problems.

The nurse safeguards the client's right to privacy by judiciously protecting information of a confidential nature.

The nurse acts to safeguard the client and the public when health care and safety are affected by incompetent, unethical, or illegal practice of any person.

The nurse assumes responsibility and accountability for individual nursing judgments and actions.

The nurse maintains competence in nursing.

The nurse exercises informed judgment and uses individual competence and qualifications as criteria in seeking consultation, accepting responsibilities, and delegating nursing activities to others.

The nurse participates in activities that contribute to the ongoing development of the profession's body of knowledge.

The nurse participates in the profession's efforts to implement and improve standards of nursing.

The nurse participates in the profession's efforts to establish and maintain conditions of employment conducive to high-quality nursing care.

The nurse participates in the profession's effort to protect the public from misinformation and misrepresentation and to maintain the integrity of nursing.

The nurse collaborates with members of the health professions and other citizens in promoting community and national efforts to meet the health needs of the public.

Reprinted with the permission of the American Nurses' Association.

issued by the ANA are general statements of the content of nursing practice. Intended to ensure the quality of nursing practice, the ANA standards are written by the different practice divisions of the ANA. Many speciality nursing organizations have developed their own standards or have worked with the ANA in the development of the ANA standards. Standards have been used by individual nurses and nursing departments of health-care agencies as resources for developing nursing audits and peer review systems. Both activities are examples of nurses regulating and evaluating their own practice.

Certification. A third self-regulatory activity by private nursing organizations is certification. One example is ANA certification (see Table 10–8). Available to individual members of the

ANA, certification means that a registered nurse has successfully completed an examination process beyond the state licensure examination, which indicates that the nurse has a higher level of competency of nursing within a speciality area. Information about requirements for taking the examinations can be obtained by writing to the ANA practice division that gives the particular exam.

Not only is certification a sign of having achieved an advanced competency rating but it also is a sign of having passed the scrutiny and evaluation of peers. In addition, as the trend increases for nurses to receive direct reimbursement for services, certification may be a necessary step for that reimbursement. Insurance companies, the Federal government, other third-party payors, and private individuals may see certification as a measure of an individual's ability to deliver services and, hence, require it before a nurse would be eligible to receive funding for services provided.

Clients' Rights and Responsibilities: Best Interests of Clients

Although clients who enter institutions because of illness may be dependent on others for care and assistance, they continue to maintain rights that existed prior to entering such a facility. Clients, on entering an agency, assume responsibilities toward that agency, such as abiding by its rules and regulations or financial obligations.

A general rule is that every adult (defined in most states as at least 18 or 21 years of age) is competent unless, through a formal legal proceeding, it is determined that the individual is not competent. In the latter situation, a guardian usually is appointed to make all decisions for the incompetent person. In addition, a guardian may be appointed to make only medical, financial, or contractual decisions. The guardian or parent of an individual under 18 or 21 years of age sees to the rights and responsibilities of the child and is deemed to act in the best interests of the incompetent child.

Every individual possesses rights and obligations. All hospitals accredited by the Joint Commission on Accreditation of Hospitals (JCAH) are accountable to the American Hospital Association's (AHA) Bill of Rights (see Table 10–9), therefore nurses are also accountable for

TABLE 10–8. CERTIFICATION IN NURSING SPECIALTIES

Certification Programs	Number of Nurses Certified as of March, 1985
• Community Health Nursing	1388
• Adult Nurse Practitioner	3770
• Family Nurse Practitioner	4363
• School Nurse Practitioner	430
• Gerontological Nurse	2462
• Gerontological Nurse Practitioner	466
• Maternal and Child Health Nursing	246
• Child and Adolescent Nurse	429
• High-risk Perinatal Nurse	233
• Pediatric Nurse Practitioner	1006
• Medical-Surgical Nurse	3660
• Medical-Surgical Clinical Nurse Specialist	490
• Psychiatric and Mental Health Nurse	4211
• Adult Psychiatric and Mental Health Clinical Nurse Specialist	1904
• Child Adolescent Psychiatric and Mental Health Clinical Nurse Specialist	207
• Nursing Administration	4052
• Nursing Administration, Advanced	793

From ANA Certification Catalog, 1986.

TABLE 10–9. AMERICAN HOSPITAL ASSOCIATION PATIENT'S BILL OF RIGHTS

1. The patient has the right to considerate and respectful care.
2. The patient has the right to obtain from his physician complete current information concerning his diagnosis, treatment, and prognosis in terms the patient can be reasonably expected to understand. When it is not medically advisable to give such information to the patient, the information should be made available to an appropriate person in his behalf. He has the right to know by name, the physician responsible for coordinating his care.
3. The patient has the right to receive from his physician information necessary to give informed consent prior to the start of any procedure and/or treatment. Except in emergencies, such information for informed consent should include but not necessarily be limited to the specific procedure and/or treatment, the medically significant risks involved, and the probable duration of incapacitation. Where medically significant alternatives for care or treatment exist, or when the patient requests information concerning medical alternatives, the patient has the right to know the name of the person responsible for the procedures and/or treatment.
4. The patient has the right to refuse treatment to the extent permitted by law and to be informed of the medical consequences of this action.
5. The patient has the right to every consideration of his privacy concerning his own medical care program. Case discussion, consultation, examination, and treatment are confidential and should be conducted discreetly. Those not involved in his care must have the permission of the patient to be present.
6. The patient has the right to expect that all communications and records pertaining to his case should be treated as confidential.
7. The patient has the right to expect that within its capacity a hospital must make reasonable response to the request of a patient for services. The hospital must provide evaluation, service, and/or referral as indicated by the urgency of the case. When medically permissible a patient may be transferred to another facility only after he has received complete information and explanation concerning the needs for and alternatives to such a transfer. The institution to which the patient is to be transferred must first have accepted the patient for transfer.
8. The patient has the right to obtain information as to any relationship of his hospital to other health care and educational institutions insofar as his care is concerned. The patient has the right to obtain information as to the existence of any professional relationships among individuals, by name, who are treating him.
9. The patient has the right to be advised if the hospital proposes to engage in or perform human experimentation affecting his care or treatment. The patient has the right to refuse to participate in such research projects.
10. The patient has the right to expect reasonable continuity of care. He has the right to know in advance what appointment times and physicians are available and where. The patient has the right to expect that the hospital will provide a mechanism whereby he is informed by his physician or a delegate of the physician of the patient's continuing health care requirements following discharge.
11. The patient has the right to examine and receive an explanation of his bill regardless of source of payment.
12. The patient has the right to know what hospital rules and regulations apply to his conduct as a patient.

(Reprinted with permission of the American Hospital Association, copyright 1975.)

We, the Council on Human Rights of the Maryland Nurses Association, in order to promote increased knowledge and understanding of the rights and responsibilities of all registered nurses, have developed The Bill of Rights for Registered Nurses. We propose that this Bill will aid in educating consumers and health care professionals about the rights of registered nurses, as well as their corresponding responsibilities. Therefore, we submit the Bill of Rights for Registered Nurses as a positions statement of the Maryland Nurses Association.

The Nurse Has a Right:

To practice according to the Maryland Nurse Practice Act

To make independent nursing judgments

To question any delegated medical order or any plan of care that may cause possible harm to the patient/client or others

To refuse to carry out any delegated medical order or any plan of care that may cause possible harm to the patient/client or others

To pursue quality continuing education

To teach individuals and groups health care practices that facilitate treatment, prevent illness, and provide optimal wellness.

The Nurse Has a Responsibility:

To assume personal accountability for individual nursing judgments and actions which consider the individual value systems and the uniqueness of each patient/client

To implement the nursing process in providing individualized nursing care

To safeguard the patient/client and the public from incompetent, unethical or illegal health care practices

To refuse to perform any nursing action which will jeopardize the patient/client or the public, and the obligation to communicate the rationale to the proper authority

To avail one's self of opportunities which will broaden knowledge and refine and increase skills

To educate the patient/client and the public

Employment

To competitive hiring and promotion which is based on knowledge and experience and which is unrestricted by consideration of sex, race, age, creed, or national origin

To realistic assignments that can assure the patient/client quality care that includes safety, dignity, and comfort

To negotiate salary and individual conditions of employment

To work in a safe and adequately equipped environment

To work with qualified, competent nursing personnel

To periodic, fair, objective evaluations by peers

To pay increases based on demonstrated performance

To due process whenever accused of unethical, incompetent, illegal, or unqualified practice or of prejudicial or inappropriate conduct

To be an advocate for the patient/client and the public when health care and safety may be affected by incompetent, unethical, or illegal practices

To representation by a negotiator in labor matters

To maintain competence and prepare one's self adequately for promotion

To evaluate one's own work environment and to communicate and document unrealistic workloads through appropriate channels

To make known individual convictions and preferences prior to hiring

To assess, evaluate, document, and correct unsafe conditions and to communicate such information to the appropriate authority promptly

To objectively document and report to appropriate authorities evidence of competent, as well as incompetent performance and to evaluate, inform, counsel, and teach nursing personnel when indicated

To participate in the development of reliable and valid evaluation criteria for peer review

To maintain competence, incorporate new techniques and knowledge, and continuously upgrade the quality of health care

To participate in the planning, establishment, and implementation of procedures to ensure due process

To be alert to any instances of incompetent, unethical, or illegal practices by any member of the health care system and to take appropriate action regarding these practices

To select and utilize a knowledgeable and impartial negotiator

Figure 10–2. The Bill of Rights for Registered Nurses, Maryland Nurses Association.

Professional

To receive support from the nursing profession at all levels

To belong to an autonomous nursing organization

To have expert testimony supplied by the nursing organization for both legal actions and legislative issues

To full and equal representation on all decision-making bodies concerned with health care

To be involved actively in the political decision-making process at all levels of the government

To participate in activities that contribute to the ongoing development of the profession's body of knowledge

To be an active member and to participate in the nursing organization's effort to implement and improve standards of nursing

To provide knowledgeable, objective, articulate expert testimony

To provide knowledge, active, and effective collaborating with members of the health professions

To be knowledgeable, active, and effective in the legislative process by direct involvement, effective education and selection of representative legislators, lobbying, and creating citizen awareness in promoting local, state, and national efforts to meet the health needs of the public

Figure 10–2. (continued)

seeing that clients' rights are protected. Most rights in the AHA bill are legally enforceable, meaning that legislation or judicial opinion exists that establishes each right as one that the law will enforce.

Nurses' Rights and Responsibilities: Best Interests of Nurses

The delivery of nursing services is not an effort where only one group's interests should be observed. Nurses have rights and responsibilities that balance and complement those of others, including clients.

One bill of nurses' rights and responsibilities was written by the Maryland Nurses Association (MNA) (Fig. 10–2), developed by the MNA Council on Human Rights, and approved by the Board of Directors. This bill describes nursing rights and responsibilities according to different relationships (for example, the nurse and the client, and the nurse and employer).

Progress in a profession is related to the control of practice and standards within the profession. Nurses, therefore, should take an interest in defining standards of practice, delineating a code of ethics, and studying how laws affect the nursing profession.

SUMMARY

Nursing practice is governed by many legal and ethical concepts. Many law concepts have a direct relationship to nursing practice; therefore, it is important for nurses to have some basic knowledge of these laws. There are five major sources of law in the United States and they are intertwined.

Many laws affect nursing practice because the legal system is designed to protect the rights of individuals and groups. Laws are classified into two major areas: criminal and civil law. Criminal law involves conduct considered harmful to society as a whole, whereas civil law concerns the rights of individuals. Most litigation involving nurses has been civil in nature and in the areas of: torts (negligence and malpractice) and contracts.

Nurses enter into contractual agreements with both clients and agencies, and also are involved with keeping client records. Nurses should be familiar with charting policies and the importance of keeping accurate and thorough records.

Informed consent is another area that involves nurses. They should be aware of the facts of obtaining this type of consent and specific agency policies regarding informed consent.

Professional nurses are accountable for their practice to state and professional organizations as well as to clients, families, agencies, and themselves. Nurses have many standards by which to judge themselves, for example: licensing laws, continuing education, ANA Standards of Practice, and codes of ethics.

For nursing to continue to emerge as a health-care profession, nurses must become involved in formulating standards of practice, enforcing codes of ethics, and participating in legislation.

Study Questions

1. List and discuss the specific nursing tasks or functions that carry the greatest legal risks.

2. What is the difference between a nurse's personal liability and her responsibility as an employee of the institution?

3. Discuss the advantages and disadvantages of a professional nurse obtaining professional liability insurance.

4. What is the nurse's role in interpreting and ensuring the patient's bill of rights?

5. Can a nursing student be sued?

6. What should a staff nurse do if he or she observes a member of the health-care team performing what is judged to be an incompetent or unethical activity?

7. Locate your state practice act and regulations. What is the scope of nursing practice under the act?

References

1. Loy Wiley, "Liability for death: Nine nurses' legal ordeals," *Nursing '81,* (September 1981): 34–43.

2. M. Hiller, and V. Beyda, "Computers, medical records, and the right to privacy," *J Health Polit Policy Law,* (March 1981):463–87.

3. American Nurses' Association code for nurses, with interpretive statements (Kansas City, Mo.: American Nurses' Association, 1976, 1985).

4. American Nurses' Association, Committee on Ethics, *Guidelines for Implementing the Code for Nurses* (Kansas City, Mo.: American Nurses' Association, 1982).

Annotated Bibliography

Bagwell, M., and Clements, S. 1985. *A Political Handbook for Health Professionals.* Boston: Little, Brown. Reviews the political process, legislative process, and lobbying methods. Guidelines and strategies for increasing political clout and shaping the law are given.

Beauchamp, T., and Childress J. 1983. *Principles of Biomedical Ethics,* 2nd ed. New York: Oxford University Press. Taking a fresh approach to ethical principles, these authors discuss theory, initially, and each of four principles: autonomy, nonmaleficence, beneficence, and justice. Relationships, ideals, virtues, and integrity also are discussed.

Campazzi, B.C. 1981. "Nurses, nursing and malpractice litigation." *Nurs Adm Q* 5(1):1–18. This article summarizes the content of almost 400 negligence cases involving nursing over a 10-year period.

Christoffel, T. 1982. *Health and the Law.* New York: Free Press. This reference reviews law and the legal system and public health law and discusses the impact of law on clinical practice.

Davis, A., and Aroskar, M. 1983. *Ethical Dilemmas and Nursing Practice,* 2nd ed. New York: Appleton-Century-Crofts. This book addresses topics such as abortion, informed consent, dying and death, behavior control, mental retardation, client rights, and professional ethics. Examples of ethical dilemmas are discussed.

Hemelt, M., and Mackert M. 1982. *Dynamics of Law in Nursing and Health Care,* 2nd ed. Reston, V.: Reston Publishing Co. This text outlines doctrines and principles of law related to negligence, contracts, defenses, and damages. Over 30 situations are analyzed from legal perspectives.

Murchison, I, Nichols, T, and Hanson, R. 1982. *Legal Accountability in the Nursing Process,* 2nd ed. St. Louis: C.V. Mosby. Placing the discussion of legal accountability in a unique context, that of the nursing process, these authors focus on the nurse practice act, legal grounds for disciplinary action, the reasonably prudent nurse, and rights of patients. Many cases are used as examples.

Northrop, C. 1984. "Current states of nursing litigation." *Nurs Econ* 4 (November–December):427. Reviews cases involving nursing practice for an 18-month period from considering lower and higher court decisions.

O'Rourke, K., and Barton, S. 1981. *Nurse Power, Unions and the Law*. Bowie, Md.: R.J. Brady. This text provides a much-needed discussion on collective bargaining and the politics of nursing. Sample contracts and forms are included.

Wing, K. 1985. *The Law and the Public's Health*, 2nd ed. Ann Arbor, Mich.: Health Administration Press. Covers many important topics in health-care law, including power of the state governments, privacy, social welfare, antitrust, malpractice and hospital liability for denial of medical care.

Chapter 11

Accountability

Helen Foerst

Chapter Outline

- Objectives
- Glossary
- Introduction
    Accountability Defined
- Standards of Care
- Quality Assurance
    Concept and Purpose
    Methodology
    Nursing Quality Assurance
- Credentials
    Licensure
    Certification
    Accreditation
- Professional Literature
    Purposes
    Encouraging Accountability
    Accessing the Literature
    Nursing Journals and Periodicals
- Continuing Education
    Trends in Continuing Education
    The Continuing Education Unit
    Professional Associations and Continuing
    Education
    Accreditation of Continuing Education
    Mandatory Continuing Education
- Summary
- Study Questions
- References
- Annotated Bibliography

Objectives

After completion of this chapter, the reader will be able to:

▶ Define the terms in the glossary
▶ Describe the evaluation and processes of the nursing profession's accountability as society and health care changes.
▶ Discuss standards development and how standards ensure quality of care
▶ Relate standards and their application to the nursing process
▶ Discuss the purposes of communicating nursing knowledge through written materials
▶ Name three forms of credentials and describe how they influence the quality of nursing care
▶ Discuss the concepts of quality assurance and nursing's basic approach in developing assessment methodology
▶ Identify the sources of nursing information
▶ Describe how technology facilitates literary endeavors
▶ Describe the nursing profession's historical perspectives, philosophy, and goals on continuing nursing education
▶ Delineate individual, professional, and employer responsibilities for continuing education
▶ Discuss the relationship between continuing education and competence in practice

Glossary

Accreditation. The process by which a voluntary, nongovernmental agency or organization appraises and grants accredited status to institutions, programs, or services that meet predetermined criteria.

Certification. A process by which a nongovernmental agency or association certifies that an individual licensed to practice a profession has met certain predetermined standards specified by that profession for specialty practice.

Contact Hour. A unit of measurement that describes 50 minutes of an approved organized learning experience.

Continuing Education. Planned, organized learning experiences designed to augment the knowledge, skills, and attitudes of nurses for the enhancement of nursing practice, education, administration, and research, to improve health care to the public.

Continuing Education Unit (CEU). Ten contact hours of participation in an organized continuing education experience that meets the criteria established by the National Task Force, including sponsorship, capable direction, and qualified instruction.

Credentials. Certification by a qualified agent that individuals or institutions have met minimum standards at a specified time.

Criteria. Predetermined elements against which aspects of the quality of an activity or service may be compared.

Effectiveness. The extent to which preestablished objectives are attained as the result of an activity.

Evaluate. To ascertain or fix the value of, or worth of. To examine and judge, to estimate, appraise, assess, assay, rate.

Factor. Any of the component parts instrumental in determining the nature of the complex. Something that actively contributes to the production of a result.

Implement. To carry into effect, fulfill, accomplish. To provide with the means for carrying into effect or fulfilling. To provide a definite plan or procedure to ensure the fulfillment of.

Inservice Education or Staff Development. An educational program planned by an agency to assist employees in becoming increasingly knowledgeable and competent in fulfilling role expectations within that specific agency. The two terms often are used interchangeably, but staff development usually includes out-of-agency activities.

Norms. Numerical or statistical measures of usual observed performance.

Nursing Audit. The end review of the client care record to secure measurements of quality of a comprehensive set of components of nursing care.

Objectives. Criteria by which one measures the degree to which the purpose is achieved. The statements are made in terms of results to be achieved rather than methods to be used.

Orientation. The means by which new staff are introduced to the philosophy, goals, policies, procedures, role expectations, physical facilities, and special services in a specific work setting. Orientation is provided at the time of employment and at other times when changes in roles and responsibilities occur in a specific work setting.

Peer Review. A process or technique by which people secure observations associated with behaviors of equals.

Quality. The distinguishing characteristics that determine the value, rank, or degree of excellence.

Quality Assurance. The accountability of health personnel for the quality of care provided.

Standard. An agreed-upon, established, or expected level of performance or excellence.

Value. A principle or quality that is intrinsically desirable. To rate or scale in usefulness, importance, or general worth. To consider or rate highly, prize, esteem.

INTRODUCTION

Scientific knowledge is being generated, distributed, and assimilated into our technological society with staggering rapidity. The delivery of health-care services is becoming an increasingly complex endeavor in a rapidly changing society. A health professional's knowledge base and skills are the result of rigorous preparatory education that must be constantly expanded and updated. Individuals and employers are accountable to the public for the quality of practice offered. This accountability has placed emphasis on the establishment of quality controls, peer review, certification of health professionals, continuing education, and the production of professional literature.

Nursing can point with pride to a long history of growth, development, commitment to quality client care, and accountability for the services rendered. The record of accomplishment in fulfilling this obligation has kept pace with scientific and technological achievements, changes in health-care needs of society, and constantly changing patterns of medical and health care.

This chapter presents an overview of accountability and standards of practice, the professional nursing literature, and aspects of continuing education for nurses. Accountability is examined in terms of the development and implementation of standards of nursing practice and nursing education. The evolutionary processes for assuring accountability are discussed. The nursing literature is discussed in terms of nursing's responsibility to document its expertise and of the nurse's responsibility to be familiar with the literature. The professional accreditation of programs offering nursing education and agencies offering nursing services and the certification of nursing practitioners are emphasized. Contemporary trends in achieving accountability highlight peer review and quality assurance programs.

Accountability Defined

Accountability is an obligation to reveal, explain, and justify what one does or how one discharges one's responsibilities. Within a job or work situation, areas of responsibility include the purposes, principles, procedures, relationships, results, and incomes and expenditures. Applied to nursing, accountability can be defined as the process by which individual or group behavior is explained, analyzed, and justified in relation to established standards.[1] Accountability involves personal and professional responsibility. The individual's and the profession's **values** are integrated in concepts of accountability. As health care and professional practice have changed, concepts of accountability have expanded. Efficiency and effectiveness were of special importance in the 1950s. Economical performance and proper productivity were elements of accountability. In the 1960s the concept of appropriateness was emphasized. Goals, policies, values, and the relative benefits of the various health-care systems and professional practices were questioned and stressed. Although quality was a basic tenet of the health professions throughout the century, it became the principal conviction and the motivation for refining old and developing new measures of accountability in the mid-1970s. All of the standard measures of accountability that had been developed for assuring quality, such as licensure, accreditation, certification, continuing education, as well as those related to functional performance, were scrutinized. An unprecedented effort was begun to develop definitive measures of quality for establishing standards of care.

STANDARDS OF CARE

Standards of care are the basic framework of accountability. **Standards** are the attributes of good care. The development of nursing standards and measures of good care can be traced to Florence Nightingale. Standards were implicit in her untiring efforts to provide for better nursing and care of the sick. They also were reflected in her perception of nursing as an art and as a trained profession. The search for indicators and measures of quality care has its origins in the Nightingale systematic evaluation of care and study of the ways in which nursing care was provided.

Webster defines a standard as that which is set up and established by authority as a rule for the measure of quantity, weight, extent, value, or quality. A standard is further defined as an accepted or established rule or model having a recognized and permanent value. A nursing standard measuring quantity, for example, would be the number of nurses that should be available to provide good care. A nursing standard measuring quality would be the training or education essential for those nurses to render care.

Standards have several major characteristics. Two basic elements used in their development are **criteria** and **norms**. Criteria are rules for performance and the degree of achievement of the expected outcomes (specified in the criteria of the standard). Norms are predetermined expected levels of performance or achievement, usually the average or median achievement, that can be expected of a large group.

A criterion in the quantitative standard for the number of nurses needed by the nation to provide care would be a ratio of the number of nurses to the population to be served, for example, 560 nurses per 100,000 people. The norm would be a reasonable goal, established by averaging the ratios attained among the several states, that is judged capable of achievement—for example, 300 nurses per 100,000 population. A criterion of the qualitative standard for the training and education of nurses providing care would be the number that ideally should be prepared at the baccalaureate level, for example, one-half of all nurses. The norm would be established by examining the capability of nursing schools to prepare a prescribed number or percentage of nurses with baccalaureate degrees, for example, one-fourth of all nurses. Standards and criteria set **objectives** and goals for desirable attainment. In addition, they provide a basis for improvement and measurement of the degree to which the goals are met.

Quality, **effectiveness,** and efficiency are inferred, judged, and measured by established standards and criteria. Different approaches and methods are used for establishing standards. Essentially, they are based on existing good practices that can be used as models. Methods for developing and establishing standards have evolved from basing criteria on the experience and judgment of what constitutes good practice to conducting surveys and studies of nursing activities to develop measures of good practice. Increasingly, research is being conducted and provides the criteria for standards development. All of the methods have their limitations and can be criticized. Most standards and criteria require and reflect some degree of value judgment and philosophy of the particular group of experts involved in their development.

The earliest standards of care were derived from experience. They were based on policies and procedures and patterns of practice in given situations and institutions that were judged to lead to the provision of good care. They addressed particular aspects of care and nursing activities or the qualifications and functions of the practitioners delivering care. When there were fewer types of services and nurses and care was less technical, standards were simple measures of quantity, quality, and performance based on concepts of the role of nursing. They were abstract sets of criteria for elements of nursing practice and indicators of competence or quality and guidelines for practice that nursing leaders accepted as attainable. Performance could be evaluated, and progress and achievement measured, by comparison to the recommended standards such as:

- Criteria for educational programs
- Levels of educational attainment
- The function of each level of nursing personnel
- Staffing ratios or number of nurses required for client care

One of the primary responsibilities of a profession is to develop and maintain its own standards. The professional nursing organizations assumed responsibility for the development of the standards by which the services of nurses could be evaluated late in the eighteenth century. The first step was the establishment of the organizations themselves. The first standards were those for membership in the organizations. The criterion was that members be graduates of training schools. One of the major objectives of the early state organizations was legislation for the registration of nurses, which they saw as the first step in the betterment of the nursing profession. The first state law requiring the registration of nurses was passed by North Carolina in 1903, followed by New Jersey in the same year. The New Jersey law stated:

> any graduate nurse deserving to practice the profession of a trained nurse must first obtain a license (upon presentation of a diploma and 50 cents) from the clerk of the county in which such applicants reside.[2]

The registration acts set standards for the quantity and quality of training for practice. In the New Jersey law the diploma was to be awarded by a training school connected with a hospital of the state where at least two year's practice and theoretical training is required.[3]

Standards of performance also were embodied in the early permissive licensing statutes. Only registered persons were authorized to use the particular title or official designation specified in the legislation. Unregistered persons were not prohibited from working in the nursing field but could not use the title. The licensing laws were meant to protect the public and the registered nurses from incompetent practitioners.

Between 1903 and 1923, 48 states passed nurse practice acts and established state boards of examiners who inspected schools and administered compulsory examinations for graduates of approved schools. The practice acts have been amended as nursing practice changed. Most acts are now mandatory, requiring all who nurse for monetary compensation to be licensed. The nurse practice acts incorporate statements on the function of the nurse or the nature and scope of nursing practice.

The professional associations developed other means for their members or practitioners to judge one another as professionally competent and to evaluate the quality of their services. The evolution of today's standards of care is reflected in definitions of nursing, in statements on the functions and qualifications of nurses, and in manuals and guidelines for practice. *The National Organization for Public Health Nursing 1912–1952: Development of a Practice Field* records one organization's development of standards for nursing services and education and changes in those standards as the practice and education of public health nurses evolved.[4]

In 1916, the National Organization for Public Health Nursing (NOPHN) developed and issued its official definitions of public health, district, visiting, school, and industrial nursing. *The Visiting Nurse Manual* was published. It contained daily nursing routines, nursing care techniques, and specific information on the care of medical, surgical, pediatric, maternity, and chronically ill clients. The manual was

regarded as the basic standard for public health nursing. Standards for the qualification of nurses in public health work were issued in the same year, to be enforced by 1930. These are recognized as the first official minimum educational qualifications to be set by the professional nursing organizations. These qualifications were: high school graduation, completion of nurse training, state registration, and a minimum of four months of field experience in public health nursing. The standards were waived for those nurses who graduated from training schools before 1920. The NOPHN upgraded and revised its statement of the qualifications for public health nurses every five years. The 1935 standards, for example, called for staff nurses with one year's postgraduate education in public health nursing, and the 1950 standards, for baccalaureate preparation.

An official *Public Health Nursing Manual* was published in 1926.[5] It was to serve as a general guide for practice and included procedures and techniques of care and practice in clinics, schools, homes, and industry. The manual was revised in 1932 and 1939 and was recognized as the standards guidebook for public health nurses for 25 years. The development and revision of standards also included periodic redefinitions of public health nursing, official descriptions of the various kinds of public health nursing services, and the functions of public health nursing. The 1931 statements contained objectives and functions based on age, disease, and practice setting. The 1936 and 1941 statements added emphasis on a general approach to care. The independent functioning of nurses and the assessment of health problems, care planning, and evaluation were stressed in the 1949 statements. Changes in definitions and functions were, naturally, related to changes and new developments in nursing practice.

Many of the original and revised definitions of nursing and functions and qualification standards resulted from various studies of nursing. They were views of what was required as recommended in studies of nursing practice and nursing education. Over the years, broad-based studies of nursing, the surveys of nursing activities, and research on elements of client care have provided knowledge of nursing practice, services, and client-care needs on which standards were based. The purpose of these studies was the improvement of nursing practice. Some examples of these efforts will be described.

The Goldmark Report of 1923—a study of nursing and nursing education—set goals for the educational preparation of nurses in administration, supervision, and instructor positions, and for public health nurses.[6] Initiated to study the status of public health nursing and propose training for nurses' preparation, the report assessed the entire fields of nursing service and nursing education. The work is recognized as the first in which actual observations of nursing practice were made in order to develop recommendations.

The Committee on the Grading of Nursing Schools of the National League of Nursing Education issued two study reports in 1934. One report recommended and set standards for the educational preparation of faculty in nursing schools—that they be registered nurses with special training and experience in particular fields of nursing.[7] Entrance requirements for students—that they meet the entrance requirements of a good college—were also recommended. The second report, *An Activity Analysis of Nursing,* distinguished nursing functions from non-nursing duties.[8] Conclusions on what every nurse should know and do became criteria for judging a competent nurse.

A natural progression in the development of standards were studies in the particular settings where standards are applied. In 1937, the National League of Nursing Education conducted a study in 50 general hospitals to find out how well clients were nursed.[9] The hours of nursing care provided clients by graduate nurses, students, attendants, and ward helpers were obtained. The time provided was analyzed in terms of type of hospital, service, and shift. Recommendations suggested minimum hours of bedside service per client in each 24 hours for medical, surgical, obstetric, and pediatric units. The number and kinds of personnel needed and their hours of employment were included.

In the mid and late 1940s, the profession began efforts to rigorously validate its nursing care standards by more in-depth studies of nurse staffing and the utilization of nurses. In 1948,

the National League of Nursing Education selected 22 hospitals in the New York City area that were reported to be well managed and providing quality nursing care. An extensive study was made of nurse:client ratios in these hospitals.[10] It was determined that, on the average, each client received 3.5 hours of nursing care per day, of which two-thirds was provided by registered nurses and one-third by nursing aides, practical nurses, and others. This ratio, based on existing good practice in hospitals, became a model for the delivery of nursing services and a standard for staffing mix in hospitals for many years.

Another step was the development of techniques and instruments for measuring the nursing care requirements from which levels of client care and nurse staffing could be determined in acute-care settings. Clients in these settings were classified in care groups according to the intensity of illness and need for care. For example, clients who could feed, bathe, and dress themselves would be placed in one group; those who needed to be bathed, dressed, and fed in another. The purpose of the earliest client classification instruments was to determine the number of nursing personnel required and how staff should be allocated to care for these clients. Client classification systems provided norms for staffing. Various tools and guidelines for their use were developed to classify clients in hospitals and nursing services.[11–13] More than 40 different methods have been developed.[14] The client assessment associated with classification provided indications of care needs that helped to strengthen standards development. As client classification and other assessment tools for appraising client-care needs were developed and refined, they were used in conjunction with and as part of care planning and evaluation. Well defined client-care standards reflect the nursing process.

Many corollary efforts led to the development and refinement of nursing-care criteria, models of nursing practice, and nursing practice standards. One effort and source of professional impetus was the American Nurses' Association's (ANA) Code of Ethics.[15] The code was adopted in 1950 and was revised in 1960, 1968, and 1976. It identified acceptable areas of nursing practice, conduct, and relationships. The code of ethical standards supports high-quality maintenance nursing care and the establishment, and improvement of nursing practice and client care standards. The eighth standard in the code speaks to the nurse's responsibility to participate in standards development: "The nurse participates in the profession's effort to implement and improve standards of nursing." The ANA Code items and interpretative statements can be found in Chapter 12. The ANA Code for nurses and its interpretative statements reflect the concepts of responsibility and accountability as they apply to contemporary nursing theory.

As the professional association for public health nurses from 1912 to 1952, the NOPHN established standards and guidelines for the practice of public health nurses. The ANA, as the professional organization for registered nurses, is concerned with all matters pertaining to their practice. The first standards were developed for private duty nurses in 1916. Since then, the ANA periodically has defined nursing and established, revised, and published new standards. In the 1950s, the ANA conducted a full study on the functions of nursing and issued publications on the functions, standards, and qualifications of various nurse positions, such as general duty nurses, office nurses, and industrial nurses.[16]

In the 1966 reorganization of the ANA, divisions of practice were established for the advancement of practice in the fields of medical-surgical nursing, maternal and child health nursing, psychiatric and mental health nursing, geriatric nursing, and community health nursing. These divisions and the Congress of Nursing Practice were charged with establishing standards of nursing practice in their fields of concern.[17] Generic standards and standards developed in the special fields of nursing by the five divisions were published by ANA in 1973 and 1974 in separate booklets. A list of these standards and others in subspecialty areas published later are listed in Table 11–1. Also see references 18 to 34 for the source documents. The standards are guidelines for adaptation by individual nurses to clients in particular nursing situations for development of the care plan and to appraise the effectiveness and excellence of care. They were specifically designed to be used as

TABLE 11–1. ANA SPECIALTY GROUPS WITH STANDARDS OF PRACTICE

ANA Specialty Group	Year Established
Standards for Nursing Practice	1973
Cancer Nursing Practice Outcome Standards	1979
Cardiovascular Nursing Practice	1981
Community Health Nursing Practice	1981
Emergency Nursing Practice	1975
Geriatric Nursing Practice	1973
Gerontological Nursing Practice	1973
Maternal-Child Health Nursing Practice	1973
Medical-Surgical Nursing Practice	1974
Neurological and Neurosurgical Nursing Practice	1977
Orthopedic Nursing Practice	1975
Operating Room Nursing Practice	1975
Pediatric Oncology Nursing Practice	1978
Perioperative Nursing Practice	1981
Psychiatric-Mental Health Nursing Practice	1973
Rehabilitation Nursing Practice	1977
Urological Nursing Practice	1977

part of the nursing process. The standards outline assessment factors or criteria for:

- Collection of data about the health status of the individual
- Nursing diagnosis derived from the health status data
- Formulating goals for nursing care
- Developing the plan for nursing care to meet the goals
- Implementation of the nursing care plan
- Evaluating the plan and client response to care
- Reassessment, rediagnosis, setting new goals, revision of plan of care

The standards provide assessment factors focused on physiological functions, elements of care, and client goals for the speciality or subspeciality fields of practice. For example, in the standard for cardiovascular nursing practice, the assessment factors on data for health status include pulmonary, vascular, and circulatory criteria.[25] They must be applied to the specific client with arrythmias, congestive heart failure, or acute myocardial infarction.

It should be noted that many of the speciality standards were developed in cooperation with the speciality nursing organization concerned. For example, the *Standards of Nursing Practice: Operating Rooms* were joint endeavors of the ANA and Association of Operating Room Nurses (AORN).[29] The AORN prepared and published for its members an implementation case study to interpret the standards and illustrate how they are used, and republished the standards in 1978.[35] Examples from the hypothetical case for each of the seven standards explain how the criteria are applied to the client situation.

In publishing the generic and speciality standards in 1973 and 1974, the ANA pointed out that the standards were only an initial step toward measuring quality of care. Work was begun immediately on developing a system or model for use with the standards to assure the quality of care rendered. The model was published by ANA in 1975 in *A Plan for Implementation of Standards of Nursing Practice*. Work in developing standards and means for their application to the actual practice of nursing is never completed. Standards must be continuously refined, modified, and revised. Means for implementation must be explored to keep them relevant to nursing practice and to assist nurses in being accountable for care given.

QUALITY ASSURANCE

The nation's health goals of the 1970s focused on assuring the quality of health care. Federal initiatives and legislation promoted the development of formalized systems and programs for the appraisal of the quality of care rendered in health-care institutions and agencies. Efforts were intensified in all health fields to establish procedures and surveillance methods for assuring quality care to be performed jointly by professional colleagues as an ongoing activity of their practice.

Quality assurance in health care connotes the accountability of health personnel for the quality of care they provide. The term implies a commitment to improve care and to upgrade professional practice. To address its accountability and responsibility for quality assurance, nursing, in cooperation with other health disciplines, undertook expanded and intensified research, evaluation, and demonstration projects for the development of the building blocks and tools for implementing quality assurance and control programs. Among others, standards and criteria development, peer review, certification, and accreditation were areas of study. These processes of quality assurance are described in this section.

Concept and Purpose

The Social Security Amendments of 1972 (Public Law 92–603)[36] mandated the establishment of Professional Standards Review Organizations (PSROs). PSRO legislation provided the underlying concept of quality assurance programs. PSROs, through practicing physicians, were to assume responsibility for reviewing the appropriateness and quality of medical care paid under Medicare, Medicaid, and Maternal and Child Health Programs. Medical care was to be reviewed to determine if it was: 1) necessary; 2) consistent with professionally recognized standards of care; and 3) provided in the least costly setting possible. PSRO legislation, in effect, extended and involved the care of all clients regardless of their health-care payment plan. The law recognized that health care is provided by a wide variety of health-care disciplines and called for the involvement of nonphysician health-care practitioners in the review process. It directed that review of care provided by nonphysician practitioners should be performed by their peers in cooperation with PSRO committees, including the ongoing revision of norms, criteria, and standards. The PSRO legislation accelerated the development of quality assessment methodologies and fostered the standardization of review activities.

The purpose of a quality assurance program is to **implement** a systemic means of evaluation and control to assure the delivery of quality care. A quality assurance program defines, **evaluates** and measures quality in terms of explicit operational objectives and focuses on the outcomes of care. It documents whether the actual service provided matches predetermined criteria of excellence for providing care. Continuous corrective actions are taken to secure improvement when care is found to be deficient.

Methodology

The concept of **quality** is difficult to define and its measurement is complex. In 1966, Avid Donabedian made an extensive analysis of methods for appraising medical care and suggested an approach for assessing quality.[37] Donabedian proposed that for the purpose of measurement, the structures, process and outcomes of care were the determinants of quality. This approach has been widely accepted and embraced in developing standards and methods of measurement of the quality of care.

In 1972, medicine, in conjunction with the American Hospital Association, described the critical components of a quality assurance system as development of standard measurements of quality of care, surveillance and evaluation of care provided, and corrective action.[38] The system involves a continuous cycle of five steps not unlike the steps in carrying out the nursing process:

- Standards and criteria development
- Description of the actual care provided
- Review and evaluation—does the care provided equal the standards?
- Corrective action
- Reassessment

Nursing Quality Assurance

Building upon its tradition in standards development and evaluation of nursing practice and nursing programs, the nursing profession refired and adapted their quality assessment methodologies for the development of quality assurance models and programs. Embracing the concepts of Donabedian and Slee, the American Nurses' Association refined the profession's nursing practice criteria and standards and developed guidelines and a model for quality assurance.[39]

A nursing quality assurance program evaluates the quality of the results of the nursing component of health care. Although other approaches have been developed and are used, the basic approach to nursing quality assurance is evaluation of the structure, process, and outcomes of care in relationship to the nursing process. The major focus for measurement is outcomes of care, but the relationship of structure and process to outcomes of care is recognized as essential to identifying deficiencies so that improvement of quality can be achieved.

The ANA defined these three determinants of quality for developing criteria for measurement as follows:[40]

- *Structure* considers the purpose of the institution, agency, or program. It includes organizational characteristics, fiscal resources and management, qualifications of health professionals and other health workers, and physical facilities and equipment.
- *Process* focuses on the nature, sequence of events, and activities in the delivery of client care and the extent to which they help clients reach specified health-care goals.
- *Outcome* refers to the end results of nursing care and measurable change in the state of the client's health.

The ANA model for quality assurance is shown in Figure 11–1. The ANA publishes a *Quality Assurance Workbook* to facilitate the implementation of a quality assurance program.[41]

Other models have been developed with variations on the basic framework. The Veterans Administration has developed a nursing process model for a decentralized nursing service.[42] The model uses nursing unit monitoring programs for the continuous documentation and review of the quality of nursing care based on predetermined standards. This model includes strategies for interdepartmental coordination and collaboration of unit quality assurance programs. The Duke University Hospital nursing assurance model uses a nursing process-and-outcome approach as the framework for its methodology.[43]

The development of quality measurement tools and control methods has been a concern of nursing since the 1950s. Many of the methodologies developed over the years are used singly or are incorporated into today's nursing quality assurance programs. Examples of some of these methods for appraising the quality of

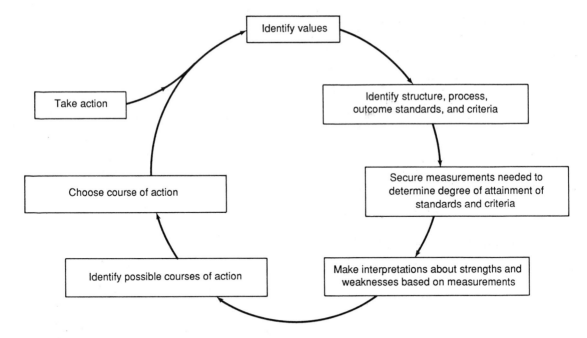

Figure 11–1. Model for quality assurance: Implementation of standards. *(Adapted from Norma Lang, A Model for Quality Assurance in Nursing, 1974, with participation—Reprinted from A Plan for Implementation of Standards of Nursing Practice [Kansas City, Mo.: American Nurses' Association, 1975], 15.)*

care that entail use of carefully developed measures are:[44]

- *Stater Nursing Competencies Rating Scale*
  Measures the competencies displayed by a nurse under observation in nurse–client interactions
- *Quality Patient Care Scale*
  Measures the quality of nursing care being received by the client while care is ongoing.
- *Nursing Audit*
  Measures the quality of nursing care received by a client after the cycle of care has been completed and the client discharged through examination of the client record

The development of instruments and tools for the measure of quality and methodologies for nursing care assessment is ongoing. Nursing is giving increasing attention to quality nursing care research. Research is focused on defining quality in nursing practice, identifying indicators of quality, developing criteria and conceptual frameworks for assessment, and testing new approaches for evaluation and **peer review.** As nursing practice changes and new specialities

emerge nursing will be motivated and challenged to further its research for designing relevant assessment procedures.

CREDENTIALS

The use of **credentials** is an important aspect of quality assurance, whether applied to healthcare institutions, educational programs, or to health professionals. Nursing has historically used various methods of establishing credentials to monitor and maintain quality of care. The 1979 Study of Credentialing in Nursing defined and described the process of establishing credentials and its mechanisms:

> Credentialing refers to the processes by which individuals or institutions, or one or more of their programs, are designated by a qualified agent as having met minimum standards at a specified time.[45]

The credentials concept supports the premise that accreditation mechanisms for programs or individuals are designed to ensure quality care for the public they serve. Accreditation processes are methods for maintaining standards of education and service and for stimulating continued self-improvement. The three major mechanisms of establishing credentials for nurses, nursing education, and nursing services are the licensure of nurses, the certification of practitioners of nursing specialties, and the accreditation of programs offering nursing education or agencies offering nursing services. Nursing has been a leader in establishing credentials, particularly in licensure and accreditation for nursing education, which can be traced to the early 1900s. Over the years, the scope and processes of establishing credentials in nursing have been modified and the systems strengthened to keep pace with health-care needs and changes in nursing practice and nursing education.

Licensure

Licensure in nursing is a complex mechanism. It is defined and described by the profession as:

> Licensure is a process by which an agency of state government grants permission to individuals accountable for the practice of a profession to engage in the practice of that profession and prohibits all others from legally doing so. It permits use of a particular title. Its purpose is to protect the public by ensuring a minimum level of professional competence.
>
> Established standards and methods of evaluation are used to determine eligibility for initial licensure and for periodic renewal. Effective means for rescinding or modifying the licenses of individuals involved in acts of professional misconduct, incompetence and/or negligence are employed.[46]

Requirements for licensure are contained in the rules and regulation of state nurse practice acts and are not necessarily uniform in the various states. Some states also set requirements for advanced or specialty practice. State boards of nurse examiners set the standards in each of the states and jurisdictions. A national examination, developed and prepared by the National Council of State Boards of Nursing, is in use in most of the states and jurisdictions. The mechanism for nurse licensure assesses initial competence for the general practice of nursing and grants a credential for entry into practice. The license is a "life-long license," since no evidence of competence in current practice is required for renewal. The major weakness of nurse licensure, as it currently exists, is the failure to ensure continuing competency and personal accountability for practice. The legal aspects of licensure and the Nurse Practice Acts are discussed in Chapter 10.

Certification

Certification recognizes that quality care is directly related to the caliber of the professionals rendering services.

> Certification is a process by which a nongovernmental agency or association certifies that an individual licensed to practice a profession has met certain predetermined standards specified by the profession for specialty practice. Its purpose is to assure various publics that an individual has mastered a body of knowledge and acquired skills in a particular specialty.[47]

Certification in nursing has developed mainly as a voluntary professional mechanism for establishing credentials. The professional nursing organizations develop and administer the certification programs in nursing.[48] The goals of certification among the organizations are very similar. They usually include:

- Assessment of advanced knowledge and skills
- Demonstration of excellence in practice
- Encouragement of professional growth
- Assurance of the public's welfare
- Standardization of the qualifications necessary for specialty practice
- Advancement of the knowledge and standards of the specialty

The objectives, however, may differ and are generally of two types:

- To recognize and encourage personal achievement and superior performance, e.g., the certification programs of the ANA
- To set entry criteria to practice in the field and denote minimum competence for practice

in the specialty, e.g., the certification programs of the American College of Nurse Midwives

Standards for certification are based on the acquisition of knowledge and skills that exceed the minimum required for R.N. licensure and require periodic assessment to ensure continued competency. The eligibility requirements for initial certification generally include:

- Basic nursing education: A bachelor's of science, nursing, or higher degree may be required
- Current R.N. licensure
- Completion of an accredited educational program in the specialty of specified length or a reasonable substitute meeting professional educational guidelines for the specialty
- Experience in the specialty of specified duration and recency—commonly two years immediately prior to application

The standards and eligibility requirements for renewal of certification are, for the most part, identical to those for initial certification. Some certification programs offer the option of substituting documented **continuing education** credits obtained during the period of certification in lieu of taking a recertification examination, e.g., the ANA certification program. The recertification interval is usually three to five years.

Autonomous boards of the professional organizations administer the certification programs and confer and revoke certification. The process of certification includes an evaluation of the candidate's knowledge, competence, and excellence in practice. The procedures of the process and sequence are as follows:

- Application: Candidate files an application submitting evidence on each of the eligibility requirements
- Determination of eligibility: Application is reviewed by the certifying organization; credentials are assessed and rated
- Testing and assessment of knowledge: If requirements are met, candidate is registered for a scheduled examination and successfully completes a national examination
- Endorsement by colleagues and evidence of clinical performance: References are re-

quested from persons familiar with candidates practice and educational achievement
- Evaluation of evidence: The certification board evaluates all the evidence and makes a decision
- Certification is conferred

As compared to licensure, certification in a specialty field in nursing is relatively new. The American Association of Nurse Anesthetists (AANA) began its certification program in 1945; the American College of Nurse Midwives (ACNM) in 1971. In response to the increasing specialization of nursing practice and demand for quality in services, the ANA began the development of a certification program in 1970.

The ANA's divisions of practice defines the scope of practice and standards for certification for advanced practice in each specialty, based on the guidelines of the Congress for Nursing Practice. In May, 1974, the ANA offered its first certification examination to recognize professional achievement and excellence in the practice of nursing in the area of geriatric nursing and pediatric nursing in ambulatory care settings. Proficiency examinations in psychiatric/ mental health nursing were administered in September of 1974.[49] The ANA certification program now includes 15 specialities in clinical nursing practice and two in nursing administration.[50] The Association is planning for development of generalist nursing certification for registered nurses and for testing in special areas of practice proficiency for these generalists.[51]

Specialty nursing organizations have developed certification programs in increasing numbers as the specialties in which nurses practice have emerged. Other professional societies have also developed certification programs that recognize nurses' qualifications for practice in various specialties. Certification programs for nurse specialties are shown in Table 11–2. Detailed requirements for each specialty are available on request from the professional organizations.

Accreditation

Concept and Purpose. **Accreditation** is a peer review mechanism in which recognition for meeting or exceeding established standards of

TABLE 11–2. NURSING SPECIALTY CERTIFICATION PROGRAMS

Programs Sponsored by American Nurses' Association	Programs Sponsored by Specialty Nursing and Other Professional Organizations
Community Health Nurse	Critical Care Nursing
Adult Nurse Practitioner	Emergency Room Nursing
Family Nurse Practitioner	Enterostomal Therapy
School Nurse Practitioner	Hemodialysis Nursing
Gerontological Nurse	Infection Control
Gerontological Nurse Practitioner	Intravenous Therapy
Maternal and Child Health Nurse	Neurological Nursing
Child and Adolescent Nurse	Nurse Anesthetist
High-Risk Perinatal Nurse	Nurse-Midwifery
Pediatric Nurse Practitioner	Nursing Home Administration
Medical-Surgical Nurse	OB/GYN Practitioner
Clinical Specialist in Medical Surgical Nursing	Inpatient Obstetric Nurse
Psychiatric and Mental Health Nurse	Neonatal Intensive Care Nurse
Clinical Specialist in Adult Psychiatric and Mental Health Nursing	Neonatal Nurse Clinician
	Oncology Nurse
Clinical Specialist in Child and Adolescent Psychiatric and Mental Health Nursing	Occupational Health Nursing
	Operating Room Nursing
Nursing Administration	Post Anesthesia Nurse
Nursing Administration Advanced	Pediatric Nurse Practitioner
	Rehabilitation Nursing
	Urological Nursing

American Nurses' Association, Center for Credentialing, Kansas City, Mo., The Specialty Nursing Organizations and Professional Organizations, September 1986.

quality is granted to education and service programs, institutions or agencies.[52] The accreditation concept has two significant features:

- Agencies, institutions or programs conduct ongoing evaluations of the educational experiences or services they offer and are judged by an accrediting body as to their compliance with established standards
- Accrediting bodies assist institutions and programs in evaluating and improving the quality of their activities

The general purposes of accreditation are to:

- Foster excellence through the establishment of standards, criteria and guidelines for service or educational institutions and programs
- Promote improvements in service or educational institutions or programs
- Help ensure institutional or program objectives and accomplishments appropriate to societal educational and service needs
- Identify for various publics information about acceptable service or educational institutions or programs for decisions about their use

- Ensure adequate educational preparation of practitioners and high-quality nursing services

The importance of accreditation is that it signifies that a nursing service or education program that attains accreditation is of high quality and meets criteria of excellence. Maintaining accreditation stimulates continuous efforts to correct deficiencies, improve programs, and keep them abreast of current knowledge and practices.

Overview. Accreditation in nursing had its origins in the early 1900s when nursing began the development of its standards for education and practice.[53] The foundation of accreditation in nursing education was laid with the passage of state nurse licensure laws and the appointment of inspectors of nurse training schools. In the 1920s, the ANA and NOPHN developed statements on the qualifications and functions of nurses and procedure manuals and guidelines for practice. The studies of nursing and nursing education set goals for upgrading nursing schools and improving the practice of nurses.

The Goldmark Report, *Nursing Schools Today and Tomorrow*, and *An Activity Analysis of Nursing* were stepping-stones to the establishment of professional accrediting services in the late 1930s. During the 1930s, the NOPHN, the National League of Nursing Education (NLNE), the Catholic Hospital Association, and the Association of Collegiate Schools of Nursing (ACSN) become involved in various accrediting services. The first national accreditation service was established in 1945. The services of the NOPHN, NLNE, and the ACSN merged to form the National Nursing Accreditation Service (NNAS). The service became part of the NLN when it was formed in 1952 by merging the NLNE, ACSN, and NOPHN.

Types of Accreditation. There are two types of accreditation: institutional and program. Institutional **accre**ditation applies to an entire institution or agency, e.g., a university, a hospital, often referred to as general accreditation. Program accreditation applies to a unit of an institution or agency, e.g., the nursing school in a university or a nursing department of a hospital. Program accreditation is referred to as specialized or professional accreditation. In nursing, professional accreditation usually refers to accreditation by the recognized accrediting bodies of the professional nursing organizations or nongovernmental agencies, e.g., the ANA and NLN. Two kinds of institutions can be accredited, i.e., nursing education and nursing service. Accreditation is a function of both voluntary nongovernment and governmental agencies.

Governmentally imposed regulations under the state nurse practice acts govern the practice of nursing and set minimal operating standards for nursing schools within each of the states. State boards of nurse examiners accredit or approve schools and programs in initial nursing education. This approval assumes that the minimum standards for nursing education for qualifying graduates for licensure and certification are met as specified in the regulations for state nurse practice acts. The state approval or accreditation of a nursing school is one of the eligibility requirements for voluntary or professional accreditation.

In the *voluntary*, nongovernment sphere,

the NLN accredits programs of education for nursing practice in practical, diploma, associate, baccalaureate, and master's programs. The professional nursing organizations recognize the NLN as the national professional accrediting agency for nursing education. The United States Department of Education and the Council on Postsecondary Accreditation recognize the NLN as the official accrediting agency for nursing education programs. NLN accreditation identifies programs eligible for Federal financial support. The ANA accredits continuing education programs and certificate (less than a degree) programs for the preparation of nurse practitioners.

The nursing profession, over the years, has focused its accreditation endeavors on nursing education to upgrade and improve nursing practice. Program or professional accreditation of nursing services is less developed. The NLN with the American Public Health Association (APHA) accredits home health agencies and community nursing services.[54] This program was begun in the late 1960s and is administered by the NLN.

Nursing services in hospitals are accredited as part of the institutional accreditation of the Joint Commission on the Accreditation of Hospitals (JCAH) which was formed in 1951. The focus of institutional accreditation is on quality client care. All client care services in the institution are evaluated. JCAH also accredits the following health-care facilities of which nursing services are a component:

- Psychiatric facilities
- Substance abuse treatment and rehabilitation programs
- Community mental health centers
- Organizations providing services for the mentally retarded and developmentally disabled
- Long-term care facilities
- Ambulatory health care organizations
- Hospice programs

Criteria and Standards. The nursing profession sets and promulgates the standards for nursing education and nursing service programs. The accrediting agencies apply the standards to the type of institution or program seeking accreditation and develop criteria and guidelines for self-study, appraisal, and review. The early accreditation standards focused on the structure of an institution or program.[55] They were concerned with the physical plant, its safety and functional efficiency. Standards were set for organizational structure and administration and their potential effectiveness and for personnel qualifications and procedures. It was assumed that if these standards were met the institution or program was sound. Later, evidence of compliance and more objective measurement of quality were added to the standards, e.g., matching personnel qualifications with capability and audit or record review. The PSRO legislation and the development of quality assurance programs stressed the need for increasingly rigorous accreditation programs. Accreditation criteria and standards have been broadened to include objective measures of process and an evaluation system that places emphasis on the assessment of outcomes. Today, the standards of accreditation require that institutions and programs have an effective quality assurance program for accreditation.

Accreditation Process. Institutions and programs meet requirements for accreditation through peer review and self-regulation. The major aspects of the accreditation process are self-study by the institution or program seeking accreditation and the site visit and review process of the accrediting body. The stages of the process are:

- Eligibility
- Application
- Self-study and report
- Site visit
- Evaluation by the accrediting body's board of review
- Continuing self-evaluation

The self-study is the most critical procedure in the accreditation process. The self-study requires an evaluation of all aspects of a program and provides for evaluative input from all of the staff. It allows for an assessment of progress in attaining program objectives and reveals strengths and weaknesses. The self-study gives directions for improvements and for future planning. The self-study report is the primary document used by the site-visit team and the review board in the appraisal of a program for accreditation.

The review board makes the final decision on accreditation. In general, the actions of a review board are approval, disapproval, or deferral. Recommendations for improvement may be made by a review board whether or not approval is granted. Approval is granted for a specified period of time, usually four to six years. Continued approval is based on periodic reevaluation. Lists of accredited programs are published by the parent organization of the accrediting body. For example, the NLN publishes lists of accredited programs yearly in *Nursing and Health Care* and issues pamphlets listing accredited programs. The list of NLN accredited practical nursing programs appears in the February issue, diploma programs in the September issue, and baccalaureate and master's degree programs in the June issue.[56-58]

In the case of deferral of accreditation, the program or institution is notified and may be given an opportunity to correct the deficiencies and be revisited and reassessed after a specified interval. When a program or institution is disapproved there is usually an appeals process for review of the board's decision. These procedures allow a program or institution to work for accreditation that signifies it has met a level of acceptable quality.

The mechanisms of licensure, certification, and accreditation are viewed by the nursing profession as being interdependent in influencing and upgrading the quality of nursing care. Licensure standardizes nursing care at a safe level. Accreditation promotes excellence in nursing education and nursing services. Certification is dependent on both demonstrated competence in practice and the high quality of nursing instruction of accredited programs of study.

PROFESSIONAL LITERATURE

Nursing produced and evaluated its own professional literature at an early date. Writing was perceived as a professional responsibility—an obligation inherent in accountability. To share and communicate expertise and valuable information with others was a mark of professionalism and influenced publication productivity. This philosophy persists today. The professional literature is as diverse as the nursing profession. The topics are inexhaustible. The literature is disseminated through journals, periodicals, books, texts, and reports that speak to nursing theory processes and document its studies and research efforts. To facilitate the use of the literature, nursing has produced reference guides, manuals, handbooks, indexes, dictionaries, and bibliographies.

Purposes

The professional literature serves many purposes. Writing ability and communication through the written medium is important in every facet of nursing. In general, nursing publications are used to communicate two types of information, focusing on:

- The issues, trends, or beliefs related to nurses and nursing practice
- The clinical or theoretical knowledge basis of nursing and reporting of technical and scientific methods

The literature is intended to enhance nurses' knowledge in clinical practice, education, administration, and research. It promotes the application of that knowledge in nursing practice. The hope is to effect change and to keep nursing practice relevant to trends in health care. The purpose and effectiveness of the nursing literature are illustrated in the following examples from its development and trends.

The first publications for nurses in the United States were textbooks published in 1878 and 1879 by groups of nurses in the early schools of nursing. These schools were operated mainly to train workers for the parent hospital. The first two textbooks were handbooks written for the graduate practicing nurses and the student apprentices in the Bellevue and Connecticut Training Schools for Nursing. They were small, compact manuals or guidebooks covering the complete system of nursing in these insitutions.

The *American Journal of Nursing* (AJN) published its first issue in October, 1900. The golden anniversary issue credited the journal with exerting great influence on laying the foundations of nursing.[59] As an important medium of nursing communication and unification, the *Journal* furthered the development of professional organizations. It provided a forum for the exchange of nurses' ideas and was a "source of information about the art and technic of nursing care." By nurturing concerted action and concern for the quality of care offered the public, nursing practice was secured and improved.

The impact that the written word and a nursing literature can have on the political process in nursing is implied by Kalisch and Kalisch in their book *Politics of Nursing*.[60] Letters, telegrams, and written policy statements on legislative issues of concern to nursing are used to influence the position and action of key lawmakers on pending legislation. The well-written and literate testimony of the professional associations and other nursing pressure groups can be an effective means of influencing the votes of legislators on proposed laws that involve nursing.

Encouraging Accountability

The commitment of the nursing profession to producing its own literature includes responsibility for preparing nurses to write and publish. To encourage literary endeavors benefiting nursing, instruction in developing writing skills and in the publishing process is included in many nursing education programs. Continuing education workshops also offer this instruction. Texts and journal articles address the criteria and pitfalls in manuscript preparation. Hospital nursing services are instituting programs to encourage writing for publication by nurses at the clinical practice level. Authorship promotes nursing excellence through communication and learning across practice settings. In addition to instruction in writing skills, these programs often include a journal club. Journal clubs stimulate writing and publication. Here, the content, writing style, techniques, and professional impact of journal articles are reviewed and criticized by groups of nurses. Topics for publication are identified and publication goals reinforced. All of these efforts are deliberate means to foster the essential communication of nursing knowledge through the written medium.

Efforts to develop the writing skills of

nurses and provide knowledge of the publication process in part help to ensure quality in the nursing literature. But nursing literature is also, in large part, subject to the criteria and standards of publishers. It is generally accepted in the scientific community that the most highly valued articles and information materials are those of publishers that use a refereed process for evaluating the quality of manuscripts. A refereed process usually uses three or more experts and consultants in the subject area or professional field to review manuscripts for acceptance or rejection. It is a professional peer review process that influences and develops excellence in literary endeavors.

Writing also has many recognized values for the author. It requires review of the current literature, keeps one abreast of professional trends, and promotes learning. In addition, in many education programs in institutions of higher education, writing and publishing are **factors** in promotion, tenure, and career advancement. One standard used to measure the quality of academic activities is the number of articles published in reputable journals.[61] Publishing is seen as a professional responsibility, and the "future of the profession depends on it."[62]

Accessing the Literature

Rapid advances in science and technology and changes in health-care delivery quickly outdate current information and knowledge. On the other hand, modern technology facilitates both the preparation of literary materials and their access. Critical reading is essential to maintaining competence and lifelong learning. This assumes an awareness of pertinent journal articles and new nursing literature. Selection of journal and reference materials appropriate to learning needs is equally important. Knowledge of the sources of professional information, the use of library resources and reference services, and the development of discriminating reading and writing habits and skills are of paramount importance.

Knowledge of and access to the literature is important for its ready use by nurses to help improve the quality of their practice. Knowledge and review of the literature is essential to teachers so that they are fully informed about their subject matter and are up-to-date in their field of instruction. Search and study of the literature is required by researchers to develop and formulate their research topics and methods. Nursing theories are generated from study of recorded and reported nursing information. Nursing also must perpetuate its literature to continuously develop the profession's scientific body of knowledge.

Recognizing the importance of access to the literature, the nursing profession has furthered the development of nursing bibliographies, indexes, abstracting services, and other library resources. Three excellent examples of library resources for nursing information are the following nursing indexes. The *International Nursing Index* is a periodically updated bibliography, published quarterly since 1966, with an annual cumulative edition.[63] Articles in 200 nursing journals are included. Subjects are classified according to a system developed with the National Library of Medicine (NLM). Libraries across the country participating with NLM in the dissemination of health and scientific information use or modify this classification system to fit their users.[64] Libraries make titles in the index available through a computerized information retrieval system.

The *Cumulative Index to Nursing Literature* was first published in 1956 and indexed topics in major English language nursing periodicals. It was the only nursing literature index from 1960 to 1965. In 1967, it added indexes from the publications of the national nurses' associations, and in 1972, those of the state nurses' associations. Since 1977 it has expanded coverage to include selected periodicals for certain allied health professions and changed its name. Today the *Cumulative Index to Nursing and Allied Health Literature* is still a valuable source of information on topics in nursing journals and periodicals. In addition, it contains lists of books, films, filmstrips, recordings, and pamphlets.[65]

The *Nursing Studies Index,* prepared by Virginia Henderson and a Yale University staff, is recognized as the foremost index for nursing literature for the period 1900 to 1959.[66] Its four volumes are an annotated guide to research reports, studies, biographies, and historical materials about nurses and nursing reported in English language books, periodicals, and journals for the first 60 years of the twentieth century. It is the single most important resource for locating historical materials on nursing practice, education, administration and research, and the development of the nursing profession. Included are the sources of trend data and information on nursing personnel, services, agencies, institutions, and programs.

Libraries across the country are a valuable resource for obtaining clinical and health information. The development of better library resources for nursing has been promoted by the Interagency Council on Library Resources, an advisory body of representatives of 19 agencies and organizations, including the ANA, the NLN, the American Hospital Association, and the U.S. Public Health Service. It has encouraged improved library services and makes information on library resources available to nurses. The major data base on literature in the nursing field is available from the NLM. Data bases contain information available in a printed index or in a series of printed indexes. Through the use of the computer for storing and retrieving information, libraries have access to vast resources of information. Computerized information and retrieval systems now make it possible for nurses and other health professionals to obtain reference materials and current professional literature at their own location. The most highly developed international system is that of the NLM. The data bases are searched for subscribing libraries in two ways: on-line and off-line. On-line means that interaction with a computer is direct through the use of a terminal connected by telephone to the computerized document-retrieval system (Fig. 11–2). Off-line means that processing is at a computer center, and information is mailed to a patron or library.

The NLM system includes several data bases pertinent to nursing. These include the following[67]:

- MEDLINE (Medical literature analysis and retrieval system)
  Covers nursing, medicine, dentistry, and allied health literature since 1978 and some citations since 1975. It includes journals in the *International Nursing Index* and *Hospital*

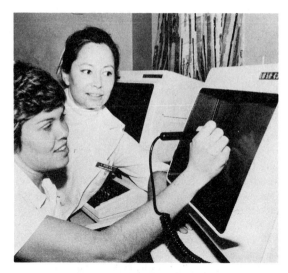

Figure 11–2. On-line computer services allow direct access to reference materials. (Photo courtesy of Norwalk Hospital, Norwalk, Connecticut.)

Literature and *Index Medicus.* Available online at a subscribing library or institution
- MEDLARS (Medical Literature Analysis and Retrieval System)
  Covers the same indexes as MEDLINE off-line from 1966 to 1969. MEDLARS went online in 1970 and was named MEDLINE
- AVLINE (Audio visual catalog on-line)
  Titles, medium type, description, terms, audience level, rating, price, and source of audiovisuals, covering all aspects of health science including nurse–client relations, nurse practitioners, nursing audit, nursing care, nursing staff, legal aspects of nursing, and pediatric nursing, since 1975
- HISTLINE (History of medicine on-line)
  Author, title, and source of historical information on medicine and other health sciences, individuals, drugs, diseases, institutions, and professions, since 1970
- CATLINE (Catalog on-line)
  Author, title, and source of books and serials in the NLM's catalog, covering biomedical, dental, and nursing literature, as well as popular works related to the health sciences by or for laymen

The NLM system also includes other computerized data bases on BIOETHICS (bioethics),

CANCERLIT (cancer literature), CANCER PROJ (cancer research projects), and HEALTH (health planning and administration) that have important information of use to nurses.

The NLM retrieval system includes a network of cooperating regional medical libraries that have on-line capability. Eleven major institutions have been designated regional medical libraries (Table 11–3). These libraries coordinate request for on-line accessibility through a communications network. The regional medical libraries also serve as a resource for obtaining other clinical and health information. The approach to the regional medical library system varies from state to state. Materials, documents, and reference services are, preferably, solicited first through the local resource: university, hospitals, medical, or health science library. In areas without a local contact point, the regional library may be approached directly.

Nurses should be familiar with two important resources for the reports of government-sponsored research and reports by the Federal agencies, their contractors or grantees, or special technology groups. The Federal Depository Library System includes some 1400 libraries nationwide. These libraries receive free and stock Federal publications of their choice. Most have the major government publications in the science and health fields. Local libraries have information on the location of the Federal Depository Library in your area.

The National Technical Information Service (NTIS), a component of the U.S. Department of Commerce, is another central, permanent source of scientific and professional literature of government-sponsored origin.[68] The NTIS contains a data base of 45 files arranged by specialty areas. Of interest to nurses are references to nursing literature in health planning organization and management that includes nurse manpower and nursing services planning. The volumes in the nurse planning information series are shown in Table 11–4. The NTIS acquires, screens, synthesizes, disseminates, and makes available other specialized documentary material on nursing, as well as methodological information on a wide variety of topics relevant to nursing.

There are, of course, many other reference collections and sources of useful informational materials pertinent to nursing. Only a small number have been discussed for illustrative purposes and to encourage further inquiry. It is

---

TABLE 11–3. REGIONAL MEDICAL LIBRARIES: LOCATION AND GEOGRAPHIC COVERAGE

New England Region (Conn., Maine, Mass., N.H., R.I., Vt.), Francis A. Countway Library of Medicine, 10 Shattuck St., Boston, Mass. 02115

New York and Northern New Jersey Region (New York and the 11 northern counties of New Jersey), New York Academy of Medicine Library, 2 East 103 St., New York, N.Y. 10029

Mid-Eastern Region (Del., the ten southern counties of New Jersey, and Pa.), Library of the College of Physicians, 19 South 22 St., Philadelphia, Pa. 19103

Mid-Atlantic Region (D.C., Md., N.C. Va., W.Va.), National Library of Medicine, 8600 Rockville Pike, Bethesda, Md. 20014

East Central Region (Ky., Mich., Ohio), Wayne State University Medical Library, 4325 Brush St., Detroit, Mich. 48201

Southeastern Region (Ala., Fla., Ga., Miss., Puerto Rico, S.C., Tenn.), A.W. Calhoun Medical Library, Emory University, Atlanta, Ga. 30322

Midwest Region (Ill., Ind., Iowa, Minn., N.D., Wis.), John Crerar Library, 35 West 33 St., Chicago, Ill. 60616

Midcontinental Region (Colo., Kans., Mo., Nebr., S.D., Utah, Wyo.), University of Nebraska Medical Center, 42nd St. and Dewey Ave., Omaha Nebr. 68105

South Central Region (Ark., La., N.M., Okla., Tex.), University of Texas Southwestern Medical School at Dallas, 5323 Harry Hines Blvd., Dallas, Tex. 75235

Pacific Northwest Region (Alaska, Idaho, Mont., Oreg., Wash.), University of Washington, Health Sciences Library, Seattle, Wash. 98105

Pacific Southwest Region (Ariz., Calif., Hawaii, Nev.), Center for the Health Sciences, University of California, Los Angeles, Calif. 90024

TABLE 11–4. VOLUMES IN THE NURSE PLANNING INFORMATION SERIES

1. Accountability: Its Meaning and Its Relevance to the Health Care Field
2. Nursing Involvement in the Health Planning Process
3. The Problem-Oriented System: A Literature Review
4. Patient Classification System: A Literature Review
5. Nurse Practitioners and the Expanded Role of the Nurse: A Bibliography
6. Comparative Analysis of Four Manpower Nursing Requirements Models
7. Nursing-Related Data Sources: 1979 Edition
8. Relationship between Nursing Education and Performance: A Critical Review
9. Nurse Staffing Requirements and Related Topics: A Selected Biography
10. Home Health Care Programs: A Selected Bibliography
11. Community Health Nursing Models: A Selected Bibliography
12. Quality Assurance in Nursing: A Selected Bibliography
13. Continuing Education in Nursing: A Selected Bibliography
14. A Classification Scheme for Client Problems in Community Health Nursing
15. Prospectives for Nursing: A Symposium
16. Computer Technology in Nursing
17. Factors Affecting Nurse Staffing in Acute Care Hospitals: A Review and Critique of the Literature

important to learn how to access these sources in order to understand the full scope of services available to you for lifelong learning.

Nursing Journals and Periodicals

Nursing journals and periodicals are one excellent resource for keeping abreast of trends in the nursing profession and advancing practice. As the needs for clinical and health information expanded and accelerated, the scope and availability of nursing journals greatly increased. Between 1900 and 1963, 20 major nursing journals were published. The number increased significantly in the next 20 years, as nursing became more specialized. One guide to nursing literature published in 1980 lists 60 major nursing journals alone.[69] If nursing and health related journals are added, the resources number well over 200.[70]

Today, nursing journals reflect the nature of health care, the contemporary knowledge explosion, technical advances, and the need of

nurses for information. Nursing journals have a specific audience and address particular practice interests and specialities. Both the *American Journal of Nursing* (AJN) and *Nursing Research* carry articles for clinical application. The AJN articles have a "how to" approach, whereas the focus in *Nursing Research* is conceptual and scientific.

The professional journals and newsletters are featuring more and more articles on the nursing journals. These articles primarily address publishing opportunities for nurses, journal audiences, and the referee process. They are intended to provide manuscript guidelines and help nurse authors understand publishing practice.

Elizabeth Swanson and Joanne McCloskey, associate professors at the University of Iowa College of Nursing, conducted surveys of the nursing journals in 1977, 1982, and 1986.[71–73] The number of nursing journals (whose audience was 50 percent nurses) included in the three surveys increased from 22 in 1977 to 47 in 1982 and to 72 in 1986. As can be expected, the 1982 and 1986 surveys showed that the journals with the largest circulation were those related to general practice. The three leaders, with a combined total circulation in 1986 of more than 1.10 million, were *Nursing 85*, the *American Journal of Nursing*, and *RN Magazine*. The journals in the specialized fields of nursing practice are more than 50 percent of the nursing journals. They have a low circulation but are significant in the coverage of major specialties and the scope of nursing literature.

The *American Journal of Nursing, Nursing '88* (the title changes annually to reflect the current year), and *RN* offer a broad selection of information on nursing in general. The intended audience differs, however. The *American Journal of Nursing* is the official journal of the American Nurses' Association. It reports, for its membership, important trends, issues, problems, and events of professional concern across the entire spectrum of nursing. It includes important legislation and legal decisions at the Federal and state levels, a periodic directory of organizations, a book review section, and articles and programmed instructions in the nursing practice fields. *RN* also reports on nursing trends, issues, concerns, and practice. It is directed, however, to the nurse who gives direct client care and particularly to those nurses who received their basic preparation in the diploma school of nursing. *Nursing '88*, whose subject areas present easy-to-read selections on clinical practice for nurses in direct-care settings, provides excellent information on practice conerns and employment information for staff nurses, such as employee relationships, staff development, and continuing education.

The speciality nursing journals serve as sources of original information on the role and functions of nurses and the art and science of nursing in the particular practice fields. These journals usually feature regular sections devoted to news briefs, book reviews, continuing education programs, trends and issues in the practice fields, and reports on current studies and research with implications for their practice. Those publications that are the official journals

of the special professional nursing societies also feature news on formal organization business, meetings, and members. The organizations' positions on issues and updates on state and Federal legislation of interest to the membership also are included. The journals of the national organizations may carry information and news from or related to their regional or state constituent organizations. The journals focused on the special fields of nursing have value for the specialized information needs of nurses who want to keep abreast of nursing practice, the issues, problems, and conflicts in their fields of practice.

Table 11–5 illustrates more fully the various focuses of the nursing journals in the four tracts of administration, education, clinical practice, and research. The list is not intended to be all-inclusive. *Lippincott's Guide to Nursing Literature* annotates the contents and sub-

---

TABLE 11–5. SELECTED PROFESSIONAL NURSING JOURNALS

Administration
The Journal of Nursing Administration
Nursing Administration Quarterly
Nursing Economics
Nursing Management

Education
Journal of Continuing Education in Nursing
Journal of Nursing Education
Nurse Educator
Nursing and Health Care
Journal of Nursing Staff Development

Research
Advances in Nursing Science
Nursing Research
Research in Nursing and Health
Western Journal of Nursing Research

General Practice
American Journal of Nursing
The Nurse Practitioner
Nursing '88
Nursing Life
RN
Topics in Clinical Nursing
Nursing Clinics of North America

Specialty Practice
American Journal of Infection Control
AORN Journal
Cancer Nursing
Oncology Nursing Forum
Cardiovascular Nursing
Critical Care Nurse
Focus on Critical Care
Heart and Lung
Journal of Emergency Nursing
Geriatric Nursing
Journal of Gerontological Nursing
Journal of Nurse-Midwifery
American Journal of Maternal/Child Nursing (MCN)
Journal of Pediatric Nursing
Journal of Nephrology Nursing
Issues in Mental Health Nursing
Journal of Psychosocial Nursing and Mental Health Services
Orthopedic Nursing
Today's O.R. Nurse
Public Health Nursing
Rehabilitation Nursing

Professional Development
Computers in Nursing
Image
Imprint
International Nursing Review
Journal of Professional Nursing
Nursing Outlook

From: Swanson and McClaskey, "Publishing opportunities for nurses," Nurs Outlook, (September/October 1986): 232–33.

ject areas of the current nursing jounrals.[74] The *Cumulative Index to Nursing and Allied Health Literature,* the *International Nursing Index,* and Henderson's *Nursing Studies Index* help nurses gain access to journal articles on specific subject matter. New journals are still being published periodically and are not included in journal reference lists until they are updated. *Nursing Economics Business Perspectives for Nurses,* published its first issue in July 1983.[75] Anthony J. Jannetti, Inc., who also publishes *Pediatric Nursing, Orthopaedic Nursing, The Pediatric Nurse Practitioner,* and *Occupational Health,* advertised the new journal as meeting an unaddressed need for communicating information about the economics of nursing and the business management aspects of nursing and health care. The audience is nurse executives in middle- and upper-level-management positions and nurse consultants who need specific knowledge on the fiscal aspects of nursing service. The regular subject and content areas include: economic issues, markets and marketing, change and innovation, resource management, politics and policy, legal briefs, ethics and values, executive forum, personal finance, and nursing connections. *Nursing Economics* is viewed as a resource for business management skills development and as contributing to the furtherance of the nursing profession in policy and decision making related to the business management, legal, and economic aspects of nursing.

In 1986 to 1987, two nursing publications were issued to address and provide information on issues of major concern to nurses in the areas of quality assurance and psychiatric nursing. The *Journal of Quality Assurance* is issued quarterly and provides relevant information on standards of practice, monitoring practices, and quality cost considerations. The *Archives of Psychiatric Nursing,* published six times a year, disseminates knowledge on psychiatric and mental health nursing theory, practice, and research. It is imperative that nurses be aware of the current journal sources and become familiar with their subject and content areas in order to select the materials that will best meet their information needs. The need for careful selection of relevant articles and well-developed reading habits cannot be overstated. This is an ongoing process of professionalism that can have considerable influence on requirements for changing and improving practice.

CONTINUING EDUCATION

Medicine, health care, and nursing are no longer static but continue to change. Competence in practice and individual accountability for the quality of services rendered demand a commitment to continued learning on the part of all health professionals. This commitment implies continuous self-development based on periodic review and updating of one's knowledge. Planned appropriate continuing education throughout the professional career is now seen as one way of ensuring maintenance of quality practice.

The term **continuing education** came into common use in the past 20 years, and connotes a life-long learning process that builds on the previously acquired knowledge and skills. Continuing education means continuous updating of knowledge and skills required for practice. The underlying premise is that the quality of health care depends to a large degree on the knowledge, skills, and attitudes of practitioners. The content and structure of continuing education must be flexible to meet the practice and career goals of practitioners. Continuing education is defined differently by various health professions. Different concepts of which training or education activities constitute continuing education stem from the different requirements for basic preparation for general and specialized practice. Continuing education for nurses is broadly defined or interpreted as education of the individual beyond basic preparation for the practice of nursing that promotes the development of nursing knowledge and skills for the continuing enhancement of nursing practice.[76] Continuing education for nurses is directly related to the scope of nursing practice and professional growth. It is most often job-related. Nursing does not have one universally accepted approach to basic preparation. Hence, participation in formal degree education is considered as continuing either from diploma or associate degree, to baccalaureate degree, to advanced degree, or to specially designed clinical programs. Included also are programs for advanced preparation in administration, education, and research.

Orientation programs for employment and on-the-job training are not regarded as continuing education unless they fill or update an identified gap in knowledge or skills. For example, if the analysis of **nursing audit** data identifies a knowledge deficiency among the group of nurses providing care in a given situation, an on-the-job training or **inservice education** program designed to correct that knowledge deficiency would be considered continuing education. Continuing education for nurses that meets criteria established and recognized by the nursing profession may include:

- Academic courses, with or without credit, offered by educational institutions, professional associations, or consumer groups
- Inservice education programs offered by the employer
- Self-directed study or clinical practice based on identified professional nursing needs

Trends in Continuing Education

The continuous upgrading of professional competence is a priority tenet of the profession of nursing and its organizations. The early role of the professional organizations in continuing education is evidenced in the publication of the nursing journals that contained articles on clinical nursing practice. The *American Journal of Nursing* and the *Public Health Nurse Quarterly,* from their initiation in 1900 and 1913, respectively, were intended to be sources of information about the art and technique of nursing care.[77,78] Signe Cooper and May Hornback, leaders in continuing education in nursing, in their book *Continuing Nursing Education,* trace educational efforts that could be identified as continuing education back to the early 1900s.[79] The alumnae associations of the first schools of nursing offered educational programs for their members as early as the 1870s. Hospitals, in the early 1900s offered postgraduate programs for nurses, such as postgraduate programs in maternity nursing. The early university schools of nursing in the 1920s began to provide credit

and noncredit courses for updating knowledge and skills and keeping nurses abreast of practice. The schools of nursing were committed to continuous learning and offered a variety of continuing education programs throughout the 1930s, 1940s, and 1950s.

Continuing education took on national significance in the 1960s. As the need became more and more evident, Federal monies were appropriated for continuing education. The Health Amendments of 1959 included aid for nurses enrolled in short-term courses.[80] The program began in February 1960 and in two years had made 200 grants to institutions for short-term courses and had enrolled approximately 13,000 nurses.

The development of regional medical programs under the Heart Disease, Cancer and Stroke Amendments of 1965 (Public Law 89-239) was a significant impetus for continuing education in the health fields.[81] The purpose of the program was education, research, training, and demonstration in the fields of cancer, stroke, kidney, and related diseases in order to improve the quality of care for clients with these diseases. The intent of the law was to diminish morbidity and mortality associated with these chronic diseases, the "principal killers." This was to be done by disseminating knowledge about them from researcher to practitioner, and by Regional Medical Programs (RMPs) emphasizing continuing education for physicians, nurses, and other health professionals through cooperative arrangements among health agencies and their staffs. The RMPs supported the hiring of a large number of the most competent professionals in heart disease, cancer, and stroke, who demonstrated a variety of approaches to health-professional training and continuing education and the dissemination of knowledge by telecommunications. Its coronary care training and demonstration projects are credited with training 12,000 nurses in coronary care and expanding the number and effectiveness of coronary care programs.

Continuing education is now well established as a professional responsibility and is supported and provided by educational institutions, the professional societies, and a wide variety of health agencies and commercial interests. Continuing education today is not traditional education or the transmission of knowledge from master teacher to learner. It is based on problem-solving concepts and approaches for initiating actions that will produce changes required in nursing and health-care systems. Continuing nursing education addresses specific learning needs and permits the learner to identify problems. It is intended to provide mechanisms to help the learner solve problems and become more effective and productive in work situations. Continuing education in nursing tends to deal with new roles for nurses, new and innovative health care and services, and the additional knowledge and skills required for specialized areas of practice.

The Continuing Education Unit

In general, continuing education is viewed as an educational offering not awarded academic credit. Therefore, a system for recognizing credits for continuing education was devised. In 1968, more than 30 interested agencies established a national task force to develop a uniform unit to identify, measure, and recognize individual efforts or accomplishments in noncredit continuing education. The task force developed the **continuing education unit** (CEU), defined standards for continuing education, and set operational procedures and guidelines to implement the CEU mechanism.[82]

The continuing education unit (1.0 CEU) is defined as " 10 **contact hours** of participation in an organized continuing education experience under responsible sponsorship, capable direction, and qualified instruction." The CEU provides a common measure for accumulating data on noncredit continuing education training or a universal way of recording completed courses and continuing education activities. Today, the CEU has been adopted by colleges, universities, professional societies, and government and industrial training centers across the country as a basis for award of certificates of continuing education. Licensing boards, certification bodies, professional societies, and other institutions that may require verification of continuing education also use the CEU for recording purposes. The CEU is well suited to computer recording and retrieval of continuing education information. The ANA, the National

League for Nursing, the AORN, and the state nurses' associations have recognized the CEU but tend to use the contact hour as the basic unit, for recording purposes, for their continuing education programs.

The criteria and guidelines specified by the National Task Force on the Continuing Education Unit are the essential elements of sound education programs. They include:

- Sponsoring organization with an identifiable educational unit, to assure that educational objectives are met
- Professional staff qualified to administer, coordinate, and conduct continuing education
- Appropriate educational facilities and instructional aids
- Capability to plan, design, conduct, and evaluate a program or activity in response to the educational needs of a large group
- A system for recording and verifying awarded CEUs

The CEU is not to be awarded for work experience, orientation courses, community service, publication of articles, committee meetings or assignments, self-study, or research projects.

No organization has authority over another in the awarding of CEUs. It is expected, however, that agencies that choose to use the CEU meet the criteria and guidelines prescribed by the National Task Force on Continuing Education Units. The CEU does not connote the accreditation of continuing education programs or single offerings. The use of the CEU, rather, implies "approval," meaning that the program or offering has been evaluated by the agencies or institutions concerned as meeting the national task force criteria for awarding CEUs.

The accreditation of sponsors or providers of continuing education is vested with the accrediting bodies of educational institutions. The total nursing program is accredited, not individual courses or separate departments within the nursing program structure, e.g., the Department of Continuing Nursing Education. The National League for Nursing accredits schools of nursing. The ANA accredits providers of continuing education, such as the state nursing associations, military and government services, and commercial providers.

Professional Associations and Continuing Education

When the need to make opportunities for continuing education available to all types of health personnel became widely recognized in the early 1960s, the professional organizations took the initiative in instilling in their membership the importance of continuing education. The need was discussed at professional meetings, at conferences, and in educational groups. Various programs for furthering continuing education endeavors were developed. The associations have issued statements on continuing education for nurses; developed standards and guidelines for the individual nurse, nursing services, nursing education programs, and the employers of nurses, and established programs for the accreditation of continuing education.

The nursing profession takes the position that the ultimate responsibility for both short- and long-range continuing education rests with the individual nurse. The responsibilities are diverse and include identification of one's continuing education needs, making these needs known to the employer and providers of continuing education, taking the initiative to seek continuing education activities to meet the identified needs, sharing the information obtained from the continuing education activities with the employer and colleagues, and accepting responsibility for an evaluation of continuing education activities.

The professional accountability for continuing education extends to nursing education institutions and programs. Nursing schools are charged with professional responsibility for instilling in students the desire for continuing self-education and for providing continuing education opportunities that meet prescribed educational standards. The standards were developed for all providers of continuing education. They apply the sound principles and criteria for planning, implementing, and evaluating educational courses for the adult learner. The employer's responsibility for continuing education for nurses is seen primarily as accountability to the health-care recipient. The employer is expected to facilitate continuing education for nurses through the establishment of policies that stimulate and encourage nurses to participate in continuing education. It is further recommended that employers provide the time and finances for appropriate continuing education outside the institution or agency. In addition, employers should hold the participants accountable for the application of learning to the practice situation.

Accreditation of Continuing Education

To help assure quality in continuing education, the ANA developed a voluntary national system of accreditation of continuing education activities in nursing. As defined by the ANA, "accreditation of continuing education in nursing is the process whereby the Association, through designated approving bodies, grants public recognition to continuing education activities which meet certain established educational standards as determined through initial and periodic evaluations."[83] Through the accreditation program, the ANA provides for the implementation of the standards at the national, state, and local levels and encourages sponsors to continually improve the quality of offerings.

The ANA Council on Continuing Education developed specific standards and criteria for continuing education. Through the National Accreditation Board and regional accrediting committees, the criteria are used for accreditation and approval of providers of continuing education. The standards for continuing education provide for a professional nursing judgment as to the quality of continuing education offerings. The standards are based on sound educational principles and include the following factors[84]:

- Assessment of learning needs
- Design of educational offerings
- Implementation of education designs
- Objectives of the educational programs or offerings
- Teaching strategies and methodologies
- Evaluation of outcomes and process
- Record keeping
- Organizational resources and financing

The ANA accreditation mechanism emphasizes self-regulation and collaboration between all levels of the ANA and other national organizations and agencies that sponsor continuing education activities. Continuing education activities that are approved and conducted by ANA accredited organizations are transferable.

Being based on common standards and criteria, all ANA-accredited organizations recognize continuing education programs or offerings of another ANA-accredited organization. This reciprocity is particularly helpful, since continuing education may be acquired from diverse sources and in widely dispersed locations. Most state boards of nursing administering mandatory continuing education licensure regulations and laws also recognize continuing education sponsored by ANA-accredited organizations as meeting their mandatory requirements. The ANA periodically publishes a directory of its accredited organizations and approved offerings.[85] This directory is most useful in identifying accredited sponsors of continuing education.

Mandatory Continuing Education

An issue of significant concern to all health professions that generated considerable debate in the early 1970s was that of mandatory versus voluntary continuing education. Mandatory continuing education is prescribed attendance at a set number of practice-related courses, or a set number of hours of continuing education within a given period of time, in order to maintain licensure. The contention was that mandated continuing education would maintain and ensure professional competence.

As of January 1, 1986, 12 states and Puerto Rico required mandatory continuing education for nurses. In these states, legislation had designated the state board of nursing as the official state agency to control and assure the competence of nurses through continuing education. The underlying rationale is to protect the public by upgrading nursing practice. The premise is that by requiring the nurse to participate in continuing education, learning will result, and practice will be changed and improved. The states' mandating continuing education for relicensure and the particular state requirements are shown in Table 11–6.

Today there is little disagreement about the value of continuing nursing education. The technical advances in continuing education for nursing and its increased accessibility in the past ten years have unlimited potential for assisting in professional growth. Continuing nursing education substantially contributes to expanding

TABLE 11–6. MANDATORY CONTINUING EDUCATION REQUIREMENTS BY STATE

State	Continuing Education Requirement
Registered Nurses	
California	30 hr/2 yr (6 hr home study permitted)
Colorado	20 hr/2 yr (no limit on home study)
Florida	24 hr/2 yr (no limit on home study)
Iowa	30 hr (first renewal) 45 hr/3 yr thereafter
Kansas	30 hr/2 yr (6 hr home study permitted)
Kentucky	30 hr/2 yr
Massachusetts	15 hr/2 yr
Minnesota	30 hr/2 yr
Nebraska	20 hr/5 yr (or 75 hr/5 yr if less than 200 hr of practice in the 5-yr period.
Nevada	30 hr/2 yr (6 hr home study permitted)
New Mexico	30 hr/2 yr
Puerto Rico	45 hr/3 yr
Washington	15 hr/1 yr
Nurse Practitioners	
Alaska	30 hr/2 yr
Idaho	60 hr/2 yr
New Mexico	100 hr/2 yr
Mississippi	40 hr/2 yr
New Hampshire	20 hr/2 yr
Oregon	100 hr/2 yr

From: "What you need to know about licensing," Nursing Opportunities 1986 (Oradell, N.J.: Medical Economics Co., 1986), 15.

knowledge, correcting deficiencies, and promoting excellence. The necessity for completing a required number of hours of attendance at "approved" courses or offerings and submitting the proper forms to ensure continuing licensure or certification, however, is still fraught with controversy.

The relative significance and outcome of the process of mandatory continuing education is subject to question and, as yet, the process has failed to reveal evidence of the usefulness and worth.

The real underlying issue in the value of mandatory continuing education is evaluation of the outcomes of continuing education and the proven effects on nursing practice. "Approved" continuing education offerings, courses, or programs incorporate planned methods of evaluation. The most common evaluation tools are pencil-and-paper tests on the information learned about each course objective and participants' satisfaction ratings on the methods of course presentation, the learning environment, and the facility or instructors. What is lacking, in terms of mandatory continuing education, is effective ways for evaluating the participants' changed behavior and improvements in nursing practice as a result of the learning that may have taken place. Collaborative relationships need to be established between the continuing education and nursing service entities concerned, so that evaluation can take place in the client-care setting. Individual goals in continuing education need to be part of nurses' career development and progression plans and their ongoing performance evaluations. Only then will the question of mandatory continuing education be resolved. Today, however, continuing education remains as a career requirement of every health professional.

SUMMARY

Accountability is assuming responsibility for one's own decisions and actions. In relation to nursing, the concept is not new and, as a mark of the profession, has been a characteristic for two centuries. The evaluation of accountability in nursing has kept pace with the changing society and an increasingly complex health-care delivery system. The profession has continually delineated methods for guiding nursing practice and evaluating nursing performance and provided means for changing and improving patterns of practice. Five of these major efforts have been discussed—standards, quality assurance, credentialing mechanisms, the nursing literature, and continuing education.

Standards development in nursing began in the early 1900s with the enactment of state nurse practice acts that established criteria for the training of nurses and their performance. The early standards were based on experience and judgments of what constituted good practice and care. Nursing standards were later embodied in manuals and guidelines for practice and statements on the function and qualifications of nurses. In their progressive develop-

ment, standards were based on studies of nursing practice and nursing education that provided knowledge on nursing practice, services, and client-care needs. The nursing process began to be reflected in nursing standards in the late 1940s. Today, nursing standards are increasingly derived from research and incorporate means for measuring the quality of care.

Quality assurance has been a concern of nursing since the 1950s, and the development of instruments and tools measuring quality nursing care is ongoing. In recent years increasing attention has been given to this area by nursing research. Another important aspect in the quest for quality in nursing is credentialing. The use of credentials in nursing in evidenced by licensure of individual nurses, certification of nurses in clinical practice, and accreditation of educational institutions and programs.

The nursing profession has promoted quality in practice and the application of its standards and accountability through the simultaneous development of its nursing literature. The development of nursing's theoretical, clinical, and technical literary materials and media has kept pace with the increasing sophistication in clinical practice, education, administration, and research. Communication expertise has been augmented by deliberate endeavors to encourage and prepare nurses to write and publish. Today, the nursing media are impressive and include thousands of journals, periodicals, books, texts, reports on practice experiences, and documents on studies and research efforts. The contents are as diverse as the nursing profession. To facilitate the use of the literature, nursing has produced reference guides, manuals, handbooks, indexes, dictionaries, and bibliographies. Access to the literature is being made easier by computerized storage and retrieval systems. Nursing's literary resources are evidence of its accountability.

A highly emphasized part of nursing's accountability is continuing education for nursing. The enhancement of nurses' knowledge to keep nursing practice relevant to trends in health care has been a long-standing professional goal facilitated by postgraduate education and short-term courses. Continuing education and life-long learning is now viewed as a requirement for maintaining competence in practice. This recognized need has given rise to special programs for the continuing education requirements for licensure and accreditation programs for the sponsors and providers of continuing education.

Study Questions

1. Identify and discuss three ways in which the nursing profession has helped to assure quality of care in a rapidly changing society and increasingly complex health-care delivery system.

2. What is the relationship between ANA's standards for nursing practice and the nursing process?

3. What are the mechanisms for establishing credentials?

4. How do credentials influence the quality of nursing?

5. Select a special nursing practice field and develop a care plan for a hypothetical case using the nursing practice standards for that particular field.

6. What is quality assurance? Why is it important?

7. Name two purposes of the nursing literature and describe how it benefits the nursing profession.

8. Select a nursing topic for a term paper and list three or four library resources you would use to identify literature citations relevant to your topic.

9. Discuss the scope of the nursing journals. What are the major differences and similarities of the journals? Who are the various audiences?

10. List two or more retrieval systems for assessing citations and abstracts from the nursing literature.

11. What is the philosophy and position of the nursing profession on continuing education?

12. Why have states enacted laws requiring mandatory continuing education for the relicensure of nurses? What are the issues and answers?

13. What is the significance of the CEU? How is it used?

References

1. Stanley J. Matek, *Accountability: Its Meaning and Its Relevance to the Health Care Field* (Hyattsville, Md.: Department of Health, Education and Welfare, Pub. No. (HRA) 77–72, September 1977), 4.
2. Sara Erickson, "Spotlight on history" *New Jersey Nurse* (January/February 1983): 9.
3. Ibid.
4. M. Louise Fitzpatrick, *The National Organization for Public Health Nursing, 1912–1952: Development of a Practice Field* (New York: National League for Nursing, 1975), 48, 53–54, 101–103, 119, 126, 185–186.
5. The National Organization for Public Health Nursing, *Manual of Public Health Nursing, 3rd ed* (New York: Macmillan Co., 1939).
6. Committee on the Study of Nursing, *Nursing and Nursing Education in the United States* (New York: Macmillan Co., 1923).
7. Committee on the Grading of Nursing Schools, *Nursing Schools Today and Tomorrow, Final Report* (New York: National League of Nursing Education, 1934).
8. Committee on the Grading of Nursing Schools, *An Activity Analysis of Nursing* (New York: National League of Nursing Education, 1934).
9. The National League of Nursing Education, The Committee on Studies, *A Study of Nursing Service in Fifty Selected Hospitals* (New York: The National League of Nursing Education, 1937).
10. National League of Nursing Education, Department of Studies, *A Study of Nursing Service* (New York: The National League of Nursing Education, 1948).
11. John P. Young, *A Method for Allocation of Nursing Personnel to Meet Inpatient Care Needs* (Baltimore, Md.: The Johns Hopkins Hospital, Operations Research Division, 1962).
12. E.W. Jones, B. J. McNitt, and E.M. McKnight,

Patient Classification for Long-Term Care: User's Manual. (Department of Health, Education and Welfare, Pub. No. (HRA) 74-3107, December 1973).

13. Doris E. Roberts and Helen Hudson, *How to Study Patient Progress*, U.S. Public Health Service Pub. No. 1169 (Washington, D.C.: Government Printing Office, 1964), 121.

14. Myrtle K. Aydelotte, "State of knowledge nurse staffing methodology," *Research on Nurse Staffing in Hospitals, Report on a Conference.* U.S. Department of Health, Education, and Welfare, Division of Nursing (Washington, D.C.: U.S. Government Printing Office, 1973), 11.

15. American Nurses' Association, *Code for Nurses with Interpretive Statements,* rev. (Kansas City, Mo.: The American Nurses' Association 1976).

16. American Nurses' Association, "ANA statements of functions, standards, and qualifications," *Am J Nurs* 56, (July 1956): 899.

17. American Nurses' Association, *Bylaws As Amended* (Kansas City, Mo.: The American Nurses' Association, 1974), 21–25.

18. American Nurses' Association, *Standards. Nursing Practice* (Kansas City, Mo.: The American Nurses' Association, 1973).

19. American Nurses' Association, *Standards, Maternal-Child Health Nursing Practice* (Kansas City, Mo.: The American Nurses' Association, 1973).

20. American Nurses' Association, *Standards. Community Health Nursing Practice* (Kansas City, Mo.: The American Nurses' Association, 1973).

21. American Nurses' Association. *Standards. Psychiatric Mental Health Nursing Practice.* (Kansas City, Mo.: The American Nurses' Association, 1973).

22. American Nurses' Association, *Standards of Medical-Surgical Nursing Practice* (Kansas City, Mo.: The American Nurses' Association, 1974).

23. American Nurses' Association, *Standards. Geriatric Nursing Practice* (Kansas City, Mo.: The American Nurses' Association, 1973).

24. American Nurses' Association, *Standards of Gerontological Nursing Practice* (Kansas City, Mo.: The American Nurses' Association, 1976).

25. American Heart Association Council on Cardiovascular Nursing and American Nurses' Association Division on Medical-Surgical Nursing Practice, *Standards of Cardiovascular Nursing Practice* (Kansas City, Mo.: American Nurses' Association, 1975).

26. American Nurses' Association Division on Medical-Surgical Nursing Practice and Oncology Nursing Society, *Outcome Standards for Cancer Nursing Practice* (Kansas City, Mo.: American Nurses' Association, 1979).

27. American Nurses' Association Division on Medical-Surgical Nursing Practice and Emergency Department Nurses' Association, *Standards of Emergency Nursing Practice* (Kansas City, Mo.: American Nurses' Association, 1975).

28. American Nurses' Association Division on Medical-Surgical Nursing Practice and Association of Neurosurgical Nurses, *Standards of Neurological and Neurosurgical Nursing Practice* (Kansas City, Mo.: American Nurses' Association, 1977).

29. Association of Operating Room Nurses and American Nurses' Association Division on Medical-Surgical Nursing Practice, *Standards of Nursing Practice: Operating Room* (Kansas City, Mo.: American Nurses' Association, 1975).

30. Orthopedic Nurses' Association and American Nurses' Association Division on Medical-Surgical Nursing Practice, *Standards of Orthopedic Nursing Practice* (Kansas City, Mo.: American Nurses' Association, 1975).

31. American Nurses' Association, Division on Maternal and Child Health: Nursing Practice, and the Association of Pediatric Oncology Nurses, *Standards of Pediatric Oncology Nursing Practice* (Kansas City, Mo.: 1978).

32. American Nurses' Association Division on Medical-Surgical Nursing Practice and Association of Operating Room Nurses, *Standards of Perioperative Nursing Practice* (Kansas City, Mo.: American Nurses' Association, 1981).

33. American Nurses' Association Division of Medical-Surgical Nursing and Association of Rehabilitation Nurses, *Standards of Rehabilitation Nursing Practice* (Kansas City, Mo.: American Nurses' Association, 1977).

34. American Nurses' Association and American Urological Association, *Standards of Urological Nursing Practice* (Kansas City, Mo.: American Nurses' Association, 1977).

35. Association of Operating Room Nurses, "From standards into practice," *AORN J* (October 1978): 603–42.

36. U.S. Public Law 92–603 (Section 249F).

37. A. Donabedian, "Evaluating the quality of medical care," *Milbank Mem Fund Q* (July 1966).

38. V.N. Slee, "How to know if you have quality control," *Hosp Prog,* (Jan 1972): 38.

39. American Nurses' Association, *A Plan for Implementation of the Standards of Nursing Practice* (Kansas City, Mo.: The American Nurses' Association, 1975), 14–25.

40. Ibid., 16.

41. American Nurses' Association, *Quality Assurance Workbook* (Kansas City, Mo.: The American Nurses' Association, 1976).

42. Ruth A. Braulick, Jose R. Coronado, Evelyn Heil, et al. "On the Scene: Audie L. Murphy Memorial Veterans Hospital," *Nurs Admin Q*, (Spring 1983): 15–45.

43. "On the scene: The Duke University hospital experience in QA," *Nurs Admin Q* (Spring 1977): 7–50.

44. Kathryn S. Chance, "The quest for quality: An exploration of attempts to define and measure quality nursing care," *Image*, (June 1980): 41–45.

45. American Nurses' Association, *The Study of Credentialing in Nursing*, vol. I, the Report of the Committee (Kansas City: Mo.: The American Nurses' Association, 1979).

46. Ibid., 64.

47. Ibid., 67.

48. Janet L. Fickeissen, "Getting certified," *Am J Nurs 85*, (March 1985): 266–69.

49. American Nurses' Association, *The American Nurse*, (January 1974): 1.

50. American Nurses' Association, *The American Nurse*, (February 1986): 9.

51. Ibid., 7.

52. American Nurses' Association, *Study of Credentialing*, 33–36.

53. Inez G. Hinsvark and Helen Dorsch, "The role of credentialing in the educational preparation for nursing practice," *The Study of Credentialing in Nursing: A New Approach*, vol. II, Staff Working Papers (Kansas City, Mo.: American Nurses' Association, 1979), 1–7.

54. Lucie Y. Kelly, *Dimensions of Professional Nursing*, 4th ed. (New York: Macmillan Co., 1981), 559.

55. John D. Poterfield, "The external evaluation of institutions for accreditation," *Quality Assurance of Medical Care*, Monograph DHEW Pub. No (HSM) 73-7021 (U.S. Department of Health, Education and Welfare, Health Services and Mental Health Administration, Regional Medical Programs Service, 1933), 121–26.

56. "Practical nursing programs accredited by the NLN, 1985," *Nurs Health Care,* (February 1986): 105–108.

57. "Diploma programs in nursing accredited by the NLN, 1986–1987," *Nurs Health Care* (September 1986): 402–05.

58. "Baccalaureate and master's degree programs in nursing accredited by the NLN, 1986–1987," *Nurs Health Care* (June 1986): 332–38.

59. Editorials, *Am J Nurs 50*, (October 1950):583–85.

60. Beatrice J. Kalisch and Philip A. Kalisch, *Politics of Nursing* (Philadelphia: J.B. Lippincott Co., 1982), 332–36.

61. Elizabeth Swanson and Joanne C. McClaskey, "The manuscript review process of nursing journals, *Image*, (October 1982): 72–75.

62. Margretta Styles, "Why Publish?" *Image*, (June 1978), 29.

63. American Journal of Nursing Co., *International Nursing Index* (New York: Quarterly and annual circulations 1966 to date).

64. Katina P. Strauch and Dorothy J. Brundage, *Guide to Library Resources for Nursing* (New York: Appleton-Centruy-Crofts, 1980), 400–02.

65. Glendale Adventist Medical Center Publications Service, *Cumulative Index to Nursing and Allied Health Literature* (Glendale, Calif.: Bimonthly with yearly cumulation, 1961 to date.)

66. Viriginia Henderson, ed., *Nursing Studies Index* (Philadelphia: J.B. Lippincott Co., Vol. 1 (1900–1929); Vol. 2 (1930–1949); Vol. 3 (1950–1956): Vol. 4 (1957–1959).

67. Jane L. Binger and Lydia M. Jensen, *Lippincott's Guide to Nursing Literature. A Handbook for Students, Writers, and Researchers.* (Philadelphia: J.B. Lippincott Co., 1980), 209–15.

68. Strauch and Brundage, *Guide to Library Resources*, 27.

69. Binger and Jensen, *Lippincott's Guide to Nursing Literature*, 267–68.

70. American Journal of Nursing Co. *International Nursing Index*, 1982.

71. Joanne C. McClaskey and Elizabeth Swanson, "Publishing opportunities for nurses: A comparison of 100 journals" *Image*, (June 1982): 50–56.

72. Swanson and McClaskey, "The manuscript review process."

73. Elizabeth Swanson and Joanne McClaskey, "Publishing opportunities For nurses," *Nurs Outlook*, (September/October 1986): 227–35.

74. Binger and Brundage, *Lippincott's Guide to Nursing Literature*, 72, 82, 85, 118, 130–31.

75. Anthony J. Jannette, Inc. *Nursing Economics Business Perspectives for Nurses* (July/August 1983): 1–60.

76. American Nurses' Association, Council on Continuing Education *Continuing Education in Nursing: An Overview* (Kansas City, Mo.: The American Nurses' Association, 1979).

77. Fitzpatrick, *Public Health Nursing*, 31.

78. Editorials, *Am J Nurs 50*, (October 1950): 5.

79. Signe Skott Cooper and May Shiga Harnback, *Continuing Nursing Education.* (New York: McGraw-Hill Book Co., 1973), 19–34.

80. U.S. Department of Health, Education, and Welfare, Public Health Service, *Toward Quality in Nursing Needs and Goals,* Report of the Surgeon General's Consultant Group on Nursing, PHS Pub No. 992 (Washington DC: US Government Printing Office, 1963), 41.
81. U.S. Department of Health, Education, and Welfare, Public Health Service, Health Resources Administration. *Health in America,* DHEW Pub. No (HRA) 76–616, (Washington, DC: U.S. Government Printing Office, 1976), 111–13.
82. National University Extension Association, *The Continuing Education Unit,* The National Task Force on the Continuing Education Unit (Washington, DC: The National University Extension Association, 1974).
83. American Nurses' Association, *Accreditation of Continuing Education in Nursing, State Nurses' Associations, National Specialty Nursing Organizations, Federal Nursing Services, State Boards of Nursing.* (Kansas City, Mo.: The American Nurses' Association, 1975), 2.
84. Ibid., 20–23.
85. American Nurses' Association, *Directory of ANA Accredited Organizations, Approved Programs/Offerings, and Accredited Continuing Education Certificate Programs Preparing Nurse Practitioners* (Kansas City, Mo.: The American Nurses' Association, periodically updated).

Annotated Bibliography

American Nurses' Association. 1979. *The Study of Credentialing in Nursing: A New Approach,* vol. I., the Report of the Committee, Kansas City, Mo.: American Nurses' Association. This report presents the background and conclusions of the Study of Credentialing in Nursing. The study was undertaken to address all aspects of the credentialing of institutions and individuals in the occupation of nursing, including accreditation, certification, licensing, degree designation, and other forms. The study was inaugurated in 1976 by the American Nurses' Association through the appointment of an independent study committee. The report includes sections on the origins of the study, the participants, the purposes and methods, a summary of findings, derived principles and positions, and proposals for future directions. A plan for follow-up and implementation appears as an addendum to the report.

American Nurses' Association. 1979. *The Study of Credentialing in Nursing: A New Approach,* vol. II, Staff Working Papers. Kansas City, Mo.: American Nurses' Association. This supplement to the Report of the Committee contains the working papers of the staff and consultants on background information and analyses and principles and perspectives on credentialing issues in nursing today. Addressed are the major issues of credentialing in preparation for nursing practice, job market issues, the politics of credentialing and the bases for committee recommendations and a new credentialing system.

Binger, J.L., and Jensen, L.M. 1980. *Lippincott's Guide to Nursing Literature. A Handbook for Students, Writers, and Researchers.* Philadelphia: J.B. Lippincott. This book is a guide to timely nursing journals, relevant non-nursing periodicals, and selected references for nurses unfamiliar with the literature. The format allows students, the practicing nurse, educators, administrators, and researchers quick access and practical step-by-step assistance in identifying pertinent sources and using relevant journals and references more effectively. The guide features use of the library, steps in literature search and surveillance, computerized literature processes, and how to prepare journal articles and manuscripts. It includes a profile of current nursing journals, indexes and abstracts, a list of statistical information resources, and guides and directories on writing and editing. The guide is intended to facilitate the use and dissemination of nursing literature for independent study and continued learning, for instruction, for writing, and for research.

Duke University Hospital Nursing Services, 1980. *Quality Assurance: Guidelines for Nursing Care,* Philadelphia: J.B. Lippincott. This book describes the quality assurance program of the Duke University Hospital Nursing Service. It details the quality assurance program strategies that let every nurse know the nature and extent of client outcomes to strive for and the related care clients should receive. Criteria and standards are defined for specific client populations. Measurement and operational methods for evaluating the quality and the impact of nursing interventions on the outcomes of care are presented.

Johnson, B.C., Dungca, C.V., Hofmeisler, D, and Wells S.J. 1981. *Standards for Critical Care.* St. Louis: C.V. Mosby. This text includes concise descriptions of potential problems, assessment factors, expected outcomes, and recommended nursing activities for more than 60 clinical problems. Introductory materials provide a brief rationale for the standards and suggested activities for care plans.

Mason, E.J. 1984. *How to Write Meaningful Nursing Standards.* New York: Wiley. Designed as a workbook, this text provides step-by-step methods for writing nursing process, outcome, and content standards. Specific examples of actual standards are provided. A design for writing nursing standards for a unit, division, or health-care agency is included.

Meisenheimer, Claire Gavin, ed. 1985. *Quality Assurance: A Complete Guide to Effective Programs.* Rockville, Md.: Aspen Systems Corp. This handbook is a comprehensive practical guide to quality assurance in health care. It provides information and tools for designing a cost-effective program, to evaluate ongoing programs, to prepare reports and to asssess learning needs. Information on the effects of quality assurance programs on consumers as well as how to improve programs is included. The role of the computer in quality assurance is also described.

National League for Nursing. 1981. *Guide for the Development of Nursing Libraries.* New York: The National League for Nursing. This guide for the evaluation of the nursing library may also be used for setting up or further developing nursing library resources and services. The characteristics, functions, administration, operation, and evaluation of the nursing library are succinctly outlined and briefly discussed. Topics covered include the library policies, budget, physical environment, collections, and staff, as well as the technical sources—namely, cataloging and classification, indexing, and abstracting, and computerized retrieval. A bibliography is appended.

Strauch, K.P., and Brundage, D.J. 1980. *Guide to Library Resources for Nursing.* New York: Appleton-Century-Crofts. This is a guide for all persons involved in nursing on the usefulness of library resources and tools to the nursing profession. It features general information on the library's functions, services, and use, and current library materials in nursing. Included are both general reference sources and annotated lists of books in selected nursing topics as well as a list of periodicals and audiovisual materials in these subject areas. The names of medical, nursing, and allied health publishers are in the appendix.

Chapter 12

Ethical Aspects of Nursing

Elsie L. Bandman
Bertram Bandman

Chapter Outline

- Objectives
- Glossary
- Introduction
  Definitions
  Distinctions between Philosophy, Religion, and the Law
- Importance of Ethics to Nursing
- Major Ethical Orientations
  Rational Paternalism
  Libertarianism
  Love-based Ethics
  Natural Law
  Egoism
  Utilitarianism
  Absolute Principles
  Justice-based Ethics
- Moral Principles and Values in Nursing
  Paradigm Case Argument
- Professional Accountability
  Role of the Nurse as Moral Agent
  Development of Moral Judgement
- Ethical Issues in Nursing
  Clients' Rights
  Nurses' Rights
  The Right to Life
  Abortion
  The Right to End Life
  Behavior Control
  Technology
- Conclusions
- Summary
- Study Questions
- References
- Annotated Bibliography

Objectives

After completing this chapter the reader will be able to:

▶ Define all the terms in the glossary
▶ Discuss the importance of ethical study by nurses
▶ Discuss several differences between philosophy, religion, and law
▶ Describe common ethical issues surrounding client care
▶ Discuss reasons for nurses' participation in shared decision making
▶ Explain moral decisions based on major ethical theories and principles

Glossary

Advocacy. The principle of speaking for or working on behalf of the claims and rights of individuals or groups; in particular, giving support to those who are disadvantaged and vulnerable because of illness, disability, age, ethnicity, or socioeconomic status.

Agape. A love that is spiritual in nature; the Christian "love of God" and love of others in the name of God.

Altruism. Having concern for the welfare of others; the quality of selflessness.

Autonomy. The quality of being self-determining and independent; in the context of ethics, the capacity to understand ethical alternatives as the rational basis for moral choice; to be an autonomous person means to be rational and self-legislating and free of external control as the basis for moral choice.

Beneficence. Doing good by helping clients or patients in constructive ways toward positive goals.

Egoism. The ethical doctrine that morality has its foundation in self-interest; the belief that an individual's interest in self is the just and proper motive for human conduct.

Ethics. The discipline dealing with the ideas and premises for how people think about and believe in what is good or bad, right or wrong, moral or immoral.

Fidelity. The principle that includes the duty to tell the truth and to keep promises based on respect for self and for others as autonomous persons.

Libertarianism. The viewpoint that reflects a belief in free will for individuals; freedom of action and thought.

Morals. Statements or convictions, judgments, and modes of conduct based on ethical beliefs.

Nonmaleficence. The quality or condition of not doing any harm.

Pluralism. A condition of society in which numerous distinct ethnic, religious, or cultural groups coexist within one nation; also refers to a doctrine that reality is composed of many ultimate substances.

Utilitarianism. The philosophical doctrine that considers usefulness as good, worthwhile, and the criterion of action.

Utility. The condition or quality of being useful.

Value. An idea or belief that a person holds in high esteem; something of worthy and desirable quality.

INTRODUCTION

The concept of nursing ethics is being given increasing attention in professional nursing publications, in continuing education agendas for nurses, and in basic nursing education curricula. This focus reflects a growing acknowledgment of the many roles nurses play in health issues that involve questions of ethics and values.

Definitions

To understand the concept of ethics and its importance to nursing and health care, several terms need to be clarified. **Morals** are beliefs or principles that people use to distinguish between good and bad, or right and wrong. One author views morals as the "shoulds" and "oughts" or "should nots" of life, culture, society, and religion.[1] These traditional beliefs about right and wrong are derived from a combination of religious values and family, school, and various other social institutions. **Values** connote desirable beliefs that are held in high esteem and may serve as a guide to behavior. Similar to morals, values are personal and meaningful affirmations that come from an individual's experiences of family life, school, friends, religion, economic status, and culture. Values contribute significantly to the developmet of a person's goals, attitudes, and feelings.

Ethics is the discipline of morals in a broad sense, or a system of morals in a particular sense. Ethics are often expressed as a "Code of Ethics," which is an organized system of morals, such as those set forth in a formal statement by a professional organization. Ethics is concerned with the "why" of moral belief, e.g., what are the reasons behind an individual's particular moral principles? Ethical theory, a branch of philosophy, is the study of general ethical principles and their application and justification to moral problems.[2] When these theories and principles are applied to problems in health care, the process is called bioethics, a type of applied ethics. The application of general ethical principles to moral problems that arise in nursing is called nursing ethics. However, the same general principles of ethics apply across professional and nonprofessional fields as well.

Given the distinctions between all of these terms as defined above, it is important to realize that there are numerous viewpoints among philosophers and scholars on how to define ethics and morals. Also, in general usage, people may apply many of these terms interchangeably. For nurses, the significance of making specific distinctions among ethics terms is important primarily to the extent it enhances appreciation and understanding of bioethical issues and assists in providing a framework of knowledge within which morally appropriate actions or responses can be distinguished.

Distinctions between Philosophy, Religion, and the Law

Morality and law are different but with overlapping areas. The law is a codified set of rules enacted by society over time that both prescribes and forbids particular behavior by its citizens. For example, the law requires that drivers stop for red lights and stop signs and that nurses be licensed. The law forbids killing, stealing, and rape. The overlap is in those areas of behavior considered both immoral and illegal, such as murder. In this area, law and morals have the same general purpose of applying an agreed-upon set of rules enabling people to live together harmoniously in pursuit of their own aims and desires without infringing on others.[3] Law and ethics, however, can differ radically. What is legal at a given time, such as slavery and discrimination as to race, sex, ethnicity, and age, is clearly in conflict with moral principles of respect and autonomy. The issue of homosexuality is a current issue with differing or conflicting moral and legal positions.

Religion and ethics are not conceptually identical. Ethics can exist without religion and religion can exist without ethics.[4] Clouser provides us with one view of the distinction between religion and ethics as follows: First, ethics must have universal appeal through a basic set of rules that rational persons would agree are moral and worth following by everyone.[5] Religion and theological precepts are accepted as a matter of faith, rather than reason, by groups of believers. Clouser's second point is that religion demands special acts of its adherents, such as the Roman Catholic prohibition of all forms of reproductive technology for infertile couples. In contrast, general ethics approaches such issues from a rational point of view with universal applicability.[6] Clouser's third point is that religion, unlike ethics, may motivate people to be moral by inspiring and rewarding moral behavior.[7] In contrast, ethics consist of theories and principles that justify actions. It is a discipline in and of itself. Philosophy, of which ethics is one branch, is translated from Greek meaning "love of wisdom" or "the love of exercising one's curiosity and intelligence."[8] A short definition that substantially follows Plato's definition of philosophy is "that department of knowledge which deals with ultimate reality, or with the most general causes and principles of things."[9] Ethical theory, as described earlier, is a branch of philosophy from which the terms bioethics and nursing ethics are defined.

IMPORTANCE OF ETHICS TO NURSING

The goal of nursing is to protect, promote, and restore health, prevent illness, and alleviate suffering. As the main providers of care, comfort, and therapeutic interventions, nurses are moral agents and client advocates in the health-care delivery system. The most fundamental value in nursing is respect for persons' autonomy and the right of self-determination. Health is valued as a means to a meaningful life in which the client is the primary decision maker.[10]

Arguments in nursing ethics may consist of nursing metaphors and slogans (such as, holistic nursing is treating the whole patient), which, along with ethical, religious, scientific, and legal premises, are intended to imply practical nursing ethics conclusions. The schema of a nursing ethics argument may be found in Table 12–1.

Self-regulation is a characteristic of an accountable and mature profession.[11] "Each nurse inherits a measure of the responsibility and trust that have accrued to nursing . . . , as well as the corresponding obligation to adhere to the profession's code of conduct and relationships for ethical practice."[12] Within nursing practice, education, and research, nurses make decisions that are based on moral principles and that have moral consequences.

The aim of nursing is "to conserve that which is of value to every individual—the optimum functioning of all body systems and of the whole as an integrated unit."[13] Through advances in science and medical technology, the nurse participates in therapeutic interventions that control vital functions necessary to life, in organ transplants, in genetic and in reproductive

TABLE 12–1. SCHEMA OF A NURSING ETHICS ARGUMENT

Nursing metaphors	Jones, the client, is a whole person rather than a disease carrier.
	The nurse is an autonomous agent and client advocate, not an instrument or servant of the physician.
Nursing slogans	Treat the whole client, not the disease.
Nursing ethics principle	"The most fundamental" principle to "justify nursing actions" is "respect for persons"[a]
Nursing case	Jones is a Jehovah's Witness, a competent adult client, who refuses blood transfusions.
Nursing ethics decision	Therefore, assist Jones in refusing a blood transfusion.

One could, however, mount the following nursing ethics counterargument with a shift in only one premise:

Nursing metaphors	Jones, the client, is a whole person rather than a disease carrier.
	The nurse is an autonomous agent and client advocate, not an instrument or servant of the physician.
Nursing slogan	Treat the whole client, not the disease.
Nursing ethics principle	"The nurse does not act deliberately to terminate the life of any person." [a]
Nursing care	Jones, a Johavah's Witness, refuses blood transfusions. Failure to transfuse will result in death.
Nursing ethics decision	Therefore, do not assist Jones in refusing a blood transfusion.

[a]American Nurses' Association, *Code for Nurses.*

engineering, and in human experimentation involving innovative drugs and treatments. Nurses strive to meet the human needs of sick individuals for care in ways that enhance the personhood and the humanity of all those involved in the care."[14]

Nurses seek to do good. Good intentions, however, are not enough. Demonstrably, lack of knowledge of moral choices may cause harm. Reasons for choosing one option rather than another need to be examined in relation to moral considerations of usefulness (utility), universality, human rights, and justice. In a pluralistic culture made up of individuals with many different values, moral agreement among care providers and consumers is not always desirable or possible. Nurses need to be part of the necessary process of deliberation that surrounds moral issues, problems, and dilemmas in healthcare delivery. Knowledge of ethics, therefore, is indispensable to the nurse who seeks to participate responsibly and intelligently on a moral basis in doing that which is good in daily practice and in everyday life. Nursing ethics incorporates this knowledge and this process of deliberation from the perspective of nursing. How does one decide between contradictory nursing ethics conclusions? To answer this question, we consider aspects of the *American Nurses' Association Code for Nurses,* its implications for ethics; some functions of an ethical theory in nursing; some models of morality in nursing; some principles and values in nursing ethics, such as autonomy, beneficence, **fidelity** and nonmaleficence; and some criteria for judging an ethical theory in nursing.

The *Code for Nurses* (Table 12–2) provides a synopsis of both legal and ethical practices. Conversely, it is clearly ethical to respect a client's confidentiality, engage in autonomous behavior, practice beneficence and nonmaleficence, tell the truth, keep promises, and treat clients and colleagues fairly.[15] But within these broad parameters of what is both legal and ethical, it is at times difficult to draw the line. For example, if a client is dying and in apparently extreme pain, to what extent should a nurse use pain-relieving procedures that may hasten death?

MAJOR ETHICAL ORIENTATIONS

To try to resolve ethical problems and dilemmas, one initially appeals to one of several ethical orientations. Each has its moral principles, standards, and ethical theory along with nonethical premises, metaphors, and slogans. The premises of an ethical orientation, taken together, are intended to imply and also to help justify a practical ethics conclusion.

TABLE 12–2. CODE FOR NURSES

1. The nurse provides services with respect for human dignity and the uniqueness of the client unrestricted by considerations of social or economic status, personal attributes, or the nature of health problems.
2. The nurse safeguards the client's right to privacy by judiciously protecting information of a confidential nature.
3. The nurse acts to safeguard the client and the public when health care and safety are affected by the incompetent, unethical, or illegal practice of any person.
4. The nurse assumes responsibility and accountability for individual nursing judgments and actions.
5. The nurse maintains competence in nursing.
6. The nurse exercises informed judgment and uses individual competence and qualifications as criteria in seeking consultation, accepting responsibilities, and delegating nursing activities to others.
7. The nurse participates in activities that contribute to the ongoing development of the profession's body of knowledge.
8. The nurse participates in the profession's efforts to implement and improve standards of nursing.
9. The nurse participates in the profession's efforts to establish and maintain conditions of employment conducive to high quality nursing care.
10. The nurse participates in the profession's effort to protect the public from misinformation and misrepresentation and to maintain the integrity of nursing.
11. The nurse collaborates with members of the health professions and other citizens in promoting community and national efforts to meet the health needs of the public.

From the American Nurses' Association.

Rational Paternalism

According to rational paternalism, an authority knows best, providing it is really wise. Often enough, there are true applications of authority figures knowing best. Parents, nurses, physicians, lawyers, teachers may actually know what to do to help someone. A given nurse, in particular, may know best that Smith, aged 77, a fragile, elderly client, needs a locking waist belt because he is unsteady when walking or standing. The question arises, however: Even if an authority figure knows best regarding what is good for a given client, such as Smith, what about Smith's **autonomy** or self-determination rights? Doesn't Smith have a right to decide what happens in and to his or her body?

Libertarianism

The difficulty of rational paternalism in dealing justifiably with cases involving recognition and respect for a client's autonomy and self-determination rights leads one to another ethical orientation, **libertarianism.** A major principle of libertariansim is the uncompromising liberty of the individual. Libertariansim says in effect: "Leave me alone." Its major thrust in health care is to guard against "unjustified interference" with an individual's will. On libertarian grounds, a Jehovah's Witness has a right to refuse a blood transfusion, even if the conse-

quence is death to that client. The decision is the client's exclusively, providing only that the client is of sound mind.

A major contribution of libertarianism to health-care ethics is the enunciation of the principle of "informed consent." According to this principle, a central plank of patients' bill of rights and an important assumption of the *Code for Nurses* in protecting nurses' rights, no one may perform a procedure on a client without that client's fully informed consent.

There are obvious but different difficulties with both paternalism and libertarianism. An authority figure doesn't always know best. Even if one does, to rely on an authority figure other than oneself divests an individual of self-responsibility and precious decision-making powers. But an individual may need the help of others. To make decisions on one's own may be ill-advised and against a client's own best interests. To ease the difficulty of choosing what to do in a given case, there are, fortunately, still other ethical orientations. These models are like overlapping circles (Fig. 12–1). Each model expresses its values along with an attempt to justify these values in nursing care.

Love-based Ethics

St. Thomas Aquinas, for example, used the metaphor that life is a gift of great value as a reason

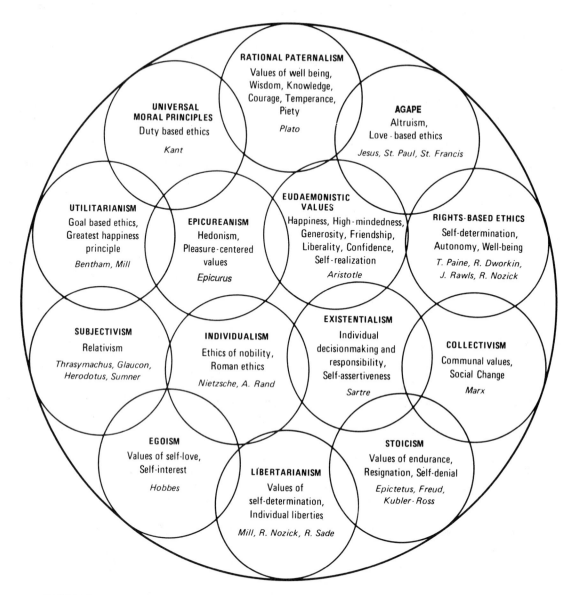

FIGURE 12–1. Models of Morality in Nursing Practice. *(From: E. L. Bandman and B. Bandman, Nursing Ethics in the Life Span* [East Norwalk, Conn.: Appleton-Century-Crofts, 1985], 41.)

for never taking any human life through murder or suicide.[16] He used principles of love found in the Christian religion to attempt to justify respect for life, regardless of cost or consequences. This Christian love is known as **agape.**

Natural Law

Aquinas, moreover, contributed to an important concept in ethics, the idea that there is a law above and beyond any civil law, namely "natural law." One may appeal to natural law to test the moral worth of a civil law. Aquinas argued that abortion, masturbation, homosexuality, euthanasia, suicide, homicide, and usury (making excess profits) were violations of natural law. In current society and in Roman Catholicism appeals to natural law are made to confront the unnaturalness of abortion, reproductive technology, homosexuality, and withholding or terminating artificial feedings.

There are, however, difficulties with natural law, such as: Who decides what is in accordance with natural law? How effective can inflexible stipulations be? How does one decide between conflicting health-care values? What shall a nurse do in the face of a terminal client's desperate wish to be helped to die by withholding or terminating gastric feedings?

A way to test the principle of the sacredness of life is to bring tough cases against it, such as deciding whether to save the life of a hopeless infant with trisomy 18 or a comatose ten-year-old child.

A further rejoinder to the concept of agape comes from the ancient Greek philosopher Aristotle (384–322 B.C.). According to some proponents of agape or **altruism,** one can be happy even though one is hungry, poor, disadvantaged, ugly, deformed, and lacking in health. For in the altruist view, real happiness consists in the next life, one that is eternal. Aristotle's rejoinder is contained in a profoundly commonsensical insight that one cannot be happy without good health, reasonable wealth and good looks. Generally, beautiful, handsome, healthy, and wealthy people are happier than poor, unhealthy, ugly individuals. Hardly anyone would choose to be in the latter category.

Egoism

The difficulties with valuing love of others under all conditions gives rise to an alternative model of morality, championed by various proponents throughout history. This model is called **egoism.** It proposes that people are oriented by self-love. According to Thrasymachus, a philosopher who argued for egosim, concern for others is hypocrisy. He claimed that people naturally love themselves, and justice is defined according to the interests of those who have power.

A modern egoist, Thomas Hobbes (1599–1679), argued that self-preservation is the primary drive in human nature.[17] The only basis on which people come together to form social institutions and contractual arrangements is to achieve more peace and greater opportunity for self-interest. Otherwise, life would be like a jungle, where it would be a "war of all against all."[18] In the egoist view, whatever a nurse does is done out of self-interest.

Utilitarianism

A modern effort to combine the strengths and also minimize the weaknesses of altruism and egoism is found in **utilitarianism,** especially the works of Jeremy Bentham (1748–1826) and J.S. Mill (1806–1873). The desired goal here is the "greatest happiness of the greatest number," sometimes identified with majority rule and happiness for the majority. To Bentham, a hedonic calculus was intended to measure human qualities as a basis for ethical decision making. All humans are governed by two masters, pain and pleasure, the desire for the latter and the avoidance of the former. Out of this concept, Bentham developed his "calculus."

The way to evaluate pain and pleasure is to consider seven criteria in what is now regarded as a cost-risk-benefit ratio. In coming to any decision, one asks the expected cost, the risk, and the benefit. Bentham's criteria for calculating pleasure and pain are[19]:

- Intensity
- Duration
- Certainty or uncertainty
- Propinquity or remoteness
- Fecundity
- Purity
- Extent

An example of the application of these criteria is the fulfillment of sexual desire. It is considered to be one of the most important of human interests.

To these criteria, J.S. Mill added that of quality of life, which is intended to include contemplation and esthetic experiences. "Actions are right," Mill held, "if they tend to promote happiness, wrong if they tend to produce the reverse of happiness."[20]

Mill attempted to prove utilitarianism as follows. The reason that an object is visible is that people see it; a sound is audible because people hear it. "In like manner, . . . the sole evidence . . . that anything is desirable is that people . . . desire it."[21] In inferring that what is desired is therefore desirable, Mill commits the "is-ought fallacy." For X to be desired does not imply that X is desirable. For example, that hospital administrators desire nurses to work double shifts does not imply that for nurses to do so is desirable.

An application of utilitarian ethics in health care is the triage principle. Here, three groups of people in need of health care are sorted into those who will recover on their own, those who are likely to die, and those for whom health care and nursing intervention may make a difference. A utilitarian-oriented nurse would choose to work with the latter group and ignore the needs of the first two.

Absolute Principles

Difficulties with applying utilitarianism account for the appeal of absolute moral principles, expressed in modern times in Immanuel Kant's ethical theory. Kant (1724–1804), a great moral philosopher, distinguished hypothetical imperatives (if-then, conditional imperatives) from categorical imperatives (absolute principles). With if-then, conditional imperatives, one decides one's goals or wishes and the means to achieve these goals. A nurse may say, "If I want to help Mrs. Welch, I will make frequent visits to her bedside."

A categorical imperative commands a person, without qualifying, and prescribes what that person must do as a moral agent. The categorical imperative says to act on that rule that ought to apply to all people in similar circumstances, without exception. Three features of a categorical imperative are that it assumes freedom of the will of a moral agent, it is universally binding, and it consists of an action that a "rational impartial spectator" would take.[22] Kant cites five examples[23]:

1. Suicide is always wrong, for if everyone who felt like it commited suicide, there would be no human race left
2. Keeping promises is right. Breaking them is wrong. Social institutions depend on people, including nurses, to fulfill their promises
3. Always develop your talents to the utmost of your ability

4. Always help those in need
5. Always tell the truth

Finally Kant states an important substantive principle to always treat oneself or another as an end, "never as a means only."

Clearly, some examples Kant cites are easier to defend than others. There are conflicting values, such as always to keep promises, that are not easy to resolve. But Kant's ethics appeal to those who believe one should act on principle rather than for expedience. Furthermore, Kant's ethics favor equality, justice, and fairness, in contrast to utilitarianism. Kantian ethics place great value on respect and respect for clients. Kant's principles provide a welcome rejoinder to defenders of the wanton disregard of clients and nurses alike that prevails in much of health-care delivery.

Justice-based Ethics

The difference between utilitarian and absolute principle ethics involves a conflict between inclination and obligation: Utilitarianism champions inclination, and Kant's absolute principles favor obligation. J. Rawls has attempted to provide an effective synthesis of both utilitarianism and absolute principle ethics. To Rawls, justice as fairness is uncompromising. Slavery, exploitation, and servitude are never made right, no matter how many people may vote for retaining these negative social institutions and values.

Rawls arrives at the idea of justice as a central principle through a powerful thought experiment, called "the veil of ignorance."[24] Everyone is to imagine not knowing one's biologic, social, economic role, place, and identity in the world. Imagine that we do not know whether we will be born smart or dull, healthy or unhealthy, white or black, rich or poor, male or female, beautiful or ugly. Under this "veil of ignorance," what rules would we all agree to live by? Rawls suggests that we would choose two principles. The first is that we would want all people to have equal liberties. The second principle, in three parts, is that social and economic inequalities are justifed only if they (1) help the least advantaged; (2) serve the advantage of all; and (3) if offices are open to all on a basis of equality of opportunity.[25]

The Rawlsian conceptual enterprise has an

important role in health care and in nursing, in particular. Rawls has tried to bring together two important values, need and merit.

There are difficulties in implementing Rawlsian priorities as to need and merit in health care on a just basis. However, appeal to justice as fairness uncompromisingly rules out certain socially profitable practices, such as a two-class health-care delivery system (one for the rich and one for the poor), racism, sexism, abuse and disrespect of clients and of nurses. Rawls's aim is to demonstrate justice as equal access to the "primary goods" of life, such as power, money, and the means for achieving good health. To Rawls, "justice is to social institutions what truth is to systems of thought. Rawls's work brings home to health-care ethicists, including nurses, that there can be no ethics without justice, and that justice is to ethics what health care and nursing care are to a good life.

MORAL PRINCIPLES AND VALUES IN NURSING

Some ethical values and principles are explicitly cited in the *Code for Nurses* as well as in general bioethics literature. These include the principle of autonomy, showing respect for an individual's rational exercise of freedom. A second principle is that of **beneficence,** meaning that nurses aim to do good in all their work with clients. Another ethical principle is that of **nonmaleficence,** which counsels nurses to avoid harming or injuring clients.

There are these further values cited by the *Code for Nurses.* Nurses are urged to show respect for a client's privacy and confidentiality; express loyalty; and treat clients justly and fairly.[26] Moreover, nurses are explicitly urged to **advocacy** for their clients' interest and safety if these are threatened in any way. The Code creates the picture of an ethical nurse as a caring, principled, intelligent, purposeful, highly trained nurse, who does her or his best to help clients achieve optimal health care.

Paradigm Case Argument
One form of argument for evaluating ethical orientations in nursing is the appeal to a para-digm case argument or to a standard example. A standard example is found in Aquinas's argument that "life is a gift" or in the principle of autonomy, which propounds that if one has rights at all, one has a right to decide whether to give informed consent to what is done in and to one's body. With the help of such moral principles as autonomy, beneficence, nonmaleficence, and the right to self-determination, one may expose such evils as those that occurred at Tuskeegee or Willowbrook, where harmful research was performed without the informed consent of subjects. Such procedures may then be identified as violations of clients' rights and therefore as immoral. With the help of oaths, formal declarations, and manifestos, like the *Code for Nurses,* one can identify moral ideals and standards in health care that are laudatory models for nursing practice.

Lastly, the ethical, caring, intelligent, highly trained nurse, knowledgeable in nurse–client ethics, will have to be autonomous also, and try to answer the continuing question, "How can I make a difference?" Only by combining thought and action in complex ways does a nurse fulfill the potential to be a professional, humanistic, and ethically sensitive nurse.

PROFESSIONAL ACCOUNTABILITY

Role of the Nurse as Moral Agent
As clinicians and coordinators of client care, nurses are key figures in promoting a moral climate for both consumers and providers of health care. More than any other health professionals, nurses are in continuous contact with clients, their families, and significant others. Nurses witness expressions of clients' most intimate feelings of fear, despair, hope, and regret. Family relationships become obvious as family members interact regarding necessary decisions related to the illness and choices of treatment, prognosis, costs, and values. Clients, their families, and significant others trust nurses to share relevant information and experience in clarifying the problematic situation and in moving toward resolution. Nursing is identified as doing good with and for people who are sick or well. Nurses are regarded as moral agents who do good by meeting universal human needs for

nursing care, and through practice that enhances the worth and dignity of every individual involved in that care.

Thus, nurses are universally regarded as having good intentions. Good intent, however, is not enough. Knowledge of ethical theories and principles or ignorance of them can be the cause or source of good or harm. Reasons for choice or refusal of treatment need to be critically examined. Knowledge of ethical theories and principles, therefore, is as indispensable to nurses in daily practice as is scientific and technical knowledge related to the illness. Unexamined values and beliefs, subject to intensely subjective past experiences, are insufficient guides to choice and to action—whether professional or personal.

One of the hallmarks of a profession is the development of a code of ethics. The code indicates the profession's acceptance of the responsibility and trust granted to it by society in return for professional autonomy and self-regulation. Thus the nurse is professionally accountable. The nurse has the obligation to protect the health and the safety of the client and the public.

> The nurse's primary commitment is to the health, welfare, and safety of the client. As an advocate for the client, the nurse must be alert to and take appropriate action regarding any instances of incompetent, unethical, or illegal practice by any member of the health care team or the health care system, or any action on the part of others that places the rights or best interests of the client in jeopardy.[27]

To be effective as client advocate, the nurse needs awareness of institutional policies and procedures, nursing standards of practice, reporting and management processes for handling questionable practice at local and state levels, and functions of licensing boards, professional organizations, and other authorities. Nurses should participate in professional review processes, such as quality assurance, peer review, client care, nursing practice, and ethics committees based on established criteria with stated purposes for making recommendations to improve the quality and safety of nursing and health-care delivery. Legally constituted licensing bodies are a further resource for protecting the health and safety of the client and public from unsafe and unethical practitioners or systems.

The concept of accountability implies being answerable for what one has done or not done, both commissions and omissions. To be accountable means to provide a rational explanation to self, clients, co-workers, colleagues, the community and society for individual acts, judgments, and quality of practice at any point. This requires that the nurse be competent, knowledgeable as to relevant new therapies, theories, and research, and ethical concepts and principles underlying practice. When the client's needs are beyond the nurse's competence and knowledge, consultation, collaboration, help, and relief must be sought from appropriate sources to ensure safe, ethical, legal nursing and health care for clients and the public.

Development of Moral Judgment

A recent contribution to the theory of moral development is the psychological-philosophical work of Lawrence Kohlberg. He identifies three levels and six stages of moral development through which humans grow. Level I is called Preconventional and has two stages: Stage 1 is behavior oriented by fear of punishment and obedience to authority; Stage 2 is instrumental and relativistic ("You scratch my back and I'll scratch yours."). Level II is called Conventional and has two stages: Stage 3 is behavior characterized by seeking approval, as in a "nice girl, nice boy" rating; Stage 4 is behavior that confirms to "law and order." Level III is called Postconventional and describes autonomous, principled behavior: Stage 5 is behavior oriented to the concept of a social contract, a constitutional–legal orientation; Stage 6 is behavior oriented to universal ethical principles (Table 12–3).

Kohlberg's analysis has advantages and drawbacks. An advantage is that Kohlberg gives an argument against relativism and subjectivism. A second advantage is Kohlberg's suggestion of parallel intellectual and moral growth. Thus he suggests that brighter individuals are more apt to reason at a higher moral level.[28] A third advantage of Kohlberg's analysis is his contention that organized discussion of moral

TABLE 12–3. STAGES OF MORAL DEVELOPMENT

Premoral Period:
The concept of morality has no operational meaning from birth to early childhood.

I. Preconventional Level

The child is responsive to cultural rules and labels of good and bad, right or wrong, but interprets these labels in terms of either the physical or the pleasurable consequences of action (punishment, reward, exchange of favors), or in terms of the physical power of those who announce the rules and the labels.

Stage 1: The Punishment and Obedience Orientation
The physical consequences of action determine its goodness or badness regardless of the human meaning or value of these consequences. Avoidance of punishment and unquestioning deference to power are valued in their own right.

Stage 2: The Instrumental Relativist Orientation
Right action consists of those means that satisfy one's own needs and sometimes the needs of others. Human relations are viewed in terms of the marketplace. Fairness, reciprocity, and sharing are interpreted in a practical way. Reciprocity is a matter of "You scratch my back and I'll scratch yours."

II. Conventional Level

At this level, maintaining the expectations of the individual's family, group, or nation is perceived as valuable in its own right, regardless of immediate and obvious consequences. The attitude is not only one of conformity to personal expectations and social order, but of loyalty to it, actively maintaining, supporting, and justifying the order and of identifying with the persons or group involved in it.

Stage 3: The Interpersonal Agreement or "Good-Boy, Nice-Girl" Orientation
Good behavior is that which pleases or helps others and is approved by them. There is much conformity to stereotypical images of what is majority or "natural behavior." Behavior is frequently judged by intention; "he means well" becomes important for the first time. One earns approval by being "nice."

Stage 4: The "Law and Order" Orientation
There is orientation toward authority, fixed rules, and the maintenance of the social order. Right behavior consists of doing one's duty, showing respect for authority, and maintaining the given social order for its own sake.

III. Postconventional, Autonomous, or Principled Level

At this level, there is a clear effort to define moral values and principles that have validity and application apart from the authority of the groups or persons holding these principles and apart from the individual's own identification with these groups.

Stage 5: The Social Contract Legalistic and Utilitarian Orientation
Right action tends to be defined in terms of general individual rights and standards that have been critically examined and agreed upon by the whole society. Aside from what is constitutionally and democratically agreed upon, the right is a matter of personal and relative "values" and "opinion." The result is an emphasis on the "legal point of view" and changing the law toward gaining "the greatest happiness for the greatest number." Beyond this legal realm, free agreement and contract is the binding element of obligation. This is the "official" morality of the American government and constitution.

Stage 6: The Universal Ethical Principle Orientation
Right is defined by the decision of conscience in accord with self-chosen ethical principles appealing to logical comprehensiveness, universality, and consistency. These principles are abstract (the Golden Rule, the Categorical Imperative). At heart, these are universal principles of justice, of the reciprocity and equality of human rights, and of respect for the dignity of human beings as individual persons.

Adapted from L. Kohlberg, "Stages and aging in moral development—some speculations," Gerontologist, (Winter 1973), 497.

principles and behavior can positively influence moral growth and development.

The difficulties with Kohlberg's analysis are that even if his account of moral development is accurate, it does not imply or justify how one ought to behave. It is fallacious to suggest that what is is what ought to be. There are, for example, many practices in nursing, such as working double shifts, that ought not to exist. A second criticism of Kohlberg's analysis is that the right decision may be reached at a lower rather than a higher level of reasoning. The moral hierarchical method of arriving at universal moral principles is not necessarily "the valid and sound view in all cases."[29] Lastly, Kohlberg has not been able to show that moving through these stages of moral development from self-centeredness and obedience to acting on universal principle is the way to achieve the highest stage of morality. "If Kohlberg were successful, he would show that ethics is a true and valid answer. This . . . has not been shown."[30]

ETHICAL ISSUES IN NURSING

Clients' Rights

The American Hospital Association approved *A Patient's Bill of Rights* with the expectation that its use would increase client-care effectiveness and satisfaction. The Association recognized that although "a personal relationship between physician and patient is essential for the provision of proper medical care, the . . . relationship takes on a new dimension when care is rendered within an organizational structure [when] the institution itself has a responsibility to the patient."[31] In its first provision, the Bill affirmed the client's right to considerate and respectful care. This right is extended in later provisions to knowing what hospital rules and regulations apply to the client role and to the examination and explanation of the hospital bill, regardless of who pays. The second, third and fourth provisions are significant. These acknowledge the client's right to receive from his physician the necessary information to give informed consent including "the specific procedure and/or treatment, the medically significant risks involved . . . the probable duration of incapacitation . . . medically significant alterna-

tives for care or treatment . . . the name of the person responsible."[32] The client then has the right to refuse treatment and be informed of medical and legal consequences. The client has the further right to be informed of human experimentation affecting his care or treatment with the right to refuse participation in such research. Provisions 5 and 6 speak to the client's right to privacy and confidentiality of communication, records, case discussion, consultation, examination and treatment. Provisions 7, 8, and 10 refer to the client's right to secure reasonable responses to requests for service, to receive information and explanation regarding transfers and referrals, and "the right to expect reasonable continuity of care . . . what appointment times and physicians are available and where . . . of the patient's continuing health care requirements following discharge."[33] The Bill ends with the disclaimer that "No catalog of rights can guarantee . . . the patient the kind of treatment he has a right to expect." The message appears to be that "hospitals have many functions to perform and, therefore, are very busy places, but we'll show concern for the client . . . his dignity as a human being and try to defend the rights of the client"[34] (Fig. 12–2).

Nurses' Rights

One function of the American Nurses' Association code of ethics is to elevate the profession of nursing by clearly investing nurses with rights and correlative responsibilities. These rights enable nurses to care more effectively for clients by protecting rights that cannot be entrusted solely to physicians. Nurses' rights empower nurses to act on behalf of clients and for nurses' own right of conscience as well as against other professionals, if necessary to protect the safety and health of clients.

Irrespective of the particular health problem, the nurse respects the worth and dignity of each human being and "therefore, must take all reasonable means to protect and preserve human life. . . ."[35] However, if the nurse is "ethically opposed to interventions in a particular case because of the procedures to be used, the nurse is justified in refusing to participate."[36] Abortion and such reproductive technologies as artificial insemination, in vitro fertilization, im-

Statement on A Patient's Bill of Rights
American Hospital Association, 1972

The American Hospital Association presents A Patient's Bill of Rights with the expectation that observance of these rights will contribute to more effective patient care and greater satisfaction for the patient, his physician, and the hospital organization. Further, the Association presents these rights in the expectation that they will be supported by the hospital on behalf of its patients, as an integral part of the healing process. It is recognized that a personal relationship between the physician and the patient is essential for the provision of proper medical care. The traditional physician–patient relationship takes on a new dimension when care is rendered within an organizational structure. Legal precedent has established that the institution itself also has a responsibility to the patient. It is in recognition of these factors that these rights are affirmed.

1. The patient has the right to considerate and respectful care.
2. The patient has the right to obtain from his physician complete current information concerning his diagnosis, treatment, and prognosis in terms the patient can be reasonably expected to understand. When it is not medically advisable to give such information to the patient, the information should be made available to an appropriate person in his behalf. He has the right to know by name, the physician responsible for coordinating his care.
3. The patient has the right to receive from his physician information necessary to give informed consent prior to the start of any procedure and/or treatment. Except in emergencies, such information for informed consent should include but not necessarily be limited to the specific procedure and/or treatment, the medically significant risks involved, and the probable duration of incapacitation. Where medically significant alternatives for care or treatment exist, or when the patient requests information concerning medical alternatives, the patient has the right to such information. The patient also has the right to know the name of the person responsible for the procedures and/or treatment.
4. The patient has the right to refuse treatment to the extent permitted by law, and to be informed of the medical consequences of his action.
5. The patient has the right to every consideration of his privacy concerning his own medical care program. Case discussion, consultation, examination, and treatment are confidential and should be conducted discreetly. Those not directly involved in his care must have the permission of the patient to be present.
6. The patient has the right to expect that all communications and records pertaining to his care should be treated as confidential.
7. The patient has the right to expect that within its capacity a hospital must make reasonable response to the request of a patient for services. The hospital must provide evaluation, service, and/or referral as indicated by the urgency of the case. When medically permissible a patient may be transferred to another facility only after he has received complete information and explanation concerning the needs for and alternatives to such a transfer. The institution to which the patient is to be transferred must first have accepted the patient for transfer.
8. The patient has the right to obtain information as to any relationship of his hospital to other health care and educational institutions insofar as his care is concerned. The patient has the right to obtain information as to the existence of any professional relationships among individuals, by name, who are treating him.
9. The patient has the right to be advised if the hospital proposes to engage in or perform human experimentation affecting his care or treatment. The patient has the right to refuse to participate in such research projects.
10. The patient has the right to expect reasonable continuity of care. He has the right to know in advance what appointment times and physicians are available and where. The patient has the right to expect that the hospital will provide a mechanism whereby he is informed by his physician or a delegate of the physician of the patient's continuing health care requirements following discharge.
11. The patient has the right to examine and receive an explanation of his bill regardless of source of payment.
12. The patient has the right to know what hospital rules and regulations apply to his conduct as a patient.

No catalogue of rights can guarantee for the patient the kind of treatment he has a right to expect. A hospital has many functions to perform, including the prevention and treatment of disease, the education of both health professionals and patients, and the conduct of clinical research. All these activities must be conducted with an overriding concern for the patient, and, above all, the recognition of his dignity as a human being. Success in achieving this recognition assures success in the defense of the rights of the patient.

Figure 12–2. A Patient's Bill of Rights. *(From: the American Hospital Association, Chicago, Ill., copyright 1972.)*

plantation, and surrogate motherhood are morally repugnant to some nurses. Such nurses should communicate their refusal well in advance so that other arrangements for nursing care can be made. Some states, such as New Jersey, protect the "right of conscience" to refuse participation in abortion procedures. In case of emergency, however, the nurse has the duty to protect the client's safety until other sources of nursing care are provided. Otherwise, the nurse is abandoning the client, a serious moral and legal act and omission. Similarly, the nurse has the right to violate the client's right to privacy if the safety of clients or of innocent parties is in danger, as in threatened suicide or homicide.

Since the nurse's primary obligation is "to the health, welfare, and safety of the client,"[37] the nurse has both the right and the duty to protect the client from "any instances of incompetent, unethical, or illegal practice by any member of the health care team or the health care system, or any action on the part of others that places the rights or best interests of the client in jeopardy."[38] The nurse has the right to call the physician's attention to the possibility of harm to the client. The nurse has the right to report potential or actually harmful practices to the appropriate authority within the employment setting without fear of reprisal and according to established procedures. If harmful practices are not corrected, the nurse has the right to report these practices to outside authorities, such as professional misconduct bodies connected to licensing boards and relevant professional organizations. The nurse has the right to participate in review mechanisms based on stated criteria, purposes, and processes that serve to safeguard clients and the quality of nursing practice. Nurses have the right to refuse physician's orders and employing agencies' directives, since neither relieves the nurse of accountability for judgments made and actions taken or not taken. The nurse has the right to refuse to carry out a specific function "if the nurse concludes that he or she lacks competence or is inadequately prepared to carry out a specific function."[39] The nurse has the right to seek consultation and collaboration from qualified sources.

In research participation, the nurse has the right to obtain information about the purpose, design, and the methods of research, as well as the informed consent statement and institutional review board status for the protection of human subjects, as the basis for acceptance or refusal.

Nurses have the moral and legal right to participate in collective bargaining agreements for determining conditions of employment essential to effective nursing care. Nurses have the right to actively participate in decision making and policy formation at all levels and arenas to secure a just distribution of health-care and nursing resources as a "basic right of all people."[40]

The Right to Life

Alternative models of morality guide the nurse in the care of clients for whom the right to life is an issue. Models of morality are like overlapping circles. "Each model sets out its values along with an attempted justification to some decision-making aspect of nursing."[41] St. Thomas Aquinas's concept that human life is a gift, never to be destroyed, supports the view that all life is sacred. This principle is used against the practice of abortion and suicide. This principle is also used by nurses and others to save the lives and to treat infants at all cost, even with multiple physical and neurological defects and a prediction of very poor and burdensome quality of life.

The libertarian model holds that individuals have the right to decide what happens in and to their persons and bodies. Using the libertarian model, the 42-year-old woman who is pregnant for the first time decides for herself whether she will continue the pregnancy and under what conditions. Similarly, the person with a serious, life-threatening illness, such as AIDS, has the right to all care and treatment in the course of the disease—irrespective of the cost and the certain, fatal outcome—on the basis of an egoist model of self-preservation first.

The universal moral principle that prohibits suicide or the taking of any life is expressed in Kant's concept that "an act is good if everyone ought, for rational reasons and in similar circumstances, to act in the same way without exception. . . . On the basis of this categorical imperative . . . Kant formulates a substantive principle, which is to act so that one treats oneself or any other person always as an 'end' and never as a means only."[42] Kant's universality principle holds that everyone is to be helped to live without regard for other people's desires, convenience, pleasure, inclination, or cost. Everyone would be treated rationally and impartially in the same circumstances. No life is to be taken, and everyone is to be respected.

According to R. Dworkin, individual rights are held equally, and the function of the state is to protect those rights.[43] Dworkin distinguishes between a right to equal shares or equal treatment in distributing health-care resources that people do not have and a right to equal consideration and treatment as equals that he claims they do have. In this view, everyone would have equal consideration necessary to health-care support.

Abortion

The decision to terminate an unwanted pregnancy or a pregnancy in which the fetus is seriously deformed is a decision of great responsibility. Ethical arguments provide justification for ending the pregnancy either in terms of the woman's right to her own body, her own self-preservation interests, the greatest happiness of the greatest number of her family affected by an additional person, the best interests of the child damaged by a disadvantaged social situation, severe disability, or the injustice of a pregnancy conceived in violence, rape, or incest.

The ethical arguments favoring abortion are against the argument that the right to life is absolute and sacred. The counterargument is that the fetus is likened to the acorn. Acorns are not oak trees, nor is the fetus any more than a potential person. That fetus's right to life, if, for the sake of argument, the fetus is granted personhood at conception, does not outweigh the mother's right to decide what happens in and to her body, to her person, and to her life.[44]

To the charge that a woman engaging in sexual intercouse is at least partly responsible for her pregnancy, J. J. Thomson points to the statistical evidence of less than 100 percent effectiveness of contraceptives. She compares an unwanted pregnancy to the burglar climbing in an opened window. Neither have a right to the use of the house. The use of another's body, as in pregnancy, is not guaranteed in the right to life.

The counterargument to Thomson's view of the woman's right to her own body, person, and life from the right-to-life movement is Aquinas's statement that "Life is God's gift to man and is subject to His power who kills and who makes to live."[45] Another counterargument to abortion is that the pregnant woman is really two persons. "The fetus has the same moral status as a mother, and therefore the same right to live. This means abortion is not morally justifiable; even in cases that threaten a mother's life."[46] The difficulty with this argument is that human life as a set of conscious acts is made equal to the undeveloped state of the mind of the fetus. A further argument is that since women generally carry on the rearing of children and provide the right to a full human life, they should have the decision-making role in continuing or terminating pregnancy.

There are other perspectives on abortion besides its being a woman's right to decide what happens in and to her body, or that a fetus has a right to life. An abortion may also be mandated by a society or family that perceives the need for population controls. An abortion may be a tragedy to a woman affected by it, and in some cases, an abortion may be a relief. In any event, a fetus does not have an undisputed right to life.

The Right to End Life

The right to end life includes both the issue of suicide and that of withholding or terminating life-support treatments and measures. Suicide and refusing life-saving therapy are sometimes regarded as equally moral assertions of the right to one's body, person, and life. The counterargument is that most suicides are related to a sense of hopelessness and helplessness. Therefore, a paternalistic moral position, supported by Kant's categorical imperative to save all life and never destroy it, would require the nurse to thwart the suicide attempt.

Altruistic ethical principles and the wish to spare loved ones further anguish and financial burdens are sometimes cited by the elderly as another basis for suicide or refusing life-support treatments. For example, artificial feeding through intravenous or gastric tubes is now widely debated as a medical treatment to be refused or as an essential of life, like air, universally provided.

There is now virtual agreement, supported by Living Wills that protect both the client and the health provider and given legal status in some states, that the rational adult client can refuse even life-saving treatment such as gastric tube feedings. The Living Will is the legal expression of the rational person's "refusing in advance futile prolongation of dying if they become terminally ill with no hope of recovery."[47] Families may give proxy consent for voluntary euthanasia, a merciful death, if this is the explicit, documented wish of the client who may now be unable to insist that his or her wishes be respected.

The written order not to resuscitate is both moral and legal if it is the expressed wish of the competent, rational adult client. In 1986, the Judicial Council of the American Medical Association stated that it would be ethical for physicians "to withhold all means of life-prolonging medical treatment, including artificial nutrition and hydration, from irreversibly comatose patients even if death is not imminent and where there is adequate medical confirmation of the diagnosis. . . . In treating a terminally ill or irreversibly comatose patient, the physician should determine whether the benefits of treatment outweigh its burdens. . . ."[48] This position is based on the utilitarian model of the greatest happiness for the greatest number, calculated in terms of benefits and costs. Clearly, the costs of human suffering and the futile allocation of limited resources used in the care of these persons outweighs the benefits to the individual, the family, and to society. This position has not received universal endorsement from religious groups because it permits withholding artificial feedings. Nevertheless, the trend appears to be increased public, judicial, and legislative support for the right to die.

Behavior Control

The ethical problems associated with behavior control have increased along with the effectiveness of the technology. The technology includes powerful psychotropic drugs, behavior modification programs, electroconvulsive therapy, psychosurgery, and various psychotherapies. The intent of these therapeutic measures is to alter behavior. The therapeutic agent, therefore, usually the staff nurse, functions as "double agent," working both to protect society from client behavior that deviates from societal norms and as a therapeutic agent for the client. This may create conflicts of interest because what may be for the greatest good for the greatest number, society, may not be good for the individual client. For example, a psychotropic drug may effectively tranquilize the client but may also cause irreversible, highly disturbing side effects, such as involuntary facial grimacing and tongue movements. Thus, the behavior control satisfies the demands of society but not the client's desires. Choice of action has been effectively taken from the client, a major loss of liberty rights.

The concept of dangerousness has been particularly difficult to determine, even though it is still used to justify commitment to mental institutions. In the past, the diagnosis of committing harm to onseself or others was overused. The result was that people were institutionalized, largely untreated, except for the use of psychotropic drugs, and totally deprived of their freedom for most of their lives. The pendulum has swung to the opposite extreme. There is now so much protection of mentally ill people's civil liberties and rights to refuse treatment as to constitute a threat to their safety and well-being from lack of treatment and the food, clothing, and shelter they may need and cannot secure for themselves. The dilemma is to protect mentally disabled individuals from unwarranted coercion while protecting their rights to receive treatment in order to restore their autonomy.

Technology

The prevailing ethical principle regarding the use of technology has been: If it helps, use it. Little thought or research has been dedicated to evaluating technology on the basis of effectiveness, its impact on society, the ethical implications of its use, and its cost in relation to benefit. Each phase of organ transplant, for example, raises profound ethical issues in client selection, of criteria of human worth, equality, and justice. Bias as to socioeconomic class, education, intelligence, sex, age, and ethnicity may be operating unfairly in recipient selection and organ donation.

A further ethical issue concerns the cost:benefit:risk ratio of all technology. If scarce resources, including nursing personnel, are allocated to exotic technology that benefits only a few while low-cost high-benefit hypertension screening and treatment programs, for example, are ignored, the utilitarian principle of the greatest happiness to the greatest number and the principle of justice as fairness are violated.

Issues of the quality of life that is saved by the use of high technology are further considerations in the cost:benefit:risk calculation. Renal dialysis is a case in point. The program now reaches about 100,000 clients annually and costs billions of dollars. The dialysis machine, like the respirator, sustains life when there is no hope of regaining health. Senile and comatose clients are transported by ambulance to dialysis centers three times weekly for treatment that can only prolong a life that has lost its quality and purpose, all on the grounds of the right to health care. Critics hold that for these irreversibly and terminally ill clients, implementation of the right to health care is unwise, unkind, and a waste of resources. The allocation of limited resources to maintain futile treatment for a life without quality versus the individual's right to life at any price is the central issue in the use of high technology. Societal decisions related to the morality of the universal use of technology are needed.

CONCLUSIONS

Ethical issues relevant to professional nursing practice are an ongoing challenge. The individual nurse, acting as a responsible member of many overlapping groups, i.e., the nursing profession, society, religious groups, and social organizations, has a responsibility to formulate and follow a coherent set of moral values that constitute his or her personal ethics. The values that individual nurses hold determine modes of conduct, both personally and professionally, that are the criteria for action and for morally

judging themselves and others. These personal values, in some percentage, are always going to conflict with the values of other persons and of institutions, necessitating a logical approach based on moral reasoning rather than learned values.

There are often no straightforward yes or no answers in situations of moral or ethical concern. When nurses are called upon, as care givers, teachers, or colleagues, to formulate their best judgment about an ethical issue, the ability to reach a reasonable conclusion will depend upon a number of factors. One of the most important of these is the ability to think logically and critically, combining one's own personal ethical convictions with a sensitive appreciation of others' ethical convictions. Gaining competence in this area is not automatically learned through experience or maturity but can be enhanced by deliberate pursuit through self-examination and discussions with others.

Thinking about one's own personal values and ethical beliefs, and delineating them in some organized and meaningful way is more complicated for some than others, but is not an easy task for anyone. This process is often referred to as *values clarification*. Values clarification can be an enlightening and positive experience that is facilitated by reading about ethics and understanding many of the concepts and ideas presented in this chapter. The outcomes of such an inquiry, and the consciousness gained, will inevitably serve to foster professional growth and confidence in one's practice of nursing.

SUMMARY

This chapter provides the learner with essential concepts derived from theories of ethics and the ANA code of ethics applicable to nursing practice. As the main providers of health care, nurses can and ought to be moral agents and client advocates in the health-care delivery system. Good intentions are insufficient guides to action. Knowledge of major ethical orientations includes analysis of rational paternalism, libertarianism, love-based ethics, egoism, natural law, utilitariansim, absolute principles, and justice. Principles of autonomy, beneficence, and rights can be derived from overlapping theories.

Important issues in ethics, such as clients' and nurses' rights, abortion, the right to life, the right to end life, behavior control and technology are discussed from the perspective of nursing and competing ethical theories. Emphasis is placed on the nurse's role as a participant in ethical decision making affecting client care and nursing practice, based on an overview of essential theoretical and practical knowledge.

Study Questions

1. Who is (are) the primary decision maker(s) in health care? Who ought to be the primary decision makers and on what ethical grounds can that be justified?

2. What are the advantages and disadvantages of shared decision making?

3. Nurse Smith cares for Mr. Jones, aged 94 and without relatives and friends except for the nursing staff in the long-term facility in which he has resided for the past eight years. Nurse Smith and other nursing staff have had a long, close, and affectionate relationship with Mr. Jones. He suffers a cardiac arrest in the midst of morning care. What would you advise Nurse Smith to do, based on which ethical theories and principles?

4. What are the strengths and weaknesses of utilitarian ethics in relation to DRGs, treating seriously defective babies, and treating mentally disabled persons?

5. Compare the provisions of the *Code for Nurses* and *A Patient's Bill of Rights* in relation to client participation, clients' rights, nurses' autonomy, nurses' participation, advocacy, and shared decision making.

6. Critically examine the ethical issues in surrogate motherhood, organ transplant, the artificial heart, lung cancer associated with smoking, obesity, and free health care from the perspective of absolute principle, utilitarianism, justice, and love-based ethical theories.

References

1. J.E. Thompson and H.O. Thompson, *Bioethical Decision Making for Nurses* (Norwalk, Conn., Appleton-Century-Crofts, 1985), 6.
2. T.L. Beauchamp, "Ethical theory and bioethics," in T.L. Beauchamp and L. Walters (eds.), *Contemporary Issues in Bioethics*, 2nd ed. (Belmont, Calif., Wadsworth Publishing Co., 1982), 1.
3. K.D. Clouser, "Some things medical ethics is not," in S. Gorovitz and Ruth Maklin (eds.), *Moral Problems in Medicine*, 2nd ed. (Englewood Cliffs, N.J.: Prentice-Hall, 1983), 36.
4. Ibid.
5. Ibid., 36–37.
6. Ibid., 37.
7. Ibid.
8. J. Passmore, "Philosophy," in P. Edwards (ed.), *The Encyclopedia of Philosophy*, vol. 6 (New York: Macmillan and The Free Press, 1967), 216.
9. Ibid., 217.
10. American Nurses' Association, *Code for Nurses with Interpretive Statements* (Kansas City, Mo.: The American Nurses' Association, 1985), i.
11. Ibid., 7.
12. Ibid., iii.
13. E.L. Bandman and B. Bandman, *Nursing Ethics in the Life Span* (East Norwalk, Conn.: Appleton-Century-Crofts, 1985), 2.
14. Ibid., 2.
15. American Nurses' Association, *Code for Nurses*, 1.
16. E.L. Bandman and B. Bandman, *Nursing Ethics in the Life Span*, 41.
17. T. Hobbes, "The leviathan," in W.T. Jones, F. Sontag, M.O. Beckner, and R.J. Fogelin (eds.), *Approaches to Ethics*, 3rd ed. (New York: McGraw-Hill Book Co., 1977), 182.
18. Ibid.
19. J. Bentham, *"Morals and legislation,"* in W.T. Jones, F. Sontag, M.O. Beckner, and R.J. Fogelin (eds.), *Approaches to Ethics,* 3rd ed. (New York: McGraw-Hill, Book Co., 1977), 260.
20. J.S. Mill, *Utilitarianism* (New York: Liberal Arts, 1957), 6.
21. Ibid., 44.
22. I. Kant, *Fundamental Principles of the Metaphysics of Morals,* (New York: Liberal Arts, 1949), 38.
23. Ibid.
24. J. Rawls, *A Theory of Justice* (Cambridge, Mass.: Harvard University Press, 1971), 136–142.
25. Ibid., 302.

26. American Nurses' Association, *Code for Nurses,* 4.

27. Ibid., 6.

28. E.L. Bandman and B. Bandman, *Nursing Ethics in the Life Span,* 52.

29. Ibid., 52.

30. Ibid., 52–53.

31. American Hospital Association, *A Patient's Bill of Rights. (Chicago, Ill., 1975).*

32. Ibid.

33. Ibid.

34. Ibid.

35. American Nurses' Association, *Code for Nurses,* 2–3.

36. Ibid., 3–4.

37. Ibid., 6.

38. Ibid.

39. Ibid., 11.

40. American Nurses' Association, *A National Policy for Health Care* (Kansas City, Mo.: The American Nurses' Association, 1977).

41. E.L. Bandman and B. Bandman, *Nursing Ethics in the Life Span,* 41.

42. Ibid., 49.

43. R. Dworkin, *Taking Rights Seriously* (Cambridge, Mass.: Harvard University Press, 1978), xi.

44. J.J. Thomson, "A defense of abortion," *Philos Public Affairs* (1971), 47–66.

45. St. Thomas Aquinas, "The sin of suicide," in R. Abelson and M.L. Friquegnon, eds. *Ethics for Modern Life,* 2nd ed. (New York: St. Martin's Press), 1982, 25.

46. E.L. Bandman and B. Bandman, *Nursing Ethics in the Life Span,* 132.

47. Society for the Right to Die: *Handbook of 1985 Living Will Laws* (New York: The Society for the Right to Die, 1976), 5.

48. Ibid., 11–12.

Annotated Bibliography

Bandman, E.L., and Bandman, B. eds. 1986. *Bioethics and Human Rights: A Reader for Health Professionals.* Lanham, Md.: University Press of America. This book clearly defines and seriously addresses many of the complex bioethical issues that have direct implications for nurses, physicians, and all professionals practicing in a health-care setting. Fifty-two contributors, of whom 21 are women, include philosophers, physicians, lawyers, nurses, and leaders in the field of bioethics who represent a wide variety of cultural and ethnic backgrounds. The contributors present opposing viewpoints on important topics to provide a broad base of information and guidance for professionals and a stimulus for lively and thoughtful discussion by students.

Bandman, E.L., and Bandman, B. 1985. *Nursing Ethics in the Life Span.* East Norwalk, Conn.: Appleton-Century-Crofts. This book addresses the issue of the nurse's role in evaluating the moral problems that occur throughout the life span of clients. Ethical principles are applied through a developmental framework beginning with the procreative family and ending with the dying patient. Models of nurse–client–physician relationships are analyzed as well as approaches to making ethically justifiable decisions based on nursing strategies, guidelines, and canons of critical reasoning.

Curtin L., and Flaherty, M.J. 1982. *Nursing Ethics: Theories and Pragmatics.* Bowie, Md.: R.J. Brady Co. This book presents a view of ethics as involved with interactions between nurse and patient or client. The authors emphasize, as an integral part of all practice, recognition and respect for the rights of others and the use of logical reasoning in addressing issues and conflicts in relationships.

Davis, A.J., and Aroskar. M.A. 1983. *Ethical Dilemmas and Nursing Practice,* 2nd ed. East Norwalk, Conn.: Appleton-Century-Crofts. A scholarly overview of the main ethical issues in nursing from a philosophical and a broad social policy perspective.

Murphy, C.P., and Hunter, H. 1983. *Ethical Problems in the Nurse–Patient Relationship.* Boston: Allyn and Bacon. A book of contributions by 16 authors, including nurses, philosophers, and lawyers, with a focus on the ethical issues of the nurse–client relationship.

Part III

Concepts Related to Communication

This section presents concepts related to developing a nurse–client relationship and professional relationships in general. These concepts include ethnicity, communication, client teaching, change theory, and the research process. Since communication is vital to the formation of the nurse–client relationship and the nursing process, it is essential that these concepts be considered carefully.

Cultural variability and ethnicity are discussed in this section as broad areas that may require unique knowledge to carry out the nursing process. Communication as a component of culture is addressed and examples of nursing actions are highlighted as they have implications on establishing a nurse–client relationship. Methods of establishing a means of communication are discussed in this chapter as well.

Communication has a theoretical basis, and the chapter on communication introduces the reader to several models and then focuses on how to use the nursing process to communicate effectively.

The chapters on client teaching and change theory discuss aspects of communication used by nurses to assess health behaviors and maintain the health status of individuals, families and groups within the context of the health-care system.

Research is the process by which the scientific body of nursing knowledge is formulated, established, and disseminated through time. It is included in this section as a form of communication among professional nurses, between nurses and other health-care providers, and between nurses and their clients.

Selected clinical applications are given in these chapters, to provide examples of how the nursing process is used in each concept area. For nurses to effectively interact with clients, families, and groups, they must know how to communicate first, and then use that knowledge to provide holistic nursing care.

Chapter 13

Culture, Health, and Illness

Joan M. Roche
Janet-Beth McCann Flynn

Chapter Outline

- Objectives
- Glossary
- Introduction
- Biocultural Perspectives
- American Values
- Culture and Cultures
- Family, Group, and the Life Cycle
- Food
- Religion
- Disease and Illness in Cultural Context
    Sick Role
    Healers and Healing
- The Nursing Process
    Assessment
    Planning
    Implementation
    Evaluation
- Conclusions
- Summary
- Study Questions
- References
- Annotated Bibliography

Objectives

At the completion of this chapter, the reader will be able to:

▶ Define the terms in the glossary
▶ Describe the relationship of culture to prevalence of disease and illness
▶ Describe the differences between culture and cultures
▶ Identify and discuss American core values that serve as standards for behavior
▶ Describe the relationship of culture to health behaviors, beliefs, and practices
▶ Discuss the concept of culture shock
▶ Describe a cultural assessment
▶ Incorporate the cultural assessment in the nursing care plan

Glossary

Core Values. Values that are central to a specific culture.

Cultural Relativism. A perspective through which cultures are viewed as different and acceptable. There is no attempt to define inferior or superior cultures.

Culture. A set of standards for perception, belief, evaluation, communication, and action (Goodenough, 1970).

Culture Shock. A state of anxiety precipitated by the loss of familiar signs and symbols of social intercourse when one is suddenly immersed into a cultural system markedly different from one's home or familiar culture.

Cultures. Groups of people who share similar beliefs, attitudes, values, and practices.

There may be more variability within cultural groups (intracultural) than between groups (intercultural).

Ethnocentrism. The judging of other cultures by the standards of one's own cultural heritage. There is an implicit or explicit tendency to view one's own culture as the superior one.

Intercultural Variability. Differences between cultures.

Intracultural Variability. Differences within a culture.

Sick Role. A set of behaviors expected of people who are ill.

Social Roles. A series of expected behaviors that are culturally acceptable.

Stereotyping. Assuming the presence of a particular characteristic or set of characteristics in a member or members of a group without consideration of individual traits. Stereotyping is not based on objective assessment and is frequently derogatory.

Subcultures. Groups within a larger society sharing the overall culture but each with many of its own distinctive life-styles, beliefs, and values. In the United States, teen-agers are often considered as a subculture.

INTRODUCTION

All groups of people confront similar issues in adapting to their environments. These issues are fundamental to the maintenance of the group and of its individual members. They include providing for nutrition, shelter, care, and education of children, division of labor, social organization, health maintenance, and control of disease. Human beings are characterized by the ability to devise cultural solutions to meet these needs, and it is this ability to adapt to varying environments using cultural means that is responsible for their success as a species.

Understanding of the cultural dimension of humans is derived from the field of anthropology. Cultural anthropologists use a comparative approach in studying groups of people, through which they attempt to understand both similarities and differences among human groups. This knowledge, in turn, contributes to our under-standing of humanity as a whole. Anthropology also is characterized by a holistic view of both culture and humans. Cultures are very complex, consisting of facets that relate to all aspects of life (Fig. 13–1). Cultures are systems in which all parts are interrelated. Events in the system do not occur in isolation. Changes in one part of the system result in changes in others. The wholeness of the human being is emphasized in the awareness that human interaction is with a total physical and social environment. Human behavior has meaning in the context of the environments with which the individual interacts.

The cultural basis of human behavior has great importance for the practice of nursing. With anthropology, nursing shares a holistic view of humanity. Almost all facets of culture have an impact on nursing practice. Some of these facets have more weight than others, however (Fig. 13–2).

Both anthropology and nursing are concerned with adaptation. Anthropologists seek to understand the process of adaptation and the role of culture in adaptation. Roy has defined the purpose of nursing as that of fostering client adaptation.[1] In attempting to achieve this purpose, "the system of the person and his inter-

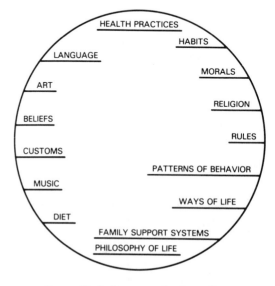

Figure 13–1. Components of a culture.

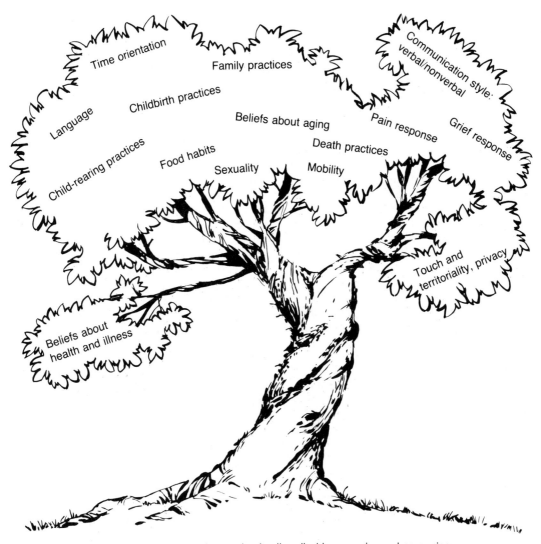

Figure 13–2. Selected aspects of culture that have an impact on nursing.

action with the environment are the units of analysis of nursing assessment. . . .Manipulation of parts of the system or the environment is the mode of nursing intervention."[2] Whereas anthropologists focus on understanding culture in terms of a group of people, nurses use cultural information to understand and assist individual clients, their families, or groups in achieving optimum health.

BIOCULTURAL PERSPECTIVES

Over millions of years, humankind has demonstrated that it can adapt successfully to a number of environments. Through the mechanism of culture, human beings have lived in natural environments that are hospitable and inhospitable, in diverse settings, such as mountains, deserts, islands, fertile plains, and, more recently, complex industrial settings. Temperate, hot, and cold climates require different strategies for living, and human beings have devised them.

We shape and, to some extent, are shaped by our environment. The occurrence of specific genotypes (genetic makeup) and phenotypes (visible traits) result from both biological and cultural adaptation. An example of this is an individual who receives genetic instructions for blood type O from one parent and for blood type A from another. The individual will show a visible trait of blood A (phenotype) and genetic instructions for both A and O (genotype).

Through time, and in all environments, humankind has coped with disease and illness. Prehistoric fossil remains show the presence of arthritis, trauma, and tooth decay. In the historic record, there is evidence of epidemics of smallpox, bubonic plague, and influenza. There is a staggering array of health problems around the world today. Diseases of poverty and malnutrition persist in industrialized as well as in nonindustrialized countries. Famines and droughts still take an enormous toll on human life and health.

The absence, presence, and severity of disease in a population are indicators of human adaptation. Through a process of long-term adaptation, the occurrence of selected genes can provide an advantage where specific health threats exist. One of the most striking examples of this process is seen where malaria occurs. Malaria continues to be a life threatening disease in large areas of the world. Populations that inhabit these regions are at continuous risk for the disease. In many of these populations, biological adaptation has taken place with the appearance of the sickle cell trait in recessive form. A proportion of such populations will be disabled or die because of inheriting these genes from both parents; others will suffer similar consequences from malaria. Individuals carrying this trait, however, have some protection from the disease and can live to produce another generation. Under environmental conditions in which the threat of malaria does not exist, the adaptive significance of the trait is overlooked, and the problem of transmission of sickle cell disease becomes highly visible.

In the United States and other industrialized nations, the health picture has changed considerably in the last 50 years. Advances in both the prevention and treatment of disease have almost eradicated certain diseases or disease outcomes. Smallpox, for example, has been eliminated. Improvements in sanitation, the discovery of antibiotics, and a wide variety of public health programs are twentieth century accomplishments that have had an impact on the infectious diseases. Polio, diphtheria, and pertussis rates decreased dramatically as vaccination programs were implemented. The pneumonias and other bacterial diseases have become more manageable with antibiotic therapy. With all of these improvements, however, new health threats have emerged. Legionnaire's disease, acquired immune deficiency syndrome (AIDS), Reye's syndrome, and other "new" diseases continue to appear, indicating that the process of human adaptation to the environment is an ongoing one.

As many of the infectious diseases of the past have yielded to modern science, new health problems have emerged. Acute illness still ranks as a significant factor in the demand for health and medical services, but there has been a shift toward an increase in the incidence and prevalence of chronic diseases and chronic illness.

Chronic disease and illness are long-term processes in which therapeutic goals are aimed at the control of symptoms and disease rather than at cure. Diabetes, hypertension, and cardiac and pulmonary disease are examples of these processes. Chronic diseases are most apparent in industrialized countries and can be considered a pattern of disease for those environmental settings. In general, these problems seem to be linked to cultural and social factors, such as stress, lack of exercise, smoking, overcrowding, and overeating. All of these are thought to lead to altered health states.

AMERICAN VALUES

The United States is a land of diversity. Geographically, the area is large with vast differences in climate and terrain. The people represent a variety of life-styles and ethnic traditions. There are differences in foods, accents, values, and forms of work and play. Some of the differences are obvious; others are subtle and less easily recognized.

All inhabitants of the United States have, even if in distant generations, ancestors who migrated to this country from other parts of the world. Areas from which people have migrated have changed over the centuries. In the historic past earlier groups came primarily from the European countries. More recent populations have come from Latin America, Africa, and Asia. They have come as immigrants, refugees, and so-called "illegal aliens." In the early years of this century, the United States was described as a melting pot. This term implies that immigrants, by assimilation and acculturation, somehow became American and lost their cultural identity. However, the popular notion has been challenged, as the reality of our cultural pluralism has been recognized. The 1960s and 1970s were decades of increasing awareness of ethnic identity and pride.

Ethnic groups share characteristics such as language, dialect, values, food habits, customs, and a sense of distinctiveness as a group. Census data indicate that 5.4 percent of the people in this country were born outside the United States, and 10.9 percent claim another ethnic heritage along with their American one.[3] At a minimum, 106 ethnic groups have been identified within the United States.[4]

According to Murray and Zentner, many different orientations and value systems operate in a society at one time, but only one orientation dominates in any given period. Currently in the United States, middle class orientation and values are dominant.[5] Examples of these values can be seen in Table 13–1.

Within this rich diversity, **core values** are central to the American culture. Self-reliance has been identified as a core value with which all other values are connected. This does not mean that any or all individuals are, or can be, totally self-reliant. However, it is the ideal by which people evaluate and are evaluated. Self-reliance manifests itself, in part, in a fear of dependence on others and in the belief in individual freedom.[6] In everyday life, expressions like "pulling one's self up by one's bootstraps" and "standing on one's own two feet" indicate the importance of individual achievement.

TABLE 13–1. EXAMPLES OF THE DOMINANT MIDDLE-CLASS VALUES IN THE UNITED STATES

1. Speed, change, progress, activity, and efficiency
2. Personal achievement, occupation, financial and social status, self-reliance
3. Youth, beauty, health
4. Science and technology
5. Materialism and consumerism
6. Group conformity
7. Competitive and aggressive behavior
8. Mobility
9. Pursuit of leisure
10. Equality

From Ruth Beckmann Murray and Judith Proctor Zentner, Nursing Concepts for Health Promotion, 2nd ed. (Englewood Cliffs, N.J.: Prentice-Hall, 1979), 342.

The belief that individuals should work for a living is another American core value. Individuals believe that hard work and industry will lead to the "good life." Many immigrants also hold this value, since one of the reasons they came to America was to have a better life. They work hard at menial jobs and struggle to learn the language and educate themselves and their families.

American culture is characterized by a vast array of manufactured products, a concentration of populations in urban settings, and high-level technology. Values associated with American culture have been described as those of the middle class. There is an emphasis on material goods and on systems that support comfort in life. These include electricty, central air conditioning and heating, and ease of transportation. The success of individuals and groups is, to a great extent, measured by the possession of material goods and a comfortable life-style. Success and achievement also are measured by level of education and by occupation, although to a lesser extent; these alone do not always guarantee high status.[7]

The belief in opportunities for all persons is an American ideal. The value of equality for all, or egalitarianism, is one that has not become a reality for some individuals or groups. Ethnic minorities, women, and handicapped persons have had limited access to paths that traditionally have brought material success. This commitment to equality is often expressed in an informal approach to others, overlooking differences in age or prestige. For Americans, there is frequently an attempt to establish relationships on a first-name basis almost immediately.[8]

Another American core value is the value of romantic love and free choice of spouse. Building on this value is the value of each married pair to establish its own household in which to raise children. Owning one's own home is an American dream.

The health-care system reflects the norms and values of American culture. There is an emphasis on cleanliness and efficiency. The technology is sophisticated, encompassing diagnostic, monitoring, and treatment aspects of care. The orientation to time is defined by the clock, and routines are established for specific hours of the day and night. Clients are seen by appointment during specified times. In inpatient facilities routines for physical care, medications, and treatments are scheduled by the clock. Meals are served according to a schedule rather than when individuals are hungry and timing may not conform to individual preferences for eating. Visiting hours are regulated, and there are restrictions on children's visits. In some instances, only immediate family members, such as spouse or parents, may visit. There is much variation in these patterns, however, and not all agencies reflect the same degree of efficiency and technology. Values are meaningful for those who hold them, and often they are accepted without question.

Values are a part of a pattern of living, and because of this, they change slowly. Nurses cannot change a client's values quickly. Any open attack on an individual's value system is likely to be deeply resented, and the lines of communication may be cut.

All individuals, regardless of their cultural orientation, tend to view their own values as superior to those of others and may even attempt to have others accept their value systems. In nursing, it is important to respect clients' values and to use a sensitive, diplomatic approach if it is necessary to present them with other values. The decision to incorporate new values into an existing set of values should be worked out mutually and ultimately left to the individual involved.

CULTURE AND CULTURES

Human beings are characterized by the need to live in social groups. **Culture,** used in a very broad sense, is a people's way of living, or a design shared by a group or groups of people. Culture, however, does not exist in and of itself, but can be inferred only from the behavior of people. Culture has been defined as a set of standards for perception, belief, evaluation, communication, and action.[9] While humans have the inherent capacity for culture, the specific cultural standards differ from group to group. In every society, culture is learned through both explicit and implicit means. It is shared by the members and is transmitted from one generation to another.

Culture has material and symbolic aspects. Material dimensions include objects, clothing, tools, and forms of technology. The symbolic realm consists of language, ritual, values, norms of behavior, religion, kinship systems, and other nonmaterial content.

Symbolic systems help to organize one's life and social relations. Material aspects of culture would be the importance of a car to a teen-ager; the object itself carries with it implications of power, adulthood, and freedom. The symbolic domain of ritual allows for culturally prescribed approaches to life passages. Events such as marriage, childbirth, and death typically are surrounded with culturally appropriate rituals. Culture provides solutions for everyday life situations and problems. While the repertoire of solutions varies from culture to culture, there is a regularity to human existence in every society, to which humans respond with culturally defined behavior.

Anthropologists make a distinction between culture, the design for living, and cultures. **Cultures** are groups of people who share similar beliefs, attitudes, values, and practices that form a common design for living. Where groups occupy territories spread over a wide geographic area, there may or may not be continuity of a particular culture. Boundaries between cultural groups may be difficult to identify, and what appears to be all one culture may, in fact, be several. Native Americans often are presumed to be one culture but are actually many different cultures. There are differences in language, in customs, and in means of using the environment for life-sustaining needs. These are known as **intercultural variability,** that is, differences between cultures.

There may be differences within any one culture. Individuals or groups of individuals do not consistently conform to cultural norms and standards in the same manner. Child-rearing may vary from family to family in matters of expressions of affection, discipline, play, and other aspects of child care. Adherence to religion and religious practices may vary within groups. Food preferences and eating patterns also may differ. Reasons for such differences include individual preferences, economic status, religious beliefs, role, social standing, age, and sex. Each member can and does choose options for behavior from the whole of the existing cultural content. In any culture, the options may be limited or broad, but social sanctions are used for behavior that is perceived to fall outside the norms of the culture. Differences within a culture are called **intracultural variability.**

In every cultural group, members are socialized with the expectation of participation in the life of the group. Individuals are exposed to the norms, values, and behaviors appropriate for the particular culture of which they are members and for their specific roles within that culture. In every culture, there are expectations of what is appropriate. For instance, the roles of women vary from culture to culture, but in each, there is a role or are roles appropriate within the context of that culture. Roles appropriate for one culture do not readily transfer to others. Some adaptation on the part of individuals and groups is necessary in situations of culture change or migration to other environments.

Many times when individuals move to another country, community, or neighborhood, or are admitted to the hospital, they experience a phenomenon known as culture shock. Kramer defines **culture shock** as a state of anxiety precipitated by the loss of familiar signs and symbols of social intercourse, when one is suddenly immersed in a cultural system markedly different from one's own.[10] Verbal and nonverbal cues in the environment are misleading, because they are misinterpreted by the individual. Responses may be wrong, inappropriate, or totally lacking. Research in this area has found that individuals suffering from culture shock undergo several stages of behavior. The first phase has been called the "honeymoon phase." In this phase, individuals are frequently fascinated with the new culture. Friends and family often act as buffers or translators for the newcomer, and he has no real interaction with the new environment. The newcomer is excited and desires to learn more about the new culture. In this sheltered cocoon, the new culture looks interesting and rosy. Soon, however, a new reality emerges. Familiar cues, such as rewards, sanctions, and role behaviors, are lost, and the honeymoon phase terminates. The individual becomes disenchanted.

The disenchantment phase begins when individuals come "into daily contact with conflicting values and ways of doing things for which appropriate skills, interpersonal cues, and responses are lacking."[11] Minor details that did not bother the individual earlier may cause the person to lash out bitterly. Rejection of the culture and regression of behavior can be observed during this phase. The desirability of the past home environment, family, and friends suddenly assumes enormous proportions. Individuals feel the need to be nurtured and protected in an environment in which they have some control. Preoccupation with the past and an idealization of the home culture is also common. Loneliness is experienced, and contact and extra reassurance from friends and family are required. Contact by means of telephone and mail becomes central to the individual. If this phase continues, it can become maladaptive, because it arrests the progress of self-discovery and growth. The individual in this second phase of culture shock may begin to reject self. The individual may feel a failure, that he or she cannot cope, and that he or she should not have made a move into a different culture. The person may assume blame for every mistake that occurs and may feel defeated when imminent success is not evident. Behavior may be aggressive or hostile, and the person may feel depressed or extremely fatigued.

The third phase is the resolution or recovery phase, which is the beginning of a positive adaptation. There is a marked reduction in tension. Individuals are able to see the lighter side of the situation and are capable of objectively evaluating the new culture. Individuals then are able to interpret the verbal and nonverbal cues of others more accurately in the host culture.

Effective function is the last phase in the process. This is the highest level of adaptation, and not all individuals reach this stage. In this phase, individuals become as comfortable in the new culture as in the old. Responses can be made in appropriate ways, and there is a high degree of understanding of the new culture. The old ways are not forgotten or given up, but are adapted to meet the new environmental requirements. Individuals are able to grow and change in a healthy, meaningful way.

Not all aspects of a culture are shared with all members. Age and sex influences exposure to cultural content, and specialized knowledge, such as healing practices, may be known to only a few members. Partly as a result of differing participation in the overall culture, **subcultures** may emerge. These are groups within the larger culture that, while sharing the overall culture, have distinctive beliefs, values, and in some instances, life-styles. They also may have a specialized language that facilitates communication within the group. As an example, the hospital has been described as a subculture. It demonstrates a system of values, a belief system regarding care for the sick, a specialized language, and norms of behavior for its various members including its client population. Other subcultures in the American culture might include teen-agers, professional athletes, the entertainment industry, and the military.

One's own culture, because it is familiar, seems right to its members. It defines the ways to perceive, to act, and to assign meaning and value to one's actions and the actions of others. Behaviors, communication styles, and person-to-person interaction styles observed in other cultures often seem strange, as might actual encounters with individuals from other cultures. Encounters with individuals from other cultures provide an opportunity for appreciating the variety of responses in human situations. Because one's own cultural standards seem right and others seem strange, there is the possibility of misunderstanding. Other cultures may be perceived negatively and thought to be inferior to one's own. The judging of other cultures by one's own standards is known as **ethnocentrism**.

Stereotyping is another form of cultural misunderstanding. It occurs when people assume the presence or absence of characteristics in members of other cultural groups. They may be labeled "lazy," "stoic," "dirty," or as having various other traits. Stereotyping is not based on objective assessment of others but, rather, results from preconceived notions. In order to provide holistic, individualized care to clients, families, or groups, nurses must take care not to stereotype clients on the basis of cultural orientation.

One anthropological perspective for understanding human behavior in various cultures is known as **cultural relativism**. This approach is different from ethnocentrism, in that norms and behavior are viewed in relation to their specific cultural contexts. The approach emphasizes that cultures cannot be evaluated as better or worse; cultures are just different. It assumes that differences are an adaptation to specific physical, cultural, or social environments. For instance, in Western civilizations the preferred form of marriage is monogamy. This is not so in some areas of the world, where polygamy is the norm. In these societies, there are economic, cultural, and social factors that support and encourage polygamy's continuation. It is as difficult for an individual coming from such a heritage to understand the Western custom as it is for Westerners to appreciate polygamy.

FAMILY, GROUP, AND THE LIFE CYCLE

The pattern of living in every culture has a regularity of its own. Human beings everywhere order their social relations so that they can live together effectively. Mutually understood behaviors are a necessary part of this. A series of **social roles**, i.e., expected behaviors that are culturally acceptable, is found in every society. Only when these reciprocal behaviors are understood and respected can the purposes of the society be carried out. Individuals are socialized into the role behaviors appropriate for membership in the group. In every society, for example, there are culturally approved role expectations for men and women. Role expectations also differ based on age and social status and, even in the so-called primitive cultures, can be extremely complex.

The basic unit of organization in every society is the family. In its simplest form, this is composed of mother and child; in most societies the father is the male individual who socially fulfills the role but he need not be the biological father of the child or children. In some societies, the mother's brother is responsible for the upbringing of the children, and the mother's husband (who may be the biological father) has the same responsibility for his sister's children. In all societies, the mother–child unit is part of a larger group through which economic, educational, and affective needs are met.

In all cultures, kinship systems determine the relatedness of people. These systems are part of the larger design for living and include ties of marriage and descent. Kinship may be based on biological ties, which are culturally determined to be important, and on social ties, in which no biological tie is present or necessary. Kinship may be reckoned along the maternal line only, the paternal only, or along both lines. Residence patterns often reflect the larger kinship systems, with married children living with either the wife's family or the husband's family or establishing independent households.

In Western culture we consider the nuclear family, mother–father–children, to be the standard. Cross-culturally, however, this is not the most usual arrangement, and family structures take many forms. (The reader is referred to Chapter 30, Family Systems, Concepts, for further discussion on family structures.)

All human groups note the biological processes of life with culturally acceptable behaviors. The life cycle—representing stages in the process of maturation starting with birth and ending with death—is a universal human experience. Progress through the various stages—infancy, childhood, puberty, adulthood, and old age—involves role changes that are significant for the individual and the group. Not all cultures identify stages in the same way, and there may be specific distinctions within stages. For instance, in the United States, we separate the stages of childhood into infancy, toddler, pre-

school, and school age. In some cultures, where breast-feeding lasts up to two years, infants are defined as children when they are weaned. Cultural definitions of adulthood—when it is achieved and how it is socially recognized—also vary cross-culturally.

Movements from role to role through the life-cycle are accompanied by rituals that emphasize the importance of these changes. Rites of passage serve to separate the individual from his or her earlier status, allow for a transitional period before moving to another and, finally, become incorporated into the new status.[12] In many cultures, progress from adolescence to adulthood occurs at the time of marriage, i.e., a permanent economic and social arrangement between male and female. Culturally prescribed behaviors, such as an engagement period that concludes with marriage, surround these events in most societies.

Through infancy, childhood, and adolescence, the individual is being prepared to become a competent adult in his or her own culture. The process of enculturation, the transmission of cultural knowledge from one generation to the next, is the means through which this is accomplished. Childhood is a time of intense learning. Children are expected to learn language, appropriate behaviors toward parents, relatives, other societal members and the opposite sex, social norms, systems of values, beliefs, and religion, and a view of self, group, and the world. Positive and negative sanctions are used by parents, other caretakers, and the peer group to ensure conformity to cultural standards. Both the natural social sanctions of ridicule and gossip and supernatural sanctions, in the form of roots and ancestors, are used.

With the onset of puberty, another turning point in social development is reached. Roles change as the child moves toward adulthood. Rituals and ceremonies mark this step in the life cycle. The ritual confirms to the group and to the individual that this stage in social development has occurred. Although it usually coincides with the physiological changes associated with puberty, there is some variation among cultures in this regard.

Frequently, socially recognized adulthood comes with parenthood. Everywhere there is considerable attention given to matters of pregnancy and birth. In societies where diets are inadequate and health care is poor or lacking altogether, miscarriages and high infant mortality are common. Everywhere there are limits on the behavior of pregnant women and on newly delivered women. Taboos related to food, sexual activity, bathing, and a variety of other behaviors are culturally developed ways of ensuring a successful outcome of pregnancy—a healthy infant and mother. When miscarriage, stillbirth, or fetal death occurs, a violation of taboos may be identified as the reason, and the unfortunate woman may be subject to anger or scorn from her family and group members. Labor and childbirth are processes that, in all cultures, demand the support and presence of designated people. In some cultures, the midwife and the woman's relatives assist her. In professional health-care systems, physicians, nurses, and technical staff assist in delivery, and family are only rarely present. In the United States in recent years there has been movement away from a depersonalized approach to labor and delivery, and the inclusion of the father and sometimes the siblings is encouraged in the events surrounding childbirth. Professional nurse midwives are increasingly in demand, and some hospitals have homelike "birthing" rooms in addition to the traditional delivery room.

Adulthood also can be divided into stages, and these vary among cultures. Chronological age may indicate the stages. Events such as the marriage of children or the birth of grandchildren can mark passage from one stage to another. Old age is only one of these stages. In some cultures, old age carries considerable weight and is recognized and rewarded. The elderly are honored members of the group. In the dominant American culture, with its emphasis on youth, many people go to considerable pains to conceal their increasing years by undergoing face and body lifts and using makeup and hair dye.

Death is a biological fact. It is, for the living, primarily a social fact that requires some major readjustments. Humankind has devised many rites, ceremonies, and rules for prescribed and prohibited behaviors concerning the inevitability of death. Death separates the living from the dead. In societies where the dead are respected as ancestors, they continue to exist, but in a changed relationship to the group. Almost universally, there is a belief in some form of continuation of the person. Expected behaviors surrounding death define how mourners should behave and how others in society relate to the dead individual's kin. Mourning periods are culturally defined in terms of length, and ritual acts announce their termination. Funeral customs, despite their variations in form, must be suited to two goals: appropriate disposal of the body and assistance to the mourners in reordering their lives and relationships. Cross-culturally, funeral rites reflect the status of the dead person; those of higher status are accorded more elaborate rites, and the period of mourning may be extended.

FOOD

One of the main tasks facing all social groups is that of providing adequate nourishment for its members. The survival and continuation of the group and of its individual members depends, to a great extent, on successful strategies for meeting this need. Cultures around the world have met this need in a variety of ways. There are hunters and gatherers who feed themselves successfully from the plants and animals in their environments. In these societies, most individuals have some role in the acquisition or preparation of food. Other societies depend on subsistence farming in addition to relying on naturally occurring foods. In the industrialized nations, such as the United States, relatively few individuals are involved directly in the production or distribution of food, and only a small portion of the land is used in the production of food for the majority of the people. In these countries, most food is acquired by means of a cash economy, and a large variety of foods is usually available.

Human nutritional needs are those of adequate calories, protein, carbohydrates, fats, vitamins, and minerals. Nourishment is a physiological need. Food is a cultural definition, and from the environment in which we live, we select substances for use as food. Only a portion of all the available nutritional possibilities are defined as edible. What is considered to be edible is defined differently in cultures around the world. Substances considered to be edible in one culture may be inedible in others. Examples of this are numerous. Shellfish are avoided by some cultural groups but are routinely consumed in others. In India, cattle are considered to be sacred and are never slaughtered for food; in American culture, beef is one of our principal meats. Other substances, such as insects, snakes, cats, and horses, are used as food in many cultures but are rejected by Westerners.

Within the category of edible food, there are many distinctions. Food may be considered fit for animal consumption but not human. Foods may be acceptable for adults, but not for children. Conversely, foods may be thought necessary or suitable for children but partially or totally avoided by adults. For instance, in American culture, milk is seen as a requirement for children, but most adults do not routinely drink it. This is largely the result of culturally learned attitudes. However, adults in some cultures, including some Native American Indians and Oriental people, are deficient in lactase, an enzyme necessary in the digestion of milk, and are unable to tolerate it.

Food taboos are common throughout the world. Some are the result of religious dogma, but the origins of many are unknown. Taboos associated with animal flesh and animal products are numerous. Muslims and Jews do not eat pork; other groups avoid beef. Food taboos often are associated with pregnancy and the postpartum period. Some cultural prohibitions of certain foods during pregnancy are based on notions that the child will be marked or harmed in some way, e.g., eating strawberries will result in red birthmarks on the baby. Where food taboos involve foods for which no comparable nutritional substitutes exist, the consequences for health can be severe. Kwashiorkor, for example, is a disease that occurs when young children do not receive adequate proteins, in both quantity and quality, to meet their maintenance and growth needs. The disease results in a lack of normal development. Called the "second child disease," it is frequently seen in children who have been weaned because of a second pregnancy of the mother. The word *kwashiorkor* comes from the Ghan language and, literally translated, means "the sickness the older child

gets when the baby is born."[13] In some African societies with dietary taboos on milk and meat, kwashiorkor in children is common. Even in the United States, each year a number of cases of this condition are reported.

Beliefs and customs about food differ from culture to culture but exist in some form in every culture. Foods may be described as "good for you" in that they promote or maintain health. In some cultures specific foods are of enormous importance and are consumed at all or most meals. Among these are rice in the Orient and yams in parts of Africa. In areas where Western culture has been introduced into tribal cultures, foods such as white bread and refined sugars have prestige value and are often consumed in place of traditional foods. The replacement of breast-feeding with bottle-feeding for infant nutrition in many societies (often with disastrous consequences) is one example of recent influences of prestige in changing traditional practices.

There are many social and symbolic aspects of food and food habits. Eating is a social behavior, and it involves prescribed rules all over the world. For example, timing, content of meals, and norms for who eats with whom in each society. In some cultures, women and men eat separately. In industrialized countries, employers and employees do not usually eat together. The sharing of food has expressive functions in maintaining social ties. Celebrations and feasts are activities in which food, often elaborate and in great amounts, enhances group solidarity. Important events and rituals, such as marriages and funerals, are frequently accompanied by food.

RELIGION

All human societies have some set of beliefs that can be defined, in a broad sense, as religious. No one definition of the term "religion" can be used in all cultures. Religion is the means humans use to deal with forces and beings that are not visible in the material world. These include gods, spirits, good and evil, angels, ghosts, and other unknown powers. In some cultures, invisible beings are part of the "real" or natural world, and in others they are assigned to the realm of the supernatural.

Religion functions to help humankind deal with life events and situations that are beyond its control. Problems of disease and illness are commonly handled in religions. It offers an explanation of why things happen, as well as culturally prescribed religious behaviors to manage them. Religion defines the natures of good and evil. For many cultures, the term *magicoreligious* is a useful one. These systems include aspects of magic that can be used for good and evil, and witchcraft, which is always seen as harmful.

Religious rituals may be quite simple or extremely elaborate. Rituals contribute to group solidarity and, at the same time, reinforce the beliefs of the systems. Beliefs also are reinforced by trances, visions, or dreams. Systems of religion reflect and are embedded in the larger cultural system. Sacred myths describe the origin of humankind and how human life came to be. In all cultures, even simple tribal societies, religious systems are complex sets of beliefs.

The great religions of the world today, e.g., Buddhism, Christianity, Judaism, are institutionalized. They are characterized by unique buildings, writings, and ritual specialists. However, religion, whatever its external aspects, serves as a universal solution for fundamental human problems.

DISEASE AND ILLNESS IN CULTURAL CONTEXT

In every society, illness is a matter of concern. It disrupts social relationships and threatens the overall functioning of society. All cultures are similar in that they have some systematic approach to treating disease and caring for the sick. They are different in the specific ways in which disease and illness are caused, diagnosed, and treated. The health beliefs and practices of any society are an integral part of the total cultural system. Illnesses found in one culture cannot always be understood in another cultural system. For example, *susto,* an illness caused by fright, is widely recognized among Latin American peoples. It is a cultural reality for which

causes and treatment can be identified, but it has no counterpart in Western medicine.

Western medicine is one system of health beliefs and practices. It is a biomedical approach in which disease is identified primarily through objective measurements. Identification of disease-causing organisms and abnormal laboratory values are a major part of the system. Disease may not be synonymous with illness and may be present without the knowledge of the individual or other societal members. For example, hypertension, often called a silent disease, is an example of these distinctions. An individual may be hypertensive without being aware of it, but on the basis of elevated blood pressure reading, be medically diagnosed as hypertensive, and, therefore, considered "diseased" by biomedical criteria. However, it is likely that the individual will present no disturbance in his work, family, or social life; he will not exhibit behaviors associated with being "ill." Illness is a cultural and social definition describing an inability to function in usual roles and activities.

Non-Western cultures have other beliefs regarding causes of disease and illness. One view is a personal one, in which the affected individual perceives self and is perceived as a victim. Illness results from the actions of human or supernatural beings and is intended for that individual alone. These beings may be sorcerers, evil spirits, ancestors, gods, or other beings whose existence is acceptable in the cultural context. Another view is based on notions of equilibrium. Health is maintained under conditions of equilibrium between opposite elements; illness results when equilibrium is disturbed. Balances of heat and cold figure prominently in these systems. The definition of hot and cold is primarily symbolic rather than physical. In Latin America "hot" causes of disease include emotional upsets, such as anger or exposure to the sun; they are treated with "cold." A similar distinction appears in traditional Chinese medicine, in which the forces of yin and yang interact. Yin represents the positive, which includes heat; yang represents the negative, which includes cold. In both cultural systems, it is believed that treatment with the substances containing the opposite element restores equilibrium and cures the individual.[14]

Sick Role

Every culture has ways of caring for those members who are, by cultural definition, ill. Persons who are ill and those who care for them reflect role expectations and behaviors. One way of describing these expectations is the **sick role**. It is not known whether or not this model, based on Western cultural norms, can be useful in cross-cultural understanding of illness as a universal human experience. The role has four components[15]:

- The sick person is exempted from his or her usual responsibilities
- The sick person is unable to return to health through his or her own efforts and must seek assistance
- The sick person should wish to recover
- The sick person must cooperate with treatment

The ill person and the healing and caring persons are involved in a set of reciprocal behaviors. The situation of providing nursing care is one in which role behaviors can be illustrated. The nurse assesses the client on the basis of behavioral cues provided by the client. These behaviors may include those related to physical activity, verbalization, eating, interaction with family members and health professionals, and health maintaining and promoting behaviors exhibited by the client and his family. Similarly, the nurse's evaluation of client responses to nursing intervention is based on changes or alterations in these behaviors that indicate the effectiveness of the intervention. When behavioral norms are rooted in the nurse's cultural background, the standard of measurement may not be culturally appropriate for the individual client.

Commonalities and differences were identified when sick role expectations were examined in the United States and India. Both American and Indian nurses believed their clients should trust them, should be cooperative, and should ask questions about their care. However, there were differences in the degree and timing of independence that was expected of their respective clients. The American cultural emphasis on independence and self-help was evident in an expectation of early independence. The Indian cultural orientation toward interdependence and destiny led to a different set of norms for behavior. Indian nurses expected their clients to take a less active role in treatment than did the American nurses. Expected client behaviors in each culture were norms held by both nurses and clients, not by either group alone.[16] These, then, are implicit and reciprocal understandings that guide both care givers and sick individuals in therapeutic situations.

Healers and Healing

The professional health system of the Western world is characterized by a variety of specialized roles. The roles include those of nurse, physician, dietitian, social worker, and an array of other therapeutic and technical roles. These are usually full-time professional roles for which lengthy training is required. Practitioners generally wear clothing that defines their roles and the types of tasks they accomplish, for example, scrub outfits required in operating rooms. The system is large, complex, and usually, depersonalized. Treatment is privately done in offices, clinics or hospital rooms.

In both Western and non-Western societies, traditional systems and traditional healers exist. Traditional healers are often called indigenous curers or indigenous healers. Other titles include shaman, medicine men or women, and among the Navajo, "singers." In these systems, and in the various folk traditions, religion and medicine often are blended. They are systems of belief and practice that have their own internal logic and are imbedded in the larger culture of which they are a part. Herbs, rituals, massage, and medicines are some of the therapeutic tools. Culturally defined diseases, such as the "evil eye," are known to be outside the curing ability of professional health practitioners and are referred to traditional healers. Conversely, diabetes and other chronic diseases usually are not referred to traditional healers.

In many nonliterate societies, today as in the past, the traditional healer carries out vital functions in curing disease and in maintaining social solidarity. The healer acts as a judge where illness is believed to be caused by the breaking of taboos or other socially unacceptable behavior. Illnesses caused by the supernatural or by witchcraft are also within the realm of the healer's power. Healing rituals are generally performed before the client's family or the whole community. They serve to cure disease and to correct the life events that led to the illness, thereby reestablishing social stability. The body–mind distinction, so apparent in Western thought, is not reflected in traditional systems.

In the United States today, there are many folk systems and healers. Native American Indian systems, the black folk tradition with its "root" medicine, and Spanish-American folk medicine are only a few of those routinely used. Spiritualists, faith healers, herbalists, and local curers offer alternative approaches. These jobs are not full-time occupations, as in the case of professional practitioners, and are frequently based on a calling from a higher power.

In order for nurses to work effectively with individuals, families, and groups of different cultural orientations, cultural concepts must be assessed and incorporated into the nursing process.

THE NURSING PROCESS

Due to the great diversity of ethnic backgrounds in the United States, the cultural aspects of care have always been an important part of health-care delivery. Some of this diversity is due to the underlying philosophy of individuals and some may be due to types of ethnic background. Today, cultural aspects of health care are even more important. Mobility, poverty, and world turmoil bring more immigrants to America every day in search of a new life. These immigrants need to be channeled into the health-care system for illness prevention, immunization, health teaching, health maintenance, and medical care. No other country in the world has so many different cultural groups, each with its own beliefs, values, practices, and life-style. Many of these are congruent with the dominant society, but some are not. In order to provide comprehensive health care, nurses need to be knowledgeable about components of culture and how these components affect behavior, expectations and adaptation. Knowledge about many cultures is desirable, but it is especially important to learn about those that are prominent locally.

Nurses are able to provide comprehensive care through use of the nursing process. Nurses need to be aware that cultural heritage may influence behavior related to health and illness practices, and therefore should make a careful assessment of cultural background and needs.

Assessment

Although each culture has unique features, some cultural universals can be identified and specifically assessed. These include language, religion, rituals, health perceptions and practices, nutrition, family systems, birth and death practices, time orientation, privacy, territoriality, and touch. Cultural assessments and planning strategies are essential to providing comprehensive nursing care. In assessing an individual holistically, the nurse should systematically gather information regarding cultural orientation (Fig. 13–3). It is suggested that the culturally relevent data be gathered by the primary nurse assigned to the client. The nurse may wish to proceed slowly with the data gathering, perhaps in two or three sessions over a few days. In this way, the information gathering is not as threatening. This tool may be used selectively along with other assessments, and some parts may be omitted totally.

Communication. When people do not speak English well enough to express their needs or understand what is said, they may become highly stressed and anxious. Alternate means of communication may need to be used including: flash cards, nonverbal behavior, use of translator, or printed material, such as pamphlets or booklets. These printed materials can be obtained from a number of agencies, such as the American Diabetes Association, the American Cancer Association, and others. Translations on flash cards can be made in most high school or college language departments. Frequently, the nursing service office has a list of people who can act as translators. In large cities, embassy offices may be contacted for a reference list of translators. Family members also can be asked to visit at specific times to act as translators. It is important to keep three things in mind when dealing with individuals who do not speak English:

- Assess how much English is known
- Speak to the patient in English, since communication is a natural process
- Use nonverbal communication

Inability to communicate also complicates the teaching–learning process. It is impossible to teach a client, family, or group if a common language cannot be found, or if literature in the client's language is not available. An interpreter will be necessary in situations like this. When this situation arises, it is important to locate an interpreter who will interpret what is said literally by both the client and the nurse. If it is not tactful to ask a client certain types of questions—for example, about birth control—an interpreter who will rephrase the questions in an acceptable way is needed.

Another issue related to culture and language involves asking the client, "Do you understand?" rather than assessing a change in behavior or evaluating learning in a more concrete manner. In some cultures, it is considered rude to say "no," so the individual may respond "yes," even though he or she doesn't understand. Later, the client may be too embarrassed to ask for further information or to question nurses on other aspects of health data.

Religion. Religion has an impact on many aspects of clients' lives. Brownlee writes,

> Health workers who come from cultures where religion receives very minimal attention may not fully realize the profound effect religion may have on the lives of patients from strongly religious backgrounds. Religion may affect a people's values, beliefs, practices . . . a . . . whole concept of health and illness and influence the health care that they receive.[17]

Health Perception. "Some cultures view illness as a punishment from God for sinful acts. Others may regard illness as the work of malevolent persons who want to see them suffer . . . others are convinced that illness is caused by evil spirits, and as a result they can receive help only from spiritualists or witch doctors."[18] Prevention and cure are often closely related to the way that the cause of the illness is perceived. If the cause is perceived as punishment, cure and comfort measures may be refused. Other steps may be taken, such as lighting candles; bargaining with God, saints, or spirits; fasting; or using tradtional items. Clients may prefer a faith healer or shaman to deal with illness.

Health–Illness Practices. Another important factor to be considered in a cultural assessment is health–illness practices. It is important to find out the individual's perception of health. Many times it means not the absence of disease but the ability to work in the face of pain or illness. Clients who believe that illness is caused by God as punishment may be difficult to educate about illness prevention.

Further illness behaviors may include self-diagnosis, self-medication and medication exchange with friends. If these do not produce a cure, a physician may be seen. Many cultural groups feel that the health-care system will not be helpful for them and they seek alternatives, such as folk medicine, herbs, and folk healers.

Many culturally defined illnesses are cured by a knowledgeable adult in the family, a close friend, or a curandero or curandera (persons who practice folk medicine). Western medical care is not believed to be helpful for these illnesses but may be sought if traditional healing practices have not been effective.

The Native American also has culturally related illness practices. Prevention or curative rituals may be performed in order to restore the body's harmony with nature. Medicine men or women traditionally fill this role. Curative rituals may include sprinkling cornmeal, singing, dancing, and sand painting.

For the Chinese, health is defined as a normal flow of energy. This life energy is kept in balance by the forces of yin and yang, and when an imbalance occurs, there is illness.

Nutrition. Many nutritional habits are based on religious beliefs. For example, the Orthodox Jewish diet forbids shellfish, pork, and meat and dairy products during the same meal, and there are special requirements for handling, storing, and using dishes, utensils, and pots. The heads of men are covered when eating. These beliefs stem from the time of Moses and are still held today.

Name _____ Age _____ Sex _____ Marital Status _____

Address _____ Phone _____

Religion (specify denomination) _____ Clergy _____

Education level _____ Occupation _____

Communication
Language spoken at home _____ Does patient speak English? Yes _____ No_____
If yes, how much? Few words _____ Basic vocabulary _____ Speaks fluently _____
Does patient read English? Yes _____ No _____ If yes, how much? _____
Can a family member (or friend) speak English? Yes _____ No _____
Can that person stay with the patient to interpret? Yes _____ No _____
If yes, when? (hours) Sun _____ M _____ T _____ W _____ Th _____ F _____ S _____
Can another person act as translator? Yes _____ No _____ Who _____ Phone _____
Does patient reach out to touch? Yes _____ No _____
Does the patient pull away when touched? Yes _____ No _____
Does the patient touch health-care givers? Yes _____ No _____

Religious Beliefs
Is Baptism permitted? Yes _____ No _____ If so, by whom? _____
Under what circumstances? _____
Will the patient permit blood transfusion? Yes _____ No _____
Will the patient accept medications? Yes _____ No _____
If only specific types, which types? _____
Do religious leaders have a role in prevention or treatment? _____
What rituals are necessary? _____ Circumcision? Yes _____ No _____
How are religious artifacts disposed of? _____

Health Perception
Prevention: Related to religion? Yes _____ No _____
Do any beliefs contradict those of health-care agency? Yes _____ No _____
If yes, what? _____
Do any beliefs coincide with health-care agency? Yes _____ No _____ If yes, what? _____
How is health-care system perceived? _____
Illness: Will of God? Yes _____ No _____ Predestined? Yes _____ No _____
 Evil spirits? Yes _____ No _____ Evil eye? Yes _____ No _____
What rituals or practices are necessary to restore health? _____

Health-Illness Practices
What medications and folk medicine treatments, regimens, etc., is patient using? _____
_____
Where are these purchased? _____
Who prepares them? _____ Who administers them? _____
Is the patient permitted by his physician to continue taking these preparations? Yes _____ No _____
Who treats the sick in the patient's family? Grandmother _____ Faith healer _____ Medicine man _____
Does patient ask for pain medicine or exhibit stoicism? _____
What are cultural beliefs about the experience of pain? _____
Belief as to what caused the disease process the patient is exhibiting? _____
What is the patient's outlook for the future? _____
Disposal of amputated limbs _____
Physical care and comfort: Skin care _____ Hair care _____ Bathing _____
What are practices concerning prevention of illness? _____

Figure 13–3. Cultural assessment tool. *(From Janet-Beth McCann Flynn, copyright 1980.)*

Nutrition
Ethnic preference _____ Cultural/Religious taboos _____
Holiday and festive occasions _____ Who prepares food at home? _____
If necessary can someone bring special foods? Yes _____ No _____ Who _____ Phone _____
Has diet been modified by illness? Yes _____ No _____
Likes _____ Dislikes _____

Time Orientation
Does patient need to be reminded of appointments? Yes _____ No _____

Territoriality
Does patient stand close to others? Yes _____ No _____ Far away? Yes _____ No _____
Does patient retreat to room _____ bed _____ for privacy?
Does patient pull covers over face _____ turn away _____ draw curtains _____?

Privacy
Will patient allow physical examination? Yes _____ No _____
   By person of opposite sex? Yes _____ No _____
Will patient remove his/her clothes? Yes _____ No _____
Does another family member have to be present? Yes _____ No _____
Any special considerations of personal belongings? _____

Family
Who makes decisions? _____ Relationship _____
Who makes health decisions? _____ Relationship _____
Can patient make own health decisions? Yes _____ No _____
Does patient have to consult with the decision makers? Yes _____ No _____
Do family health beliefs or practices conflict with hospital/clinic health teaching and practices?
   Yes _____ No _____ If yes, describe _____
_____
Effects of illness or hospitalization on other members of household _____
_____
What hours are best for various family members to visit? _____
_____

Death (section is optional)
What are dominant practices? _____
Deathbed confession? Yes _____ No _____ Last rites? Yes _____ No _____
Who is to be called? Family _____ Clergy _____
Will bedside ritual be required? Yes _____ No _____
Are there measures to ward off death? Yes _____ No _____
Where does patient/family want the patient to die? Home _____ Hospital _____ Other_____
Who should be with patient at the time of death? _____
What is the role of the family members in the death of patient? _____
What are the preparations for burial? _____
Who performs these? _____
Additional comments, observations, and assessments _____

Figure 13–3. (continued)

Diets in some cultures are chosen for their health-maintenance quality. If these diets are not followed, it is believed that a disequilibrium will occur and result in sickness. If hot foods and cold foods are not balanced, the individual may become sick. Examples of these cultures include Mexican, Native American, and Chinese. What makes a food hot or cold is not its temperature but is defined by beliefs about the food themselves.

Food produces "feelings of security and happiness . . . used as a link to friendship, . . . pleasure . . . and as a symbol of religious belief."[19] In the assessment phase of the nursing process, nurses should be aware of the holistic effect of food on clients and the relationship of food, religion, and ritual.

Time Orientation. Most middle-class Americans tend to be future oriented. Some cultural groups may appear to be present oriented because of a focus on their immediate situation or need. It is important to recognize this, especially when planning future care, clinic visits, and other health-oriented activities such as immunizations. Time orientation within a 24-hour period is also important to assess. Americans tend to "live by the clock" and instructions to take a pill at 8 A.M. and at 8 P.M. are meaningful. In some cultures, other timed events, such as bedtime or sunrise, may be more meaningful.

Territoriality. Territories are fixed areas around individuals that are unconsciously learned. Territoriality is a form of nonverbal behavior and is generally influenced by culture. E. T. Hall, an anthropologist who studied the use of space, divided the space individuals use into four measurable distances: intimate, personal, social, and public.

Entering a person's intimate or personal space can be disturbing to that person. Individuals in some groups stand very close to each other while others do not. Territoriality should be viewed holistically because of the many opportunities health workers have for violating this cultural norm.

Touch. Americans are not a group who touch a great deal or who like to be touched. Many clients, however, touch and like to be touched. Greeting persons without touching them may be interpreted as dislike or rejection in some cultures.

Privacy and Modesty. In many cultures, modesty and privacy are supremely guarded. Nurses and other health-care workers often are preoccupied with "getting a job done" and may overlook the client's need in this regard. In some cultures modesty is extremely important for women. Women of the Mexican-American, Arab, and Gypsy cultures are some examples of this, as are Orientals and other Easterners. Violations of a person's need for privacy can generate anger and resentment, as well as noncompliance with treatments and therapy. It is, therefore, very important that nurses identify and respect the need for privacy and modesty.

Family. Another cultural facet to be explored is the family structure and role definition. The family is important to all clients. In some cultures, the kin network is extensive, and individuals have close emotional ties to large numbers of people. In most cultures a specific member of the family is designated as the decision maker. It may be the breadwinning male or the oldest female, depending upon the culture. Also, the decision maker for family matters may differ from the individual who makes the health-related decisions. The person who decides if the sick child will return to the clinic for follow-up should be identified and included in the teaching plan. If that person is not involved, follow-up may not be carried out. Because the person who makes decisions about health is the person who influences the health practices of the family or group, it is very important for the nurse to identify this person.

If the client is terminally ill, cultural variations of death and dying should be assessed. This may be done by questioning the client, the family, religious persons, or by consulting the literature. In some cultures, death is never directly discussed, so assessment of this should be done with the utmost sensitivity.

At the conclusion of the nursing process, nursing diagnoses are formulated. Some examples of nursing diagnoses based on a cultural assessment might be:

- Impaired communication related to a language barrier
- Potential noncompliance related to cultural beliefs
- Knowledge deficit related to language barrier

After the nursing diagnoses have been prepared and written on the care plan, the planning phase of the nursing process begins.

Planning

The nursing care plan is based on the data gathered during the assessment phase. As it is developed it is written on the client's chart or cardex. Concepts related to cultural orientation should be incorporated into the plan in order to be individualized.

When using the cultural assessment as a guide to prepare the plan, several things need to be considered. If the client does not understand English, planning for an interpreter is essential. If the client is literate in his or her own language, written materials in that language can be gathered. Also, some of the major drug companies have small booklets providing translations of medical and nursing terms in several languages.[20,21] These may be obtained by writing to the various companies or consulting a patient education specialist.

If religious leaders have a role in rituals or services, they need to be incorporated into the plan, for example, an American Indian medicine man or woman.

Knowing the client's perception of disease causality is essential in planning care. Any behaviors associated with this perception should be incorporated. If pain and disease are viewed as punishment, providing information regarding the disease process and pain medication may be required.

Planning for health and illness practices is also helpful. The health-care team needs to be consulted in planning in this area. If clients wish to take folk medicines or herbs, the pharmacist should be consulted to establish the origin of the medicine or herb in the event it may be contraindicated. If these alternative herbs and folk medicines are to be incorporated, then a source must be established.

If rituals are performed at the bedside using materials held in high regard to peoples of ethnic groups, it should be determined who should handle and remove them. Many times, it is the person or persons who placed them around the client, but in some instances the nurse or the housekeeping department may remove any materials. This aspect should be confirmed by the client and the persons performing the service and incorporated in the plan.

Nutritional aspects of culture need to be taken into account when planning client care. This is generally an interdisciplinary plan with the agency nutritionist acting as the consultant. Frequently, institutional foods can be adapted for special requirements. Most hospitals, for example, have kosher dinners with disposable dishes and utensils to meet kosher clients' requirements. Family and friends can be consulted, and plans to bring food from home can be made.

In terms of space, touch, and privacy, steps can be planned so as not to violate the client's sense of territory or privacy. If nurses are aware that this is a real problem, extra time can be allotted to allow for more privacy. Privacy also should be assured if the client is to have a religious ceremony or folk-healing ritual.

Finally, clients' families should be incorporated into the plan. Times for visiting can be scheduled so that nurses have time to interact, assess, and teach. If appropriate, the family decision maker should be sought out and asked to participate in the care and planning as well as in the decision making.

During the planning phase, time limited goals, objectives, and outcome criteria should be formulated and written on the care plan (see The Teaching and Learning Process, Chapter 15). These, too, should reflect the cultural components of health and illness.

Once the plan, with goals, objectives, and outcome criteria, has been formulated, the third phase of the nursing process can begin.

Implementation

Implementation is the dynamic process of carrying out the plan. The first step is establishing a trusting relationship with the client, family, or group. This requires freedom from judging them based on ethnocentric standards. In order to form a nurse–client relationship, a means of communication must be established.

Folk medicines and herbs can be prepared by the nurse if necessary and administered with other medicines ordered by the physician. Folk healers may wish to assist during the implementation phase of the plan and, when possible, should be encouraged to do so. Traditional beliefs can be supported in this manner and incorporated into the Western mode of health care.

Nurses need to be culturally sensitive to all aspects of the nursing care plan as they work with the wide variety of clients from many ethnic groups seen in the health-care system today. During the implementation phase, evaluative data are gathered regarding the effectiveness of the plan. This leads to the fourth and final step of the nursing process, the evaluation of the plan and care.

Evaluation

Evaluation is an ongoing process that weighs the outcomes of the plan. Client behaviors are measured and evaluated using the goals, objectives, and outcome criteria that were formulated during the planning phase. If some aspects are not working, then a reassessment of the client situation is in order. It is important to note that many cultural differences between people are extremely subtle and not easily identified. When these cultural nuances take the form of attitudes and feelings rather than overt behaviors, the nurse may have difficulty evaluating and pinpointing specific causes of the misunderstandings. The cause may be a global mistrust of nurses or the whole health-care system, for example, and this fact may never be isolated, particularly in the hospital setting, where contact is episodic and brief. Consultation with family and friends is very helpful in the evaluation phase and can provide the nurse with further assessment information. The nursing care plan then can be revised.

CONCLUSIONS

Culture is a primary stretegy in adapting to the physical and social environment. The presence or absence of disease is a measure of adaptive success to specific environmental situations. In all cultures, human beings have sought solutions to disease and illness.

The inclusion of cultural concepts in the knowledge base used by the nurse is needed for effective nursing care. It broadens the nurse's understanding, not only of the significance of cultural traditions in regard to health and illness, but of human behavior itself. It leads to a recognition of both the uniformity and diversity found in cultures and of how humans seek solutions to universal experiences and problems.

Nurses need to become culturally sensitive when delivering health care and should promote this awareness in other health-care professionals. In order to do this, there are several things nurses can do:

- Become knowledgeable about individual cultures
- Examine their own beliefs, values, and practices
- Indicate interest in the client's culture
- Show respect for client values and beliefs
- Avoid ethnocentrism
- Avoid stereotyping
- Base nursing actions on a cultural as well as a physical assessment

The challenge for all nurses who seek to provide quality, holistic nursing care is to increase their knowledge of cultures and to use the nursing process accordingly. In order to promote health, nurses must care. In order to care, nurses must continue to learn. Many times, clients themselves can be the best teachers. Nurses need to open their hearts and their minds to all clients in order to be culturally sensitive, so that, through a mutual sharing, the best possible care can be provided.

SUMMARY

Culture is defined as people's way of living, or a design for living shared by a group of people. Cultures are groups of people that share similar beliefs, attitudes, values, and practices.

The cultural basis of human behavior has great importance for the practice of nursing. Nurses use cultural information to understand

and assist individuals, families, and groups in achieving optimum health.

With the exception of Native Americans, all inhabitants of the United States have ancestors who migrated to this country from other parts of the world in the past several hundred years. Areas from which people have migrated have changed over the centuries. While earlier groups came primarily from the European countries, more recent populations have come from Latin America, Africa, and Asia. They have come as immigrants, refugees, and illegal aliens. In the early years of this century, the United States was described as a melting pot. This term implies that immigrants, by assimilation and acculturation, became American and lost their cultural identity. The 1960s and 1970s brought increasing awareness that pride in past ethnic identity persisted through several generations.

Ethnic groups share cultural characteristics, such as language, values, food habits, customs, and many others. Values play a central role in any cultural group and are defined by the group. Many authors feel that in the United States today, middle-class values are dominant. A few examples of these include change, progress, achievement, youth, cleanliness, beauty, technology, materialism, and equality.

Values are meaningful for those who hold them, and they are generally accepted without question. It is crucial for nurses to identify and respect clients' value systems.

When individuals move to another country, they frequently experience a phenomenon known as culture shock. Culture shock has four phases: honeymoon, disenchantment, resolution or recovery, and effective functioning.

Ethnocentrism and stereotyping are types of cultural misunderstandings. These behaviors should be avoided by health-care providers, or holistic care will not be possible.

The fundamental and basic unit of any culture is the family. How the family is defined and oriented is dependent on cultural orientation. An accurate view of the role of the family in the life of the client is important information for the nursing process.

Food plays an important role in all cultural groups, serving to nourish and sustain the group. Food has many social and religious functions as well. Many groups avoid certain types of foods, and these are culturally defined.

All groups have some type of religion that helps them deal with life events and situations that are beyond their control. Problems of disease and illness are commonly handled within a religious context. Religion offers an explanation of why things happen, as well as culturally prescribed religious behaviors to manage these events.

Cross-culturally, in every society, illness is a matter of concern. All cultures are similar in that they have some systematic approach to treating disease and caring for the sick. They are different in the specific ways in which disease and illnesses are defined, caused, diagnosed, and treated. Within the framework of illness, all cultures have an expectation of the way the ill behave. This is called the sick role, and it is culturally defined.

Many cultures have persons who care for the sick in traditional fashions. They may be shamans, medicine men or women, curers, or singers.

Inclusion of cultural concepts in the nursing knowledge base is essential for carrying out the nursing process. Cultural sensitivity is largely a learned behavior, and learning resources include the client, family and friends, other professionals, and the general and scientific literature.

Study Questions

1. Discuss the meaning of culture and cultures.

2. How does culture relate to adaptation?

3. Define and discuss culture shock. How might it affect client behavior?

4. List several American core values.

5. Why is stereotyping a hazard to the nurse–client relationship?

6. Interview a person from another culture, using the assessment tool.

7. Describe several potential client problems related to cultural heritage.

References

1. Sr. Callista Roy, "The Roy Adaptation Model" in Joan P. Reihl and Sr. Callista Roy, eds., *Conceptual Models for Nursing Practice*, 2nd ed. (New York: Appleton-Century-Crofts, 1980), 183.
2. Ibid., 179.
3. U.S. Bureau of the Census, *Statistical Abstract of the United States, 1982–1983*, 103rd ed. (Washington, D.C.: U.S. Government Printing Office, 1982).
4. Stephen Theernstrom, Ann Orlor, and Oscar Handlin, eds., *Harvard Encyclopedia of American Ethnic Groups* (Cambridge, Mass.: Belknap Press of Harvard University Press, 1980), xi–ix.
5. Ruth Beckmann Murray and Judith Proctor Zentner, *Nursing Concepts for Health Promotion*, 3rd ed. (Englewood Cliffs, N.J.: Prentice-Hall, 1985), 342.
6. Francis L.K. Hsu, "American core values and national character," in Francis L.K. Hsu, ed., *Psychological Anthropology* (Cambridge, Mass.: Schenkman Publishing Co.), 248–250.
7. Conrad M. Arensberg and Arthur Neihoff, "American cultural values," in James P. Spradley and Michael A. Rynkewich, eds., *The Nacirema* (Boston: Little, Brown, & Co., 1975), 364–365.
8. Ibid.
9. Ward Goodenough, *Description and Comparison in Cultural Anthropology* (Chicago: Aldine Press, 1970), 98.
10. Marlene Kramer, *Reality Shock* (St. Louis: C.V. Mosby Co., 1974), 4.
11. Ibid., 5.
12. Arnold Van Gennep, *The Rites of Passage* (Chicago: University of Chicago Press, 1960, originally published in 1908).
13. Lucille F. Whaley and Donna L. Wong, *Nursing Care of Infants and Children*, 3rd ed. (St. Louis: C.V. Mosby Co., 1987).
14. George M. Foster and Barbara Gallatin Anderson, *Medical Anthropology* (New York: John Wiley & Sons, 1978), 53–65.
15. Talcott Parsons, *The Social System* (New York: The Free Press, 1951).
16. Patinhara Pokkiarath Bhanumathi, "Nurses' conceptions of 'sick role' and 'good patient' behavior: A cross-cultural comparison," *Int Nurs Re* 24, (1977), 20–24.
17. Ann Templeton Brownlee, *Community, Culture, and Care* (St. Louis: C.V. Mosby Co., 1978), 156.
18. Barbara Kozier and Glenora Erb, *Fundamentals of Nursing*, 2nd ed. (Menlo-Park, Calif.: Addison-Wesley Publishing Co., 1984).
19. Marie Branch and P.P. Paxton, *Providing Safe Nursing Care for Ethnic People of Culture* (New York: Appleton-Century-Crofts, 1976), 174.
20. *A Language Guide for Patient and Nurse* (Indianapolis, Indiana: Eli Lilly and Co.).
21. *Breaking the Language Barrier* (Morris Plains, NJ: Warner-Chilcott).

Annotated Bibliography

Brink, P.J., ed. 1976. *Transcultural Nursing: A Book of Readings.* Englewood Cliffs: Prentice-Hall. A selection of readings intended to raise the consciousness of nurses on cultural aspects of patient care in relation to childrearing, value systems, research methods, and language.

Capers, C.F. 1985. Nursing and the Afro-American client. *Top Clin Nurs* 7(3):11–17. This article presents an overview of the health, beliefs, and practices for this group of clients. Clinical implications are described.

Clark, A.L. 1978. *Culture, Chidbearing, Health Professionals.* Philadelphia: F.A. Davis. This book presents an overview of the childbearing practices for persons from nine selected cultures. Also presented are cultural reviews for the selected cultures.

Clark, A.L. 1981. *Culture and Childrearing.* Philadelphia: F.A. Davis. This book focuses on nine selected cultural groups, one of which is the Native American culture. The other chapters include a brief description of other selected cultures and describe the child-rearing practices of each group.

Fong, C.M. 1985. Ethnicity and nursing practice. *Top Clin Nurs* 7(3):1–10. This article describes cultural diversity and its implications for the nursing process.

Foster, G.M. and Anderson, B.F. 1978. *Medical Anthropology.* New York: Wiley. A comprehensive overview of a number of themes related to a cultural dimension of health and illness. A central perspective is that all health-related behavior is an adaptive strategy in all cultures.

Grasska, M.A. and McFarlane, T. 1982. Overcoming the language barrier problems and solutions. *Am J Nurs* 89(9):1376–79. This excellent article discusses some of the pitfalls of using translators to ease communication and offers solutions.

Grosso, C., Barden, M., Henry, C. and Vieau, M.G. 1981. The Vietnamese American Family . . . and grandma makes three. *Matern Child Nurs J* 6:177–80. A case study is presented and solutions to the client problems are suggested.

Harwood, A. 1981. *Ethnicity and Medical Care.* Cambridge, Mass.: Harvard University Press. This book presents several cultural orientations and provides guidelines for culturally appropriate health care.

Louie, K.B. 1985. Providing health care to Chinese clients. *Top Clin Nurs* 7(3):18–25. This article briefly describes the Chinese, their beliefs, and customs. It covers cultural health beliefs and outlines an initial culture assessment.

Mardiros, M. 1984. A view toward hospitalization: The Mexican American experience. *J Adv Nurs* 9(5):469–78. Observations made on a large medical-surgical inpatient unit in the southwestern U.S. indicated the specific concerns Mexican-Americans experienced during their hospitalization.

Melesis, A.I. 1978. The Arab American in the health care system. *Am J Nurs* 81(6):1180–83. Expectations of health care are quite different for the Arab-Americans who do not so much expect personal care as an effective cure. This article describes the origin of the Arab culture and how it affects behavior. Relevant nursing interventions are offered.

Spradley, J.P. and Rynkiewich, M.A. 1975. *The Nacirema.* Boston: Little, Brown. A collection of readings of American culture describing values, social life, customs, and acculturation.

Theernstrom, S., Orlov, A., Handlin, O. eds. 1980. *Harvard Encyclopedia of American Ethnic Groups.* Cambridge, Mass.: Belknap Press of the Harvard University Press. An extensively researched work containing essays, maps, and detailed information on 106 ethnic groups.

Wood, C.S. 1979. *Human Sickness and Health.* Palo Alto, Calif.: Mayfield. A biocultural perspective of human societies in which disease is viewed as a critical element in environmental stress and adaptation. Topical areas include nutrition, malaria, syphilis, and women and reproduction.

Chapter 14

Communication

Rose Kurz-Cringle

Chapter Outline

- Objectives
- Glossary
- Introduction
- Human Communication Theory
  - Relation to Behavioral Science Theory
  - Communication Models
  - Types of Communication
- Communication and the Nursing Process
  - Factors Facilitating Communication
  - Specific Communication Techniques
  - Nurse–Client Relationship
- The Nursing Process
  - Assessment
  - Planning
  - Implementation
  - Evaluation
- Summary
- Study Questions
- References
- Annotated Bibliography

Objectives

At the completion of this chapter, the reader will be able to:

▶ Describe the elements of the communication process
▶ Describe the ingredients in the Berlo human communication model
▶ Describe the characteristics of effective communication
▶ Identify selected communication techniques used by others that facilitate communication
▶ Identify selected communication behaviors that inhibit communication
▶ Explain the concept of a helping relationship
▶ Describe the phases of the professional nurse–client relationship
▶ Describe the significance of communications skills in the nursing process

Glossary

Attitudes. Consistent responses to a particular set of circumstances or individuals that has both an intellectual and an affective component.

Consummatory Communication. Communication that is intended solely to fill time.

Dysfunctional Communication. Communication that interferes with the development of a meaningful relationship because it is either unclear or deliberately disrespectful of the receiver.

Effective Communication. Communication that is understood by the receiver as it was intended by the sender.

Empathy. The capacity of one individual to share the feelings of another at the moment the feelings are experienced.

Instrumental Communication. Communication that is intended to assist with the accomplishment of a goal.

Kinesics. Communication through the use of body movement.

Language. A systematic means of communicating ideas using signs, sounds, gestures, and marks that have agreed-upon meanings.

Sign. A motion, mark or other representation that announces a situation or event.

Symbol. A motion, mark, or object that represents some other motion, mark, or object.

Sympathy. The quality of being affected by a situation that involves others.

Therapeutic Communication. Communication that is intended to assist another person to change his or her way of communicating.

INTRODUCTION

Modern civilization has evolved as a result of activities undertaken by human beings working together. Human beings are able to work together because they can communicate. The word *communication* symbolizes the process by which information, feelings, and ideas are transmitted to other organisms. All living things communicate because communication is essential for survival.

Plants and animals have a system of communication that enables them to survive by adapting to the environment. The buzzing of the bee communicates its presence to other animals and serves as a warning to them to avoid its painful sting. The odor of flowers in the spring signals to the bee the presence of the nectar and the pollen that the bee needs as food to survive. The plant that bears the flower needs to have its pollen distributed in order to perpetuate itself. These types of communication are called signs. A **sign** is a discrete motion, action, or mark that indicates a presence or condition. Human beings, as well as plants and animals, use signs in their communication with each other.

Some types of animals have developed a variety of sounds to communicate various messages. The meow of an angry cat has a different tone and intensity from the meow of a cat signaling its plan to jump on its owner's lap. This is known as *presymbolic communication*. In addition, human beings have developed a complex system of symbolic language. A **symbol** is something chosen to represent something else. It is an object used to typify an abstract idea. It may be a concrete object such as the cross, which is a symbol of Christianity, or the star of David, which symbolizes Judaism. The symbol itself may be abstract. Words are abstract. They represent reality in a conceptual way.

Prehistoric human beings communicated with pictures and diagrams. We do not know eactly how and when these pictures were converted to sounds. The development of the alphabet enabled people to represent these pictures with combinations of letters and to attach specific sounds to specific combinations of letters. This is how word symbols developed. Humankind's unique ability to store these symbols in memory and to recall them has enabled it to develop an efficient means of communication.

The spelling of words and the way they are organized into thoughts is **language.** In different parts of the world, the alphabet and methods of spelling and organizing words differ, thus, we have languages. Human beings use language to interact with one another in a way that has enabled them not only to master the environment, as animals have, but to alter it. To an English-speaking individual, the word "rain" symbolizes moisture falling from the sky. The ability to store this word in the brain and to recall it when it is not raining has enabled human beings to alter what happens to the environment as a result of rain. They have built shelters to protect themselves from rain. They have built cisterns to save rain. They have built dams as a protection from flooding caused by too much rain, and they have learned to use the energy of flood water to create hydroelectric power. None of this could have occurred if humans were only aware of rain while it was happening, as is the case with lower animals.

Pictures and symbolic objects are still an important part of human communication. The ease with which people travel to different parts of the world where different languages are used has increased the importance of picture symbols in the modern world. The outline of a man or

a woman on a door in a public building communicates the presence of sanitary facilities for men and women regardless of the language. The outline of a wheelchair at a parking spot indicates that it is reserved for the handicapped.

Playing the "Star Spangled Banner" at public events in the United States symbolizes loyalty and pride in our country. Flying the flag in front of a house is a way the owners express patriotism. The U.S. flag is an example of an object that can be either a symbol or a sign depending on the context. The U.S. flag flying on a warship symbolizes that the ship is part of the U.S. Navy. If the flag is flown upside down, that is a sign that the ship is in distress. In the first instance, the flag represents the abstract idea of ownership. In the second instance it announces the concrete need for help.

Human communication is a dynamic process that has no starting or ending point. It is so much a part of all aspects of modern life that any method of separating out a particular aspect for study is necessarily artificial. The three broad categories described by Borden[1] will be used in this chapter. These are intrapersonal, interpersonal, and public communication.

Intrapersonal communication includes all the activities within the person related to communication. These are the way the person receives messages, decodes, and synthesizes them, and uses this information to encode and transmit a response. To do this requires the use of all the senses and thinking mechanisms of the brain.

Interpersonal communication refers to all of the situations in which individuals communicate directly with each other. Individuals communicate with each other through the use of verbal and nonverbal messages. *Verbal messages* are the words we hear or see in writing. *Nonverbal messages* are the sounds, sights, and odors we hear, see, or smell.

Interpersonal communication occurs in one-to-one or group situations, as in a classroom, a committee meeting, or at a party. It does not occur in situations where individuals are in direct contact but cannot respond to each other, such as occurs between the clergy and the congregation in a church service or the lecturer and the audience at a public lecture. These latter two would be classified as *public communica-tion*. In addition to the above, public communication includes the impersonal dissemination of information through the media. The distribution of notices in a hospital or of educational materials through the mail are further examples of public communication.

Nurses are concerned primarily with intrapersonal and interpersonal communication. The effectiveness of the nursing process is dependent on the nurse's ability to communicate with other people. The nurse must be able to be understood and to understand what the client is communicating through verbal communication and the observation of nonverbal communication. As a care giver, the nurse must be able to communicate with the recipients of that care. During even the simplest procedures, the client needs to know what may be expected. In the use of highly specialized technology, the client's cooperation is equally important. If the client is unconscious, the nurse must be able to communicate effectively with other members of the health team in order to plan and implement care. The nurse's function as a health teacher also requires a wide range of communication skills. If the nurse becomes a nursing educator, the communication network will include students, clients, and coworkers. The nurse in management has a broader range of individuals with whom to communicate. The nurse-manager communicates vertically with supervisees and senior administrators. The nurse-manager communicates horizontally with peers and with representatives of other departments and other agencies. In all these situations, the nurse may be involved in one-to-one communication or in small-group communication.

HUMAN COMMUNICATION THEORY

The study of human communication blends theory and knowledge from psychology, sociology, anthropology, mathematics, and linguistics.

Relation to Behavioral Science Theory

Before World War II, inquiry into human communication occurred in academic speech and language departments where attention was directed toward the structure of communication. At the same time, psychologists were studying the meaning of behavior. Human communication is the process that gives meaning to behavior. Thus, the understanding of human communication requires a blend of knowledge from these two disciplines.

Two concepts from Freudian psychoanalytic theory continue to be relevant to the understanding of communication theory.[2] One is the concept of levels of awareness. The other is the concept of the agencies of the mind.

According to Freud's theory, mental activity occurs at three levels of awareness. The *conscious* level is the level where the least amount of activity occurs. Nonetheless, it includes all of the mental activity in the awareness of the individual at the moment. The second level is the *preconscious*. This level contains all the information an individual can recall at will. Two old friends reminiscing will find themselves recalling events that neither has thought about in years. This is an example of mental activity stored at the preconscious level. The third level of awareness is the *unconscious* level. This level stores all the events and relationships from the past that shape a person's behavior. Mental activity in the unconscious mind continuously influences the individual's conscious behavior, even though the actual material cannot be brought into consciousness. For example, most people have had the experience of feeling uneasy or frightened when summoned to see someone of authority, such as a school principal or a supervisor at work. If the individual does not recall an immediate reason for the summons, the reaction may be motivated by previous misdeeds and their consequences, which are stored in the unconscious mind.

The agencies of the mind are the id, the ego, and the superego. The id is the reservoir for all the instinctual, uninhibited urges. It operates completely at the unconscious level. Instinctual urges satisfy needs such as hunger without regard to any other conditions. Totally uncontrolled rage when frustrated is an example of an urge experienced in the id.

The opposing counterpart to this agency is the superego. The superego consists of all the acquired socially sanctioned attitudes and behaviors. These include the desire to be considered lovable, the feeling of obligation to those who care for us and of responsibility to those who are dependent upon us. The superego operates at the conscious and preconscious level. The id and superego are constantly tugging at each other. It is the ego that serves the function of mediating between these two extremes and produces the behaviors that constitute the compromise. The ego becomes that part of the personality that is revealed to others. It operates at both the conscious and preconscious levels and is the person with whom others communicate. The concept of the ego has been greatly expanded by recent theorists, but the term continues to be used with its original meaning.

Theories of gestalt psychologists also have contributed to the understanding of human communication. *Gestalt* is a German word meaning pattern or configuration. This school of psychological thought developed in the early twentieth century in opposition to the mainstream psychological inquiry at the time. Psychological study then was concerned with the structure of the mind and the location of various mental processes. The gestalt psychologists insisted that to understand any phenomenon, it must be examined as a whole. The parts may be separated and analyzed, but the total determines how a phenomenon is perceived. A simple way to say this is, "The whole is different from the sum of the parts."

In the field of human communication, the significance of any one interaction cannot be determined by analyzing each ingredient individually. Each interaction, as in the following example, must be examined as a gestalt.

A bereaved widow recalled a card she received from a friend that simply stated, "What can I say?" If one analyzes just the language content of that message, it clearly doesn't say much. The legibility of the handwriting, the quality of the paper, the reason for using the mail rather than a face-to-face communication could all be examined, but these analyses would not explain the significance of the communication. The significance is that it was perceived as a very kind expression of sympathy.

Gestalt psychologists were concerned with the mental activity of the individual. Systems theorists have expanded upon gestalt concepts to apply to all living things.

The process of intrapersonal communication follows very closely the systems theory model described in Chapter 5. The messages an individual receives can be considered the input. The throughput includes all of the components involved in processing that message. The responses the individual makes become the output. The concept of feedback in systems theory is an essential component of the communication process. Each individual needs feedback to determine if the communication has reached its destination and been perceived in the manner intended. Only in this manner does one know if one's communication system is working effectively.

In a larger system, consisting of groups of living things, communication is the process by which an essential element, information, enters the system. Communication between the elements must occur if transformation is to take place. Thus, the communication process may be a system and a subsystem, an element of a larger system.

Communication is a dynamic process. It has no starting or ending point and no single objective. A young woman talking to a small group at a party may have several objectives: to help the hostess keep the party moving, to find out if anyone needs additional refreshments, and to come to the attention of a young man in a nearby group. Responses may come from her immediate group or from outside that group. The young woman who is the source, or initiator, of the communication may use responses in the situation as messages for the hostess or for the individuals who are served, the guests. If the young women succeeds in any of her objectives, she may become the content of messages sent the following day from several different sources. Similarly, a nurse talking with two clients in a semiprivate room may be interested in helping them become acquainted, gathering data about the clients to include in a care conference, and determining their self-care level. The output of this conversation may influence two separate additional groups: the nurse's communication network in the hospital, and the clients in their communication networks. The characteristics of a network are:

every unit in a network does not interact with every other unit, the units do not have clear boundaries, the only common characteristic is the relationship to the ego or pivotal center around which the network exists.[3] From the two examples above, the application of network theory to the communication process is evident.

Communication Models

A model that can be applied to any form of communication is the Shannon–Weaver Model[4] shown in Figure 14–1. This model was developed by two mathematicians. The basic components are essential to the process of communication in plants and lower animals, in human beings, and even in electronic equipment.

The simple example of the wish to communicate disapproval can be used to demonstrate how the model applies to human communication. The wish originates in the human being represented as the information source. That person will decide which channel to use to transmit the message. The channel will determine the form of the message. A verbal signal "Please Stop" may be used, or facial muscles may be used to transmit a nonverbal message. The information source encodes the message and sends it out from the transmitter. The message becomes the signal that must get past the noise source to the receiver. The noise source may be any type of outside interference with the signal reaching the receiver. In human communication it may be a visual distraction that causes the receiver to look away and not see the nonverbal signal. It may be loud sounds that interfere with hearing, or it may be an overwhelming emotion, such as fear, that interferes with comprehension. In an electronic system, just as with people, it could be a failure at the energy source or it could be static, literally. In the print media, noise could take the form of a failure of the press to reproduce some words, blurring of print, or even large colorful illustrations that distract from the content. For communication to occur, the message must get past the noise source to the receiver. The receiver must be capable of decoding the message so that it can be understood at its destination.

Through the process of communication, human beings reveal themselves to one another.

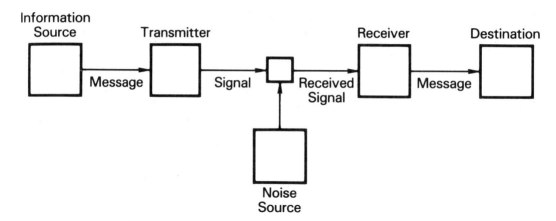

Figure 14–1. General communication system. *(From C. Shannon and W. Weaver, The Mathematical Theory of Communication (Urbana, Ill.: University of Illinois Press, 1949), 5. Reprinted with permission.)*

How much is revealed, to whom, when, and why are determined by the uniqueness of the individual and the context in which the communication occurs. Berlo's source-message-channel-receiver model (SMCR) is an attempt to develop a comprehensive model that includes all the ingredients that influence each single act of communication[5] (Fig. 14–2).

Source. In this model, the source is the person who originates the idea for the message. The characteristics of the person that influence the message are that individual's communication skills, attitudes, knowledge, the social system in which the individual exists, and the culture in which the communication occurs.

Communication skills are the tools for

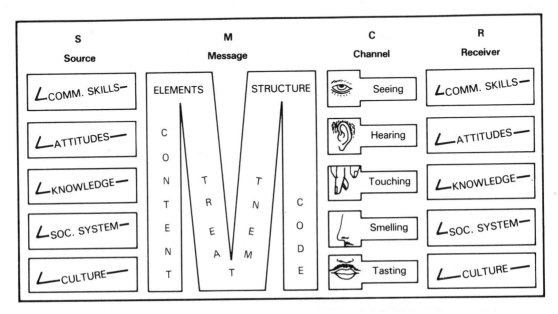

Figure 14–2. A model of the ingredients in communication. *(Reprinted with permission from David K. Berlo, The Process of Communication (New York: Holt, Rinehart & Winston, 1960), 72.)*

transmitting the message. These include: speaking, writing, preverbal uttering, gesturing, and moving. The specific tools selected by the source will be determined by that person's special abilities or deficiencies. An individual with an extensive vocabulary will have choices of words to use. A person who is just learning the language may have to use gestures to supplement a limited vocabulary.

Attitudes have both cognitive and affective components. They are formed by a combination of something a person believes and feelings about that belief. As one matures, one develops attitudes about self, other people, and abstract concepts. A person's attitude toward self is an integral part of that person's behavior and will be reflected in communications with others. Attitudes toward other people may be individualized to a particular person or they may be generalized to a group or class. Generalized attitudes toward people are called stereotypes or prejudices. An example is "poor people are lazy." A person with that attitude will surely find that it influences communication with poor people. Attitudes about abstract concepts may have developed as a result of personal experiences with the concept or as the result of absence of personal experiences. For example, many people in the United States have attitudes about different political systems, even though they have only had personal experience with one. These people cannot believe that any form of government other than our own is acceptable. The more one can learn about the basis of one's attitudes, the more able one will be to change those that interfere with effective communication.

The amount of knowledge the source has about the subject of a communication will influence that communication. When one wishes to make another person understand something, a thorough understanding by the source will aid in the process. If the source is seeking additional information, the communication will be different from the way it would if the source were trying to hide a lack of information.

Social systems have developed to provide the structure and order human beings need to work together harmoniously. These systems develop around defined goals. In the family, for example, one goal is the care and nurturing of children. In the health-care system, the goal is the provision of services needed to maintain or restore the health of numerous subsystems of the population. Within each system, roles are assigned to the members of the system, and norms of behavior are established. The norms of behavior and the assigned roles both determine communication patterns. New members learn these patterns through the process of communication. Communication is essential for the social system to function.

In the health-care system, the nurse's assigned role influences how the nurse communicates with clients. It also influences how that communication differs from the nurse's communication with the physician. Norms of behavior influence such things as the appropriate use of slang or the appropriate time to lower one's voice.

The culture from which the individual originates determines the system of symbols used to communicate. Alphabets and language differ between cultures. The use of sign language in the form of gestures and facial expressions varies in different cultures. People of oriental extraction are often considered "inscrutable" because of their apparently unchanging facial expression. It is easier for us to comprehend the words of someone from a western culture whose "eyes flash with anger" or "eyes light up with joy." Each culture also has its own norms of behavior or customs. For example, in some cultures a woman does not speak unless she is specifically addressed. In the North American culture, men greet each other by shaking hands. In some other cultures, men embrace.

All five of these ingredients—communication skills, attitudes, knowledge, social system, and culture—are influencing the source simultaneously as the desired message is encoded.

Message. The message exists as the concrete product of the communication process. Everything that exists is composed of elements and structure. These are present in every system. The elements are the parts; the structure is the manner in which they are assembled. Because it exists, the message must be composed of elements and structure. Three other factors involved in the message are the content, code, and treatment. The content and code form the legs of the **M**. Both content and code must receive treatment for a message to be formed. The content of the message is the idea the source wishes to communicate. The content consists of elements. The code is a way of organizing symbols to make them meaningful. Language is one form of code. Nonverbal communications, such as facial expressions, are another. Different expressions, such as a raised eyebrow, communicate different things. The decisions the sender makes about which codes to use constitute the treatment of the message and determine the message's final structure. A young mother communicating with her baby wishes to show her love for her baby. The message is encoded for the sense of sight (the smiling face) and touch (the encircling arms). The hug and the smile are the treatment of the message. A kiss could have been used instead. The final structure of this message is a young woman smiling with her arms encircling her baby.

Channel. The channels for receiving messages are the five senses. Most human communication is received by the eyes and the ears. Animals rely more heavily on their senses of smell and taste. Dogs are used to help track lost people and retrieve the hunter's quarry because of their highly developed sense of smell. Human beings use their senses of smell and taste together with other senses. A person may notice a distinctive odor but be unable to identify it until the origin becomes known. Nurses need to use their sense of smell when they are assessing a client. Problems such as alcohol intoxication or the presence of infection are communicated by a distinctive odor.

Apparently, the human sense of sight is the dominant one. Individuals frequently make decisions based on what they see. We look at vegetables in the market and decide how they will taste. We look at another person and make a judgment about that person's personality on the basis of what we see. The sense of sight is strong enough to distort the sense of hearing and touch. A person may assume a rumbling noise comes from a truck in clear view when, in fact, it is thunder.

The sense of touch is used less often as a means of communication than are seeing and hearing. In interpersonal communication, it is used primarily to express emotions. Individuals

use touch to increase their knowledge of an object, an animal, or person's body. Nurses use their sense of touch to learn about a client's body during the assessment phase of the nursing process. Touch is also used in the implementation of nursing care. Touch may be used to identify the site for an injection. Touch in the form of massage has a healing effect on sore or stiff muscles. The psychological effects of touch can be an important therapeutic tool of the nurse.

Perception, or how the message becomes encoded in the brain of the receiver, starts with the neurophysiological equipment of the individual involved. The relative health of the sensory organs will influence the perception of a message. The physiological structure is a combination of inherited tendency, general nutritional state, and the presence or absence of diseases that may have resulted in impairment. Myopia, or nearsightedness, is an example of an inherited perceptual impairment. A diet that is insufficient in vitamin A also can result in visual impairment. Scar tissue in the middle ear, as the result of childhood infections, can cause hearing impairment.

Past experiences also influence perception. People are much more likely to perceive what they expect to perceive, based on their past experiences. An individual who has been watching boats sail gracefully past may not immediately realize it when one of the boats overturns. When a person is told that an elderly friend who has been seriously ill has died, that person will perceive the message rather quickly. If the person is told that an apparently healthy elderly friend has died in an accident, that person may ask to have the message repeated.

The physical and psychological state of both the source and the receiver influence the perception of the message. A headache or fever can interfere with perception. Angry feelings not dissipated after a heated argument can interfere with perception of new stimuli. Perception is most accurate in physically healthy, relaxed individuals who are able to focus their entire attention on the message.

Receiver. The same five factors that influence the source influence the receiver. These are communication skills, attitude, knowledge, social system, and culture. Similarity between the source and the receiver in these areas will improve communication. Sensitivity to differences in these ingredients will improve communication.

A nurse who is the child of first-generation Americans and who grew up in an ethnic neighborhood in a city in the Northeastern United States will differ primarily in knowledge from a client who grew up in the same type of community. Similarities in communication skills, attitudes, and culture will help overcome the communications barrier created by the social system. A nurse from a middle-class suburb of a southern city, whose family has been in this country for several generations, will come from a very different culture with different attitudes and different communication skills. Sensitivity to social and cultural differences will improve communication with the client. Sensitivity on the part of the client to these differences will increase the chances for effective communication between them.

Types of Communication

Verbal and Nonverbal Communication. Human communication is both verbal and nonverbal. Verbal communication includes any expression in a common language. These expressions are made through speech, writing, or their counterparts, listening and reading. Ability to articulate and to understand the language is essential to interaction in human society. Without the ability to use language communication, a person cannot acquire knowledge, work, or socialize. Factual information is usually transmitted verbally. We also use words to transmit emotional information, but the affective or feeling component of an emotional message is usually transmitted nonverbally.

Thus, the full meaning of any communication is not grasped if the nonverbal elements are ignored. Nonverbal communication includes preverbal sounds, body movement, facial expression, physiological activities, and the use of space and time.

Preverbal sounds are used to express the range of human emotions. A scream for help and a shout for joy are both preverbal sounds. The ability to communicate in this manner precedes the ability to form language and is thus considered more primitive. It is the language of the id in Freudian theory.

Body movement is a significant form of communication. The way a person stands or sits and the movements of hands and feet as the person stands or sits all communicate something about the person and the message being communicated. A rigid posture with muscles in a continuous semiflexed state is used to communicate fear or physical discomfort. It also may be used to convey anger or respect. Hand and foot movements can be used to enhance a verbal message. A slouching, careless stance can communicate boredom, disrespect, or low esteem. Leaning toward the other person conveys interest in the communication. These concepts are illustrated in Figure 14–3.

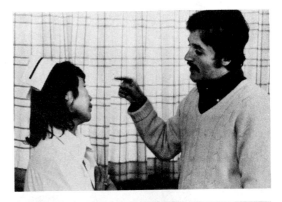

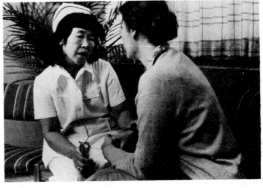

Figure 14–3. Body posture and movement are ingredients of communication in both these pictures.

The use of structure and movement in the form of dance as a means of communication began in primitive times. It may have preceded the development of language. As human beings perfected the use of language, less attention was paid to nonverbal methods of communication. In recent years, interest has rekindled for the study of body movement as a form of communication. The term used to describe this form of communication is **kinesics.**[6]

Facial expressions are usually in harmony with body movement. They are listed as a separate category because they can change when changes in the individual's body movement may be imperceptible. Both body movement and facial expression are less under the conscious control of the individual and, therefore, more likely to be the authentic message when not consistent with the verbal message. A person who scowls while saying "Everything is O.K.," is communicating that everything is not O.K.

Physiological activities, such as rumbling sounds from the abdomen or coughing, communicate information about the health state of the individual.

The way individuals use *space and time* in their interactions with others is a form of communication. When a person returns a telephone call as soon as it is received, this communicates a wish to be involved with the caller. The reason for the involvement may be positive or negative. Allowing time to elapse before returning the call indicates that the caller has a low priority in the receiver's frame of reference. Hall, an anthropologist, studied the significance of how individuals use space and distance to communicate with others.[7] He described four relationships that can be identified by the actual physical space maintained between the participants. These are in order of closeness: intimate, personal, social, and public. These relationships are depicted in Figure 14–4.

Though actual distances vary within the context, some average figures have been developed. Intimate distance is the distance between two individuals involved in intimate activities. These are the activities related to affection, anger, and the maintenance of body integrity. The distance between two individuals in intimate communication begins with body contact and

extends about 18 inches. Nurses in their caregiving role often invade the intimate space of a total stranger. Whenever two individuals are close enough to achieve body contact, the possibility exists for one person to gain control over the other. Most people become uncomfortable when a stranger invades their intimate space, because of concern that they may lose control.

Personal distance is from 18 inches to 4 feet. At this distance, subjects of a personal nature can be discussed without concern that the other individual will gain physical control. The expression, "keeping a person at arm's length," is used to convey the wish to avoid being controlled. This is the distance usually maintained between individuals in an interview situation.

Social space is the distance from 4 to 12 feet from the individual. From this distance one-to-one communication is possible, but business of a private nature cannot be transacted. Most casual social and business transactions occur at this distance.

Public distance begins about 12 feet away from the individual, and precludes the possibility for meaningful one-to-one interaction. One individual may look at and listen to the other and may receive a clear message. It is, however, difficult to make a clear response.

The uses of time and distance, because they are measurable, are easier to assess than any other forms of nonverbal communication. In an evaluation of communication difficulties, the way time and space have been used can provide data to clarify the problem. However, communication difficulties cannot be understood and corrected unless all aspects of the situation are included.

Instrumental and Consummatory Communication. Communication can be categorized according to purpose.[8] Communication that is directed toward achieving a specific goal is **instrumental communication.** The goal may be transacting business with the bank teller or it may be comforting a friend who is ill. Social norms will dictate differences in the use of voice tone, choice of vocabulary, and body movement in these two examples, but in both situations, communication becomes the instrument to accomplish the goal. Communication that is the

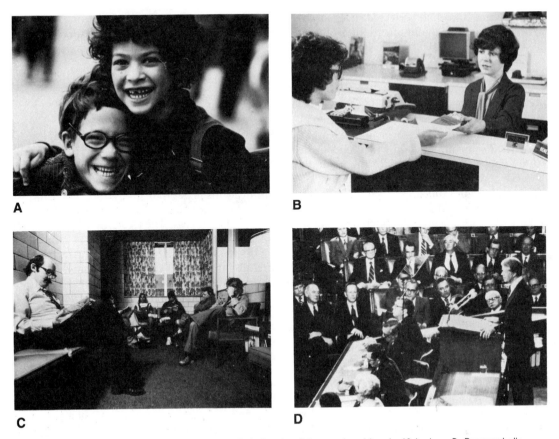

Figure 14–4. Hall's spatial relationships. **A.** Intimate distance: touching to 18 inches. **B.** Personal distance: 18 inches to 4 feet. **C.** Social distance: 4 feet to 12 feet. **D.** Public distance: 12 feet and more.

goal in itself is called **consummatory communication**. This may be in combination with some other activity, such as eating and drinking. It may be during the introductory phase of a relationship, when each party is deciding how much of him- or herself to reveal, or it may be during an unavoidable "waiting" time, such as in a supermarket line. Americans are reputed to be skilled at this form of communication. An American woman who was living in another English-speaking country reported several occasions when she felt rebuffed as she attempted to converse with someone at a bus stop or in a supermarket line. Since both of these were familiar institutions, and the language was familiar, it was the lack of response to her conversational overtures that reminded her she was in another culture. Social chitchat, or consummatory communication, with strangers was not the practice in that country.

Dysfunctional and Therapeutic Communication. **Dysfunctional communication** is the term used to describe the type of communication that interferes with the establishment or maintenance of meaningful interpersonal relationships. It is characteristic of individuals in our society who are lonely and withdrawn. The individuals are often described as neurotic or mentally ill. In some forms of mental illness, such as schizophrenia, dysfunctional communication is considered symptomatic of a thought disorder. In other individuals, it may be both the cause and effect of a lifetime of experiences of feeling misunderstood and rejected. Individuals with these types of communication problems also may have physical illnesses. Thus, such a person may be a nurse's client, regardless of the specific field of nursing involved. This is one of the reasons it is important for all nursing students to experience communicating with clients who have dysfunctional communication patterns. Much of the early scientific inquiry in the field of human communication focused on the dysfunctional communications of the mentally ill. Ruesch, a psychiatrist, developed the concept of **therapeutic communcation.**[9] He describes it as communication that has, as its purpose, changing another person's manner of communicating. Techniques of therapeutic communication are important for the nurse to be helpful to the client with dysfunctional communication. These techniques usually are taught in advanced nursing courses. This chapter addresses the problem of communicating effectively with clients who do not have dysfunctional communication patterns, since this group comprises the majority of people.

Effective Communication. **Effective communication** is perceived by the receiver as it was intended by the source. The message from the source does not need to be pleasant or positive, it simply needs to be understood as intended. Communication that enables a terminally ill person and that person's family to understand the nature of the illness and the expected consequences is effective, however heartbreaking it may be. If students are told the instructor would like to have the term papers on Thursday, then are penalized for delivering them on Friday, effective communication has not occurred. What one would like and what one expects are not necessarily the same.

Because of the dynamic nature of the communication process and the constantly shifting settings in which communication occurs, an individual can never achieve closure on the ability to communicate effectively. It is a goal toward which people can continually strive. Some individuals, because of a high degree of sensitivity to other people, and some special talent in organizing and transmitting their ideas, seem particularly gifted in effective communication. Even those

individuals may have lapses. Everyone with motivation and practice can learn to improve the effectiveness of his or her communication.

COMMUNICATION AND THE NURSING PROCESS

Factors Facilitating Communication

No nurse can fulfill the professional role without communicating with clients. There are some rather simple guidelines for facilitating the communications process in any setting. Focusing attention on the other individual is one important part of the process. The freedom of both parties to focus attention on each other is influenced by distractions in the environment: the "noise" of the Shannon-Weaver Communication Model. Physical discomfort may be one of the distractions. Two individuals outside in a blizzard will probably limit their communication to messages that assist in finding shelter. Those same two people in a crowded elevator will be distracted by the presence of other people. A quiet, well-ventilated space with comfortable seating arrangements is the physical environment that will be most conducive to their communication.

Intuitive attraction to the other person is an important facilitator of effective communication. There are some people who are instinctively drawn to each other without being able to explain why. However, in both a social and a professional role, it is sometimes necessary to communicate with people to whom one is not especially attracted. When this situation occurs, it is necessary to work harder to establish effective communication.

The social field, or *life space,* in which it occurs influences the effectiveness of the communication.[10] An individual's life space is that individual's perception of the immediate environment at the moment. This includes physical structures and objects, other people, and psychological factors. Lewin specifies these factors as the individual's goals at the moment, perceived obstacles to achieving those goals, perceived facilitators to attaining these goals, and the route one feels obliged to use.

The following example illustrates this concept:

A young woman was alone in the city at 10 o'clock at night. Her physical environment included a lighted city street, some automobiles, and a subway station. The only people in the environment were strangers. Her goal was to return to her place of lodging. She could either take a taxi or the subway. Her finances were limited, so she felt she must use the subway. The obstacles to her taking the subway included a phobia of heights, which resulted in her becoming dizzy, a very steep escalator, no police officer or woman she might approach to ask for directions to an elevator, and a lifetime of being warned about speaking to strange men. The factors facilitating her goal attainment were a strong desire to get off the street and safely to her lodging, a good command of the language spoken in that city, a knowledge of the city, and the appearance of a pleasant-looking young man who walked with a slight limp.

She perceived him as someone who might have some understanding of her distress. She approached him and asked if he could direct her to the elevator. He told her he did not know the location of the elevator in this particular subway station. When she explained her plight he suggested she ride beside him on the escalator, facing him rather than looking down. She did this and safely arrived at the bottom of the escalator. Within a few moments she was on the subway en route to her lodging.

Each individual involved in an interaction is part of two different life spaces: one's own and the other individual's. If the young man in the example above had just concluded an argument with a jealous girl friend, he might not have appeared approachable. If the young woman had not appeared genuinely distressed, he might not have responded positively to her need for help. Sensitivity to what is happening in the life space of the other individual is an important contributor to effective communication.

Clients whose ability to communicate is impaired by some physical disability, such as blindness or deafness, present special problems, but there are specific nursing techniques that can be learned to foster communication with the sight- or hearing-impaired client.

Specific Communication Techniques

There are specific modes of expression and linguistic techniques that can be learned that contribute to the effectiveness of the communications process. Some people resist learning these techniques because they think it is unnatural and will impede communication. With practice, these techniques can become part of the person's natural speech pattern. In fact, individuals who do a great deal of counseling or teaching are often accused by their families of using communication techniques in casual conversation. In most instances, these techniques have become so much a part of the individual's communication pattern that the individual is not aware of using them. The small grandson of a college professor recognized this when he remarked: "Everytime I ask Granddad a question, he teaches me a lesson."

In the previous section, the importance of focusing attention on the other party in an interaction was discussed. This requires both observation and listening. Listening requires concentrating on what the other person is saying while formulating a response. One must also observe nonverbal messages simultaneously. It is not a simple task. The nurse who continues to make the bed while talking to the client may be listening to what the client is saying but, by not observing the client closely, may be missing nonverbal cues. Some nurses become skillful at apparently doing both things at the same time. That takes a great deal of practice and a high level of sensitivity to the other person's feelings.

Along with listening and observing, the nurse needs to learn the appropriate use of silence. Nurses often feel they must be doing something for the client all the time. They even view sitting and talking with the client as a waste of time. The mere presence of another human being can be helpful. Filling time with idle chatter or meaningless activity may temporarily divert attention from stress, but it will not alter the source of the stress. Silence can be used to think about what is occurring and to devise suggestions for coping. If it appears that silence is being used to avoid a subject of conversation, there are gestures and preverbal sounds that can be used to encourage the discussion to continue.

Some people nod their head, others use sounds such as: "Um" or "Uh huh."

The giving of information either as an opening to a conversation or in answer to a client's question will assist the flow of conversation. A genuine need for information can be met at the same time that respect for the client's right to question is acknowledged. Conversely, withholding information can impede communication. Refusing to answer a question can imply that the question was inappropriate or that the nurse is not interested in the client's concerns. Introducing oneself and stating one's purpose is more than a social amenity. It is an important communication that gives recognition to the other person as an individual, and it clarifies the reason for the interaction. Individuals with health problems are usually concerned about themselves and anxious to acquire information about their condition. Legislation in recent years has protected the right of the clients to know about their condition and at the same time protected their right to privacy. The privacy protection prevents information from a health-care agency about a person's physical condition being sent to an employer without permission. In each health-care agency, how and by whom information is transmitted to the client is determined by agency policy. The nurse needs to know the policy in order to respond appropriately to client inquires. If a client asks the nurse for information the nurse is not authorized to transmit, the nurse can tell the client this and tell the client who is authorized to convey the information.

There are many specific techniques for structuring language to encourage meaningful communication. A few of the more distinct types are discussed here. Statements or questions that are *open ended* will encourage clients to express themselves fully. For example, if the client is asked for the location of the pain in the client's foot, the answer will probably relate only to the location. If the person is asked to tell you about the pain, you may be given information about the location, intensity, and duration. Verbally expressing what is perceived as the nonverbal communication encourages verbilization. Statements such as, "You appeared angry when your visitor left," will make it easier for the client to discuss the situation. *Broad openings* allow the other person to determine the direction of the conversation. "How are you?" has, unfortunately, become a stereotyped greeting with a stereotyped response, but it is an example of a broad opening. Broad openings are questions such as, "How did things go at work today?" or statements such as, "I wonder what you're thinking." *Restating* what the other person has said can be used both to clarify and to encourage continuation of the topic. This is a particularly useful technique when the subject may be anxiety-producing for both parties. If someone says, "I lost my job," the response, "You lost your job," enables conversation to continue without passing judgment on the content. It also provides feedback to the first speaker that the message has been understood. *Reflection* is the directing of the question back to the questioner. It encourages finding one's own solution to the problem. This indicates respect for the individual's ability and relieves the nurse of the responsibility for making the decision. If the client says, "Do you think this new medicine will help me?" the nurse can reply, "Do *you* think it will?"

There are choices of words and types of statements that are not only not helpful, but to the extent that they make the person feel rejected or belittled, they can be harmful.

The use of cliches is one example. "Keep your chin up," and "Better days are ahead," are two rather useless statements. "Everyone feels that way sometime," may be interpreted as belittling of the client's feelings. Direct rejection of the topic with a statement like, "Let's not talk about that," will usually end that conversation. Indirect rejection by changing the subject communicates unwillingness on the nurse's part to pursue the topic. Questions that begin with why, how, or what can be interpreted as a demand for a short answer.[11] They should be used sparingly. "Why did you let the doctor upset you?" does have a coercive quality. An exploratory statement such as, "Can we piece together the events that are upsetting you?" will enable the client to gather the data to understand the reason for the upset without pressure for a specific answer.

A persistent series of short answer questions creates the impression that the questioner is only interested in the facts, not in the person providing the facts. "Did you drink all the juice?" "Did you take your medicine?" "Do you need anything for pain?" in rapid succession will probably make the client wish the nurse would just leave. It certainly will not encourage the client to elaborate on a problem.

The following case report demonstrates how the use of these techniques enabled one nursing student to improve her communication with one client. In this case, improved communication enabled the student to make effective use of the nursing process.

Sarah Jones was a nursing student enrolled in a freshman nursing course. A major objective of this course was to enable the student to develop beginning skills in communicating with clients in different age groups and from different socioeconomic levels. For their laboratory experience, a group of students went with their instructor one afternoon a week to a sheltered housing facility for the elderly. Each student was assigned to a client to identify health problems and to plan and implement assistance with these problems within the limited scope of her own nursing knowledge.

Sarah Jones's client was Mrs. Smith, a frail, 74-year-old woman living alone in an efficiency apartment. She had no seriously incapacitating health problems at the time. She had arthritis and mild hypertension. Her apartment was simply, but comfortably, furnished. It was both neat and clean.

The following is taken from a process recording the student made immediately following her second visit with Mrs. Smith.

> *Student:* (observing a plate on the kitchen sink containing chicken bones) Did you enjoy your lunch?
>
> *Mrs. Smith:* Yes.
> *Student:* Does the management send your lunch to you?
> *Mrs. Smith:* Yes.
> *(Pause)*
> *Student:* Did you go to church yesterday?
> *Mrs. Smith:* No, it was too cold.
> *Student:* Did visitors from the church come like they usually do on Sunday?

> *Mrs. Smith:* Yes
> *Student:* Oh, who came?
> *Mrs. Smith:* (sighs) I don't remember, some people.
> *Student:* What did you do?
> *Mrs. Smith:* We prayed.
> *(Long pause)*
> *Student:* Remember you said you were afraid to get in the tub alone? I told you I could help you with a tub bath when I was here. Would you like to do that now?
> *Mrs. Smith:* Yes.
> *Student:* I'll go fix your tub.
> *(Student goes into bathroom, starts the water in the tub, and locates necessary equipment. She returns to living room.)*
> *Student:* Do you want to put on clean clothes after your bath?
> *Mrs. Smith:* Yes.
> *(Student walks toward dresser.)*
> *Student:* Where will I find your clean underwear?
> *Mrs. Smith:* In the middle drawer.
> *(Student selects clean underwear, then turns to Mrs. Smith.)*
> *Student:* Is this okay?
> *(Mrs. Smith nods her head. Student returns to Mrs. Smith's side.)*
> *Student:* I'll help you to the bathroom now.
> *(Mrs. Smith gets up without speaking. They walk together to the bathroom. Student helps Mrs. Smith undress and get into tub.)*
> *Student:* You have nice new underwear.
> *Mrs. Smith:* Uh huh.
> *Student:* Where did you get the underwear?
> *Mrs. Smith:* From my daughter-in-law.
> *Student:* That's nice.
> *(The conversation continued in this manner while Mrs. Smith bathed and dressed in clean clothing.)*

When the student discussed the interaction with her instructor, she reported feeling very tired. She felt burdened with the responsibility to learn more about Mrs. Smith. Her assessment was that Mrs. Smith had lived a financially and socially deprived life and it was not realistic to think she could engage in meaningful dialogue. The instructor pointed out that Mrs. Smith had given her fragments of information that she had not pursued. They also discussed the student's almost complete reliance on short-answer questions.

Role playing was used to recreate the situation. The student assumed the role of Mrs. Smith. The instructor used a very simple vocabulary to structure broad openings and to restate and explore conversational cues. The student observed the instructor's ability to be relaxed during silences and to use the silence to think about the interaction. After this experience the student was willing to try a different approach during her next visit with Mrs. Smith. She planned a broad opening to use during her next visit. She would begin the interaction by saying, "Last week you mentioned your daughter-in-law. Can you tell me more about your family?"

When the student arrived at Mrs. Smith's apartment she found her lying on her bed, apparently staring into space. She sat beside Mrs. Smith's bed and smiled in silence. After a few moments she said, "You look worried."

Mrs. Smith: (after a long pause) I don't know what I'm going to do.

Student: Can you tell me what's bothering you?

Mrs. Smith: It won't do no good.

Student: If I knew what was wrong, I might be able to help.

Mrs. Smith: (after a long pause) You can't do nothing.

Student: I would like to try to help.

(Another long pause. The student was beginning to feel uncomfortable. She resisted the urge to suggest she prepare Mrs. Smith's bath.)

Mrs. Smith: They told me there's not going to be any hot lunches on Saturday and Sunday. (another pause) What can I do? I don't have much appetite, but I got to eat a little something.

Student: They told you they were going to stop the hot lunches on Saturday and Sunday. What reason did they give?

Mrs. Smith: I don't know. That got me upset, I didn't hear the rest.

Student: How did you find this out?

Mrs. Smith: The lady that manages the building, she came to the door. (long pause)

Student: She came to the door.

Mrs. Smith: Yes, she said there wasn't going to be any more hot lunches in the apartments on Saturday and Sunday.

Student: What else did she say? Can you remember now?

Mrs. Smith: She said we have to come downstairs for hot lunches. You know I can't walk that far. I'm so afraid I'll fall. I used to have one of those canes with three feet on it, but its broke.

The first thing the student pursued was the information about the lunches. She helped Mrs. Smith call the manager's office. From this phone call, Mrs. Smith learned that a cold lunch of sandwich, fruit, and milk could be sent to the apartments of those residents unable to come downstairs. She became more relaxed when she learned this.

Next, they located the broken cane. Mrs. Smith told the student that her son or some member of his family called her every evening. They decided to leave the cane by the telephone, so that Mrs. Smith would remember to ask if they could arrange to have it repaired.

When the student left, Mrs. Smith was in a pleasant mood, and so was she. Improved communication had resulted in assessment of problems with which she could help. She had done some on-the-spot planning and implemented her plans. She was eager to evaluate the experience with her instructor.

Nurse–Client Relationship

The nurse–client relationship is a helping relationship, similar to the relationships members of other helping professions, such as social workers and psychiatrists, establish with their clients. The nurse–client relationship differs in function from other helping professions because of the specific functions of the nurse in society.

Initial investigations into the use of the

nurse–client relationship were done in the psychiatric setting. Distinctions were drawn between the interpersonal skills needed in psychiatric nursing and the psychomotor skills needed to carry out procedures, such as irrigating a wound, used in general nursing. Modern technological advances have placed machinery that monitors the client and administers treatments between the client and the nurse in acute-care settings. The nurse has had to acquire new skills to interpret and regulate the machinery. The machinery has not replaced the client's need for comfort, emotional support, and knowledge about the specific health problem. In order to provide this, the nurse needs to be able to establish a meaningful nurse–client relationship. When nurse and client are able to move beyond the stereotyped concept that each has of the other, a relationship can start to develop.[12] The nurse must be able to stop interacting with the client as though the person is simply a client with a nursing need to be met. The nurse must be able to perceive the client as a unique human being with a unique clustering of needs. The nurse alone cannot establish a relationship with a client who continues to perceive the nurse as the efficient, impersonal dispenser of care. The client must be able to alter this stereotyped perception of the nurse, also.

In a helping relationship, the nurse uses knowledge of human behavior, along with the ability to care about and share the psychological experience of the client, to help the client. Each relationship develops in stages. These are the introduction, including the development of trust, **empathy, sympathy,** involvement, and termination. Because of the uniqueness of individuals and of each situation, these stages do not necessarily follow an orderly progression. They may seem to occur all together in a very short time span. They may occur in different overlapping combinations. They are discussed separately to facilitate understanding of the process.

In the *introductory* stage, each individual gathers data about the other person's uniqueness. It is during this time that expectations are relinquished that the other person will behave in a certain way because that person is young or old, a man or a woman, a nurse or a client. At this time, each individual should clarify for

the other the expectation of the interaction. The beginnings can be very simple statements, such as, "I am Mary Jones, the nurse assigned to your care this evening." In that statement the nurse acknowledges her own and the client's personhood. If the nurse simply stood at the bedside and said, "Your call light is on," this would maintain the stereotyped expectations that each held. These two examples are pictured in Figures 14–5 and 14–6. Notice the different use of space, facial expressions, body movement, as well as words in each situation.

During this introductory stage, each individual also will make some decision about the trustworthiness of the other. In order to reveal oneself to another human being, one must be able to trust that other human being. Trust in this context means that each can expect truthfulness from the other and that one will not be subjected to ridicule or exposure if one reveals very private information about oneself.

Empathy is defined as the capacity to feel the psychological experience of another person as though it were one's own. It is uniquely human. It is not something that one can decide in advance to do, or a skill one can practice. When empathy occurs, both parties know it instinctively and feel closer as a result. Some individuals seem to have a greater capacity to develop empathy than others. Psychologists speculate that the ability to feel empathy develops in the anterior frontal lobes, and that this section of the brain is more highly developed in some in-

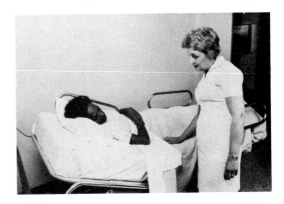

Figure 14–5. "I'm Miss Jones, the nurse assigned to your care today. I saw you had turned on the call light."

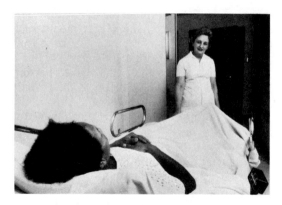

Figure 14-6. "Your call light is on."

dividual than in others.[13] It seems important that there be some similarity of experiences between people for empathy to develop. Many social support groups in our society are based on the empathetic understanding that can develop among individuals with similar problems. Alcoholics Anonymous is a well-known example. The experiences do not need to be identical. A person who has felt pride in any major accomplishment can use that feeling to empathize with the feelings of pride, for example, that a new parent experiences.

Sympathy is defined as the quality of being affected by the state of another. It is this experience that motivates one individual to help another. It can occur without empathy, and empathy can occur without sympathy. A person can wish to help someone knowing intellectually that the person is suffering. Donations to international agencies to provide relief for victims of earthquakes or floods are expressions of sympathy. If the individual does not know the victim personally, the individual cannot feel empathy. Nurses can best fulfill the nurse–client relationship when they are able to experience both empathy and sympathy for the client. An individual cannot experience trust, empathy, or sympathy without being emotionally involved. The nurse who is meeting the needs of the client in a way that permits them both to grow and change is involved.

Involvement occurs when the emotional investment essential to being helpful has been made. There are two other ways in which a

nurse may be involved that do not have a helpful outcome. These two types of involvement give the word a negative connotation. One is the solicitous involvement, which may protect the client from hurt, but also prevents growth. A nurse who will continue to spoon-feed a client with a paralyzed right arm to spare that person the struggle of learning to eat with the left hand is an example of this. The other is a distorted involvement that focuses on meeting the nurse's needs. The nurse may try to fill an emptiness in the nurse's life away from work through a relationship with a client. The client may be the same sex as the nurse, but is usually someone who lacks family or funds. The nurse may purchase needed toilet articles or clothing for the client. The client may even go to live with the nurse at the time of discharge. The relationship becomes a social relationship, and the nurse no longer is able to maintain the objectivity required in a professional helping relationship.

In the mistaken notion that these two types of behavior must be avoided at all costs, nurses used to be and are still sometimes advised to remain aloof. A nurse cannot effectively carry out the nursing process, however, by remaining aloof from the clients. If the nurse has personal problems that interfere with the ability to establish a helpful nurse–client relationship, the nurse should be encouraged to identify these problems and find appropriate solutions. A nurse whose mother is terminally ill may find it difficult to work with terminally ill clients at that time. A discussion of this with co-workers and the arrangement of assignments to avoid caring for the terminally ill temporarily may be all that is necessary. The nurse who cannot handle personal feelings while caring for the terminally ill five years after the death of a parent may have serious emotional problems that require psychiatric help.

The nurse–client relationship has an end. Closure must occur. The purpose of establishing the relationship is to facilitate the identification of client needs and the planning of strategies to meet those needs. Once those needs have been met by the nurse or alternative arrangements have been made to meet the needs, the nurse–client relationship should terminate. The effects of the relationship upon the two people will not be cancelled by the *termination*. If real growth has occurred as a result of the relationship, that growth will continue. If the client returns to the same nurse at a later time, the relationship may be much more quickly reestablished. Another hoped for result of any nurse–client relationship is that the client will feel freer to enter into a relationship with other nurses in subsequent health-care experiences.

Human beings do not like to say good-bye. This is especially true when it means giving up a rewarding experience. In most of the major languages in the world today, there are expressions that can be used to avoid saying good-bye. In English, the expression is, "So long," or "See you around." In Spanish, the expression *Hasta la vista* means "Until I see you again." Saying good-bye is an essential stage of a professional nurse–client relationship. A nurse may think this can be avoided if the client is discharged when the nurse is off duty. This type of behavior indicates a lack of understanding of the responsibility assumed when a relationship begins. Good-bye should be said the last time the nurse expects to see the client.

The termination stage is part of the relationship. It is a time to summarize what has been accomplished and to confirm that appropriate follow-up activities have been planned. It is also a time to reaffirm positive feelings. The nurse can help the client terminate if the nurse can say openly, "I wish you luck," "I have enjoyed our time together," or even, "I will miss you."

THE NURSING PROCESS

Throughout this chapter, reference has been made to the use of communication skills in the assessment of clients, the planning of nursing care, the implementation of nursing care, and the evaluation of care that has been given. These are the four steps of the nursing process that are described in detail in Chapter 7.

Assessment
The first step of the process, assessment, involves a determination of the client's health state. Assessment includes obtaining a health history, gathering information about the client's subjective complaints, and identifying objective problems. To obtain an accurate health history, the nurse must be skillful in verbal communication. The correct questions must be asked, and the client must be able to understand the vocabulary. The nurse must listen intently to what the client says and she or he must observe. Observation includes using the senses of sight, hearing, smell, and touch. It includes being alert to the client's facial expression and body movement. Specialized physical assessment measures require the use of touch to palpate parts of the body, hearing through a stethoscope, and reading gauges on instruments. The mental status of the client is obtained through observation and the use of a set of interview questions. The assessment phase concludes with the identification of the specific health needs of the client and the formulation of a nursing diagnosis. Several examples of nursing diagnoses related to the process of communication are as follows:

- Communication, impaired: verbal
- Social interaction: impaired
- Social isolation

The client's needs and the nursing diagnosis form the basis of the next step of the nursing process—planning.

Planning
Planning involves establishing goals for the client and a set of outcome criteria to determine if the goals have been met. A detailed plan of action is then prepared to attain these goals. This plan of action becomes the written Nursing Care Plan that is used by all nursing staff caring for the client. It is modified as the client's needs change. This written plan becomes a tool for communication among the staff. It must be legible and in language that everyone understands.

Implementation
The next step of the nursing process, implementation, involves putting the nursing plan into action. Whether the nurse does the actual implementation or delegates it to someone else, verbal communication is necessary. If the actions are delegated to others, the nurse must make sure they understand what they are to do. All of the nursing staff must be able to communicate with the client to allay anxiety when new treatments are introduced. Even if the treat-

ment procedures have been done before, step-by-step instructions are still necessary as the procedures are carried out. In addition to interpersonal communication skills, the nurse may use public communication materials to teach clients about their health state and to assume responsibility for their own care.

All the nurse's observations must be recorded as treatment progresses. These written records are a means of communication with other members of the health team caring for the client, such as the physician and the nutritionist.

Evaluation

In the final stage of the nursing process, evaluation, the nurse must reassess the client using all the communication skills used in the initial assessment. The data obtained in the reassessment is compared to the expected outcome criteria to determine the effectiveness of the nursing interventions. This information provides a basis for modifying the Nursing Care Plan.

The nursing process is a continuous process. The process begins again as evaluation and reassessment occur simultaneously. The use of communication skills is a continuous element of the nursing process.

Communication skills improve with experience. The nurse–client relationship can be learned only through experience. It is to be hoped that the material in this chapter will encourage nursing students to take the risks involved in developing relationships with clients. Experience, with guidance from an experienced teacher, is how everyone learns to establish mutually beneficial relationships.

SUMMARY

This chapter began with a brief review of the historic development of human communication and a description of the universality of the concept. Major contributions of the social sciences to the understanding of communication are included. Two communication models are presented. The Shannon–Weaver Model presents the components of the communication process as the source, the transmitter, the message itself, the receiver, and the destination. All outside interference in this process is considered noise.

Berlo expanded on this model to describe the ingredients that influence each of the components. The source and the receiver are both influenced by their communication skills, attitudes, knowledge, social system, and culture, when they send or receive a message. The channels that are chosen for the communication determine the structure of the message. The channels are the five senses: sight, hearing, touch, smell, and taste. The message itself is composed of elements and structure. The content of the message, the code, and the treatment interact with both elements and structure.

The structure of the communication may be verbal or nonverbal. Verbal communication is the spoken and written word. Nonverbal communication includes preverbal sounds, sights, tastes, odors, and body language. The purpose of communication may be instrumental, that is, to accomplish a specific goal, or it may be consummatory, to fill time. Individuals whose communication is described as dysfunctional are those whose methods of communication interfere with the development of meaningful relationships. The term therapeutic communication describes the technique used by health-care professionals to assist an individual whose communication is dysfunctional. Effective communication, communication that is perceived the way it is intended, is the goal toward which all health-care workers should strive.

Factors in the environment that influence communication are discussed. These include noise level, comfort, and timing. Specific interview techniques, such as the use of broad openings, reflection, and silence, are explained. The importance of the use of space, distance, and body language are elaborated upon. There is a comprehensive example of the successful use by a nursing student of these techniques with a client.

The nurse–client relationship is defined as the nurse's use of knowledge of human behavior, along with the ability to care about and share the psychological experience of the client, to help the client. The three phases of the relationship—introduction, involvement, and termination—are described as phases of any relationship, regardless of the length of time involved.

The use of communication skills and the

nurse–client relationship are elements of the nursing process. The success of the nursing process depends largely on the nurse's ability to communicate with the client verbally and nonverbally and to use written and verbal communication skills with other health-team members.

Study Questions

1. What are the five basic ingredients in the communication process according to the Shannon–Weaver Model?

2. How does systems theory relate to human communication?

3. What is meant by the term "effective communication?"

4. How many facilitative communications techniques can you identify?

5. What are the various categories of people with whom the nurse must communicate while carrying out the nursing process?

6. How does a professional helping relationship differ from a friendship? Give an example.

7. What are the general characteristics according to the Berlo Model that influence the manner in which an individual communicates?

References

1. George A. Borden, Richard B. Gregg, and Theodore G. Grove, *Speech Behavior and Human Interaction* (Englewood Cliffs, N.J.: Prentice-Hall, 1969), 5.
2. A.A. Brill, *The Basic Writings of Sigmund Freud* (New York: Random House, 1938).
3. Seymour Sarason, and Elizabeth Lorentz, *Human Services and Resource Networks* (San Francisco: Jossey-Bass Publishers, 1977), 128.
4. Claude Shannon and Warren Weaver, *The Mathematical Theory of Communication* (Urbana, Ill.: The University of Illinois Press, 1949), 5.
5. David Berlo, *The Process of Communication: An Introduction to Theory and Practice* (New York: Holt, Rinehart & Winston, 1960), 72.
6. Ray L. Birdwhistell, *Kinesics and Context* (Philadelphia: University of Pennsylvania Press, 1970), 128–43.
7. Edward T. Hall, *The Hidden Dimension* (New York: Doubleday Co., 1966), 110–22.
8. William Brooks, *Speech Communication* (Dubuque, Iowa: Wm. C. Brown Co., 1971), 121.
9. Jurgen Ruesch, *Therapeutic Communication* (New York: W. W. Norton & Co., 1961), 460.
10. Kurt Lewin, *Field Theory in Social Science* (New York: Harper and Row, 1951), 56–59.
11. Hildegard Peplau, "Talking with patients," *Am J Nurs* 60 (July 1960):964–66.
12. Sidney Jourard, *The Transparent Self*, 2nd ed. (New York: Van Nostrand, Reinhold Co., 1971), 179–207.
13. Kenneth Clark, "Empathy, A Neglected Topic in Psychological Research," *Am Psychol* (February 1980):187–89.

Annotated Bibliography

Brown, B. 1977. An innovative approach to health care for the elderly: An approach of hope. *J Psychiatr Nurs* 15(10):27–35. A warmly written description of one nurse's experience helping clients set realistic goals for themselves. The nurse was able to help the clients identify attainable goals. This enabled the clients to feel more self-confident and thus be willing to make changes in their patterns of living that resulted in an improvement in their health status.

Clark, R., LaBeff, E. 1982. Death-telling: Managing the delivery of bad news. *J Health Soc Behav* 23(4):366–80. A well-written report of research focused on the bearing of bad news by physicians, nurses, law enforcement officers, and clergy. Five communication strategies are identified and four phases of the process. Many examples are cited. This should be helpful to the beginning nurse trying to develop a personal strategy for bearing bad news.

DeVillers, L. 1982. What to do when you just can't communicate. *Nurs Life* 2(2):34–39. A helpful guide for the nurse to examine her own communication behavior when she experiences problems in communication.

Jourard, S. 1971. *The Transparent Self, Part six: A Human Way of Being Nurses*, rev. ed. New York:

Van Nostrand Reinhold. Points out how sometimes members of the helping professions use their profession to maintain distance from their clients, and gives suggestions for avoiding this behavior.

Kesler, A. 1977. Pitfalls to avoid in interviewing outpatients. *Nurs* 77(9):70–73. Common communication problems are described. To overcome the problems, easy-to-learn techniques are suggested.

Littlefield, N. 1982. A brief encounter. *Am J Nurs* 82(9):1395–99. Describes how a skilled nurse with adequate supervision entered into a therapeutic relationship. A useful article for group discussion to explore physical contact, gift giving, and relating while performing treatment procedures. Techniques used by the author would not be suitable for everyone.

Peplau, H. 1960. Talking with patients. *Am J Nurs* 60(7):964–66. A classic article that contains many suggestions to aid the beginning nursing student in the development of meaningful dialogue with clients.

Rogers, C. 1973. The characteristics of a helping relationship, in W. Bennis, Schein, E.H. Berlew, D., and Steele, F. (eds). *Interpersonal Dynamics,* 3rd ed. Homewood, Ill.: Dorsey Press. Dr. Rogers raises questions that members of the helping professions must ask themselves. As he answers these, he describes the attributes of the "helping professional."

Stewart, L.M., Dawson, D.F. 1979. Blind client sighted therapist: The interface. *J Psychiatr Nurs* 17(11):31–35. A description of the increased sensitivity to sound, touch, and smell as forms of communication for individuals who cannot see. Ways the sighted individual must modify communication patterns to accommodate the needs of those who cannot see are described.

Travelbee, J. 1971. *Interpersonal Aspects of Nursing,* 2nd ed. Philadelphia: F.A. Davis. Aids and barriers to effective communication are described in Chapter IX, entitled Concept: Communication. Chapter X, The Human-to-Human Relationship, contains a clearly written, comprehensive discussion of the nurse–client relationship, drawing heavily on existential philosophy.

Chapter 15

The Teaching and Learning Process

Janet-Beth McCann Flynn

Chapter Outline

- Objectives
- Glossary
- Introduction
- Learning
  Theories
  Principles of Learning
  Domains of Learning
  Learning Throughout the Life Span
  Barriers to Learning
  Facilitators of Learning
- Teaching
  Ethics of Teaching
  Teaching Throughout the Life Span
  Methods of Instruction
  Time, Space, Supplies, and Privacy
  Educational Tools or Aids
- The Nursing Process
  Assessment
  Planning
  Implementation
  Evaluation
- Summary
- Study Questions
- References
- Annotated Bibliography

Objectives

After completion of this chapter the reader will be able to:

- ▶ Define the terms in the glossary
- ▶ List the major theorists
- ▶ Describe the teaching process
- ▶ List methods of teaching
- ▶ Compare and contrast teaching methods for adults and children
- ▶ Compare and contrast barriers and facilitators of learning
- ▶ Discuss educational aids
- ▶ Discuss the role of the nurse in the teaching process

Glossary

Affective Domain. The area of learning that involves beliefs, attitudes, and values.

Barriers to Learning. Blocks that prevent learning.

Change Agents. Ones who facilitate change.

Cognitive Domain. The area of learning that involves the acquisition of factual information.

Facilitators of Learning. Factors that aid learning.

Goals. General statements of intent or outcome that are derived from needs identified by the nurse and the client together.

Learning. A permanent change in behavior that results from a meaningful learning experience.

Objectives. Narrow statements of intent that are derived from the goals.

Philosophy. An underlying system of beliefs that focuses an individual's thoughts and actions.

Principles of Learning. Rules under which learning occurs.

Psychomotor Domain. The area of learning that involves physical performance of skills.

Teaching. A purposeful activity based on goals and objectives in which one or more individuals provide information to one or more persons.

INTRODUCTION

Client teaching is one of the most important roles performed by nurses today. Although teaching has always been a part of the nurse's role, only in the last decades has this role been more clearly defined. These clarifications in the role of the nurse as a client teacher developed largely from nursing theories and the nursing process approach to client care. Other factors influencing the nurse's teaching role include: the American Nurses' Association's *Standards of Nursing Practice,* which describes the role of teaching as a function for all nurses;[1] *The Patient's Bill of Rights,* which indicates the client's right to know and to understand his or her diagnosis and treatment;[2] and in general, the ever-increasing base of knowledge from the biological and social sciences, education, and other fields that provide the nurse with tools and concepts that were not previously available; for example, theories of how people learn.

Nurses have been identified as the health-care providers who are most frequently involved in the assessment, planning, and implementation of the client teaching process.[3] Educating clients is extremely important in all aspects of the health-care process. Increasing a client's knowledge about a particular illness, surgery, or preventable disease can help reduce anxiety and assists the person to gain some control of the situation. The client's ability for self-care is then increased and the client has a better chance of staying healthy. Since one of the major goals of nursing is to assist individuals to achieve and maintain the highest health possible, knowledge

of the teaching–learning process is a valuable tool.

The **teaching** process, according to Redman, states that "teaching is a special form of structured, sequenced communication by which the one teaching helps another to learn."[4] **Learning** is defined as a change in behavior. These changes can be shifts in performance, knowledge, or attitudes.[5] Nurses, as **change agents,** encourage changes in behavior by providing information and promoting adaptation required in alterations of health states. In order to carry out the task of client teaching, nurses need to know how to apply the concepts of teaching and learning.

LEARNING

Theories

To examine the teaching–learning process, it is important to know how people learn. The process of human learning has been of interest to philosophers, psychologists, and educators for some time. Writings show concern for how people learn as far back as Aristotle.[6] Current theories of learning have evolved to explain how people learn, what they learn, and why they learn. In order to teach, nurses first have to be able to answer these questions and explore some of the theories of learning.

In the early development of learning theory, philosophers theorized about how individuals learn. These early theories were based on reflection, not on experimental data. Thomas Hobbes and John Locke were two early philosophers who reflected that people learn of the world through their senses and their experiences with the environment.[7]

With the birth of psychology came clinical research designed to test learning theories. Early scientific researchers included John Watson (1875–1958) and Ivan Pavlov (1849–1936).[8] Working independently, each formulated a theory of learning now called "behaviorism," the study of observable behavior. Behaviorist theory was founded on the premise that learning is based on conditioning and can be changed through careful manipulation of the environment.

Edward L. Thorndike (1874–1949) advanced the behaviorist theory.[9] He viewed the learner as passive within the environment and felt that learning could be transferred to new situations. He was concerned with the transfer of factual learning to everyday practice. He proposed that learning should be based on a careful assessment of the learner's behavior. This is an important concept and one quite relevant for nurses.

Another theorist whose work can readily be applied to nursing is John Dewey (1858–1952).[10] He believed that the outcome of learning should be clear to the learner at the *beginning* of the educational experience. He also developed the idea that the aim of education should be the growth of individuals toward independence. This idea, too, is congruent with the ultimate goal of nursing.

Stimulus–response learning theory was proposed by the psychologist B. F. Skinner, (b. 1904), whose work is based on objective laboratory observation of experimental animals.[11] He views the causes of behavior as due to both the environment and the genetic heritage. Skinner feels that most human learning is caused by environmental experiences. Within this framework, the learner is viewed as passive, reacting to stimuli, and controlled by the environment in which he or she lives. Teaching, according to Skinner, is simply the arrangement of the environment in which the individual learns.

Jerome Bruner's (b. 1915) theory adds an interesting dimension to the study of learning, because it considers how values and cultural differences affect learning.[12] He views learners as persons active within the environment, not simply reactors to it.

Robert Gagne (b. 1916) defines learning as a change in human capability that cannot be accounted for by maturation, growth, or development.[13] He writes of learning as hierarchies going from simple to complex. One must master the lower part of the hierarchy to be able to grasp the more difficult, abstract concepts and problem-solving skills at the top of the hierarchy.

No one theory explains how people learn. Each theory has strengths and weaknesses, so nurses must select the most relevant features of each to assist them in writing a comprehensive teaching plan.

Principles of Learning

The teaching–learning process is based on many rules or **principles of learning** that are drawn from the theories of learning. The nurse's ability to design a teaching plan can be enhanced if these principles are kept in mind (Table 15–1). In order for people to learn, each principle of learning must be considered.

Domains of Learning

Learning has been grouped into three distinct areas that are called domains.[14,15] The **cognitive domain** deals with knowledge and facts that require the brain to process and retain information. This domain includes sorting, storing, recalling, and applying information. The highest level of the cognitive domain encompasses problem solving and evaluating the problem-solving process.

The **affective domain** encompasses attitudes, values, and emotions. Since values and beliefs are ingrained in the unconscious and difficult to change, ethical issues are involved in changing values. Is it ethical to attempt to change someone's value system? An important factor involved in learning in this domain is to allow the client to evaluate and incorporate new learning.

The third domain of learning is the **psychomotor domain**, involving learning physical skills; for example, preparing and injecting insulin.

Learning Throughout the Life Span

As humans grow and develop, their ability to grasp ideas from their environment changes, and all of the domains of learning are affected.

Infants and young children absorb information from the world through their senses. Infants learn to distinguish their mother's voice and face from other voices and faces and begin to distinguish between their mother and themselves. Early learning occurs in all of the domains, but in infants it is most obvious in the cognitive and the psychomotor domains. Babies learn that crying brings relief from hunger, discomfort, or boredom. They learn that smiling and cooing result in getting picked up and cuddled.

Young children's thinking is concrete and based on experience, and they are incapable of

TABLE 15–1. PRINCIPLES OF LEARNING

Principle	Explanation	Nursing or Teaching Actions
Internal Principles (Those Within Each Person)		
Attitude	Accepting attitude facilitates learning.	Assess the client's attitude. Is it accepting or hostile and rejecting.
Values	A personal way of evaluating a situation based on a lifetime of experiences.	Material should be presented in a way that is congruent with the values of the learner.
Maturation	The client must be developmentally able to learn and must have the appropriate mental and physical skills.	Careful assessment of growth and development should be conducted to determine motor skill ability and psychosocial ability.
Motivation	The client must want to learn the information.	Assess the cues the client is giving. Is he questioning? Interested?
Readiness to learn	The client must be ready and willing to learn.	Assess the acceptance of the health state. Is the client ready to discuss relevant factors of illness?
Meaningfulness	The information must have meaning for the client. Can it be understood and related to previous learning?	Does the client understand the information and is it important to the life situation?
External Principles (Those From the Environment That Affect Individuals)		
Participation	The client should be an active participant in the learning process.	Encourage involvement through manipulation of materials.
Repetition	Material is more likely to be retained if it is repeated.	Use a variety of teaching materials to present the same information.
Feedback	The client will learn more effectively with continuous and prompt feedback.	Provide comments, reassurance, and other information about performance promptly and objectively.
Action	The client retains information longer if it is usable.	Provide opportunities for use of new information.
Organization	The information should be in a predetermined organized format, moving from simple to complex, and based on previous knowledge.	Assess learning needs and determine the plan before beginning.
Environment	Conducive to learning, free of distractions, well lit, and private.	Prepare the environment prior to the experience.
Physical and emotional ability	The client should be physically and emotionally able to receive the information.	Assess physical and emotional state before beginning.
Reinforcement	Positive reinforcement and encouragement should be provided.	Provide immediate feedback.

abstraction. They learn by manipulating objects in the environment. Children learn through playing and asking questions[16] (Fig. 15–1).

Older children begin to learn values, acquire knowledge, and increase psychomotor skills. The attention span is longer, and the child is able to learn from formal teaching experiences, as well as from play. Children between the ages of 7 and 11 have a basic understanding of their health state, and as they grow older and

increase their knowledge base, the ability to understand more abstract ideas increases.

Important intellectual changes occur during *adolescence*. The knowledge base of adolescents has increased sufficiently for them to be able to understand concepts. The adolescent experiences an increased interest in abstract ideas and values, such as truth, love, faith, liberty, and other concepts that cannot be seen or touched. Traditional values are questioned. Ad-

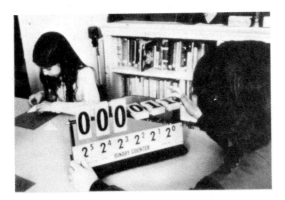

Figure 15–1. Young children learn through play.

olescents learn by seeking information, through questioning and reading, as well as by manipulating the environment. By using these methods of learning, they are able to understand relationships between ideas.

Adults have a great deal of basic knowledge and are able to think about abstract ideas. Values are well established and many psychomotor skills are highly refined. Adults are capable of learning information through reading, questioning, analyzing, and making decisions based on learning.

As individuals grow and develop, their ability to learn changes. As people experience life, they develop emotional, psychological, and intellectual strengths and weaknesses. These strengths and weaknesses affect an individual's ability to learn and are called facilitators of and barriers to learning.

Barriers to Learning

Barriers to learning are things that get in the way of learning. They can come from within the client (internal) or from the environment (external).

Internal factors are such things as present health or emotional states, previous experiences, and personal values that contribute to the way the client thinks, acts, and behaves (Table 15–2). Nurses need to look at barriers to learning. High levels of anxiety, for example, do not permit satisfactory learning. If the client is worried about impending surgery or painful treatments, learning might not be a priority.

Depression is another factor influencing learning. If the client is depressed, energy, motivation, or interest to learn may be decreased.

Negative experiences with the health-care system also can contribute to an individual client's ability to learn.

Educational level and intellectual ability both play an important part in the learning process. If clients cannot understand what is being taught, learning will not be meaningful.

Readiness to learn is another potential barrier and has two components. The first component, emotional readiness, determines the client's willingness to learn. The second component, experiential readiness, is determined by the client's past experiences, skills, attitudes, and values.[17] The two components are closely related. If the client does not understand the purpose of a treatment, motivation to learn about it may be lowered.

The client's present health state also can be a barrier to learning. If a person is so ill that

TABLE 15–2. INTERNAL AND EXTERNAL BARRIERS TO LEARNING

Internal Barriers	External Barriers
Anxiety	Environment
Depression	Time of teaching
Denial of illness, crisis, or loss	The method of teaching
Negative experience with the health-care system	The level of the material presented
Previous negative experience with the disease process	The nurse-teacher
Educational and vocabulary level	
Lack of readiness to learn	
Pain	
Fever	
Inability to accept the sick role or overacceptance of the sick role	
Values and beliefs that are not congruent with the health-care system	

activities of daily living cannot be carried out, the client may not have the energy to learn.

Inability to accept the sick role is another barrier that can affect a client's ability to learn.

Finally, if the goal of the nurse is different from that of the client, if attitudes, values, and beliefs conflict, the client may block out what the nurse is teaching.

External barriers to learning include those factors that the client may not be able to control. Environment plays an important role when barriers to learning are examined. The environment in which the teaching and learning take place needs to be controlled so that is is bright, free of noise, cool, and airy. It also should be structured so that privacy is ensured if required. Lack of family or group support can be another external barrier to learning.

The time of teaching is an important consideration. After a rest period or first thing in the morning are usually the best times for teaching. Late in the day or when the client is tired would be a poor choice.

Teaching methods need to be well chosen in accordance with individual client characteristics and needs.

Certain characteristics and approaches by the nurse also can present learning barriers. The client may not be motivated to learn if the nurse is distant, too busy, or judgmental. Failure to establish an effective nurse–client relationship also can limit a client's learning.

The nurse will be most successful as a teacher if learning barriers are assessed for each client and plans for client teaching are prepared according to individual needs.

Facilitators of Learning

Just as there are barriers to learning, there are **facilitators of learning**. A facilitator is something that aids indivudals to learn. Facilitators may be internal or external (Table 15–3). Internal facilitators include positive experiences with the health-care system, motivation and interest in the learning experience, a stable health state, and the ability to adapt to the sick role.

External facilitators include a pleasant environment conducive to learning, a supportive family, a teaching method that is based on the client's learning needs, and a supportive nurse. Every effort should be made to break down barriers and to support facilitators.

TEACHING

Teaching can be described as activities presented by a teacher that help learners to absorb new material in a structured and sequential manner. The teacher controls the learning situation and introduces information that causes the learners to change their behaviors. Teaching, therefore, is an active process and a unique form of communication.

Health teaching is an important role for the nurse. Instructing clients to carry out their own care, administer their medications safely, and perform psychomotor skills, can often make the difference between a healthy life and an unhealthy one, and in some cases may prevent severe complications or death.

Teaching is an art and although some nurses are natural teachers, others are not. Everyone who engages in teaching must first learn the formalities of the teaching process. Like principles of learning, there are principles of teaching.

Teaching is a great deal more than simply the imparting of knowledge to another. Teaching a person about a disease does not mean that

TABLE 15–3. INTERNAL AND EXTERNAL FACILITATORS OF LEARNING

Internal Factors	External Factors
Stable emotional and physical state	Environment
Positive experiences with the health-care system in the past	Family support
Positive outcomes of previous altered health states	Method of teaching
Desire or motivation to learn	The nurse
Readiness to learn	
Absence of fear, pain, fatigue	
Ability to accept the sick role and to strive to attain a higher level of health	

the person actually learns the material. Learning is the client's option. Teaching offers the opportunity for learning. Teaching involves decreasing the threat of change, and it supports changing behaviors that facilitate positive adaptation.

There are many factors that the nurse must consider before teaching. These factors relate to the nature of teaching, and they are the framework on which to build. The broadest of these is **philosophy** (Chapter 3).

Other factors arise when philosophies are considered. Nurses face several questions of philosophy with regard to teaching. One issue concerns how much and what information should be shared with the clients and how much independence clients should be allowed or should be required of them while participating in health care.[18] Other issues include: Who determines what is to be taught? How much should be taught? How much should the family participate in the learning? And who should teach the actual material? These issues are all important. In many agencies, the physician decides what is taught and when. This can present a problem for the nurse if the physician does not think that the client should know. The client, on the other hand, is questioning every available person, trying to get more information. If the nurse provides the information, he or she may be in conflict with the physician. Another issue is how much should be taught. According to Redman, this issue can be resolved "when the patient's goals and the nurse's goals are congruent."[19] These goals can be determined mutually at the outset of the teaching process. This will provide both client and nurse with a set of goals to achieve.

Another factor, family participation in the learning experience, should be established during the mutual goal-setting period. If an individual wants the family to learn about the condition or the care, they should be included.

Who should teach is an important question. In many agencies the physician might do the teaching or delegate it to the nurse or another member of the health-care team. For example, the dietitian teaches nutrition to a diabetic; an entrostomal therapist teaches colostomy care; the physical therapist teaches crutch walking and wheelchair transfer; the occupational ther-

apist might teach activities of daily living; and the nurse teaches foot care and insulin administration to diabetics.

The philosophies of learning are important to examine. They help determine the role of the nurse on the health-care team.

A number of types of goals have been discussed, and a further description of the nature of goals will help clarify their importance. **Goals** can be defined as general statements of intent of outcome derived from needs. Both the nurse the client have goals. It is important for the nurse to discuss goals with clients for them to negotiate mutual goals.[20] The client and the nurse then strive to meet these goals together in order to reach an optimum health state.

Nurses must know if clients have achieved their goal, and this can be done by using objectives. **Objectives** are narrow statements about the outcomes derived from the goals (Fig. 15–2). An objective is a statement describing a proposed change in a learner—a statement of what the learner is to be like when he or she has successfully completed a learning experience. It is a description of behavior the learner should be able to demonstrate.[21] In other words, objectives are *observable* changes in behavior.

Objectives are stated in behavioral terms, and each goal may have several objectives. Objectives are structured in terms of several small steps and are more obtainable. Each objective can be seen as a step in the staircase to health (Fig. 15–3). Each objective is followed by an

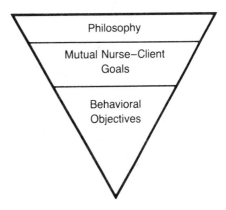

Figure 15–2. Goals and objectives can be derived from philosophy.

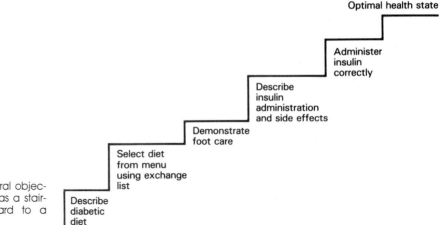

Figure 15–3. Behavioral objectives can be viewed as a staircase reaching upward to a broad goal.

outcome criterion. The outcome criterion lists the behaviors and provides a reference to a period of time. This enables the nurse to evaluate the level of success of the teaching plan. Objectives also may reflect the philosophies of the client, the nurse, and the health-care institution (Fig. 15–4), and can be united by the teaching–learning process. For example, the basic philosophy of the client, the nurse, and the health-care system is to restore the highest health state possible for the client.

Once the nurse and the client determine mutual goals, the nurse should prepare behavioral objectives and write them on the care plan with outcome criteria. If these objectives are lacking in clarity, it will be impossible to evaluate learning. In addition to this, the client can help evaluate progress as can other members of the health-care team.

The goals and objectives need to be attainable and realistic. It is the responsibility of client and nurse to keep them so. At the end of the designated time, the objective could be re-examined to discover if it was reasonable and if the behavior was attained. In an instance where the behavior change (or goal attainment) may take a long period of time, a series of progressive objectives can be written for one goal.

Another important factor to consider when writing objectives is setting priorities. Certain things are necessary to learn first for the foundation learning.

Objectives should be written in terms of behaviors so that they can be observed readily by the nurse, thus enabling evaluation of the client's progress. Mager states that "there are many 'loaded' words, words open to a wide range of interpretation."[22] Examples of these phrases include: to know, to fully understand, to have a basic knowledge, and to appreciate. What exactly do these phrases mean? What does it mean to know something? How does the nurse "know" that the client "knows." Objectives should be written so that they can be observed or measured (Table 15–4). There are a variety of ways in which behavioral objectives

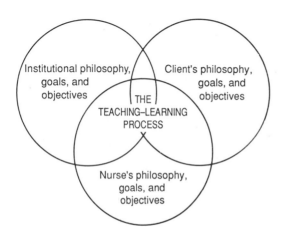

Figure 15–4. Congruent philosophies, goals, and objectives facilitate the teaching–learning process.

TABLE 15–4. LIST OF SELECTED OBJECTIVE WORDS

Weasel Words[a]	Clearly Defined Words[b]
Know	Describe
Acquire knowledge	Identify
Fully understand	Define
Realize	Compare
Be familiar with	Contrast
Appreciate	List
Value	State
Feel	Recall
	Differentiate
	Recite
	Demonstrate
	Write

[a]Words open to interpretation
[b]Words open to little interpretation

can be written. Table 15–5 illustrates some of the possibilities. A broad goal statement may precede the step-by-step behavioral objectives. Another way of writing behavioral objectives might be to list each objective without a broader goal. Or a time dimension may be added. Time, in the example used in Table 15–5, "at discharge" could mean days or weeks, and in a community setting, discharge could mean months or years. The ultimate goal of any series of mutually negotiated goals and objectives is the client's adjustment to alterations in health state, with maximum adaptation of the client and the family.

Nursing objectives may appear on the care plan, and they delineate what the nursing objectives are. Nursing objectives outline what behaviors the nurse should demonstrate. For example, a nursing goal might be stated: prevent breakdown of tissue on the feet. Individual objectives associated with the goal would outline the various steps in meeting and evaluating this goal such as:

- Wash the feet daily with mild soap and warm water
- Inspect for reddened areas
- Dry between each toe after washing
- Examine the nails of the toes for integrity and condition
- Apply lotion
- Apply powder between the toes

These are behaviors of the nurse, and in most cases they require the client's cooperation but do not necessarily involve client participation. Both nursing objectives and mutual objectives can be used simultaneously or individually, depending on the individual assessment and evaluation.

The beginning nurse may experience difficulty in distinguishing between nurse–client goals and nursing goals. A rule of thumb is to examine who is expected to perform the behavior. If it is the nurse, then it is a nursing goal. If it is the client, then it is a mutual or client goal. It takes practice and experience to be able to see the difference and to write clear, concise, appropriate objectives.

It is possible to arrange objectives in a hi-

TABLE 15–5. POSSIBLE WAYS TO WRITE BEHAVIORAL OBJECTIVES

Goal-Directed Objectives
The client will understand the diabetic diet, as evidenced by:
  Naming all foods that are not to be eaten
  Selecting diabetic diet from the hospital menu
  Describing the purpose of the diet
  Describing the symptoms of insulin shock

Behavioral Objectives
By discharge the client will be able to:
  List all foods that are not to be eaten
  Select diabetic diet from lists of foods using an exchange list
  Describe the symptoms of insulin shock
  Demonstrate proper foot care
  Differentiate between the type of insulin the client uses and other types of insulin
  Demonstrate correct insulin administration technique
  Administer own insulin
  Discuss insulin site rotation

Time-Reference Objective List
At the end of five days the client will be able to:
  Discuss administration of insulin
  List allowed foods
  Describe foot care
At the end of seven days the client will be able to:
  Demonstrate correct handling of syringe
  Draw up prescribed amount of insulin
  Observe the nurse administer insulin
  Select balanced prescribed diet from menu
  Compare and contrast insulin shock and diabetic coma
On discharge the client will be able to:
  Demonstrate correct syringe technique
  Draw up prescribed insulin dose
  Administer correctly and discuss site rotation
  Prepare weekly menu using prescribed diet
  Demonstrate foot care

erarchy from simple to complex (Table 15–6). The cognitive and psychomotor domains are arranged from simple to complex and the affective domain from mild to increasing internalization.

We are concerned with these taxonomies of learning to be able to analyze and plan what is to be taught and determine by what means it is to be taught. The nurse can use printed information for the cognitive domain. For the affective domain the nurse would use films, readings, discussion groups, role modeling, and various other techniques. The psychomotor domain could be best approached through manipulation of materials and practice.

Ethics of Teaching

Of the three domains of learning, the affective domain is usually the most difficult with which to work. How does one change a person's attitudes or values? An even more interesting question is should this be done? Is it ethical to manipulate a client? There are more practical issues, such as how does the nurse assess the affective domain? How does one write these objectives? How does one teach and evaluate learning?

Conley writes, "The hesitancy of teachers to use affective measures for evaluation of purposes stems partly from the inadequacy of ap-

TABLE 15–6. TAXONOMIES OF OBJECTIVES[a]

Cognitive Domain[b]

Knowledge
 Defines terms
 Identifies specific facts
 Recalls information

Comprehension
 Translates information into own words
 Identifies meanings of abbreviations and scientific terms
 Summarizes information
 Interprets information
 Defines implications and consequences of actions

Application
 Applies facts to situations
 Identifies steps in procedures

Analysis
 Distinguishes facts from hypotheses
 Identifies relationships between ideas and facts

Synthesis
 Describes personal experiences, ideas, and feelings
 Prepares plan of action using facts

Evaluation
 Evaluates behaviors using internal standards
 Evaluates behaviors using external standards

Affective Domain[c]

Receiving
 Awareness
 Willingness to receive information

Responding
 Responds with facts but has not internalized material

Responds with commitment
Responds with total commitment and is satisfied with the change

Valuing
 Accepts a value
 Prefers a set of values

Organization
 Places values into a framework
 Compares the relationships of values
 Identifies prominent values in the framework

Characterization by a value or value complex
 Acts consistently according to value set
 Contrasts values
 Discusses a philosophy of life
 Discusses a philosophy of health

Psychomotor Domain

Perception
 Observes skill
 Identifies and describes skill
 Recalls the skill

Readiness
 States readiness to perform skills
 Demonstrates the ability

Response
 Imitates the behavior of the skill
 Performs skill independently

Adaptation
 Adapts the skill correctly to meet own needs
 Performs the skill correctly without prior demonstration
 Performs the skill correctly after a specified lapse of time

[a]Domains of learning are ordered from simple to complex.
[b]Adapted from B.S. Bloom, M.D. Engelhart, E.J. Furst, W.H. Hill, and D.R. Krathwohl, Taxonomy of Educational Objectives: The Classification of Educational Goals. Handbook I: Cognitive Domain (New York: David McKay Co., 1956).
[c]Adapted from D.R. Krathwohl, B.S. Bloom, and B.B. Masia, Taxonomy of Educational Objectives: The Classification of Educational Goals. Handbook II: Affective Domain (New York: David McKay Co., 1964).

praisal techniques. Frequently, behaviors in the affective domain must be inferred from overt behaviors, which may or may not be valued. . . . "[23] Another factor that makes assessment of learning in this domain difficult is its very nature. This domain encompasses the value of privacy. Individuals may be uncomfortable, embarrassed, or threatened with discussion of values, attitudes, and morals. They may become offended and not wish to pursue further nursing intervention, or they may simply refuse any nursing intervention in this area. Assessment in this area is also difficult because a client may conform to the change while the nurse is observing and return to former behaviors when the nurse is not present. This is not necessarily a devious maneuver. Clients may conform momentarily because they are intimidated by authority, they may generally like the nurse and want to please but have no real belief in the change, and they adapt behavior in the nurses presence and rapidly forget when the nurse is gone. Finally, the affective domain requires that people examine their own philosophy and way of life in order to make changes. This is generally a slow procedure at best. It may take years to change attitudes and values.

The role of the nurse in teaching values or assisting clients to change values is many-faceted. First and most important, nurses should examine their own values, which can get in the way when working with another. It is important to understand that judgmental attitudes are never helpful in a helping relationship. If, for example, the client employs health practices that the nurse views as unusual or unhealthy, a values conflict is already taking place.

A third thing to consider is the ethics of the situation. Is it ethical and in the client's best interest to make a change?

The goals of teaching, in the affective domain, are the development of new sets of values that support healthful behaviors acceptable to the client and family.

Teaching in this domain is difficult. Conducting discussion groups is an excellent method for helping clients clarify their value systems. In groups with common problems, members learn from one another. They are accepted into the group easily and without judgment. Some examples of these groups include ostomy clubs, mastectomy groups, or Weight Watchers.

Involving the family can help to make changes in many instances. Another method of teaching in this domain includes active participation in the learning experience (such as role playing). Since changes in this domain take time to internalize, observed changes in behavior may be slow. This can be frustrating for nurses. Patience and the client's freedom of choice should always be kept in mind. If the client is slow to change, the nurse should focus on supporting identified strengths that will aid in positive adaptation.

Teaching Throughout the Life Span

Teaching strategies must be adapted for the level of understanding (Fig. 15–5). This is particularly true when teaching children. The first step in this process is to assess the individual child's growth, development, and level of understanding. Infants and very young children are difficult to teach, because they have not yet acquired language. At this level, the nurse might just give tender loving care to the child and provide a safe and stimulating environment. Holding, rocking, smiling, talking, singing, and providing mobiles will be effective. Health teaching of young children is generally focused on the child's mother or other caretaker.

Teaching of children usually focuses on play. Petrillo and Sanger write that, "Play is a natural phenomenon that leads to learning. . . ."[24] Concepts to be taught can be incorporated into games, puppet shows, coloring books, dolls, dollhouses, doll hospitals, group play, arts and crafts, and many other methods. Teaching children is creative and fun. A plan should be used, however, to guide the teaching–learning process in order to present the material in an orderly fashion.

Slightly older children can be allowed to manipulate syringes, intravenous (IV) tubings, alcohol wipes, empty medicine bottles, and other equipment. They can be taught to put dressings on dolls, and give them IVs and injections. Simple explanations of why the child will need to have these items should accompany the play. Art materials can be used as another medium for teaching. While the nurse and child are engaged in these activities the nurse can be

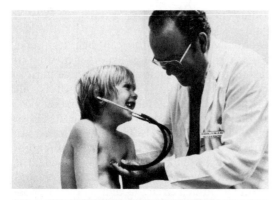

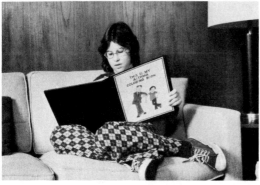

Figure 15–5. Teaching strategies must be adapted for the level of understanding.

teaching the child what to expect during procedures.

Adequate time always should be provided for tours of the hospital, treatment rooms, operating rooms, and recovery rooms. Children who are going to experience painful treatments or surgery should always be taken on tours and permitted to ask questions.

Children need constant reinforcement and repetition. Parents should be encouraged to participate in these play learning experiences, because parental support increases the child's ability, and the parents can use these methods and reinforce the learning.

Adolescents are able to understand more complex explanations, and their reading ability and vocabulary are considerably greater. They are curious about what is going on and as to the outcome of disease processes. Disfiguring diseases and conditions are very hard to deal

with at this stage of life when peer group identity is so critical to development. Emotional support and role modeling is very important. Adult and child teaching strategies can be blended effectively to produce good teaching strategies for this age group.

Generally speaking, the adult has mastered reading, conceptualizing, perceiving relationships, and many other sophisticated behaviors that come with maturity and experience. Adults can be taught using a variety of teaching methods. The teaching methods can be used alone or in combination (see the discussions of methods of instruction and educational tools below). Some examples of these include: audiovisual materials, lectures, discussion, raising questions, and use of games (Fig. 15–6).

Occasionally, special consideration has to be given elderly clients. Because the aging process may reduce mental or sensory capacities, elderly people may have difficulty learning or remembering. They may not be able to understand the nature of the condition and the need for long-term medications for a chronic condition. Older people may need more repetition of the material being taught. Teaching plans and educational tools might have to be adapted for the client who can no longer see or hear as well as in the past.

Methods of Instruction

Once goals and objectives have been developed, specific methods of instruction are selected to meet the objectives. Methods of instruction are as important as writing the goals and objectives. Teaching may evolve spontaneously during routine care when either the client or the nurse questions the other.

The quality of the nurse's interpersonal skills is very important in face-to-face teaching, as is sensitivity to the client's needs. The nurse also should be aware of medical language and attempt to avoid this when teaching, since most people do not know medical terms.

Other methods of teaching include placing the client in an identity group (Parents Without Partners, Alcoholics Anonymous [AA]) and use of audiovisual aids, self-study, or games.

The objectives generally determine what is to be taught and can determine the method to be used. Some types of information lend them-

```
G B A C K L M E C T K A B S N U T R I T I O N C A I T N
L L L T O U E J H F S Y R I N G E A K W J H G F R N R L
O O U P L K P L U K Y L P A T D S D E O E J H G W S A Y
U O C C N P S R T A S V A N P O P R J P U S E F Y U H R
C D B D O N E P L U S J I P R S O G F L Y C U C U L J F
F S I E P S O S T O Q I N S F T L J U U T P T A I I T G
B U O A U O E F G G P D M F E W Y K T S K E E R E N R H
K G O N N N R G O G R D R G W Q U L Y W Z T I B R R I K
F A S T I N G B L O O D S U G A R E E I J T U O T E K L
T R K I N D K J G F T C F T F R I J C F T H Y H Y A L O
R I M M M M J K H R E C E C G E A R J G P I Q Y Q C H P
I N N A E D D D J E I E A A H U E J E H O R U D P T F W
N K I R S A C E T O N E O R Y X X K A K E S E R U I E E
K E V T P H L L I S S N V T E E E J N N T T Y A V O R R
F O U R P L U S S G F E R R S U T T E E R F A T S N Y T
O I N S U L I N S I T E R O T A T I O N I E D E W A R D
U M A U M I N R E I N S U L I N E R E R N N O S U G A R
R N B M D Y I Y T N N O M I E R P T H R E E P L U S T D
P O C N P T O U J E X C H A N G E E U W W W E W E R G K
L E A H Y P O G L Y C E M I A A A W F A T I G U E T U R
```

CARBOHYDRATES	FATS
BLOOD SUGAR	SUGAR
FASTING BLOOD SUGAR	THIRST
ONE PLUS	EXERCISE
TWO PLUS	POLYURIA
THREE PLUS	INSULIN REACTION
FOUR PLUS	INSULIN
PROTEIN	INSULIN SITE ROTATION
ACETONE	NUTRITION
HYPOGLYCEMIA	SYRINGE
EXCHANGE	GLUCOSE
FATIGUE	FOOT CARE

Figure 15–6. Games can be an effective way of teaching terminology.

selves best to one style of teaching, and some to others.

The one-to-one method of teaching requires the nurse to present the information to the client. Factual information can be presented at a level that can be understood, and the client can freely question the nurse.

Group discussion is another method of teaching. This method encourages discussion of feelings and experiences. The nurse serves as a facilitator by clarifying when appropriate. This method is appropriate when members of the group have similar needs. During the discussion, the nurse can provide information, clarify, direct, and answer questions. Group discussion occasionally brings out some individual client's erroneous thinking.

Lecture is another common form of teaching and probably the one most familiar. Lecture consists, basically, of one person presenting factual material to others. Many hospitals have lectures for mothers-to-be on basic child care. This type of presentation does not require much interaction between the lecturer and the learner, but it can be effective when there is a need to present a number of facts to a large group of people.

Role playing, a more involving type of learning experience, is a teaching–learning technique in which the client consciously pretends to be someone else for a brief period of time. It is a type of playacting in which the client attempts to understand how the other person feels or reacts. This way of teaching tends to give insight that had not previously existed into a situation. Role playing helps individuals to understand what another person is feeling and is a most effective teaching method in the affective domain.

Role modeling is a technique for teaching in the affective domain. It provides teaching by example, and the nurse serves as the model to be copied. This technique works very well with children and adolescents, or with persons who are unfamiliar with the information. It is important to note that the nurse frequently acts as a role model, whether aware or not.

Demonstration and practice are teaching techniques for the psychomotor domain. The nurse demonstrates a procedure, such as insulin adminstration, and then allows the client to manipulate the equipment, and draw up the insulin. Demonstrations may progress through several sessions until the individual is ready to self-administer the insulin. Successive meetings might consist of the client returning the demonstration from start to finish faultlessly. Demonstration as a teaching technique is generally not good for large groups, because not everyone can observe, particularly if the demonstration requires small motions, such as drawing up insulin, or small areas, such as in umbilical cord care of newborns. As with role modeling, the demonstrator must have perfect technique. For clients to learn the skill, they must practice with supervision, and it is important that the nurse ensure adequate time, space, and suppies for all members in the group.

Assessment of learning and progress is essential with technique learning. The client must be provided with feedback about progress and with support when having difficulty performing the procedure.

Other ways of teaching include self-study, audiovisual aids, teaching machines, flip charts, and programmed instruction. Generally, these are used to assist the teacher and will be discussed in the section on educational tools.

Time, Space, Supplies, and Privacy

Teaching takes more time than one would expect, so nurses need to provide a block of time sufficient for the activity. The physical environment is an important factor to consider. Adequate space and chairs are necessary for a lecture or discussion. Well-lighted, well-ventilated areas are a priority. Supplies needed for demonstration, explanation, or clarification should be chosen carefully and assembled in advance. If return demonstration is a part of the plan, then enough supplies for each individual are also necessary. Finally, some things may require privacy; for example, birth control information, or colostomy care. Drawing the curtain around a person in a busy four-bed unit may not be adequate. Another place where no one will interrupt or overhear may be more appropriate. Sometimes in our cramped health-care institutions, these places are hard to find and might mean the head nurse's office or the conference room, where privacy could be assured.

Educational Tools or Aids

Allowing clients to experience the same information through more than one method is an excellent way to repeat the information. Recent research has demonstrated that certain individuals learn better through listening, whereas others learn best when they can see the material visually. Some learn best when combining listening and viewing, and still others learn from experience only. Very few people learn from only one route, so combinations of methods are beneficial. A mother-to-be, for example, can be given a pamphlet to read on bathing an infant, followed by a film, demonstration, and finally practice on a doll. This sequence provides the individual with several experiences. This example is known as a multimedia approach to teaching. In addition to stimulating more than one sense, it also provides information through a variety of methods.

Materials such as pamphlets, booklets, printed cards, and specially prepared instructions are widely used to help meet the client's objectives. Reading ability is a factor here. Is the client able to read? Many people who cannot read are embarrassed and may not admit this problem. At what level does this client read? Does the client read English? If English is the client's second language, does she or he prefer to read in the native language? Reading materials can be given to a person to read before more formal teaching begins, followed by implementation of the teaching plan.

Another type of educational tools is the audiovisual (AV) aids. The AVs are combinations of sound and sight, and occasionally touch and smell. They bring another dimension to the teaching plan. Some examples of AV aids include slide and tape presentations, speech and slide presentations, tape cassettes, photographs, slides, pictures, and workbooks. Models or replicas of body parts are sometimes used—in much the same way "Mrs. Chase" is used to teach student nurses. These methods should always be incorporated into an overall plan.

Programmed instruction (PI) manuals are another teaching aid. These begin with simple material and become more complex as the reader progresses. They are designed so that the learner can move at a comfortable pace. Each step is designed so that the learner masters it before moving onto the next step. The nurse should be available to provide additional information or answer questions when a client is using PI.

Games can be devised by the nurse as a teaching device. The client's participation in this activity helps the incorporation of recently acquired educational material. Developing games depends on the creativity of the designers. Again, games assist in meeting learning objectives. Games are popular with adults as well as children and adolescents.

Coloring and workbooks are especially good for children. These are available from many agencies and in various languages.

Posters and atractively designed bulletin boards are also effective aids, especially when used in clinical waiting rooms and offices.

Flip charts can be used by the nurse giving a talk to a group or to an individual client. They also can be used alone before or after contact with the more formal teaching presentation.

Most of these methods can be used in the hospital, the clinic, or the home. All of them can be used by an individual client or group of clients. Many can be used for adolescents as well as adults, but the level of the content and the speed of the presentation may be altered for understanding for younger persons and for persons whose reading comprehension is somewhat slower.

THE NURSING PROCESS

According to Yura and Walsh, "The nursing process can be applied in a variety of settings; it is flexible and adaptable, permitting the nurse to use judgment and creativity in caring for the client in an organized, orderly, and systematic manner."[25] This definition of the nursing process fits nicely with the teaching process, since both are dynamic processes, and include assessment, planning, implementation, and evaluation.

Assessment

The first step in the nursing process is the *assessment* phase, in which the client is observed and assessed. The nurse identifies what the learner needs to know and specifies characteristics and behaviors of the client (Fig. 15–7). What the client needs to know can be learned by questioning, listening, and observing behaviors. The client can be asked to do a procedure while the nurse observes the techniques and provides feedback. Many times this gives the nurse a clearer picture than if the client is asked to describe the process.

Another factor is potential learning needs. For example, a person who has diet-controlled diabetes might be told that insulin administration might one day be necessary. Another example of an anticipatory learning need is that of a pregnant woman who needs to learn how to bathe and feed an infant.

Characteristics of the client can be assessed by observation. One of these client characteristics is readiness. Growth and development have impact on readiness to learn. Clients who are ready to learn will ask questions of the nurse and appear interested. Conversely, clients who are not ready to learn will not ask direct questions and will not make much effort to partic-

---

Education Assessment

Name _____ Age _____ Diagnosis _____ Date of admission _____

Address _____ Phone _____ Date of interview _____

Marital status _____ Role in family _____ Children _____

House _____ Apt. _____ Stairs to entrance _____ Stairs to bedroom _____

Occupation _____ Education level _____ English reading ability _____

Cultural orientation _____ Language spoken _____

Chief complaint _____ How long has condition been present _____

Perception of condition _____

What has physician told client re: physical condition _____

What have others told client _____

What causes symptoms _____

What prevents symptoms _____

Questions about condition _____

Compliance with previous health regimens _____

Past experience with disease and with health care _____

Ability to learn _____ Readiness to learn _____ Anxious _____ Depressed _____

Current health state _____

Family response to illness _____

Family members' interest and ability to learn _____

Physical limitations—Fever _____ Pain _____ Medications _____ Vision _____ Hearing _____

Figure 15–7. The client education assessment tool.

ipate in the care. Clients might also become restless, anxious, or depressed when topics related to their condition are raised by the nurse or they might refuse to discuss them. Frequently, people who are not ready to learn are depressed or employing defense mechanisms such as denial. Others have maladaptively accepted the sick role to receive secondary gains.

Motivation is greatest when the client is ready to learn. Self-generated motivation is called internal motivation. The learner usually learns more and retains it longer.

External motivation comes from without and is usually created by the teacher. Rewards and praise are useful in fostering this type of motivation. If the nurse is able to determine the client's internal motivation, motivation can be increased by helping the learner see relationships between factors or concepts.

If there appear to be major learning barriers or significant problems related to any part of the teaching–learning process, it may be appropriate to state these as nursing diagnoses. Examples of such nursing diagnoses follow:

- Nonadherence to medical regimen related to knowledge deficit
- Anxiety related to knowledge deficit

Planning

Once the nurse has carefully assessed the educational needs, the second phase of the nursing process begins. In the *planning* phase, what to teach, how to teach, who will teach, where to teach, and when to teach are addressed. These all can be incorporated into a broad teaching plan (Fig. 15–8) and directed by goals and objectives.

Name ———— Age ———— Culture ———— Language ———— Address ———— Phone ————

Diagnosis ———————— Others to be taught (who) ———————— Address ———— Phone ————

Goals ————————————————————

Objectives ————————————

Objective	Content to be taught (what)	Teaching method (how)	Health care provider dept. (name) (who)	Time Date (when)	Location (where)	Evaluation method	Comments and observations

Figure 15–8. A teaching plan.

What to teach is based on the nurse's assessment of the individual's knowledge base and condition. Teaching–learning relies on the health state and on the client characteristics of readiness and motivation. What to teach can be determined by what the client wants to learn and relates to readiness to learn.

How to teach is the next decision that the nurse must take. The method chosen should reflect both what is to be taught and the individual's characteristics. Methods chosen should be the ones that involve the client the most, that is, the ones that stimulate interest. The domain in which the learning is to occur also should be considered when choosing a method, because of the different methods used in each domain.

Who will teach is another consideration. Generally, the nurse and others on the health team teach clients. A teaching plan for a diabetic client might involve the physician, the nurse, and the dietician. The nurse can serve as the link between all of the departments by reinforcing what the client has learned.

In addition to the client, who in the family needs to be taught about the client's condition and care? This can be determined by assessing cultural and developmental aspects, and cognitive development. Does the client's cultural background allow health teaching? Can the mother make decisions about follow-up care, and can she implement the teaching? Developmentally, is the individual old enough to learn the material? Do the parents or caretakers need to be included in the teaching plan? Does the client understand? Can the client read? Does he or she accept the sick role? All of these questions need to be considered when developing a teaching plan.

Where to teach is another issue and fairly easy to answer. Location of teaching depends on the method to be used and on the client's condition and location. If a film, lecture, or group discussion is to be used, it is important to secure a room large enough to accommodate the group. This usually takes advance planning, because space is often at a premium in today's health-care facilities. If flip charts or programmed instruction are to be used, the bedside or the home is as appropriate as the hospital. If filmstrips are used, the bedside or home can be used as well, but this generally involves reserv-

ing a portable projector. When one-to-one teaching is done, adequate time and privacy are required, and that involves preplanning. In many instances, pulling the curtains around the bed is not enough; therefore, arranging to take the client out of the room must be considered.

The best time for teaching is when the client is free of fatigue, fever, and pain, is ready to learn, and is motivated to get well. By careful assessment, planning, and implementation, these factors can be controlled, to an extent, when both the nurse and the client have a block of time to devote to the activity.

For major teaching needs, a specific teaching plan should be written to provide an organized structure of the who, what, where, and how of teaching. The plan is written and is placed on the cardex. A plan provides for a consistent approach for the nurse, and it provides structure. When client teaching is not the highest priority or only involves a few simple points, the teaching objective is listed on the regular care plan, and a separate teaching plan may not be necessary.

Implementation

Once a plan has been written, the next phase of the process is to implement it. During the *implementation* process, the person teaching needs to rely on knowledge of the theories of learning and teaching principles. While teaching, the nurse should allow the learner to proceed at a comfortable pace, because not all people learn at the same rate. Some individuals need a great deal of repetition, whereas others can grasp difficult concepts at once. The duration of the experience should be kept to a minimum, because attention spans can be short when people are anxious or in pain, but should be long enough to present the material.

Other steps in implementation should include giving advance knowledge of the content of the teaching plan. This can be done with a written outline or by saying what will be included. Charting for the teaching plan should be done so that others know what has been taught, and providing feedback to the client is helpful so that the client knows the strengths and weaknesses of the knowledge base.

When the nurse is implementing the plan, there are specific behaviors that can be used to make the teaching plan most effective. An important feature is to know and understand the material that is to be taught. Materials should be reviewed prior to the teaching session and an outline of content prepared to guide the session. If the person teaching is unsure of some of the material, he or she may be uneasy, and this will be conveyed to the client. Equally important is the establishment of a trusting nurse–client relationship. A good communication technique is essential for teaching. Making the client feel at ease and allowing him or her to ask questions prior to the actual session is helpful in establishing the relationship. Make eye contact with the client or clients during the presentation. Speak in language that is easy to understand. Be specific when giving information, especially instructions. Keep the session short. Tell the learners what you will be presenting first, then present material. Place all essential information first. Use verbal headings and refer back to initial outline of what was to be discussed. Repeat information and summarize prior to conclusion. Finally, allow time for questions and provide booklets or other written materials.

Evaluation

Evaluation is a form of determining what the client has learned and how behavior has changed as a result of nursing intervention. Evaluation is a crucial step in the nursing process, because it allows the nurse to see if the plan is effective and where reassessment is necessary.

Very specific criteria are needed to determine if the client has met the goals and objectives. The major purpose of goals and objectives serves to list observable items that are expressed as outcome criteria. Did the client meet those objectives and outcome criteria? If so the material has been learned and the behavior modified accordingly. If not, the situation needs to be reassessed, the nursing plan rewritten, and the new plan implemented and reevaluated.

Evaluation also serves to redirect or refocus nursing actions. If the client has learned some of the material, the nurse can go back to the assessment phase and begin the process again.

There are a variety of ways to evaluate learning. The one that we are most familiar with is the test. A test can be written (essay, short answer, multiple choice) or oral. We also can observe the behaviors that the client has learned. This is especially true when psychomotor skills are being evaluated. One way is to use check lists that test the necessary behaviors. The client gets a score that is compared with a predetermined acceptable pass or fail rate.

Evaluation is a continuous process. Because someone can repeat a list today does not mean that he or she will be able to do it tomorrow or in a week, so we must constantly and consistently monitor the client's learning. By using a formal teaching plan and proceeding through the evaluation phase, the nurse refocuses nursing interventions and the client's learning.

SUMMARY

Teaching is a primary role of the nurse and has been recognized as such for over a hundred years. The nurse's role in teaching is to assist clients to get well and to stay well.

To comprehend the teaching–learning process, nurses need to know how and why people learn. Many leaders from the fields of philosophy, education, and psychology have developed theories of learning. By knowing the writing of several theorists, the nurse can refine a theory of teaching and develop specific theory-based teaching methods.

There are three domains of learning. The cognitive domain refers to sorting and storing information. The affective domain encompasses attitudes, values, and emotions. Ethical issues are raised when one attempts to change another person's value system. The psychomotor domain involves the learning of skills.

Learning ability and learning needs change throughout life. Learning needs are different at all levels of development.

Many factors influence the learning process, and these can be grouped into barriers and facilitators. Barriers that impede learning include previous negative educational experiences, poor psychological and physical state, values, family support systems (that are either maladaptive, nonexistent, or different from the nurse's), poor past experiences with the healthcare system, and an environment not conducive to learning. Facilitators of learning enhance the ability to learn; they include adequate education and positive experiences with the health-care system, adaptive psychological and physical states, strong family support, congruent values, and an environment conducive to learning. Both facilitators of and barriers to learning need to be assessed by the nurse in order to formulate a comprehensive teaching plan.

Most nurses must learn how to teach. Teaching is an art; before nurses can begin to teach they must reflect on their philosophy of humanism, the role that environment plays in the learning situation, who fails when the client does not learn, and what is the best method of teaching. Once this has been accomplished, the nurse and others on the health-care team determine what is to be taught and who will teach. Realistic mutual goals and objectives to guide and direct the teaching plan are written in behavioral terms wtih the expected outcome of the teaching experience stated so that changes in behavior that indicate learning can be observed. Teaching methods and content vary depending on the age of the person being taught. Simple explanations are best for children. Explanations should increase in complexity as the age of the person increases.

Methods of teaching also vary and are determined from the objectives. Methods used also depend upon location of the teaching, the type of recipient (individual or group), the resources available, and the type of material to be presented (facts, values, or skills).

In the role as teacher, the nurse uses a variety of teaching aids, including films, reading material, filmstrips, and programmed instruction. These are very valuable, in that they add another dimension to the learning experience.

The nursing process can be used as a model for client teaching. Learning needs and personal characteristics of the client are assessed, the material and method planned, a teaching plan written, the plan implemented, and the results evaluated using the objectives on the teaching plan.

It is through careful assessment and use of the teaching process that the nurse can be an effective change agent and help clients attain their highest levels of wellness.

Study Questions

1. Why is it important to know learning theory?

2. What are the three domains of learning? Give an example of each.

3. List several barriers to learning. Give examples of how nursing actions can change them.

4. Write three behavioral objectives for an obese client.

5. List four teaching methods and give an example of what could be taught by each method.

6. Why is using more than one teaching method beneficial to client learning?

7. Give examples of teaching aids. How could they be used in client teaching?

8. What is a teaching plan? Why is it necessary?

9. Devise a teaching plan for a diabetic child. Compare this plan to an adult teaching plan.

References

1. American Nurses' Association, *Standards of Nursing Practice*. (Kansas City, Mo.: The American Nurses' Association), 1973.
2. American Hospital Association, *A Patient's Bill of Rights* (Chicago: The American Hospital Association), 1972.
3. E. Lee and J.L. Garvey. "How is inpatient education being managed?" *Hospitals, 51*, (1977): 75–82.
4. Barbara Klug Redman, *The Process of Patient Teaching*, 5th ed. (St. Louis: C. V. Mosby Co., 1985), 11.
5. P. Jones and W. Oertel, "Developing patient teaching objectives and techniques: A self-instructional program," *Nurse Educ* 2, (1977).
6. Aristotle. "The golden mean," in *Classics in Ed-*

ucation (New York: Philosophical Library, 1966).

7. Virginia C. Conley, *Curriculum and Instruction in Nursing* (Boston: Little, Brown & Co., 1973), 191.

8. C. H. Patterson, *Foundations for a Theory of Instruction and Educational Psychology.* (New York: Harper & Row, 1977), 188.

9. C. H. Patterson, *Theory of Instruction*, 189–90.

10. V. C. Conley, *Curriculum and Instruction in Nursing*, 194–96.

11. B. F. Skinner, "The science of learning and the art of teaching," *Harvard Ed Rev 24*, (1954): 86–97.

12. J. S. Bruner, "Notes on a theory of instruction," in P. E. Johnson (ed.), *Learning: Theory and Practice* (New York: Thomas Y. Crowell Co., 1971), 339–63.

13. Robert M. Gagné, *The Conditions of Learning*, 3rd ed. (New York: Holt, Rinehart, Winston, 1977).

14. Benjamin S. Bloom, et al: *Taxonomy of Educational Objectives: The Classification of Educational Goals, Handbook I: Cognitive Domain* (New York: David McKay Co., 1956).

15. David R. Krathwohl, Benjamin S. Bloom, and Bertram B. Masia, *Taxonomy of Educational Objectives: The Classification of Educational Goals, Handbook II: Affective Domain.* (New York: David McKay Co., 1964).

16. William D. Rohwer, Jr., Paul R. Ammon, and Phebe Cramer, *Understanding Intellectual Development* (Hinsdalle, Ill.: Dryden Press, 1974), 2.

17. Redman, *The Process of Patient Teaching.*

18. Ibid.

19. Ibid.

20. Baccalaureate Curriculum Subcommittee, *CUA—Systems Adaptation Model.* (Washington, D.C.: The School of Nursing, The Catholic University of America, 1978, Unpublished).

21. Robert F. Mager, *Preparing Instructional Objectives* (Belmont, Calif.: Lear, Siegler, Inc., 1962), 3.

22. Ibid, 11.

23. V. C. Conley. *Curriculum and Instruction in Nursing*, 224.

24. Madeline Petrillo and Sergay Sanger, *Emotional Care of Hospitalized Children: An Environmental Approach*, 2nd ed. (Philadelphia: J. B. Lippincott Co., 1980), 159.

25. Helen Yura and Mary Walsh. *The Nursing Process*, 4th ed. (E. Norwalk, Conn.: Appleton-Century-Crofts, 1983), 176.

Annotated Bibliography

Cohen, N.H. 1980. *Three steps to better patient teaching. Nurs 80:* 72–74. The need for accurate assessment of learning needs, resources available, and the content to be taught are included in this article. It also includes a brief assessment tool to determine learning needs.

Cosper, B. 1977. *How well do patients understand hospital jargon? Am J Nurs* 77:1932–34. This brief study describes how individuals can be overwhelmed by medical language and offers some advice to avoid pitfalls.

Dobberstein, K., and Miller, A. 1985. *Timely teaching. Am J Nurs 85:* 797–804. This continuing education module is designed to enable the reader to identify teaching strategies and use of evaluative behaviors to examine teaching materials.

Kratzer, J.B. 1977. *What does your patient need to know? Nurs 77* (7):82–84. This article discusses use of a plan to direct teaching and provides an example.

Haferkorn, V. 1971. *Assessing individual learning needs as a basis for patient teaching. Nurs Clin North Am* 199–209. Use of the nursing process for teaching is the crux of this article, in which an excellent assessment tool is provided.

Jones, P., and Oertel, W. 1977. *Developing patient teaching objectives and techniques: A self-instructional program. Nurs Educ 2.* This programmed instruction stresses the importance of writing learning objectives to direct teaching. It provides space for the reader to write objectives and provides answers to help clarify problems.

Murray, R., and Zentner, J. 1976. *Guideline for more effective health teaching. Nurs 76* (6):44–53. This excellent article provides a down-to-earth format for effective teaching.

Smith, D. 1971. *Writing objectives as a nursing practice skill. Am J Nurs* 71:319–20. This classic article concisely discusses writing objectives that can be measured in terms of changes in client behaviors.

Waidley, E. 1985. *Preparing Children for invasive procedures. Am J Nurs* 85:811–12. This brief article provides information on teaching children.

Ward, D.B. 1986. *Why patient teaching fails fails fails. RN* 49(6):45–47. Six common obstacles that prevent learning are reviewed in this article, and suggestions for overcoming them are provided.

Chapter 16

Change Theory

Janet-Beth McCann Flynn

Chapter Outline

- Objectives
- Glossary
- Introduction
- Types of Change
    Facilitators of Change
    Barriers to Change
- The Nursing Process
    Assessment
    Planning
    Implementation
    Evaluation
- Summary
- Study Questions
- References
- Annotated Bibliography

Objectives

Upon completion of this chapter the reader should be able to:

▸ Define change
▸ Identify the three stages in the change process described by Lewin
▸ Compare and contrast barriers to and facilitators of change
▸ Discuss the role of the nurse as a change agent

Glossary

Active Change. Change that is planned and directed.

Barriers. Obstacles that block change.

Change. An alteration in behavior.

Change Agent. A person who effects change through intentional intervention.

Change Theory. A framework for organizing change.

Covert Change. Change that occurs without an individual's knowledge.

Evolutionary Change. A slow change over time.

Facilitators. Enhancers that support change.

Leadership. Facilitation of change through creative direction, motivation, and guidance of others toward achieving mutually accepted goals.

Overt Change. Change that occurs within a person's awareness.

Passive Change. Unplanned change that occurs as time passes.

Planned Change. A change that is approached systematically.

Revolutionary Change. A rapid and drastic change.

Spontaneous Change. A change that occurs in response to natural events.

Targets for Change. Individuals, families, groups, or subsystems within the community who have health behaviors that are not good practice.

INTRODUCTION

Throughout life, individuals grow, develop, and adapt. This process is known as **change.** Change is a natural part of life and is necessary to maintain personal equilibrium. Change occurs daily on all levels—from the cellular level, organ level, organ system, client system—to the more complex family, social, and environmental systems. Change, a dynamic process, can be subtle and continuous, like growth and development, and occur without noticeable changes in behavior. Or change can be cataclysmic, occurring overnight. Without the ability to change, individuals would be unable to adapt to change.

Teaching a client about a disease process or bodily change provides that person with an opportunity to change. Learning, by its definition, indicates an observable change of behavior.

In a role as teacher, nurses assume the role of **change agent** or leader. A change agent is a person who effects the change process through creative intentional intervention. In this role, the nurse initiates planned change. **Planned change** is change that is not accidental but is systematically assessed and carefully implemented. Planned change has goals and objectives to guide it. Effective **leadership** is essential because planned change requires the organization and participation of all persons involved in the process.

Welch states, "The ability to identify and carry out planned changes is an integral part of the role of the professional nurse."[1] For nurses to engage in the process of change, they must have the knowledge base and the skills necessary to bring about change. According to Olson, nurses should be guided by a framework for effecting the change process.[2]

One framework for planned change was formulated by Kurt Lewin and is known as change theory.[3] **Change theory** describes the process of change and identifies six components of change. The first is recognition of the area where the change is needed. The second component involves a careful assessment of the situation in order to learn what is operating to maintain a status quo (**barriers**) and what is operating to change the situation (**facilitators**). A third component is identification of the methods to be used to produce change, and a fourth is the planning of the change. A fifth involves what the person's culture identifies as a method of change, and the final component is the process of change itself.

These six components cause three distinct stages in the change process—the stage of *unfreezing,* the stage of *moving,* and the stage of *refreezing.* In the unfreezing phase of the change, the discovery that change is needed is made, and the individual is motivated to change. The second stage, moving, involves working toward the change by identifying the problem, exploring the alternatives, outlining the goals, establishing the objectives, planning, and implementing the plan. The third stage is that of refreezing, in which the new changes are incorporated into the person's behavior and are stabilized.

Lewin advanced another theory about change that includes the idea that opposing forces facilitate the change process or impede it. It is important to identify these forces in order to activate the process of change.

Since the change process is dynamic, it is important to keep in mind that none of the stages or steps in the change process are rigid. There will be flow between the steps and there is no way to determine how much time will be spent in each step. The change process may move quickly through some steps, only to stop in another phase. Nurses must use all of their skills to keep the process moving to a positive outcome.

The **target for change** can be an individual, a family, a group, or a subsystem of the community with real or potential health problems.

Change is an important concept for nurses to understand so that they can serve as change agents when working with clients, families, or groups (Fig. 16–1). In identifying the steps in the process of change, the nurse can incorporate them within the four steps of the nursing process.

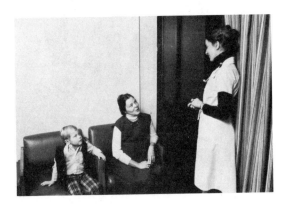

Figure 16–1. In the role of change agent, the nurse works with individuals, families, and groups.

TYPES OF CHANGE

There are several different types of change. **Evolutionary,** or developmental, change is characterized by gradual change. The stages are sequential and have identifiable characteristics. Examples of this type of change might include becoming parents or gradually becoming crippled by rheumatoid arthritis. This process is slow and does not require rapid adaptation or shift in personal goals. Because it is gradual and gives the person an opportunity to adapt, it is a less threatening form of change.

Another form of change is **revolutionary,** or haphazard, **change.** This is more rapid and drastic and may upset the equilibrium of the individual. There is a need here to alter life goals and perhaps even redesign patterns of behavior in order to cope and successfully adapt. Individuals experiencing this type of change generally have little or no warning or time to prepare. This type of change is very threatening and causes people to use high levels of energy. Defense mechanisms are often necessary to cope, and the result may be a crisis state. Some examples of revolutionary change include: loss of a limb, loss of a loved one, loss of vision (see Chapter 27), heart attack, stroke, and accidents.

Spontaneous change occurs in response to natural events. For example, the mutation of a cell. To some degree the timing of this type of change is unpredictable. Because of this, nursing intervention may be difficult.

Covert change is change that is constant and often occurs without the person being aware of it. Acculturation is a good example of covert change. **Overt change** is within the person's awareness. This type of change is generally revolutionary, and individuals may react with feelings of anxiety and apprehension. These are related to the individual's feeling of autonomy, since it may involve an involuntary change in behavior without regard for the person's feelings, needs, and desires.

Passive change occurs with the passage of time. It is like evolutionary change but generally is not planned; it just happens. **Active change,** on the other hand, is planned, and goal-directed.

Facilitators of Change

Facilitators of change are things that increase the chance of change and enhance it. Facilitators of change are much like facilitators of learning and depend on a combination of the following behaviors on the part of the client:

- Desire to change on the part of the client
- Motivation to change behavior patterns
- Positive past experience with change
- Change not perceived as a threat
- Trust in the nurse as a change agent
- Clear communication systems with the nurse and others on the health-care team
- Goals that are congruent with the health-care system's goals
- Ability to compromise to attain the above goals and to accept change
- Family support and identity-group support and acceptance
- Ability to use the health-care system and other resources available
- Dedication to change

Facilitators are extremely useful tools to use when implementing planned change. They should be carefully assessed and incorporated into the change process.

Barriers to Change

Barriers to change are factors that block effective change and can increase an individual's resistance to change. Barriers to change can be adaptive at times, and should be carefully assessed. For example, it can be important for clients to deny health-state changes for short periods of time. Barriers can lead to poor decision-making and problem-solving skills in the client's repertoire of behavior. A clear assessment of these behaviors can lead the nurse to methods of correcting them. Caution should be used when making changes because change can be disturbing to those involved. Barriers to change include:

- Desire to maintain the status quo
- Satisfaction with things as they are
- Threat of the change
- Overacceptance of the sick role
- Lack of motivation for change
- Perception of change as a threat to the self
- Perception of change as a threat to the family or group
- Negative past experiences with change
- Lack of trust in the health-care system
- Poor communication skills
- Goals that are not congruent with those of the health-care system or the nurse
- Unrealistic goals
- Traditions, attitudes, values, and culture that are not congruent with the health-care system
- Inability to compromise
- Lack of family support for the change
- Lack of cultural group support for the change
- Focusing on one point of the situation instead of seeing the whole picture
- Lack of understanding of what is needed in order to change
- Lack of ability to use health-care resources
- Lack of dedication to the change
- Fear of failure
- Expense of the change

THE NURSING PROCESS

Nurses act as change agents in almost all interactions with clients (Fig. 16–2). The nurse's fundamental role is to recognize that a change is occurring or not occurring. It is the nurse's responsibility to assess and gather data on barriers and facilitators and plan the methods of change. Change should be planned in a nonjudgmental way, taking the client's needs, wants, and values

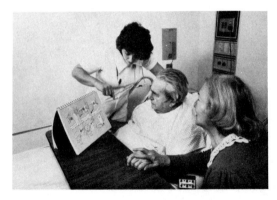

Figure 16–2. The nurse works as a change agent in many nurse–client interactions.

into consideration. Sensitivity to how much and what can be changed and not changed is a valuable asset to any nurse.

Assessment

The initial assessment will provide the data needed to determine what changes are necessary for the client to adapt. To do this, the nurse must establish a trusting nurse–client relationship based on a system of open communication. The nurse needs to assess her or his own abilities and values. Many times, a proposed change might be unrealistic for the client. For example, a client who has smoked two packs of cigarettes a day for 30 years may be unwilling to stop smoking completely. The nurse should realize the client should be persuaded to decrease smoking and establish a workable plan for the client, such as decreasing the number of cigarettes smoked until the desired number is reached.

Many times a client's beliefs and behaviors cannot be changed, for example, a religious belief about not receiving blood transfusions or taking certain medications. Trying to change behaviors that cannot be changed is frustrating for both the client and the nurse, and may destroy the nurse–client relationship. Sometimes one change in a client's system leads to another. Occasionally behavior assessed as unchangeable may begin to change as a result. Change is viewed by many as a threat, but when a small unthreatening change is made, other changes may follow.

The nurse also should determine the ethical issues involved in the change process. Does the nurse believe that the change is in the client's best interest? Is the nurse committed to assist the client in changing behavior? (see Chapter 12).

The health state of the client must be assessed. In order to change behavior, the client must be physically able to commit her- or himself to the change.

Barriers and facilitators to change need to be carefully assessed and incorporated into the health-care plan. Change cannot be instituted or supported without knowledge of these aspects of the client's situation. It is important to assess facilitators of change, so that they can be supported and built upon. It is equally important to assess barriers to change, so that they can be modified or eliminated, or at least identified.

Most problems have more than one cause; therefore as many factors as possible should be assessed. For example, Mr. J.B., a 56-year-old disabled man with congestive heart disease and chronic bronchitis, had numerous problems. He could not read. His income was well below the poverty level. He lived in one room on the first floor of an un-air-conditioned building and served as the doorman. He kept his room spotlessly clean and prided himself on his ability to cook on his one burner hot plate. He washed his dishes in a pan of water carried from the bathroom down the hall. He rotated shifts, and on his off hours, he washed and waxed cars at the corner gas station for extra money. His activity aggravated his symptoms and caused him to be hospitalized repeatedly. He did not want to be sick and took all of his medicines faithfully. The following facilitators were assessed: a desire for change, motivation, trust in the nurse; clear communication; ability to compromise; ability to use the health-care system; and dedication to a change. The barriers included: desire for status quo; unrealistic goals, habits, values, and culture; lack of family and group support; focusing on one part of the problem; and lack of understanding of the need for change.

The nurse assessed areas for change that were then discussed with Mr. B. and established mutual goals. This initiated the unfreezing phase. The type of change was active and overt. One week later, Mr. B. had a fan, that a neighbor had given him. He was working the day shift, but was still waxing cars because he needed the money. Finally a compromise was reached. Mr. B. would rest during the day and would continue with his medications, and he would wax the cars in the early evening when it got cooler. In this way, his old routine was adapted.

The degree to which the nurse initiates change depends upon the client's present state of wellness and adaptation, understanding of the disease, the change process, ability and desire for change, the resources available, and the nurse's knowledge and ability to implement planned change. At the conclusion of the assessment phase of the nursing process, the nursing diagnoses are formulated. Examples of nursing diagnoses regarding change might include:

- Health maintenance alteration related to cultural expectations
- Knowledge deficit related to change

Planning

Planned change needs to be directed by written goals and objectives that identify how the change will occur. Objectives are written and stated in terms of observable behavior. They should state a reasonable amount of time for the change to occur. Objectives should be discussed and agreed on by the nurse and the client.

Mutual goals that could have been established with Mr. B. might include:

- The client will be free of pulmonary congestion as evidenced by absence of dyspnea, orthopnea, and cough within 24 hours
- The client can list signs and symptoms of congestive heart failure within one week
- The client is able to identify each of his medications and state its purpose within one week

Strategies for change must include the person and family, friends, or group. Level of growth and development and level of knowledge are two other factors to keep in mind when planning change. Motivation and the client's physical ability also need to be considered when planning change. All of these factors must be included in the change plan if it is to succeed.

At this stage, the problems needing change have been identified and the methods for change selected.

Implementation

Once the change has been planned, the next step is to implement the plan. Lewin's stage of moving continues throughout the implementation phase of the nursing process. Frequent feedback and open lines of communication between the client and nurse are essential. Depending on the type of change involved, implementation may be short and relatively easy to accomplish or painfully slow and difficult. As in the above case, a great deal of patience on the part of the nurse and client is often necessary and emotional support given by the nurse can make the difference between success and failure. At the conclusion of the implementation phase, the client's new behaviors should be stabilized and refrozen.

Evaluation

"Evaluation involves measuring behavior and interpreting the results in terms of desired behavior change."[4] Evaluation is always considered in terms of how the client met the written jectives in the care plan. If the client met the objectives, further changes in behavior may not be needed. If the client did not meet the objectives, a reassessment of the situation is needed, followed by plan revision and implementation.

The change process enables the nurse to help individuals or groups to change and therefore to adapt positively.

Olsen writes that:

> inaction and frustration are inevitable during the change. In order to meet the realities of the situation, persistence and flexibility are essential attributes for the nurse change agent. She must be realistic about what she can accomplish. Persistence is essential, for if the identified change fails, she must try again.[5]

Planned change is an integral part of the nurse's role. The ability to assess the need for change is essential for promoting positive adaptation.

SUMMARY

Change is a natural part of our lives, and it is necessary for humans to adapt in a dynamic environment. The nurse, in the role as a change agent, is able to bring about planned change by careful use of the nursing process.

For nurses to implement planned change, they should be guided by a theoretical framework for the change process. One framework formulated by Lewin divides the change process into three distinct stages: the unfreezing stage, the moving stage, and the refreezing stage. Lewin also proposes that there are opposing forces at work that facilitate or impede the process of change.

The target of a planned change can be an individual, a family, a group, or a subsystem of the community. The change target may have real or potential problems.

Change can occur in several ways. Evolutionary change is change that evolves slowly and allows adaptation. Revolutionary change is rapid, drastic, and does not allow for adaptation. Covert change occurs without the individual's awareness of the change, and overt change occurs within an individual's awareness. Change also can be passive or active.

Many things affect change. Things that increase the chance of change are called facilitators, and things that slow or impede change are called barriers.

Most problems with which the nurse comes into contact have more than one cause, so by careful use of the nursing process, the nurse can act as an agent of planned change.

Study Questions

1. How has your life changed since entering school?

2. Identify some barriers to change in your life.

3. Identify some facilitators of change in your present life.

4. How could you act as a change agent on your campus or community?

References

1. L.B. Welch, "Planned change in nursing: The theory," *Nurs Clin North Am 14*, (1979): 307–21.
2. E.M. Olson, "Strategies and techniques for the nurse change agent," *Nurs Clin North Am 14* (1979): 323–36.
3. K. Lewin, "Quasi-stationary social equilibria and the problem of permanent change," in W.G. Bennes, K.D. Benne, and R. Chain (eds.), *The Planning of Change* (New York: Holt, Rinehart, Winston, 1962).
4. Barbara K. Redman, *The Process of Patient Teaching in Nursing,* 3rd ed. (St. Louis: C.V. Mosby Co., 1976), 183.
5. E. M. Olson, "Strategies and techniques," 324.

Annotated Bibliography

Olson, E.M. 1979. Strategies and techniques for the nurse change agent. *Nurs Clin North Am* 14(2):323–36. The role of the nurse as change agent is discussed in this article and suggestions for potential strategies for implementing the change process are given. Three frameworks for change are presented.

Reynolds, B.C. 1980.The Nurse as a Change Agent. *Occup Health Nurs* 28:19–21. The concept of change and the nurse's role as a change agent is discussed in this article.

Welch, L.B. 1979. Planned change in nursing: The theory. *Nurs Clin North Am* 14(2): 307–21. This article describes the process of change and discusses a variety of change theories.

Chapter 17

Nursing Research

RoAnne Dahlen-Hartfield
Janet-Beth McCann Flynn

Chapter Outline

- Objectives
- Glossary
- Introduction
    Accountability
    Social Relevancy
- The Scientific Research Process and Problem Solving
- Classification of Nursing Research
    Expected Levels of Research Skills
- Historical Perspectives
- The Research Process
    Step I: The Research Problem
    Step II: The Purpose
    Step III: Review of the Literature
    Step IV: Identifying a Theoretical Framework
    Step V: Identifying the Variables
    Step VI: Formulating the Hypothesis Statement
    Step VII: Defining Terms
    Step VIII: Selecting the Research Design and Methodology
    Step IX: Specifying the Population and Sample
    Step X: The Sampling Procedure
    Step XI: Informed Consent
    Step XII: The Pilot Study
    Step XIII: Methodology and Data Collection
    Step XIV: Data Analysis and Interpretation
    Step XV: Conclusions and Implications
    Step XVI: Communicating the Results
- Evaluation of Nursing Research
- Summary
- Study Questions
- References
- Annotated Bibliography

Objectives

At the completion of this chapter, the reader will be able to:

▶ Define the terms in the glossary
▶ Describe the value of nursing research in promoting professionalism, accountability, and social relevancy
▶ Classify nursing research by purpose and method
▶ Differentiate between the roles of baccalaureate, master's, and doctorally prepared nurses in research
▶ Discuss the historical codevelopment of nursing education and nursing research
▶ Identify the trends in nursing research and its future directions for the twenty-first century
▶ Discuss the concept of informed consent
▶ Explain the steps in the research process as they relate to the beginning nurse researcher
▶ Differentiate between critiquing a nursing research study for familiarity with the research process as compared to critiquing it for use in nursing practice

Glossary

Applied Research. Research that is conducted to solve an everyday problem in practice or education.

Basic Research. Research that is designed to extend the knowledge base and test theory construction.

Bias. Any undue influence that affects the results of a research study.

Case Study. A research design method that entails an in-depth analysis of a single subject, group, unit, or institution.

Central Tendency. A statistical index of the "typicalness" of a set of scores. Most common indexes of central tendency are the mean, the median, and the mode.

Chi-square Test. A test of statistical significance that is used to determine if a significant relationship exists between two nominal level variables.

Closed-ended Question. An item on a questionnaire that is limited to the provided replies.

Coefficient Alpha (Cronbach's Alpha). A reliability index that estimates the internal consistency of a test or measuring instrument.

Confidentiality. Protection of subjects' privacy and anonymity in a study.

Construct. An abstract concept (e.g., self-concept) derived from a combination of existing theory and observations.

Construct Validity. Extent to which the research instrument measures what it was designed to measure.

Content Validity. The content of the instrument or questionnaire is determined to be representative of all possible questions or observations by a panel of judges consisting of experts in the subject area under study.

Control. To regulate and hold constant possible influences on the dependent variable under investigation.

Correlational Research. Research that attempts to determine whether and to what degree a relationship exists between two or more quantifiable variables.

Correlation Coefficient. An index that summarizes the degree of the relationship between the two variables.

Cross-sectional Design. A design that enables the researcher to observe subjects of different age or developmental stages at one point in time.

Data. Information obtained from subjects in a study.

Dependent Variable. The outcome variable of interest.

Descriptive Research. Research that identifies and describes characteristics of persons, groups, situations, or phenomena.

Descriptive Statistics. Statistics that describe or summarize the data.

Directional Hypothesis. A hypothesis that predicts the specific direction of the relationship between two variables.

Evaluative Research. A research study that determines how well a program, policy, or practice is working.

Experimental Research. A study in which the researcher controls and manipulates the independent variable and uses random selection of the subjects and assignment of the subjects to either the experimental or control groups.

Generalizable. Application of the findings from the study sample to the broader population from which the sample was drawn.

Historical Research. A type of study design that examines past events.

Inferential Statistics. Statistical methods that make it possible to make more accurate generalizations from new sets of data; these methods allow researchers to make inferences about large groups on the basis of small group findings.

Independent Variable. The variable that is believed to cause or influence the dependent variable.

Informed Consent. Voluntary participation of subjects after having been informed of the research protocol, its inherent risks and benefits, and their rights as subjects.

Mean. The arithmetic average of a group of scores.

Median. That point or score that is half above and half below the other scores.

Mode. The most frequently occurring score.

Nondirectional Hypothesis. A hypothesis that does not state the specific direction of the relationship between the two variables.

Null Hypothesis. A statement that says there is no difference between variables.

Open-ended Question. A question that does not restrict the subject to a predetermined set of responses. Freedom of reply is permitted.

Operational Definition. The definition of the variable in terms of the operations or procedures by which it is to be measured by the researcher.

Pilot Study. A study that is carried out by the researcher at the end of the design phase in order to test the elements of the design.

Population. A total membership of the group being studied.

Purpose. The aim of the research study. The research question is derived from the purpose.

Random Sample. A sample selected according to one of the procedures for probability sampling that ensures that every member of a population has an equal chance of being included in the study.

Range. The extent of the spread of scores from the lowest to the highest in a distribution.

Reliability. The degree to which an instrument consistently yields the same results when the instrument is used repeatedly.

Sample. A subset of a population selected according to predetermined criteria to participate in a research study.

Scale. A measuring instrument composed of several items that have a logical or empirical relationship to each other.

Standard Deviation. A statistical calculation to indicate how far each score in a distribution is from the group mean.

Theoretical Framework. An abstract set of interrelated propositions that present a systematic explanation about a phenomenon.

Validity. The degree to which an instrument measures what it proposes to measure.

INTRODUCTION

Research is a process whereby a subject or idea is studied critically and carefully according to a systematic plan. Close investigation of this type allows new facts to emerge and significant discoveries to be made. When this type of research-based new knowledge is added to what is already known, it is highly valued and credible, allowing for growth, change, and progress to take place.

Nursing research arises from the practice of nursing for the purpose of solving client-care problems within a given setting. Through additional research efforts, the specialized body of knowledge known as nursing science has been developed. These efforts have contributed greatly toward helping nursing in its quest to become recognized as a profession. Nursing research also assists the profession in becoming accountable and relevant to society as a whole.

Accountability

A number of factors in our society are requiring nurses to be increasingly more accountable for the nursing and health-care services they provide. In addition to being morally and ethically accountable, nurses now need to provide documented evidence regarding the need for nursing services, the method of delivery of nursing services, and the effectiveness of those services. Some of the societal factors responsible for this trend include the rise of consumerism, increasing health-care costs, and requirements of private insurance companies and governmental agencies such as Medicare and Medicaid.

The results of clinical nursing research have enabled nurse administrators to provide documentation to support not only the need for nursing services but the rationale for solving client-care problems within a given setting, validating effectiveness of specific nursing interventions toward the improvement of quality of client care, and assisting in the making of decisions about delivery systems and staffing patterns.

Social Relevancy

Nursing research helps nurses to answer very relevant questions that relate directly to the needs of clients and to nursing as a profession.

Questions such as "Of what benefit is nursing?," "How does nursing make a difference?," "Is it more cost-effective to hire registered nurses than technicians who have been trained in a narrow specialized area, e.g., operating room technicians?" are good examples of such nursing research questions. Table 17–1 elaborates on areas of social relevancy and provides examples.

THE SCIENTIFIC RESEARCH PROCESS AND PROBLEM SOLVING

The research process is a method used to seek ways to solve problems, but in addition, it is a more formal and specific process than basic problem solving. It is important for the beginning nurse researcher to be able to understand the similarities and differences between these two processes. Table 17–2 compares and contrasts the research process with problem solving.

Stetler describes research as more efficient, less prone to bias, more generalizable, and theoretically more valid than either trial or error, reliance on tradition or custom, or the opinion of the person in authority. When compared to the higher level of problem solving known as the *nursing process,* nursing research is viewed as more objective, precise, and theoretically oriented.[1]

It is equally important to know what is *not* nursing research. Nurses must be able to differentiate clearly between what is and is not nursing research—not only for their own use of information, but for the image and reputation of nursing as a scientific discipline. Nursing research is not just collecting data, reading an article, or writing up an interesting case study or protocol for plan of care. Unless monitoring for quality assurance is structured as a research study, it cannot be called nursing research either.[2]

TABLE 17–1. EXAMPLES OF SOCIAL RELEVANCE OF NURSING RESEARCH

Relevancy	Example
1. Nursing research discovers new facts about known phenomena.	Staff nurses in a nursing home used research to find out the effectiveness of a new nursing intervention on the rate of healing of the known phenomenon of decubitus ulcers.
2. Nursing research finds answers to problems that have been only partially solved by existing methods of nursing interventions.	Nursing interventions for certain types of problems that cause urinary incontinence in the older adult have been partially effective in controlling and decreasing the episodes of urinary incontinence. Experimental studies are now being undertaken to identify the effectiveness of the use of biofeedback with an individual perionometer, teaching, and Kegel exercises in decreasing the episodes of urinary incontinence in older adults.
3. Nursing research improves existing techniques and develops new instruments or products.	Before introduction of a new technique or instrument into a hospital today, nurses are pilot testing and evaluating its effectiveness and usefulness within their own setting.
4. Nursing research discovers previously unrecognized substances or elements.	The North American Nursing Diagnosis Conference Group is systematically, through various research efforts, identifying individual nursing diagnoses and their accompanying critical characteristics. Once identified, these nursing diagnoses are being validated in different clinical settings by clinical nurse specialists and nurse researchers.
5. Nursing research discovers pathways of action of known substances and elements.	Nursing research has identified a linkage between interdisciplinary communication and cooperation and mortality of clients in intensive care units.

TABLE 17–2. DIFFERENTIATION BETWEEN PROBLEM SOLVING AND THE SCIENTIFIC PROCESS

Research Process	Problem Solving
1. All elements of the research process must be precisely and explicitly described.	1. Explicitness and precision, though they may be used, are not usually required.
2. When the research data are quantitative, they are analyzed with appropriate statistical procedures.	2. Detailed statistical analysis is seldom done. Analysis is generally limited to frequency counts.
3. Elaborate pains are taken to control for factors other than variables under study.	3. Controls of extraneous factors are not imposed.
4. One of the primary aims is to ensure that findings are generalizable to a population larger than the subjects being studied.	4. The primary aim is the solution of a problem existing in the sample being studied. Little attention is given to the generalizability to the larger population.
5. Entails a written plan in sufficient detail to enable the study to be replicated and findings verified.	5. Entails no written plan and need not be replicable or verifiable.
6. There is a professional obligation to report the research findings in a professional journal or by an oral presentation at a local, regional, or national conference.	6. Findings need only be reported to those in the immediate setting.

CLASSIFICATION OF NURSING RESEARCH

Nursing research is classified by *purpose* or by *methodology*. Classification by purpose falls into two categories, **basic research** and **applied research**. *Basic research* is done solely for the purpose of theory development and refinement. It may not be immediately applicable to everyday nursing practice. *Applied research* is done for the purpose of testing theory and evaluating its effectiveness in providing solutions to practical problems.

Nursing research may also be classified according to the method used in the study. The four common methods are:

- **Descriptive research** describes what is and analyzes the findings in relation to their significance
- **Historical research** studies and examines past events
- **Correlational research** attempts to determine whether and to what degree a relationship exists between two or more quantifiable variables
- **Experimental research** involves the manipulation of an independent variable and studying its effect on other variables under controlled conditions

Expected Levels of Research Skills
Nurses have differing levels of research skills, depending on their basic educational program.

The Commission on Nursing Research of the American Nurses' Association has identified the levels of research skills that can be expected of graduates from associate degree, baccalaureate, master's and doctoral programs in nursing.[3] Table 17–3 identifies research skills that this commission outlines as important for the baccalaureate level nurse.

As would be expected, the skills of a graduate of a master's degree nursing program are at a higher level and include, in part, the following:

- Analyzing and reformulating nursing practice
- Facilitating investigative activities
- Conducting investigations for the purpose of monitoring the quality of the practice of nursing in a clinical setting

TABLE 17–3. RESEARCH SKILLS EXPECTED OF THE BACCALAUREATE NURSE

1. Reads, interprets, and evaluates research for applicability to nursing practice
2. Identifies nursing problems that need to be investigated and participates in the implementation of scientific studies
3. Uses nursing practice as a means of gathering data for refining and extending practice
4. Applies established findings of nursing and other health-related research to nursing practice
5. Shares research findings with colleagues

From the American Nurses' Association, Kansas City, Mo., 1981.

All nurses prepared at the doctoral level are well-grounded in the research process, and many nursing doctoral programs, e.g., Ph.D. programs, are focused almost entirely on research. The doctorally prepared nurse provides leadership in the design and conduct of investigations in order to evaluate the contribution of nursing activities to the well-being of clients.

It is important for each individual nurse to recognize his or her responsibility to nursing research and the appropriate role to play in it be it as a consumer of nursing research, a facilitator of others' conduct of research, user of research findings in nursing practice, or designer of his or her own research studies. Each of these roles requires certain knowledge, expertise, and experience. The beginning nurse researcher can be a consumer, facilitator, and user of research findings.

HISTORICAL PERSPECTIVES

The evolution of nursing research has been relatively slow, compared with the progress of other established disciplines. The following reasons have been cited[4,5]:

- Nursing is associated with a long history of reliance on tradition and authority
- Nursing is a practice profession and, accordingly, more emphasis has been placed on practical aspects than on inquiry and research
- There were so many pressing problems facing nursing and medicine in the early part of the century, e.g., communicable disease control, documentation of hospital nursing activities, and development of nursing education, that nursing research was afforded a low priority
- Research is synonymous with formal university education

When one examines the historical and evolutional development of nursing research, it is especially important to recognize the events that were simultaneously occurring in the evolution of nursing education. Table 17–4 provides a brief, chronological overview of historical events and the corresponding research events and focus.

In 1983, the American Nurses' Association established the first Center for Nursing Research. Its purpose is to establish coordinated nursing research programs that provide national data to policy-making bodies, administer extramural funded projects, and seek external funding for research, either by grants or fund-raising activities.

In 1986, the National Center for Nursing Research was approved by Congress and became a part of the National Institutes of Health located in Bethesda, Maryland. The purpose of this new institute is to conduct, support and disseminate information about basic and clinical nursing research. The center is intended to provide a focal point for promoting the growth and quality of research related to nursing and client care, to provide leadership to expand the pool of experienced nurse researchers, and to promote closer interaction with other bases of health-care research.

Today, nursing research is a part of all graduate programs in nursing and is increasingly introduced to students at the baccalaureate level. With the increase in the number of graduates of doctoral programs in nursing, and the support provided by the National Center for Nursing Research, research efforts in nursing can become more firmly established in the mainstream of scientific investigation.

Trends in Nursing Research. In the late 1920s, there was one nurse prepared with a doctorate in a related discipline. By the late 1950s, there were 150 doctorally prepared nurses. In the last decade, an increase in the number of nurses with academic degrees has been seen. In 1984, out of the total population of employed registered nurses (RNs) of 1,485,725, there were: 1,486 (0.1 percent) doctorally prepard RNs; 58,927 (5.9 percent) master's prepared RNs; and 355,340 (22.8 percent) baccalaureate prepared RNs.[6]

An increase in the number of doctoral programs in nursing has also occurred. In the United States before 1970, only a few doctoral programs existed (Teachers College, Columbia University, University of California; and the Catholic University of America). As of 1986, there were 43 doctoral programs in nursing.[7]

There has been a shift in those studying such factors as nursing education and nursing practice from non-nurses (such as sociologists and psychologists) to nurses. This has been accompanied by a shift in the topics of nursing research from nursing procedures, nursing ad-

TABLE 17–4. EVOLUTION OF NURSING RESEARCH

Time Span	Events	Focus of Nursing Research
1860–1890	Nursing became a formal discipline under the guidance of Florence Nightingale. During the Crimean War Nightingale worked to obtain funding and resources from England's parliament by collecting and recording detailed observations of the effects of nursing actions on the health status of British soldiers. These efforts proved successful and led to select reforms in health care. In 1860 Florence Nightingale helped to establish St. Thomas Hospital School of Nursing By 1873, the first American schools of nursing were opened and within the next 25 years, over 400 schools were established, generally in hospitals.	The beginning of research in nursing can be traced to this period through Florence Nightingale's efforts to observe and record data as she worked with soldiers in the Crimean War. These are the only recorded efforts of research in nursing during this time period.
1900–1940	In 1910 the University of Minnesota had established the first baccalaureate program in a school of nursing. The Department of Nursing Education at Teachers' College, Columbia University opened the first masters program by 1910. The Goldmark Report, published in 1923, recommended advanced preparation for nurse educators, nurse administrators, and public health nurses. The report also recommended that hospitals should hire more nurses in order to permit nursing students more time for classes. The Brown Report, published in 1948, urged research to delineate the roles of nurses with different educational backgrounds, the need for in-service education, nurse–patient relationships, and the issues of economic security for nurses.	The *American Journal of Nursing* was first published in 1910. During the first ten years of publication, five articles were published that focused on nursing research. Most nursing research conducted during this period examined nursing education to discover who were entering the programs, who were remaining, and how many were completing the program.
1940–1960	In 1952 the first nursing research journal, *Nursing Research*, was published. In 1955 the Division of Nursing, U.S. Public Health Service, established grants and fellowship programs for nursing research studies in epidemiology. In 1955 the American Nurses' Foundation was created through the American Nurses' Association to serve as a vehicle to raise, administer, and award funds for small nursing research grants. The first centers for nursing research were founded at Columbia University and the Walter Reed Army Institute of Research. As a result, a cadre of nurses were able to be trained in all facets of nursing research.	The focus of research continued to be on the nurse: Who is the nurse? What does the nurse do and how do others perceive the nurse?
1960–1980	In 1963, the Surgeon General's Report on Nursing recommended an increase in Federal support of the training of nurse researchers and the funding of nursing research. In 1968 the Mugar Library at Boston University was established as the first archive of nursing history for the purpose of fostering historical nursing research. In 1970 the National Commission for the Study of Nursing published the Lysaught Report, which recommended funds be made available for nursing research in education and nursing care.	The field of bioethics and the ethical dimensions of nursing research began to gain increased recognition and exploration during this period. The high research priorities in clinical nursing were chronic illness and decreasing the negative impact of health problems on the coping abilities of the client. Promotion of health and well-being and prevention in the highly vulnerable population groups such as the adolescent pregnant mother and the elderly received increased emphasis.

(continued)

TABLE 17–4. (Continued)

Time Span	Events	Focus of Nursing Research
1960–1980 (cont.)	The evolution and development of the nursing theories of Rogers, Roy, King, Orem, and Johnson began during this period. Primary nursing and the nurse practitioner movement gained recognition and increased usage. In the early 1970s the American Nurses' Association created the Commission of Nursing Research, which recommended the need for preparation in nursing research to begin earlier, at the undergraduate level. Several new nursing research journals began publication: *Research in Nursing and Health, Advances in Nursing Science, The Western Journal of Nursing Research, Abstracts of World Nursing Research, International Journal of Nursing Studies.*	As cost became an issue, studies in cost-effectiveness of nursing in comparison to other health-care disciplines increased in number.

ministration, and nursing education to clinical nursing practice, nursing theory, cost containment, and use of qualitative research methods. Also noted has been a shift to increased use of nursing theoretical frameworks to structure nursing research for the testing of hypotheses.

The trend to shift funding from Federal to private sources, with an increase in available funds to support nursing research has been seen. Some private funding sources include foundations, such as Russell Sage, Rockefeller, Kellogg, and the Robert Wood Johnson Foundations.

An increase in professional, regional, and scientific societies supporting nursing research has occurred, including such organizations as Sigma Theta Tau International Honor Society of Nursing, the Southern Regional Educational Board, and the Western International Commission on Higher Education. In addition, an increase has been noted in the number of schools of nursing and graduate schools in universities that provide funds to support efforts to gather research data before submission of larger grant proposals to outside funding sources.

Future Directions for Nursing Research. The Cabinet of Nursing Research of the American Nurses' Association (ANA) identified directions in the form of goals that the profession and ANA must take in directing the efforts of nursing research toward the twenty-first century.[8] Table 17–5 summarizes goals and strategies for reaching them in future nursing research.

THE RESEARCH PROCESS

The basic goal of science is to determine a factual basis of knowledge from which generalizations and predictions can be made about events. Scientific research is an orderly, purposeful, and systematic collection of measurable data that allows the investigation of presumed relationships between naturally occurring phenomena. Research is the tool used to collect the empirical data needed for validation of theoretical knowledge. The purpose of research is to seek truth, to discover solutions to problems, to generate general principles, and to establish theory by applying scientific procedures designed to increase knowledge. The research process is built on the notion of the scientific method.

There is a series of logical progressions in the framework of the scientific method. These include:

- A felt difficulty, a problem
- Definition of the difficulty
- Hypothesis formulation
- Reasoning out the consequences
- Testing the hypothesis (data collection and analyses)
- Conclusions

The steps in the research process tend to follow the basic framework of the scientific method but some of the categories are broken down into subcategories (Table 17–6).

TABLE 17–5. DIRECTIONS FOR NURSING RESEARCH IN THE FUTURE

Goal	Strategies
To ensure an increased supply of nurse scientists in research by the year 2000	Increase the ratio of doctorally prepared nurses to total population of nurses to 0.5% by 1990 and 1.0% by 1995
	Increase the ratio of doctorally prepared faculty to nursing students in schools of nursing to 15:1000 by 1990 and 25:1000 by 1995, with the ultimate aim of having all faculty within schools of nursing be doctorally prepared
	Secure additional financial support for predoctoral training fellowships to 250 in 1990 and 300 in 1995
	Secure additional funds for postdoctoral training fellowships to 50 in 1990 and 100 in 1995
	Secure additional funds for new investigator grants to 150 in 1990 and 300 in 1995
	Promote the development of established nurse scientists through midcareer development awards to 50 in 1990 and 100 in 1995
	Develop systems within the professional organizations to monitor supply, demand, and geographic distribution of nurse scientists
	Develop through the ANA, publications, and media presentations to convey the value and the nature of nursing research to the general public and health policy-makers
	Expand resources within the professional organization to monitor adequacy and use of nursing research monies and lobby for the necessary support of nursing research and research training
	Promote with private organizations the development of matching funds for nursing research
To generate knowledge of: well-being and optimum function of human beings; effective delivery of nursing services; excellence in nursing education; and the impact of the profession on health policy	Establish visible entity of contract support for nursing research, training, and related projects in nursing
	Provide financial support for intra- and extramural research: 1990, $50 million, and 1995, $75 million
	Provide small grants in new areas of inquiry: 1990—50, 1995—100
	Establish increased numbers of centers for the study of nursing practice phenomena: 1990, 5 centers, and 1995, 10 centers
	Establish intramural programs of nursing research in Federal agencies to complement work in extramural research centers
	Develop systems within the professional organization to foster and monitor private and public sector funding for nursing research
	Support interdisciplinary research by nurses with other health professions and disciplines, such as sociologists and economists
Develop an environment that supports nursing inquiry, including opportunity to initiate nursing investigations and access to subjects, personnel, research facilities, and equipment	Support laboratories and research facilities with major equipment essential for nursing investigations
	Influence accreditation policies for nursing service and educational institutions to ensure: • Socialization of undergraduate students to research careers • Preparation of baccalaureate graduates as consumers of nursing research findings • Implementation of the ANA guidelines for investigative functions of nurses in nursing services and academic institutions • Doctoral preparation for nursing in key health agencies, for those in administrative positions who are responsible for directing the progress of client care • Doctoral preparation for administrative personnel supervising nursing research in nursing practice settings
	Conduct mass media campaign through professional organization to promote the image of the nurse as a scientist: 1990, $5 million, and 1995, $10 million
To disseminate the results of nursing research to clinicians, the scientific community, the general public, and health policy-makers in order to increase the use of these results	Establish Federally supported national nursing research retrieval system for published and unpublished research
	Establish a central rapid information system for use by the academic institutions and the public

From D. Diers, Research in Nursing Practice (Philadelphia: J.B. Lippincott Co., 1979).

Step I: The Research Problem

Research begins with a study question, or what is called a researchable problem. This problem may concern clinical nursing, nursing education, nursing history, administration, ethics, or social or natural science as they relate to health or health-care delivery.

The wording of the research question will set the stage for the type of study design used. These range from a simple level of inquiry to the most complex level of inquiry or question. Donna Diers identified the four levels of inquiry in her noteworthy text on nursing research.[9]

The first level of inquiry asks the question, *"What is this?"* At this level, the researcher is concerned with identifying, isolating, and naming the factors involved. These study designs are generally known as exploratory or descriptive designs (Table 17–7).

The second level of inquiry asks the question, *"What is happening here?"* The researcher is interested in searching for and identifying relationships between factors to further describe or depict the phenomena. These study designs are still within the realm of exploratory or descriptive designs.

The third level of inquiry asks the question, *"What will happen if. . . ?"* Here, the researcher is examining and testing the association or correlational relationship between the **independent** and **dependent variables** (factors). The designs of these studies are known as correlational, experimental, predictive, or explanatory.

The fourth level of inquiry asks the question, *"How can I make something happen?"* The researcher wants to test the various prescriptions to see if the desired situational outcomes are produced.

Clinical situations provide an abundance of possible study questions, and identifying which specific problem to study can be difficult for the beginning investigator (Table 17–8). This is partly because so many questions need to be researched that it may be hard to choose between them. In other cases, there seem to be commonsense explanations, and scientific inquiry is not sought.

There are many sources of researchable problems. These include:

- The literature
- The researcher's own experience

TABLE 17–6. STEPS IN THE RESEARCH PROCESS

1. Identifying the research problem
2. Formulating the research purpose
3. Reviewing the related literature
4. Developing or identifying the theoretical framework
5. Identifying the variables
6. Formulating the hypothesis statement
7. Defining terms
8. Selecting a research design
9. Specifying the population and sample
10. Selecting the sample
11. Obtaining informed consent
12. Conducting the pilot study
13. Carrying out the methodological procedure and collecting data
14. Analyzing the data
15. Interpreting the results
16. Communicating the results

- Patterns or trends
- Other research
- Scientific interest
- Theoretical frameworks for nursing practice

Many researchable ideas can be obtained through reading professional journals and other scientific publications, a process called *searching the literature.* There is an increased tendency for nursing journals with a nonresearch focus to include an article or an abstract that describes a nursing research study. There is also an increasing number of nursing journals solely dedicated to nursing research. As a result, more and more nurses are becoming exposed to and familiar with nursing research.

In reading a reported study in the literature, the nurse researcher may want to:

- Replicate or repeat the same study in another setting
- Design a new study based upon the implications for nursing suggested by the reported study, which often include implications and suggestions for further research
- Use either the theoretical framework, instrument, sampling procedure, methods or statistics that appear to be related to his or her proposed research question

Clinical experiences offer a wealth of possible researchable questions. For example, in

TABLE 17–7. FORMULATING THE RESEARCH QUESTION

Broad Problem Area	Concepts and Variables, (Ideas and Building Blocks)
Elderly and chronic hypertension	Type of medication regime Living arrangement Presence of a caregiver Type of caregiver support system Self-care abilities of the client Self-esteem Age, sex of the client and caregiver Compliance with the medication regimen

caring for clients with chronic hypertension, the researcher may have observed that clients from different ethnic or cultural groups respond differently to this disease in the ways in which they do or do not comply with their medication regimen. This raises many questions as to why, what the different reactions are, what factors are related to these reactions, and how the nurse can intervene to increase medication compliance.

Another major source of research problems can be discovered when a *pattern or trend* is discovered. For example, a nurse might notice that persons who are given a drug exhibit a set of symptoms that are not generally associated

TABLE 17–8. CRITERIA FOR DETERMINING A RESEARCHABLE QUESTION

1. Can the question be answered by collecting observable evidence of empirical data?
2. Does the question contain reference to the relationship between two or more variables?
3. Does the question follow logically and consistently from what is already known about the topic as found in the literature and has been substantiated by research?
4. Is the question clear as to what is specifically to be studied?
5. Is the question narrow enough to be manageable for the researcher, as determined by the time allowed, the funding available, and the research qualifications and experience of the researchers?
6. Is the question able to be answered by use of ethical procedures (sampling and methods)?

From C.A. Lindeman and D. Shantz, "The research question," J Nurs Admin (January 1982):6–10.

with side effects of that drug. After further observation, the nurse may feel that there is a definite pattern, indicating that there is a definite research problem or question.

Other research that appears in the literature may serve as a springboard for ideas of research. Sometimes specific recommendations are made at the end of a study. Another person may wish to design a study to carry out those recommendations. Other studies can be replicated with a different group of subjects. Research questions may also be generated because of the contradictory results that have been reported.

Scientific interests may generate research questions. These questions are usually broader than questions directed at individual clinical situations. They may address the more abstract explanation of a phenomenon.

Step II: The Purpose

The next step in the research process is to identify the research **purpose** that describes the reason why the research is being done. It must agree with and be consistent with the research question.

Step III: Review of the Literature

Once the research purpose and research question have been identified, the next step is to determine, through review of the literature, what other researchers have done. Review of the literature involves the systematic identification, location, and reading of those materials that contain information on the research question. There are four purposes for doing a literature review:

- To help the researcher further clarify or formulate the wording of the research question
- To acquaint the researcher with what research studies have already been done in the general area posed by the research question
- To identify research methods, instruments, and statistics that may prove helpful to the researcher
- To provide the theoretical framework suitable to the research question

It may be necessary for the researcher to do several reviews of the literature at different times throughout the research process. This is necessary to determine if there have been new findings.

The number of individual journals, articles, books, and reports that are written on a selected topic may initially seem overwhelming. The librarian at the university, clinical agency, or public library is an excellent starting point. They are knowledgeable about the available resources at their library and can often assist the researcher in narrowing the search process. Such services generally include linkage with the community, state, or regional libraries, as well as the National Library of Medicine's Health Science Library Network.

A literature search is made either manually or with the assistance of the computer. The first step in a manual search is to review the various indexes to locate literature relevant to the research question. Several useful indexes for nurses include: *Index Medicus, International Nursing Index, Nursing Research Index*, and *Nursing Studies Index*. It is important to become familiar with the thesaurus of terms or subject headings that accompanies each index, for this is how the nurse-researcher will locate the references appropriate to the research question.

Many journals often print abstracts of completed research studies that can aid researchers in deciding if they should read the article or reference. This is helpful when time is limited.

Most libraries generally subscribe to one or more computerized information data bases. For a minimal fee, the researcher can request the librarian to conduct a computerized literature search. Each data base system also has a printed thesaurus that identifies the terms to be used as reference points in locating the literature relevant to the research question.[10]

Writing the Review of the Literature Section. For each reference used, notation on an index card of the complete bibliographic heading (i.e., author, date, title of the article, journal volume and number, and page number) will help organize your review and save time when writing the summary. Use the format that will guide the final report or manuscript style, for example those guidelines established by the American Psychological Association (APA).

Several examples of published research studies that have a well-developed section of review of the literature can be read as good examples to follow.

A differentiation between primary sources, those articles that are written by the person who conducted the actual study, and secondary sources, those articles that describe the study but are written by someone else other than the researcher, should be made. It is vitally important to check the primary source, because secondary source articles may contain misinterpretations or omissions.

An outline of how the literature review will be developed should be devised and used, clearly identifying how the references are linked to the research question. Be sure to present both sides of the picture objectively: those studies that support and those studies that do not support the research hypothesis. It is best to use one's own words when summarizing the information and to make an effort to keep the literature review concise but complete.

Step IV: Identifying a Theoretical Framework

The **theoretical framework** often provides the impetus and direction for the nurse researcher in identifying the research question and possible relationships of the variables. A theoretical framework can be defined as a theory-based orientation or underlying structure that gives support and clarity to a research project. The theoretical framework serves as a reference point and a basis for generalization in research. Abdellah and Levine assert "to the degree a research study can be formulated within a framework of theory, the more valuable it is in promoting the advancement of knowledge."[11]

Early nursing research was conducted without using a theoretical framework. Instead, theoretical frameworks were borrowed from other disciplines, or no theoretical frameworks were used.

As nurses searched to define and advance nursing knowledge, nursing theorists came forward and proposed various theories, frameworks, and models of nursing.

Nursing theories, frameworks, and models present systematic explanations about relationships among phenomena. Principles for explaining, predicting, and controlling phenomena are embodied within a nursing theoretical framework. These frameworks serve the purpose of:

- Making the findings of nursing research meaningful and **generalizable**
- Providing an orderly system with which to integrate facts and observations within one study or between several studies
- Providing a coherent structure of the body of nursing science that makes it easier for the clinical nurse, educator, and researcher to understand, use, and communicate within the profession and to other disciplines

Nursing theory, framework, and model provide stimulation and direction for research by guiding the researcher to develop the research questions that are subjected to empirical testing through the research process.

For nursing to continue to develop as a science, it is essential for research to spring from theory. Fawcett views research and theory as two intertwining parts that are linked to each other.[12] Theory is one side of the double helix, spiraling up from an idea; research is the other side of the helix, spiraling from the identification of the research question through the research process to recommendations. The heart of the spiral is the pairing of theory with research. In essence, theory directs research and research shapes theory.[13]

Step V: Identifying the Variables

Once the literature has been reviewed, the problem and purpose have been determined, and a theoretical framework has been identified, the variables that will become the building blocks of the study are identified.

A variable is a property or attribute that someone or something possesses. As the name implies, a variable varies. A variable differs from one person to another or from one situation to another. It can be as tangible as an individual's weight and blood pressure, or as intangible as an individual's attitude.

Variables can be discussed in several ways, depending on the qualities or properties of the variables. Variables are classified according to their relationship to the problem being investigated.[14] Two properties that variables possess are continuity and discreteness. A continuous

variable is a variable that represents a continuous progression from the smallest possible amount to the largest possible amount, with measurement theoretically possible at any point along the continuum. A continuous variable is a variable with graduated measures that may differ by infinitely small amounts.[15] Examples of continuous variables include: age, weight, height, P_{CO_2}, and P_{O_2}.

A discrete variable, on the other hand, is one for which measurement and classification are possible only in whole units.[16] Discrete variables do not progress along a continuum but are discrete and separate entities, or classes. Examples of discrete variables include: gender, number of children in a family, number of schools attended, and number of living grandparents. A true discrete variable cannot be converted to a continuous variable and can be measured only by a nominal **scale.**

Two of the fundamental purposes of the research process are: to help gain an understanding of how or why variables vary; and to determine how they are related to or differ from each other. Furthermore, because a hypothesis predicts that two or more variables are related, there are always at least two main variables under examination in a research study. These variables are known as the **independent variable** and the **dependent variable.** The independent variable is the variable that is believed to cause or influence the dependent variable. In experimental research, it is the independent variable that is manipulated. The independent variable can stand alone.

The dependent variable is the one that is presumed to be affected by the independent variable. A hypothesis is a statement that suggests that the independent variable is related to the dependent variable. See Table 17-9 for examples of independent and dependent variables.

Step VI: Formulating the Hypothesis Statement

The research hypothesis is a declarative statement that describes the nurse researcher's "hunch" about the relationship between the independent and dependent variables. It is derived from the research question. For studies, including surveys in which relationships between variables are a consideration, hypotheses are used to direct the inquiries. For research questions that are descriptive and exploratory, formulation of a research hypothesis is generally not necessary, but it is essential for higher levels of inquiry.

Hypotheses are stated in one of three formats: directional, nondirectional, or in the null-statistical form (Table 17-10).

A **directional hypothesis** states a direction of the anticipated outcomes; for example, the elderly hypertensive client with a supportive care giver has greater compliance to the medication regimen.

A **nondirectional hypothesis** does not state a specific direction; for example, there is a difference in elderly hypertensive clients with or without a supporting care giver in compliance to medication regimen.

A **null hypothesis** states that there is no difference between the variables. A null hypothesis is usually opposed to what the researcher is looking for, i.e., a difference. For example, there is no difference in the elderly hypertensive client with or without a supporting care giver in compliance to medication regimen.

The hypothesis is always reported as being either supported by the researcher's findings or rejected by the researcher's findings. A hypothesis is never proved to be "true."

Step VII: Defining Terms
The next step is to define the terms (variables) in the research question. It is important to distinguish between the conceptual and **opera-tional definitions** of the key terms. The conceptual definition is the classical or dictionary definition of the variable, which can often be derived from the theoretical framework of the study. When the variable is applied to the researcher's study, it becomes the operational definition (Table 17–11).

After the nurse researcher has defined the research question, there are certain criteria that must be applied in order to determine if the question is researchable.

Step VIII: Selecting the Research Design and Methodology
The research design provides the schema for answering the research question. It gives a plan, structure, strategy, and control that guides the researcher during the implementation and **data** analysis phases of the study. The research design, if appropriate, will decrease errors and **control** pre-existing conditions or extraneous variables that may affect the outcome or the dependent variable under study. Through this control, the nurse researcher is able to maximize the results obtained.

Survey or descriptive, experimental or quasi-experimental, **case study,** and historical designs are some of the most frequently used research designs.

Survey Research Designs. Survey research designs involve studying populations or universes based on data collected from a drawn **sample.** They are descriptive in nature and are used to

TABLE 17–9. EXAMPLES OF INDEPENDENT AND DEPENDENT VARIABLES WITHIN RESEARCH QUESTIONS

Research Problem	Independent Variable	Dependent Variable
Does the amount of alcohol consumption of a pregnant mother affect the birth weight of her infant?	Amount of alcohol consumed by the pregnant mother	Birth weight of the infant
Does preoperative teaching by the nurse reduce the level of anxiety of the child following surgery?	Preoperative teaching by the nurse	Child's level of anxiety following surgery
What is the relationship between the type of medication regimen and control of high blood pressure in the elderly?	Type of medication regimen	Control of high blood pressure in the elderly
What is the relationship between the presence and type of caregiver support system and the self-care abilities of the older adult?	Presence and type of caregiver support system	Self-care abilities and self-esteem of the elderly

TABLE 17–10. WORDING OF THE RESEARCH PURPOSE AND ITS RELATED RESEARCH QUESTION AND HYPOTHESIS

Research Purpose	Research Question and Level of Inquiry	Hypothesis
To determine the relationship of the alcohol consumption of the pregnant mother and the birth weight of her infant.	Does the amount of alcohol consumed by the pregnant mother affect the birth weight of her infant? (Second or third level of inquiry)	The birth weight of infants of non-alcohol-drinking mothers is greater than the weight of infants of mothers who consume alcohol (directional).
To compare the effects of two preoperative teaching methods by the nurse in reducing children's anxiety following surgery.	Does preoperative teaching by the nurse reduce children's anxiety following surgery? (Third or fourth level of inquiry)	There is a difference in the effects of two preoperative teaching methods by the nurse in reducing children's anxiety following surgery (nondirectional).
To determine the relationship between prescribed treatment methods, client acuity, and nursing workload.	Is there a relationship between prescribed treatment measures and client acuity to nursing workload? (Third level of inquiry)	There is no difference between prescribed treatment measures, client acuity, and resulting nursing workload (null hypothesis).
To determine the effectiveness of medication regimen in controlling high blood pressure in the elderly.	What is the most effective type of medication regimen in controlling high blood pressure in the elderly? (First or second level of inquiry)	There is no need for a hypothesis.

answer the first and second levels of inquiry with its research questions: "What is this?" and "What is happening here?" The survey design often uses a written questionnaire, interview, or observation of what people are doing. Survey research serves to collect data about defining characteristics, opinions, attitudes, or behaviors as they exist in the general population. Surveys have advantages and disadvantages as methods for gathering data. The advantages of surveys are that they:

- Can be used to gather information from a large number of subjects
- May require minimal expenditures of time, effort, and money
- Can be easily described, evaluated, and replicated
- Can be structured for computer analysis

The limitations of survey designs include:

- The possibility of low return rate
- The possibility that the questions are confusing or irrelevant
- The difficulty in storing vast numbers of questionnaires
- The difficulty in tracking data

- The tendency for responses to the questionnaire to be superficial
- No allowance for cause-and-effect study

Several types of survey designs are: evaluative, longitudinal, cross-sectional, and comparative.

The *evaluative survey* is conducted to determine what has been accomplished by a project or program. The questions most frequently asked include: "Are the results as expected?" and "Are the original purposes of the program or project met?" This method requires a sound knowledge of the evaluation process and its techniques. It involves identifying the appropriate questions to ask in order to obtain the desired information, people to be surveyed or sources to be reviewed, and, finally, the audience to whom the evaluation report will be given. An example of the use of **evaluative research** design would be to make an ongoing evaluation of the education programs within a hypertension clinic. The research questions to be answered would be: "What are the effects of the various education programs on the clients' knowledge of hypertension and medications and compliance with their medication regimen?," "What are the costs of the program and

TABLE 17–11. EXAMPLES OF CONCEPTUAL AND OPERATIONAL DEFINITIONS FOR SELECT
RESEARCH QUESTIONS

Research Question	Conceptual Definition	Operational Definition
Does the amount of alcohol consumed by the pregnant mother affect the birth weight of her infant?	Alcohol consumed: Ingestion of intoxicating product of fermentation in spirits.	Alcohol consumed: The amount of alcohol as reported by subject when questioned by means of an alcohol consumption questionnaire.
	Birth weight of infant: the amount that an infant weighs at time of birth in terms of a unit (pound, kilogram, ounce).	Birth weight of infant: weight of the baby at time of delivery as noted in medical record of mother.

how do they compare to the costs of the previous programs?," and "What are the reactions of the clients, the nurses, physicians, and other disciplines to the program?"

The disadvantage of the evaluative survey design method is that it requires a high degree of expertise and knowledge in order to design a comprehensive evaluation program. A poorly designed evaluative survey can produce a mass of irrelevant information that will make drawing conclusions difficult.

A *longitudinal survey* is conducted to collect data from the same people at more than one point in time. The purpose is to compare certain dependent variables, such as knowledge, attitudes, or adherence to a treatment regimen over time. The fundamental advantage of this type of study is that the researcher does not have to assume that different groups are comparable to designate them as representing different points of the same process. The disadvantage of the longitudinal survey design method is that changes may be caused by factors other than time. There are also difficulties in keeping subjects in the study for an extended time period. The passage of time may bring unforeseeable events, such as death or acute illness of the subject. The subject may move away or lose interest in continuing to participate in the study. All of these factors contribute to a change in sample size, which may affect the study's outcome.

A possible research question to be answered would be: "How effective is discharge planning and teaching in increasing clients' compliance to the medication regimen at 3, 6, and 12 months after discharge?"

A *cross-sectional survey* is conducted to survey several groups in various stages of development at the same time. For example, a researcher might wish to examine feelings toward hospitalization in third, sixth, and ninth graders. The disadvantage of the **cross-sectional** survey **design** method may be the inability to find an adequate number of subjects for the cross-sectional groups. Furthermore, one main limitation of this type of study is that the researcher is testing different people in the different groups, and this kind of intervention may confound the findings. The research question mentioned above could also be pursued with this type of survey design.

The *comparative survey* is conducted to compare or contrast representative samples from two or more groups of subjects in regard to the designated variables. The procedures used to obtain subjects must be carefully followed so that all subjects are as similar as possible on all variables that are not the focus of the study and also to ensure that it is as representative as possible of the population from which it was drawn.

Experimental Research Design. The *experimental research design* is considered the most rigorous and scientific of the research designs. The purpose of experimental research is to investigate cause-and-effect relationships by manipulating and controlling the treatment (independent variables) and observing or measuring the change in the dependent variable.

One of the advantages of experimental designs is that they are powerful research tools because of the rigor, precision, and control that is built into them. By using experimental designs, researchers are able to study cause-and-effect relationships or test causal hypotheses. Causal relationships are important to researchers because they allow the researcher to predict and explain.

The disadvantage of this method is that the control that is required of experimental research often creates an artificial or restrictive situation, which may become difficult for the human subjects involved in the study.

The criteria of randomization, manipulation, and control must be built into the experimental design.

Randomization consists of **random** selections of the **sample** from a total population using the method of sampling technique that ensures everyone has an equal chance of being selected from the total **population.** It also consists of *random assignment* of the subjects to either the experimental or control groups. This guarantees that each subject has an equal chance of being assigned to either the control or the treatment groups.

Control is the second criterion of experimental research. The nurse researcher attempts to eliminate all possible factors that could influence or affect the results that the manipulation of the independent variable will have on the dependent variable.

Manipulation is the third criterion of experimental research and refers to the steps that the nurse researcher takes in manipulating or varying (causing some change) the independent variable and subsequently observing its effects on the dependent variable in the experimental group.

An example of a research question suitable for the use of an experimental research design in the laboratory setting is to determine the effectiveness of biofeedback, visual stimuli, and education in controlling episodes of hypertension in the elderly.

Quasi-experimental Research Design.
A quasi-experimental research design attempts to approximate the conditions of experimental research designs in settings that do not permit control and manipulation of the variables or the randomization of the sample. Often, because of the client population or the philosophy of an institution that may view it as unethical to withhold treatment from the control group, the quasi-experimental research design is the one of choice. The quasi-experimental design has an advantage over the pre-experimental design in that it permits control for internal **validity.** There are several disadvantages of this method. These include:

- It cannot test causal hypotheses
- It may be difficult to generalize the study's findings to more than the sample group
- It is susceptible to the effects of testing and experimental conditions

An example of a research question suitable for the use of a quasi-experimental research design is to determine the effects of primary nursing on the clients' compliance to a hypertension medication regimen. Because it is necessary to implement primary nursing throughout the entire hospital, it is impossible for the nurse researcher to create the experimental and control sample groups. The alternative is to locate another hospital with similar characteristics, such as number of beds, profit-based, and the existence of a hypertensive clinic whose department of nursing does not use the primary nursing practice framework. A sample selected from this hospital's hypertension clinic could serve as the control group.

Case Study Research Design.
Case study research design is undertaken to assess specific client situations in depth. The client's medical, social, and family histories are explored. The nursing care plan, its design, and implementation are carefully analyzed and evaluated. The findings obtained by use of the case study design generally provide a wealth of information that is helpful in expanding the base of nursing knowledge.

The purpose of case study method of research include:

- Gaining insight into little known health problems
- Gaining background data for further studies
- Explaining psychosocial phenomena

This study research method is useful when exploring areas in which little is known about a phenomenon and where there have been few prior studies. For example: Psychosocial adaptation in families of AIDS clients or ethical dilemmas in providing health care for AIDS clients. Another advantage of the case study method is that it is useful in studying a process over time.

The disadvantage of the case study research design is that the findings are only applied to the subjects within the study and may not be generalizable to the total population.

An example of a research question suitable for the case study research design is to do an in-depth assessment of two clients who have been on hypertensive medication for at least one year, one of whom has complied with the medication regimen and one of whom has failed to comply with the regimen.

Historical Research Design. Historical research design uses primary sources of data, such as documents, literature, and organizational minutes, to relate past events to current or future trends, developments, or events. The passage of time often permits a more objective review of past events. There are several advantages of historical research. This research attempts to explain the reality of the past. Another advantage is that the past can be preserved by written documents. Finally, there is the potential for illuminating a current research question. The disadvantage of the historical research design is the researcher must take additional precautions to ensure that the data sources are valid and represent the true meaning of the past event, meeting, or trend.

An example of a research question suitable for the historical research design would be to examine the evolution of the role of the nurse practitioner within hypertension clinics in the Northeastern states of the United States. It would help to answer such questions as: "What are the determining factors that led to the increased use of nurse practitioners in hypertension clinics?" and "As they assumed an increased role in prescribing and monitoring medications for the clinic's clients, what were the effects on clients' compliance as compared to a physician-monitored program?"

Step IX: Specifying the Population and Sample

One of the most important steps in the research process is identifying and selecting the subjects for the study, for it is the subjects who will provide the data to answer the research question. Subjects may include clients, nurses, fellow students or members of other health disciplines. Data are generally collected from a sample rather than an entire population.

The term population means the entire set of people or objects that have common traits. An example of population is all the 200 hypertensive clients in Hospital "A." The term "sample," is a subset of the population that is selected to participate in the research study. In the above example, the nurse researcher may randomly select a sample of 50 from the above total population of 200 hypertensive clients in Hospital "A."

All researchers use sampling because it is a feasible and logical way of making statements about a larger group based on the findings from the smaller group. Researchers can then make inferences from the sample to the population if the sample-selection process was systematic.

The number of subjects needed for a sample is related to the research question that is being asked. When the research question is at the first two levels of inquiry ("What is this?" or "What is happening here?"), it is at the factor naming and relating stages; a larger sample size will be required to ensure adequate representation of the total population. When the research questions are at the third and fourth levels of inquiry ("What will happen if . . . ?" or "How can I make something happen?"), the sample size can be somewhat smaller. The randomization of the sampling procedure is the important determinant.

Subjects may be found almost anywhere, depending on the focus of the study. The sources and locations of the subjects include hospitals, clinics, nutrition sites, and physician offices. Other sites where the nurse researcher is able to obtain the type of subjects required can also be used.

Selection of subjects depends on the research question, sources of the sample, and the research methodology (Table 17-12). It is

TABLE 17–12. CONSIDERATIONS IN SELECTING A SAMPLE

- The number of subjects to be used
- Sources and location of the subjects
- Criteria or limitations for their selection
- Sampling procedure to be used
- Time available for the nurse researcher to permit obtaining the desired sample size as well as to complete the research study (e.g., the student must complete within two semesters)
- Resources of the nurse researcher become important if multiple copies of a questionnaire must be sent out to a large sample or interviews must be conducted that require extensive travel time

through the criteria, or limitations, that the nurse researcher is able to some extent control some of the extraneous and outside variables. The method of sample selection is crucial to the research design. The researcher must be concerned with how to get the most representative sample possible. For example, when concerned with compliance versus noncompliance in elderly hypertensive black clients, the sample must reflect this group.

Step X: The Sampling Procedure

How to obtain a representative sample is a question frequently asked by novice researchers. Probability and nonprobability sampling are the two major approaches. Probability sampling is the more rigorous. This requires that every member in the population have an equal or random chance of selection. In contrast, nonprobability sampling provides no way of estimating the probability that each element will be included in the study. There are several major sampling procedures that can be used by researchers. These include:

- Convenience sampling
- Quota sampling
- Simple random sampling
- Stratified random sampling
- Systematic sampling
- Cluster sampling

A *convenience sample* or *accidental sample* means choosing subjects who are convenient or readily available to the nurse researcher. The researcher will take all clients who are admitted to the medical units with the diagnosis of chronic hypertension during the study period of July and August in a given year. The limitation of the convenience sampling method is that the researcher is only able to apply the study's findings to the sample used. The findings are not generalizable to a larger population.

A *quota sample* ensures that a certain number or percentage of subjects is selected from different groups of subjects in order to obtain a more representative sample. For example, the nurse researcher may want to determine the relationship of various cultural groups to compliance of a hypertension medication regimen. The nurse researcher would determmine by the latest U.S. Census figures the percentage of the cultural groups within the total population of a given geographic area. If in the total population, blacks represented 12 percent and Hispanics represented 15 percent, the researcher would be certain to have 12 percent of the total sample number consist of black subjects and 15 percent of the total sample number consist of Hispanics.

The limitation of the quota sampling method is the difficulty in always being able to locate the predesired percentage or quota of each of the groups to be included in the final sample.

A *simple random sample* means every subject in a particular population group has the same chance of being selected. The nurse researcher uses a table of random numbers to select the sample. For example, the nurse researcher may want to conduct an experimental study on the suitability and effectiveness of use of biofeedback and education in controlling hypertension in hospitalized adults. The nurse researcher lists the total population of clients with chronic hypertension on two medical units and assigns each client a number. Using the table of random numbers (Figure 17–1), the nurse researcher closes his or her eyes and uses a pencil point to choose a number from one table. Then, moving in a systematic way—up, down, or diagonally—the nurse chooses the entire sample by picking those subjects whose numbers correspond to the table of random numbers. Those numbers that do not appear on the list of clients are ignored. The selection is stopped when the sample size is reached.

A *stratified random sample* is similar to the quota sample in that predesignated categories and respective percentages have been identified. Examples of strata of interest to nurses may include clients with certain diseases, clients of different ages, or persons who need special treatments. Random selection is used as it is described above.

Systematic sampling involves drawing a predesignated number from the population. The number is selected randomly from a table of random numbers, for example, 9; then every ninth person on the list is selected to participate. Systematic sampling generally results in a representative sample if the list does not have a built-in **bias**.

Cluster sampling requires that the population be divided into groups or clusters. Then, the clusters are randomly selected. Further, in-

dividuals from the clusters are randomly selected. Many large studies are conducted in this fashion.

Step XI: Informed Consent

Client self-determination is an important value to be respected by nurses and other health-care providers. The American Nurses' Association's Code for Nurses delineates and supports this ethical standard of self-determination as a moral right.[17]

Obtaining **informed consent** is a vitally important step in the research process. Before entering into a research study, every potential human subject must have been given a complete explanation about the study and must sign an informed consent form that contains the details of this explanation (Table 17–13). Further assurances should be given to each potential subject that the study is not harmful, that he or she may withdraw at any time, and that **confiden-**

66624	27534	66752	87631	76271	85890
12292	91687	24574	22069	72996	54352
84748	19548	19059	63168	89784	22477
68651	31747	34482	29589	96206	94916
59976	50600	33195	36384	10771	85120
21413	88889	94273	34059	48760	46861
32820	83530	57518	21576	38210	31258
75137	48809	98738	75486	97513	78997
98724	96381	84772	79889	50543	39939
69548	71705	79160	54394	17768	94793
69157	19121	71929	19782	54269	86045
96883	10244	89410	73545	58117	17843
55208	52861	62533	19998	25036	57003
61731	10033	24541	82152	27789	99840
83678	21572	61546	15029	41237	72010
73379	52589	91882	82607	26490	81039
95673	96305	22685	93092	80104	13748
50653	60803	44631	89692	26749	83230
57703	11911	38276	16590	16298	72604
69266	26913	57947	22298	18760	85202
95270	16258	11590	25085	93008	53391
11660	72973	97549	67651	87728	50718
18965	41951	71687	40767	65540	54562
49346	83818	30803	78023	63711	78978
43058	70548	20765	66420	77414	89932
67755	82535	30321	69953	93963	37593
86597	69284	64000	65895	28958	92897
13574	88434	10054	25967	67782	28047
86998	40284	31887	47074	48397	33151
84597	87512	73882	78798	53849	63674
66142	92284	65091	77342	85453	55906
42062	25426	86712	88100	40072	40119
38963	84854	61786	51553	67435	13609

Figure 17–1. Example of table of random numbers (five digits).

TABLE 17–13. COMPONENTS OF THE INFORMED CONSENT PROCESS AND FORM

Explanation of the purpose and procedures of the research study

Identification and description of the possible benefits, discomforts, or risks to the subject if they participate in the research study

Provisions for confidentiality and anonymity of the subject; *confidentiality* assures the subject her or his responses will be kept in confidence and will be unable to be linked back to the subject; *anonymity* assures the subject that the reported information about the findings of the research study will not reveal the identity of the subject

Participation in the study is completely voluntary and the subject is free to withdraw at any time without affecting subsequent type and quality of her or his care

Identification of the name and telephone number of the researcher and a person who is not directly connected with the research but is knowledgeable about the research study, to whom the subject would be able to address concerns and questions about the research study

Provision for the date and signature of the subject, the researcher, and an objective witness

---

tiality will be maintained. Further, the researcher should provide his or her phone number in the event that a subject needs further information. Health-care institutions, such as hospitals, have special committees that review research proposals in terms of ethical issues such as inclusion of appropriate informed consent procedures. These are often known as human research committees. Such committees usually have representatives from all the health disciplines and major departments within the hospital (e.g., department of nursing, medicine, radiology, pharmacy, and hospital administration). In addition, the department of nursing may have its own nursing research committee consisting of representatives from the different divisions or units, such as intensive care, medical-surgical, or obstetrics and gynecology.

Step XII: The Pilot Study

Once the nurse researcher has completed the research design (sampling procedure, sample limitations, methodology, and instrumentation), it is important to pilot test or do a mini-simulation of the research study. The purposes of doing a **pilot study** include:

- Determining the feasibility of the research study itself
- Identifying problems in the research design, data collection methods, and analysis plan
- Testing the instrument(s) to be used

As a result of the pilot study, the nurse researcher is able to make the necessary changes in the design and method before beginning the full study.

Step XIII: Methodology and Data Collection

The scientific method of inquiry is characterized by a reliance on empirical information, that is, information collected from the observable world. The scientific method allows researchers to make statements about what is true. Philosophies and theories require the researcher to seek truth in order to provide data to support or refute them.

Sources used to collect data can be documents, laboratory materials, and people. Instruments of data collection may include interviews, questionnaires, psychological tests, or physiological measurements or tests.

There are basically three methods of data collection: observation, questioning, and measurement.

Observation is a research method in which data are obtained from descriptive accounts of observations made in a field research situation. *Questioning* is a research method in which data are obtained by asking the subject questions, either verbally or in writing. *Measurement* is a research method in which data are obtained through the administration of a measuring instrument (for instance, a test) or a procedure (e.g., blood pressure) to the subjects.

There are some major factors of the observation method for data collection that the nurse researcher should consider. These include:

- The decision about who is to be observed, what is to be observed, and what to do with the data collected
- The development of an observational guide on which to record the observed data
- The identification, recruitment, and training of the research observers or assistants
- The outline of the type of subject-observer interaction: Will the subjects know they are

being watched? Will the observer be watching the actual clinical situation or an indirect version, such as in role playing or videotape

There are considerations that the nurse researcher should include when using the questioning method for data collection. The literature should be carefully reviewed to determine what others have studied and thought about the research question. The questions should be phrased so that they:

- Are clear and understandable
- Seek only one piece of information at a time
- Are free from suggestion or bias that would indirectly tell the subjects how the researcher wants them to respond
- Are grammatically correct

The nurse researcher should determine how the subjects will answer the question, either in the form of open- or closed-ended questions. An **open-ended question** permits the subject to answer the question in any manner desired. A **closed-ended question,** such as multiple choice, provides all the answers. The subjects are expected to select the answer that best reflects their response to the question.

An example of the research question that would use either the observation method or the question method is, "What are the separate clinical decisions and nursing interventions involved in helping to maintain the blood pressure of clients who have gone into shock in an intensive care unit?"

If the observation method of data collection is chosen, the nurse researcher would observe and determine the number, type, and variety of nursing interventions used. The questionnaire would consist of questions regarding the clinical decision-making processes of the nurse during this emergency situation.

There are also major factors that the nurse researcher should consider when using the measurement data collection method. These include determining if the variables (independent and dependent) are discrete or continuous.

There are four levels of measurement in statistics (Table 17–14). These are nominal, ordinal, interval, and ratio. *Nominal* is the most primitive level of measurement. The only purpose of the numbers is to identify individual entities or to classify entities in accordance to their similarities or differences in respect to a property. *Ordinal measurement* seeks to place each observation in its relative position with the others. It does not attempt to determine how far apart two observations are from each other. It is always in terms of higher–lower, or faster–slower.

For example, the nurse researcher wants to rate the discrete variable of each subject's adjustment to the chronic illness of hypertension on a four-point scale from "Excellent" through "Good," "Fair," to "Poor". The data obtained would identify those subjects whose adjustment was rated "Excellent" as being better adjusted than subjects rated "Good," and both of these groups would be consid-

TABLE 17–14. LEVELS OF MEASUREMENT FOR DISCRETE AND CONTINUOUS VARIABLES

Level	Measurement Properties	Type of Variable	Examples
Nominal	Identity	Discrete	Sex Clinical diagnoses
Ordinal	Identity Order	Discrete	Percentile norms Socioeconomic status
Interval	Identity Order Additivity Equal intervals	Continuous	Year Temperature
Ratio	Identity Order Additivity Equal intervals Absolute zero	Continuous	Distance Time Weight

ered better adjusted than subjects rated as "Fair" or "Poor." However, this ordinal data does not tell us how much better-adjusted the subject rated "Excellent" is than the subject rated "Good."

Interval measurement is the third level of measurement. This measure is sufficiently precise to enable one unit of the measure to have the same quantitative meaning at any point on the scale of measurement. Thus, one inch represents the same difference in height whether it is the inch between 5 and 6 inches or between 30 and 31 inches. The blood pressure reading is an interval type of measurement. The difference between a systolic blood pressure of 120 and 130 is the same as the difference between the systolic pressures of 140 and 150.

Ratio measurement is the highest level of measurement. It has the same property as interval measurement in that it has equal intervals. However, it goes further, in that it begins from a true zero point that represents the total absence of the quality being measured. The true zero point may be either a physical reality or a conceptual or theoretical reference point.

Selection of the Measuring Instrument. The next step in the data collection process is to select the measuring instrument. Many of these instruments can be found during the review of the literature. It is preferable, if possible, to use instruments that already have identified **reliability, validity**, sensitivity, and appropriateness.

Reliability is the basic attribute every instrument must possess. An instrument is reliable if, when it is administered twice under the same circumstances, it provides identical data. It denotes stability and repeatability.

Reliability is generally reported by the basic statistic of **coefficient alpha** (**Cronbach's alpha**). This is the reliability index that estimates the internal consistency of an instrument composed of several items or subsections. Coefficient alpha of + 1.00 indicates perfect reliability; coefficient alpha at or close to 0.00 would indicate no reliability.

Validity is another important characteristic that a measuring instrument must have. It is the extent to which the instrument actually measures what it is supposed to measure. Types of validity include **content validity, construct validity,** and concurrent validity. Content validity involves subjective judgments by experts or respondents as to the degree to which the test appears to measure what it was designed to measure. In order to obtain content validity, the instrument constructor analyzes the content of the area that the instrument is designed to evaluate and structures it accordingly. To design a knowledge test about hypertension, for example, the researcher would examine many textbooks, articles, and objectives prepared by national councils and professional organizations. From these materials the researcher determines what content should be selected for inclusion in the instrument. The researcher can also ask experts in the area to rate each test item for importance. To determine if a published instrument has content validity for the subjects in his or her research, the researcher compares the content of a course with the content of the instrument.

A **construct** is a highly complex concept that is composed of many facets that can be exhibited in a number of situations, but no one observation may be regarded as the one that explains it. Therefore, construct validity is an important type of validity to obtain. Construct validation begins with defining the meaning of the hypothesized construct in a wide variety of situations. Construct validation goes beyond the examination of the test to the theoretical basis of the construct, for example, self-concept. Therefore, construct validity refers to the degree to which a test measures the underlying theoretical explanation of the set of concepts consituting the construct. Constructs can be examined in many ways but are never definitely established.

Another type of validity that a researcher might obtain and report is concurrent validity. This refers to the extent that scores on the test can be related to scores on a similar test. Correlation between the two tests determines the concurrent validity.

Sensitivity of a measurement instrument is characterized by the ability of the instrument to make discriminations required by the research question. It should be able to detect change or evaluate differences in the change, as well as whether change has occurred.

Appropriateness is also an important characteristic and it is defined as the extent to which the sample of subjects will be able to understand and meet the demands of the instrument.

The nurse researcher might be able to locate an instrument by referring to source books that contain collections of instruments and are generally found in most university libraries. These references contain data on instruments that have been used, tested, and have reliability and validity statistics identified and described.

If a suitable measuring instrument cannot be found, the researcher may wish to create one. This type of project is only recommended for experienced nurse researchers at the master's and doctoral levels. To create a research instrument is a complex endeavor, and it may require a great deal of time and effort to construct a reliable and valid instrument.

Step XIV: Data Analysis and Interpretation

Once the nurse researcher has collected all the desired information and data from the subjects, it is time to do the statistical analysis. Identification of which statistics to use should occur at the time of selecting an instrument and designing the study method.

There are three ways to divide statistics:

- Statistics that describe the data
- Statistics that infer from the data
- Statistics that divide qualitatively into parametric and nonparametric categories

A *parameter* is a function, characteristic, or quality of the population whose concept is constant but whose value varies. Parameters are always characteristic of the universe or the population.

When there is a similar characteristic in the sample, it is called a *statistic*. Statistics help researchers by describing data, by drawing inferences to larger bodies of data, and in studying causal relationships.

Use of Elementary Descriptive Statistics. A knowledge of basic statistics is a must for the nurse researcher. This knowledge is necessary to read and interpret the findings of a reported research study. It is also necessary for the analysis of the data obtained from the research project.

Descriptive statistics are used to describe and synthesize the data that are obtained. Descriptive statistics are tools to be used for describing, summarizing, or reducing data into a comprehensive amount—the properties of an otherwise unwieldy mass of data. The first step in analyzing raw data is to use frequency distributions that will provide order for large amounts of data. Frequency counts identify the numbers within each class of observations. An example of a class of observations would be the categorical variable of sex: male and female, or the age ranges of the elderly: 65 to 75, 76 to 85, 86 to 95, over 95 years of age. A frequency distribution of the categorical variable of sex within a sample of 70 might be 20 males and 50 females.

A set of data may next be summarized into three categories:

- The shape of the distribution
- Central tendency
- Measures of variability

A *distribution* can be thought of as the way the scores fall along the x- and y-axis. The normal distribution is a theoretical distribution that allows researchers to make useful probability statements. A frequency distribution depicts the number of scores or values falling at any point in a distribution. The notion of **central tendency** helps to summarize these frequencies.

Measures of central tendency can be thought of as averages. They are characteristic representations of groups. These measures allow for comparisons between groups. The possession of a common trait of a group of items or subjects provides for the formulation of a general description of the group. This is more powerful than simply using one item or subject to formulate a description. The term used for this general characteristic is central tendency. Measures of central tendency of a set or group of scores are the most widely used statistical descriptions of data. There are three measures of central tendency. These are:

- The mean
- The median
- The mode

The **mean** is the average of a set of scores, simply the sum of the scores or values divided by the number of scores or values in a data set. The mean is the most commonly used of the measures of central tendency. The mean has two advantages. It is the most reliable and accurate of the measures of central tendency. The mean also is suitable for mathematical calculations. However, the mean has a disadvantage in that it is influenced by very high or very low scores.

The **median** is the score or value that falls in the middle of a distribution of scores. It can be thought of as the 50th percentile. The median is the second-most-often-used measure of central tendency. The calculation of the median is even easier than the mean. The scores or values are placed in rank order from highest to lowest (or vice versa) and divided at the score in the middle. An advantage of using the median is that it is less affected by extreme scores. A disadvantage is that it cannot be combined with other medians to give a combined median from other distributions.

The **mode** is that score or value that appears most frequently. The mode does not involve any calculations and can be determined quickly. It is not affected by extreme scores but may be affected by changes in the grouping of data. Other disadvantages of the mode are that it is a poor measure of central tendency, particularly in very small samples, and it cannot be used in algebraic calculations. The mode from one sample cannot be compared or averaged with a mode from another group. It is also possible that a group of scores can have no mode, or more than one mode. In a normal distribution, the mean, median, and mode all occur at the center of the curve.

The purpose of describing the central tendencies of data is to provide ways to describe how the scores group together. Measures of *variability*, on the other hand, are used to examine the dispersion of the scores. If scores in a data set are similar, there is little variability. The most frequently used measures of variability are:

- Range
- Standard deviation

The **range** is the simplest measure of variability. It is the difference between the smallest and largest scores or values in a distribution. The range is easy to compute but has many disadvantages. It is an unstable statistic in that one extreme score can change it. The range also does not account for various scores between the highest and lowest scores or values. Therefore, it is customary to report other measures of variability such as the standard deviation.

The **standard deviation** is an average of the deviations from the mean. The standard deviation is the most widely used measure of variability when the distribution is normal.

The above statistics are referred to as *univariate* (one-variable statistics). These statistics will be able to assist the researcher in describing the characteristics or variables of interest of the sample (e.g., age, sex, educational level, occupation, or scores on an attitude or knowledge scale).

Measure of Correlation. Nursing researchers may be concerned with determining the relationships or significant differences between variables (second, third, and fourth levels of inquiry). In order to do this, descriptive statistics that measure correlation are used.

The most common descriptive statistic used to measure correlation in research is the **correlation coefficient**. This statistic is used to address the question of the extent to which two variables are related to each other—to quantify the degree of relationship between variables. For example, "To what extent is attitude toward math related to math performance?," or "To what extent are cigarette smoking and lung cancer related?" These questions are answered by calculating statistics that express the magnitude or degree of a relationship.

Two variables are correlated if they tend to "go together." If high scores on one variable tend to be accompanied by high scores on another variable, then the variables are said to be correlated. Thus, the researcher can describe the degree of correlation between variables as "strong," "low," "positive," or "moderate," but these terms tend to be vague. However, if the researcher computes a coefficient of correlation between the sets of scores, the relationship can be described more explicitly. A coefficient of correlation is a statistical summary of the degree of relationship or association between two variables.[18] The correlation coefficient expresses both the magnitude and direction of the two continuous variable relationships. For example, consider bivariate-correlation of height with weight. There are two types of correlations between variables: positive correlations and negative correlations. The statistics of correlation vary from 0 through plus or minus 1. Plus or minus 1 is a perfect correlation. A positive correlation is known as a direct relationship between the variables and a negative correlation is known as an inverse relationship.

Many times correlations between variables are depicted visually. These are known as scattergrams or plots (Fig. 17–2). Each point in the graph represents one subject's scores or values on each of the variables being measured. The purpose of the scattergram is to examine the nature of the relationship between the variables. It can indicate both the direction (positive or negative) and the approximate magnitude of a correlation. The more the dots form a straight line, the higher the correlation.

The two most frequently used correlation coefficient indexes are the Pearson Product Moment Correlation Coefficient (the Pearson r) and the Spearman Rank Correlation (r_{ranks}). The Pearson r requires continuous data, such as time, height, or weight. The Spearman Rank involves ranks on each of two variables being observed.

Use of Inferential Statistics. Inferential statistics involve making predictions about a population by using a sample. Therefore, the purpose of inferential statistics is to predict or estimate characteristics of a population from a knowledge of the characteristics of a sample of the population.[19]

The most frequently used inferential statistics are the t-test, analyses of variance (ANOVA), and **chi-square test** (χ^2). These statistics help the researcher to make judgments about or generalize the findings to a larger population. Each of these tests has a specific application and can only be used with certain types of data (categorical or discrete versus continuous variables) and with certain levels of measurement (nominal, ordinal, interval, or ratio) (Table 17–15).

Calculation by hand is cumbersome and often subject to errors; therefore, nurse researchers use an appropriate software statistical package to have the computer complete the statistical analysis procedures. It is beyond the scope of this text to describe statistical formulas and steps in calculation, but many good statistics books are available in libraries.

The t-Test. The t-test is used when the researcher desires to compare two independent groups of subjects on the dependent variable of interest. For example, is there a significant difference in compliance to hypertension medication regimen between men and women, or between the experimental and control groups?

The t-test for paired samples is used on dependent or single groups when two sets of scores, such as a subject's pretest score and posttest scores, are compared. To be significant, the t-value obtained at x-degrees of freedom must be greater than the t-value identified in the statistical table for the t-test statistic.

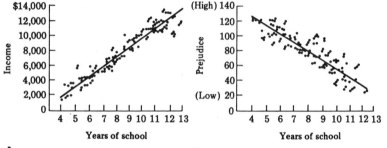

Figure 17–2. A. Scatter diagram representing a positive correlation between education and income. **B.** Scatter diagram representing a negative correlation between education and prejudice. *(From Jack Levin, Elementary Statistics in Social Research, 3rd ed., (New York: Harper & Row, 1983).)*

A   **B**

TABLE 17-15. SELECTION OF STATISTICAL TESTS

Name of Procedure	Test Statistic	Purpose	Independent Variable		Dependent Variable	
			Type	Level of Measurement	Type	Level of Measurement
t-test for independent groups	t	To test the difference between the means of two independent groups	Categorical or discrete	Nominal	Continuous	Interval or ratio
t-test for dependent paired samples	t	To test for dependent paired samples or scores, for example, pretest and posttest	Categorical or discrete	Nominal	Continuous	Interval or ratio
Analyses of variance (ANOVA)	F	To test the difference among the means of three or more independent groups of more than one independent variable	Categorical or discrete	Nominal	Categorical or discrete	Ordinal
Chi-square	χ^2	To test the difference in proportions in two or more groups	Categorical or discrete	Nominal	Categorical or discrete	Nominal
Correlation coefficient (Pearson's Product Moment)	r	To test if a relationship exists between two variables	Continuous	Interval or ratio	Continuous	Interval or ratio

ANOVA. A one-way analysis of variance (ANOVA) is an inferential statistical procedure used to test significance between three or more group means. The purpose of ANOVA is similar to that of the t-test, i.e., to compare mean scores. The difference is that ANOVA is used to compare three or *more* groups. This uses the F-ratio statistic rather than the t-test statistic. The F-ratio statistic goes a step further by looking not only at the variation between Group A, Group B, and Group C but also the variation within each group by itself. There is a table for the F-ratio statistic. Using the number of groups and degrees of freedom, the value is identified in the F-ratio statistical table. If the obtained value is greater than the tabled value, there is a significant difference between groups or within the group.

The multiple comparison procedures used in ANOVA are similar to applying several t-tests but differ in an extremely important way: The ANOVA controls the significance level to that set by the researcher.

Level of Significance. In addition to selecting the appropriate statistical test, the nurse researcher must identify the desired level of significance. The most frequently used levels of significance are 0.05 and 0.01. When the 0.05 level of significance is used, it means the researcher has identified in 95 samples that the significance is not due to chance alone but to the relationships of the variables under study. In this case the researcher is willing to erroneously reject the null hypothesis (of no relationship) 5 times out of 100. At the more conservative 0.01 significance level, the researcher has identified in 99 samples that the significance is not due to chance alone, but to the relationship of the variables under study. In this case, the researcher is willing to erroneously reject the null hypothesis only one time out of 100.

Use of Nonparametric Statistical Tests. The statistical tests in the preceding sections have summarized tests that rely on the assumptions that:

- Population distribution from which the samples were drawn was normal
- Data collected used interval or ratio level scales of measurement

Many studies, however, focus on variables that do not meet these conditions—for example, the study that ranked persons in terms of compliance, or knowledge of a disease. These data would be ordinal. Values are reported in terms of proportions and may not be normally distributed. Therefore, parametric statistics would not apply. Nonparametric statistics would be used. These statistics make no assumptions about the distribution and are known as distribution-free tests. If parametric statistics are used on data that do not meet the basic assumptions mentioned above, the statistical results will be erroneous and will lead to mistaken conclusions. Conversely, using nonparametric statistics when parametric statistics should be used will also lead to mistaken conclusions.

Chi-square. The chi-square statistic is the most frequently used nonparametric statistic. It is used when the researcher wants to test the difference in proportions of two or more groups.

The chi-square statistic sums the differences between the observed and expected frequencies under the conditions of the null hypothesis. The expected number is what would be expected by chance or according to the null hypothesis. When the discrepancy is large between what is found and what is expected would occur by chance, the chi-square statistic will be large. The researcher examines the chi-square statistical table at the desired degrees of freedom and level of significance. The obtained chi-square value must be larger than the table chi-

squared value to be significant. The null hypothesis can then be rejected and the alternate hypothesis can be accepted.

Degrees of Freedom. Degrees of freedom (df) is a statistical concept that has been introduced to control the bias resulting from using a sample instead of a population. This bias can be compensated for exactly by using the sample size (n) minus 1. This is written as

$$df = n - 1.$$

The computer will complete the computation of the statistical test and determine the degrees of freedom. This is calculated differently for each statistical test.

Use of the Appropriate Statistical Table. There is a specific statistical table for the t-test statistic, the F-test (ANOVA) statistic, the correlation coefficient (Pearson Product Moment Correlation, r) and the chi-square statistic.

Once the nurse researcher has computed the appropriate statistics, the final value is compared to the calculated value within the appropriate statistical table that identifies what value must be attained at x-degrees of freedom according to the preidentified level of significance (0.05 or 0.01).

Step XV: Conclusions and Implications

The next step in the research process is the explanation or the findings of the investigation. The researcher must be able to go beyond generalization and synthesize and interpret the results. The conclusions should follow the results and should reflect them, indicating both positive and negative findings.

Generalizations that are made have an impact on nursing practice, education, and research. The more valid the generalizations are, the more useful they are in supporting existing knowledge as well as contributing to the theory base of nursing.

The implications of the study are generally reported as recommendations. Recommendations usually suggest the impact that the finding will have on nursing and point out future research that needs to be conducted.

Step XVI: Communicating the Results

The final step of the research process is the dissemination of the research results, procedures, and insights. The purpose of communicating the results is to make them available to a wider audience.

The methods of reporting research are varied and may include the following:

- A written report
- A verbal presentation to nurses at a local, regional, national, or international conference
- An in-service presentation
- A poster session at a local, regional, national, or international research conference
- An article in a refereed research journal
- A thesis or dissertation
- An article in a nursing practice journal
- A book or monograph
- A special report
- A technical report

Each of these methods must meet certain criteria and the expectations of the audience or reviewer. The important thing is that the nurse-researcher feel a responsibility to share the information and take the time and effort to report the findings of the research study.

EVALUATION OF NURSING RESEARCH

A research critique is a critical estimate of a piece of research using specific criteria to guide the appraisal. In criticizing reported nursing research, it is important to be objective, comprehensive, and complete. There is definite skill involved in being able to criticize an article or a presenter at a research conference by identifying both the positive and the negative points of the study design and its findings. The person criticizing a study should determine what the researcher has tried to do, evaluate the strategies used, and present criteria and evidence for making judgments about the quality of the research. A critique includes comments about the information presented in the research report as well as comments about omissions.

Criticizing nursing research, first of all, pro-

vides an excellent vehicle for familiarizing the beginning nurse researcher with:

- Nursing research journals
- Research journals in other fields
- Different styles of reporting research studies, depending on the level of inquiry of the research question, the research design (descriptive, experimental), and the statistical tests used
- Each step of the research process
- Identification of instruments
- Identification of appropriate theoretical framework or statistics
- Studies to be replicated, repeated, or modified with design weaknesses altered and strengthened

Replication is seen as a most important part in the development of nursing science. By replication, nurse-researchers will be able to continue to test existing instruments and gather additional reliability and validity statistics. Replication research has many advantages for the nurse-researcher:

- It provides a specific research model to follow, simplifying the research process
- It takes less time to conceptualize and design
- It answers the call of the nursing profession for the need to replicate studies that have already been done
- It enables the nursing profession to see if significant findings are able to be replicated in other settings using different sample groups
- It enables the nurse to identify findings that would apply to nursing practice

The steps in the criticizing process are different depending upon the reason for the critique. Reading and criticizing research to become familiar with all facets of the research process require the nurse to read, evaluate, and ask particular questions about each section of the reported research. Use Table 17–16 as a guide for this type of critique.

A second reason for reading and criticizing a research study is to determine its applicability to nursing practice. This processs requires the nurse-researcher to complete a validation and a comparative evaluation before making the final decision.

The guidelines in this process are somewhat different from those outlined in Table 17–17. The results of this type of critique must enable the nurse to judge whether or not to use the findings in his or her own environment. It should also assist nurses in identifying how to implement the findings in their respective practice settings. This method of evaluating a research study is more extensive and complex than criticizing for the purposes of learning about research. However, it provides the essential link that is needed for the findings of nursing research to begin to be used in the practice setting by practicing nurses. Table 17–17 gives guidelines for evaluating research for specific clinical applicability.

TABLE 17–16. BASIC EVALUATION OF NURSING RESEARCH

I. *Problem*
Are the questions to be answered stated precisely?
Is the problem statement clear?
Is the problem researchable?
Is the problem practicable?
Are the variables identified?
Is the significance of the problem discussed and the research justified?
Are the parameters of the study identified to include limitations?

II. *Purpose*
Was the purpose stated clearly?

III. Review of the Literature
Is the cited literature pertinent to the problem?
Does it provide rationale for the research?
Are the sources ample or limited?
Are the sources mainly primary sources?
Are the sources current?
Did the material include professional journals, books, and general literature?
Are the authors experts in their fields?
Is there a logical organization of the review?
Is the relevant literature and its implications for the research problem under study summarized?
Is the theoretical framework appropriate to the research problem?

IV. *Hypothesis of Question*
Are the hypotheses to be tested stated precisely?
Are the hypotheses based on theory?
Do the hypotheses state a relationship between variables?
Are the variables identified?
Are the hypotheses defined in operational terms?

V. *Methodology*
Subjects:
Are the parameters of the study population described in order to make it clear as to what population the findings may be generalized?
Is the sampling method described?
Is there any bias introduced by this method?
Was the sample appropriate for the hypothesis or question?
Was the sample representative of the population?

Was the population adequately described?
Is the sample size appropriate?
Are the standards for the protection of human subjects adhered to?
Instruments:
Is the instrument adequately described?
Is validity addressed?
Is reliability addressed?
Is the development of the instrument, including a pilot study, described?
Design:
Is the design appropriate to the relevant theory and hypotheses?
Are proper controls included?
Does the description of the design permit replication?
Are the data gathering procedures explained?

VI. *Results*
Are results clearly and precisely presented?
Are the results organized in a logical manner?
Does the presented information answer the research question?
Are the reported statistics relevant to the research problem and hypotheses (if appropriate)?
Are the tables and figures appropriate for the presentation of the findings—complete and easy to understand?

VII. *Discussion*
Are the results discussed in terms of the original research problem?
If the hypotheses were stated, is each one addressed in the discussion of the results?
Are the findings related back to the theoretical framework that is used?

VIII. *Conclusions and Implications*
Are the conclusions that are stated substantiated by the results?
Are the implications of the findings for practice and further research discussed?

IX. *Writing Style*
Is the article clearly written?
Is it logically presented and ordered?
Is the article unbiased and written in the appropriate scientific writing format?

From M.J. Ward and M.E. Fetler, What guidelines should be followed in critically evaluating research reports, Nurs Res 28, (1979):120–25, and E.W. Treece and J.W. Treece, Elements of Nursing Research (St. Louis: C.V. Mosby, 1977), 287–88.

SUMMARY

Nursing research stems from the practice of nursing for the purpose of solving client-care problems within a given setting. Nursing research has and will continue to assist nursing in its efforts to gain recognition as a profession by becoming more accountable and relevant to society as a whole.

It is important for the beginning nurse-researcher to be able to differentiate between problem solving and the research process and to know what is and what is not nursing research. The roles of nurses in research vary according to experience, interest, and educational preparation.

The American Nurses' Association, for example, has strongly urged the undergraduate baccalaureate nursing student to be able to read, interpret, and evaluate reported research for applicability to nursing practice. There is also a need to identify nursing problems that need to be investigated, and the baccalaureate graduate nurse is often in the practice setting and in an excellent position to identify nursing problems, use nursing practice as a means to gather data, apply the findings of research to practice, and share the research findings with nurse colleagues and members of the other health disciplines. Familiarity with the specific steps in the research process and related terminology are the factors that allow this to occur.

The evolution of nursing research has been a relatively slow process in comparison to other disciplines, e.g., sociology or medicine. A great deal of progress has been made, however, in the past decade and in 1986 a National Center for Nursing Research was created by Congress as a part of the National Institutes of Health. As greater numbers of nurses are prepared at the doctoral level and interest and support for nursing research increases, the resulting body of nursing science will promote nursing more strongly as a science-based profession.

Nursing research, like all scientific research, follows an orderly, purposeful, and systematic process. Based on the scientific method, the research process is guided by a series of progressive steps.

The first step is to clearly identify the problem and state it in the form of a question that

TABLE 17–17. EVALUATING A STUDY FOR CLINICAL APPLICATION

I. *Validation*
   Are there strengths and weaknesses in the research design that invalidate the findings and conclusions? (Use of Table 17–16 is recommended at this point.)

II. *Comparative Evaluation*
   Can this study be used in the practice setting?
   How similar is the study's environment to the one in which the practicing nurse works?
   How similar are the characteristics of the sample to those of the population with which the nurse works?
   Does the nurse really need to change the current nursing practice?
      Is the nurse's current practice based on a theoretical framework of nursing and a scientific base of knowledge?
      How effective is the nurse's current practice?
      What are the successes and difficulties being encountered by the nurse?
   How likely are the study findings to be able to be implemented?
      What are the potential risks, legally and ethically, for the nurse, the fellow workers, the institution and most importantly the client?
   What decisions or changes must be made to permit use in the practice setting?
   How do the findings of the study relate to the policies and procedures of the practice setting?
   What resources are required to apply the study's findings, such as cost in time, money, and equipment?

III. *Decision Making*
   Based on the findings derived from validation and the comparative evaluation, the nurse must now decide upon applying the study's findings in the respective practice setting. The three choices are: not to apply, to apply only in expanding the nurse's cognitive approach to nursing care, or to make a direct application to the nursing practice.

From C. Stetler and M. Marram, Evaluating research findings for applicability in practice, Nurs Outlook 24 (September 1976):9.

the intended research will attempt to answer. The purpose of the research is addressed next, as the researcher cites reasons for carrying out the research and the rationale for its significance. The literature is then reviewed to identify what previous scientists and scholars have written and studied about the research topic. The literature review is recorded by the nurse-researcher in a systematic way and is later summarized in the written research proposal, as well as in the final report.

A theoretical framework is identified and explained in terms of how it relates to the research question. The next two steps involve a presentation of the variables and the hypothesis statement. Variables are specific attributes or properties contained within the research question and are those characteristics that the researcher manipulates and looks for changes (variability) in during the research process. A hypothesis is the researcher's "best guess" of what the relationship is between the variables and what the findings will turn out to be. Variables are then defined in terms of how they are to be understood and used in the research study. These research-specific definitions are referred to as operational definitions as opposed to conceptual or "dictionary" definitions.

The methodology of the research study is classified according to the type of design or plan of work the researcher intends to follow. There are a number of typical research designs that are commonly used such as surveys, experiments, and case studies. These designs can then be further classified and described in detail according to the research project. Once the design is selected, the population of subjects must be identified and the sample size decided upon. The population of subjects or objects to be studied represents the entire group or "universe" that has common traits. From this population the researcher must decide how to pick a subset or sample to be used for data collection in the research. The size of the sample and the method for choosing subjects in the sample are both very important in terms of the outcome of the research and how validly the researcher can generalize the findings to the universe of subjects.

Before the study is actually carried out, the researcher must be concerned about ethical issues and ascertain that each subject gives informed consent. Informed consent means the subject acknowledges he or she has been given an adequate explanation of how he or she will be participating in the study and what can reasonably be expected as a result of the participation, and the subject understands that he or she is free to withdraw participation at any time.

Often a pilot study is carried out before the actual research project begins. A pilot study is a small-scale version of the larger study and is done to clarify the method or "pretest" a specific tool, such as the questionnaire. This is an important step in the research process because it allows for modification and refinement, which may enhance the quality of the research.

The next step in the research process is data collection. Data can be collected by observation, questioning, and measurement, and is collected according to what is specified in the research design. The data are then organized and the findings analyzed according to statistical methods. There are numerous statistical methods, ranging from relatively simple descriptive statistics to more complex inferential statistics.

The final steps in the research process are to write up the conclusions and implications and share these results with the nursing community at large. Methods of communicating research studies include professional publications, conference presentation, and technical reporting communications.

Nursing research is evaluated by other nurses and researchers who carry out a process of criticizing the written research report or publication. Criticizing research is an art and requires discipline in looking at all aspects of the research study and making judgments based on knowledge, previous research, and adherence to research protocols, i.e., accepted methods and statistical manipulations. Research can be evaluated for the purpose of learning more about research or how well a research study has been carried out, or whether the research is applicable to a particular nursing setting.

Study Questions

1. What are the purposes of nursing research?

2. What are the steps in the research process?

3. Why should a researcher need to be aware of ethics to conduct research?

4. Identify a clinical nursing research problem. Write a problem statement and a purpose.

5. Locate, read, and write a critique of a research article from a nursing journal.

References

1. C.B. Stetler, *Nursing Research in a Service Setting* (Reston, Va: Reston, 1984).
2. Ibid.
3. Commission on Nursing Research, *Guidelines for the Investigative Function of Nurses* (Kansas City, Mo.: The American Nurses' Association, 1981).
4. P.A. Kalisch and B.J. Kalisch, *The Advance of American Nursing*, 2nd ed. (Boston: Little, Brown & Co., 1986).
5. M.A Sweeney and P. Olivieri, *An Introduction to Nursing Research* (Philadelphia: J.B. Lippincott Co., 1981), 1–16.
6. Division of Nursing, U.S. Public Health Service, *National sample survey of registered nurses* (Washington, D.C.: U.S. Government Printing Office, 1984).
7. Private communication. American Association of Colleges of Nursing, 1987.
8. American Nurses' Association Cabinet of Nursing Research, *Directions for Nursing Research Toward the Twenty-First Century* (Kansas City, Mo.: American Nurses' Association, 1986).
9. D. Diers, *Research in nursing practice* (Philadelphia: J.B. Lippincott Co., 1979).
10. R. Dahlen, C. Brundage, and B. Roth, "Easy guidelines for doing your own computerized literature search in the BRS after-dark information retrieval system," *Nurse Educ* (March–April, 1987).
11. F.G. Abdellah and E. Levine, *Better Patient Care Through Nursing Research*, 3rd ed. (New York: Macmillan Co., 1986), 107.
12. J. Fawcett, "The relationship between theory and research: A double helix," *Adv Nurs Sci* (1978):49–62.
13. E. McFarlane, "Nursing theory: The comparison of four theoretical proposals," *J Adv Nurs 5*, (1980):3–19.
14. M.A. Sweeney and P. Olivieri, *An Introduction to Nursing Research* (Philadelphia: J.B. Lippincott Co., 1981), 36–37.
15. D.B. Van Dalen, *Understanding Educational Research* (New York: McGraw-Hill Book Co., 1979), 105.
16. Ibid.
17. American Nurses' Association, *Code for Nurses with Interpretive Statements* (Kansas City, Mo.: American Nurses' Association, 1976), 4.
18. K.D. Hopkins and G.V. Glass, *Basic Statistics for the Behavioral Sciences* (Englewood Cliffs, N.J.: Prentice-Hall, 1978), 111.
19. Ibid., 3.

Annotated Bibliography

Bergstrom, N., Hansen, B.C., Grant, M., et al. 1984. Collaborative nursing research: Anatomy of a successful consortium. *Nurs Res* 33(1):20–25. This article outlines how seven researchers, living in four different geographic areas, worked successfully on a single research project. It provides insight into the research process and describes both advantages and obstacles encountered during the collaborative process.

Bush, Carol T. 1985. *Nursing Research*. Reston, Va.: Reston. This paperback text provides an overview of nursing research, including criticizing procedures, ethical considerations, and applications of research findings to clinical practice. The author believes that nursing students are capable of conducting research and offers explanations that help demystify the research process.

Brink, P.J., and Wood, M.J. 1983. *Basic Steps in Planning Nursing Research, from Question to Proposal*, 2nd ed, Monterey, Calif.: Wadsworth Health Sciences. This book provides basic, easy-to-read explanations of the steps in the research process and how to plan a research proposal. An appendix with five sample research proposals is included.

Campbell, D.T., and Stanley, J.C. 1963. *Experimental and Quasiexperimental Designs for Research*. Chicago: Rand McNally. This brief book is considered a classic in the field and provides guidelines on the essentials of a variety of experimental and quasiexperimental research designs.

Davitz, J.R., and Davitz, L.L. 1977. *A Guide: Evaluating Research Proposals in the Behavioral Sciences*. New York: Teachers College Press. This concise reference is a helpful guide to writing proposals to obtain permission from an agency to do research and to obtain funding from internal and external sources.

Flanagan, L. 1976. *One Strong Voice, the Story of the American Nurses' Association*. Kansas City, Mo.: American Nurses' Association. This reference describes the history and development of nursing research in depth and highlights, with examples, descriptions of events that occurred during select time periods.

Krone, K.P., and Loomis, M.E. 1982. Developing practice-relevant research: A model that worked. *Nurs Admin* (April):38–41. This article provides an example of how nursing research can be done in the clinical setting. The importance of collaboration between nurse researchers and nurse clinicians is discussed, especially regarding research question definition and study design.

Shelley, S.I. 1984. *Research Methods in Nursing and Health*. Boston: Little, Brown. This is an excellent integration of research and statistics and is highlighted with examples.

Welches, L., and DeJoseph, J.F. 1981. Nursing research in an acute care setting. *Nurs Admin Qu.* 5(2):38–42. This article describes how a university hospital developed an office of nursing research to stimulate and increase research activity by nurses. The point is strongly made that bedside nurses can most clearly see client care problems and are in a unique position to implement relevant research findings.

Part IV

The Human Perspective

Nursing, in a very basic and simplistic way, is an interaction between a nurse and a person where the nurse provides some type of professional, health-related assistance. This type of assistance may range from a high technology intensive care experience to a quiet talk during a home visit. Whatever the setting or type of intervention required, the nurse's effectiveness is increased by a knowledge of how persons grow and develop, how they feel about themselves as individuals, and how these lifelong processes are dynamic and affect their behavior.

This section discusses the universal concept of personhood itself, and three related concepts that enhance the understanding of personhood. The chapter on self-concept emphasizes how a person's view of himself influences and is influenced by his state of health, and how nurses can effectively use this knowledge in their practice. Sexuality is presented as an integral part of every person's life and an essential dimension within holistic nursing and health care. Aging, as a part of personhood and a concept of increasing interest to nurses and other health care providers, concludes this section. The study of aging allows nurses to gain a broader perspective of the person, to better appreciate the differences and uniqueness of individuals, and to apply the basic principles of the aging process to nursing practice.

Chapter 18

Theories of Personhood

Mary Ann Schroeder

Chapter Outline

- Objectives
- Glossary
- Introduction
- Personality
- Personhood
- Benefits of Learning about Theories of Personhood
- Selected Theories of Personhood
  Psychoanalytic Theory
  Interpersonal Theory
  Existential-Humanistic Theory
  Learning Theory
- The Nursing Process
  Assessment
  Planning
  Implementation
  Evaluation
- Conclusion
- Summary
- Study Questions
- References
- Annotated Bibliography

Objectives

After completion of this chapter, the reader will be able to:

▶ Define the terms in the glossary
▶ List the different theories regarding personality
▶ Compare and contrast each of the major theories
▶ Describe the role that events in history, philosophy, science, and changes in society have had on the development of the individual
▶ Describe the ongoing process of personhood throughout the life of the individual
▶ Discuss the application of two theories of personality to each component of the nursing process

Glossary

Accommodation. Part of the mediating process that seeks to change input.

Anxiety. Feeling that can range from extreme discomfort to being ill at ease.

Assimilation. The aspect of the mediating process in which incoming sensory data interact with what has already gone on within the brain.

Avoidance. Mechanism or process in which a situation is seen as undesirable, and the person withdraws or moves away from the situation.

Complexes. Set of associated ideas or feelings that motivates certain ways of interacting.

Congruence. State of harmony or consistency between what is said and what is meant.

Conscious. State of mind wherein readily available awareness or information exists.

Drives. Underlying forces that propel a person toward a course of action; the source of dynamics of thinking, feeling, and behaving.

Ego. Mediator between the id and superego; the part of the mind that has contact with reality.

Extroversion. The interest of the individual is directed outward, such as in seeking satisfaction in external ways.

Id. Animal instincts, innate desires.

Introversion. The individual seeks satisfaction from inner life, and interest is directed inward.

Narcissism. Self-love.

Self-disclosure. Technique in which people share honest thoughts and feelings.

Stimulus-Response. The stimulus is something that triggers a reaction; the response is that reaction.

Superego. The conscience; the way society has instructed the individual to behave.

Unconscious. State of mind when material is or has been pushed out of awareness.

INTRODUCTION

Personality and the more comprehensive concept of personhood involve the study and integration of numerous characteristics and theories. Over the years, people have been interested in such things as why people behave as they do, whether individuals can be described in terms of characteristic traits, what the relationships are between growth, development, and personality, and how we can predict the outcomes of various kinds of personality behaviors.

Theories and ideas that shed light on these kinds of questions are of great value to professional nurses. Because of the nature of the nursing process and the fact that nurses work most frequently on a one-to-one basis with people, they rely heavily on individual assessment skills and effective communication. Without a basic working knowledge of the processes of personality development and the relationship between personality and behavior, there is a great danger for faulty assessments to be made and communication to be ineffective. Appropriate planning for nursing care also can be highly dependent on personality factors.

This chapter includes material about personality theories from the social sciences, primarily psychology, and other closely allied fields. It is important to note that these theories, ideas, and concepts tend to overlap. A primary reason for this is that later theories are based on earlier ones. Also, in the general literature, there are varying opinions about the relative importance and validity of selected theories.

This chapter provides basic definitions and descriptions of selected major theories of personality and personhood and gives specific examples on how the associated concepts can be applied to nursing actions. An additional aim of this chapter is to stimulate further interest in those ideas or concepts that seem particularly useful to the reader working with clients in the clinical setting. Each subject area can be explored in greater detail, as there has been much work and research done on all of these theories. Besides gaining a better understanding of the people nurses care for, a knowledge base of personhood can foster a greater understanding of the self and the dynamics of interpersonal relationships; both are important aspects in the preparation of professional nurses.

PERSONALITY

There are many theories regarding personality and, consequently, personality has been defined in many different ways. The dictionary states that personality is the quality of being a person rather than an abstraction, thing, or lower being. Personality is not an isolated state but involves the relationship of the individual to the society. This relationship is influenced by a complex set of characteristics (such as traits, habits, attitudes, and patterns) that, in some manner, distinguish a particular individual from others.

Allport, in a definition that is almost half a century old yet seems fresh and up-to-date, states that "personality is the dynamic organization within the individual of those psychophysical systems that determine his unique adjustments to his environment."[1] There are several key thoughts in Allport's definition that seem especially relevant to understanding most theories of personality. The first idea is the use of the word dynamic, which indicates change and movement. Dynamic also means energy. It is the opposite of static, to stand still or not to move forward. Static is passive, whereas dynamic denotes action. Another concept important to Allport's definition is the word organization. Organization conveys a feeling of putting in order to make up a whole. It also means a method or model on which to look totally or as a complete overview. Organization, in this sense, is the opposite of being haphazard. The concept of systems, as expressed by Allport, connotes homeostasis and equilibrium. The various systems' balance or lack of balance is related. If there are problems in a system, the whole organism is influenced. The term unique, also part of Allport's definition, emphasizes that personality is primarily a product of an individual experience, rather than the perspective of society collectively. Finally, the word adjustment involves adaptation, development, and movement toward change. It indicates an attempt by the individual to bring things into harmony by altering positions for a more satisfactory condition.

Personality is the sum of the parts of an individual, plus an evolving pattern of relating to the world. It is an ongoing adjustment that is influenced by the society, the person's past, present, and aspirations for the future. It is a way to describe the essence of a person.

PERSONHOOD

How does the concept of personhood differ from that of personality? Once again, turning to the dictionary there are six distinct meanings of the word personality. But the term personhood is not specifically cited. Therefore, to define personhood, we must break up the word. You already have some idea of what a person is. So it is the suffix "hood" that needs further explanation. According to Webster, hood means "an instance of specific state, condition, quality, rank, character. . . ."

A theory of personhood is mingled with the philosophy of the nature of human beings. It is important to note that the spirit of the time and the view of life truly influence how the essence of the nature of a person is defined. For instance, in societies that believe people are basically good, an individual's worth is viewed quite differently from the way it is in a culture where persons are seen as inherently evil and sinful. So, too, if the major belief of society is that people have free will to choose their fate, then an individual is seen differently from individuals who reside in a culture that sees human beings as being predestined. Whatever is the predominate belief system is reflected in how the nature of humanity is defined. Most likely there will be a great correlation between a definition of the nature of human beings and the view of the person.

The current use of the term personhood conveys a spirit of dignity. People are felt to have worth. To support this position, think about what terms are linked to the suffix "hood"—knighthood, motherhood, priesthood, and maidenhood all express a rather noble view of the state of being a knight, priest, mother, or maiden.

If individuals are thought to be worthy of respect, then it follows that their desires and wishes should be considered. One modern nursing theory that capitalizes on dignity is the theory of self-care as advocated by Orem.[2] A basic tenet of self-care is that people should have control over their own health. This means a nontraditional role for health-care professionals. It emphasizes that goals should be mutually agreed upon, and that planning is jointly considered. People with health needs come to health-care providers, and together they negotiate care plans and health strategies. When people indicate needs, these must not be discounted but rather should be fully explored.

Personhood is a positive view of individuals, as people worthy of respect and dignity. The person is seen as having strengths and positive attributes that influence decisions about courses of action.

BENEFITS OF LEARNING ABOUT THEORIES OF PERSONHOOD

Why should nurses learn about various theories of personality and personhood? Nursing is a practice discipline that bases its actions on a body of knowledge. The body of knowledge regarding individuals and how they relate to others is especially important in the areas of mental health, community health, rehabilitation, and normal growth and development. It follows that if these theories are important in health and wellness, they are also important in attempting to understand disease, illness, and psychopathology. This chapter presents a multitude of theories. These theories can help to provide a better understanding of the dynamics of human behavior. They give clues to why individuals in given situations behave in a specific manner.

Along with understanding the whys of human behavior, personality theories also afford understanding about how individuals think and feel about their existence. Theories can help the nurse choose a certain course of action rather than another, based on the client's developmental stage. Knowledge of stages of growth and maturity give the nurse a basis for anticipating future needs that a client may have, as well as awareness that certain problems may occur at a given stage. Theories also provide an ideal of what the person might strive for in life goals.

One other point is that new theories are being generated continually as practitioners, theorists, and philosophers attempt to organize what they have observed in a logical fashion. A theory can provide a framework in which to conduct nursing practice.

SELECTED THEORIES OF PERSONHOOD

Theories about personality began to emerge early in the history of civilization. The theories were an attempt to make sense of or explain observations. Hall and Lindzey suggest that the early theories were generated as offspring of philosophy, and that philosophers such as Plato, Aristotle, Kierkegaard, and Locke had their own ideas of what constituted personhood.[3] According to Allport, from 400 B.C. to the 1600s, the unit of analysis for the majority of scientific material in all branches of inquiry was the Humors theory.[4] This theory categorized all phenomena according to the elements of earth, air, fire, and water. The elements then were subdivided into specific parts.

For example, if a person demonstrated a predominant mood of sadness or melancholy, it was thought that that person was under the control of "blue bile," one of the established humors. Allport goes on to state that this theory was not seriously challenged until Darwin's work, when a theory of instincts and drives emerged. Hall and Lindzey further trace the development of scientific thinking as becoming more involved with the experimental method, which Pavlov perfected. This experimental method related to personality, because ideas of motivation and situational variables came forth. At this time, case studies of individuals also enhanced the knowledge bases.

Some theories were born, disproved, and discarded. For instance, some theories, even though they sounded reasonable, did not stand up to scientific scrutiny. Specifically, during the 1940s and 1950s, William Sheldon's theory of somatotyping was very popular in attempting to explain personality makeup, based on a person's body type. Categories included the endomorph (short, fat build), the ectomorph (tall, thin physique), and mesomorph (muscular, well-proportioned). Specific personality traits such as orderliness, self-sufficiency, and cooperativeness then were postulated as being associated with each body type.[5]

The four categories presented here for consideration—psychoanalytic, interpersonal, existential-humanistic, and learning—are still considered as either valid or potentially useful. In other words, even though these theories originated in the early half of the century, there are still people who find them useful in analyzing and explaining human behavior.

Psychoanalytic Theory

Psychoanalytic theory had its beginning in the work of Sigmund Freud, an Austrian neurologist, who produced much of his work in the early decades of the twentieth century. Freud based his theory on his clinical practice. He worked with people suffering from mental disorders and published many papers about his theory. He also founded the Vienna Psychoanalytic Society, which was an important force in developing this theory.[6] Many clinicians and theorists joined Freud both physically and intellectually. Another school of thought, the neo-Freudians, broke off from the Vienna society, acknowledging that the early work done by Freud had influenced their thinking. Even today, both Freudian and neo-Freudian analysis are used in treatment.

Basic to psychoanalytic theory are the concepts of the **conscious** and **unconscious.** Consciousness is the state of the mind wherein readily available awareness of information exists. Unconsciousness is the state in which material has been pushed out of the sphere of awareness. Generally, conscious material is not anxiety-provoking, while unconscious material is emotionally charged and more likely to provoke anxiety. For this reason, it often is hidden from conscious awareness in order for the individual to be comfortable. Much has been written about the mental mechanisms that operate to help push material into the unconscious. These mechanisms, such as suppression, repression, sublimation, denial, rationalization, and numerous others, are discussed thoroughly in Chapter 26. The purpose of all these mechanisms is to reduce the discomfort of the individual.

Other concepts identified by Freud were the parts of the mind, in his structural theory. The mind is made of the **id, ego,** and **superego.**

Generally, the superego is considered the structure concerned with incorporation of parental and societal attitudes of right and wrong. It represents the values of the individual developed through the growing up process. The superego is the source of guilt feelings.

The ego has two major functions. It mediates between the id and the superego, and is the part of the mind in contact with reality. The id is involved with wants and desires. The superego is the person's conscience. The ego seeks to bring the id and superego into balance. It resolves conflict through compromise.

Bruno Bettelheim, in a recent article, redefined these terms slightly differently than do most textbooks.[7] Bettelheim contends that the original translations of Freud from the German to English distorted Freud's true meaning. Bettelheim states that the best definition of id is that part of the personality that means "it," as in a force, such as "the it" that made the person do a certain action. The "it" is something in the individual, and the person does not know what, that pulls in a certain direction. Bettelheim goes on to state that the ego is the "I," or

the conscious, rational part of the person. He indicates that it is the ego in operation when a person says "I am trying to understand why I did this." The third concept is the superego, which literally means "overself." This part of the mind is created by the person as a response to inner needs and external pressure that, Bettelheim feels, have been internalized. In the successfully adjusted person, according to the psychoanalytic school, the I, it, and over-I are in balance, and the person is in control of his "self."

Stages of development are also important concepts from Freud's theory. The psychosexual stages of development are the oral, anal, oedipal, and genital. These are the four stages through which the normal individual passes. According to this school of thought, the stages become important if a person fixates at or regresses to an earlier stage. This aspect of the theory has given rise to a jargon of descriptive phrases that can be heard about clients. For example, it is not uncommon to hear someone described as an "anal personality." The anal personality frequently demonstrates traits of excessive cleanliness or frugality. For example, people who are perfectionists about housekeeping are sometimes called anal personalities. The stage of anal development is marked by the task of toilet training, which involves attempts by the parent to get the child to control bladder and bowels. This task involves learning to eliminate feces and urine in an appropriate place and generally please significant others. The individual, according to psychoanalytic theory, becomes aware of the power he has to make another individual either happy or frustrated by the control of bodily functions. This stage is seen when the individual becomes an active force in relationships, in contrast to the earlier oral stage, in which the individual has a much more passive role. The issue of control becomes important. The psychoanalytic theory frequently uses the premise that either the function or symptoms related to the function can be and frequently are symbolic rather than actual. For instance, the symptoms manifested in the anal personality are symbolic of the functions involved in toilet training, such as giving, withholding, cleaning, and disposing.

Carl Jung, a contemporary of Freud and a proponent of the psychoanalytic theory, focused on the two major orientations of personality: **extroversion** and **introversion**.[8] Extroversion is apparent when the interest of the individual is directed outward. The extrovert seeks satisfaction in external ways. Introversion is the opposite. Introverts seek satisfaction from their own inner life, and their interest is directed inward, rather than toward people and things. Rarely, if ever, is an individual totally one or the other. Another concept that Jung identified was **complexes**. Complexes were seen as energy systems. The person has a recurring idea that frequently drains energy from the conscious personality. Examples are superiority, inferiority, mother, or father complexes. These complexes have corresponding patterns of behavior that indicate the persons' inner feelings about themselves.

Adler was another Austrian physician involved in the Freudian school. He was the first to break away from the Vienna Psychoanalytic Society, and went on to found his own analytic group.[9] *Holism* was one of Adler's major concepts. The idea of holism is that human beings must be viewed as a unit, not just a collection of parts. Adler was particularly interested in the instincts—basic motivating forces—that play a role in the decisions individuals make. He was especially intrigued when instincts seemed to be in opposition.

Two other concepts derived from psychoanalytic literature are **drives** and **narcissism**. Drives are the underlying forces that propel a person toward a course of action. Initially, the drives identified by Freud were seen quite specifically as either destructive or sexual drives. But drives can be seen as the source of dynamic thinking, feeling, and behaving.

Narcissism can best be described as self-love. Currently the concept is seen rather negatively, as someone who is self-centered and generally nonresponsive to the needs of others. Narcissism, however, is normal and expected at certain stages of life, especially in childhood. The baby, for example, is self-centered. Only when this concept is predominant in adult life is it pathological.

Many concepts have been identified by people associated with the psychoanalytic school of thought. Some of these concepts are no longer in vogue, whereas others have laid the ground-

work for subsequent theories. The psychoanalytic theory was one of the earliest of the currently used models for understanding the nature of personhood. The people who advocated this method wrote extensively. The literature is rich with clinical examples. Perhaps the greatest contribution of this theory was that it was an organized effort at defining what motivated people.

Interpersonal Theory

Interpersonal theory was, to a large extent, based on the earlier works of the psychoanalytic school of thought. The major difference was in its focus. The psychoanalytic theory's thrust was on the intrapsychic life (the internal drives, strivings, and conflicts) of the individual. The focus of the interpersonal theory was that human beings, although certainly affected by the intrapsychic life, are mainly influenced by what happens in their relationships with others. This involves the ideas advanced by George H. Mead and Eric Berne, that people not only reflect their own perceptions of their worth, but also are products of how others view them.[10, 11]

Relationships with others mold an individual's personality, thought, feeling, and behavior. For example, if a mother sees her son as naughty, most likely that is the way the child will act. Who is to say whether the acting or the perception of naughtiness came first?

Harry Stack Sullivan, an early proponent of this school of thought, defined developmental tasks not very dissimilar from the psychosexual ones of the psychoanalytic school. The central focus of the interpersonal tasks was on the reciprocal nature of need expression and satisfaction.[12] Sullivan felt that infancy was a time when the individual learns the basic cultural patterns. As the child masters language, the finer but equally important points—cooperation and socialization—emerge. Sullivan emphasized that by adolescence, either a "well-behaved" citizen had developed or the child had basic problems in his interpersonal relationships. These problems yielded a great deal of discomfort and dissatisfaction to both the individual and those who interacted with the individual.

Clarity of communication was seen by several theorists (including Berne and Virginia Satir) as one major objective in personality development. (For a more detailed explanation of this aspect, see Chapter 14).

Carl Rogers, basically an existential-humanistic psychologist, but eclectic, identified the concept of **congruence**, especially in communications, as one of the laws of interpersonal theory.[13] Congruence is seen as the state of harmony between what is said and what is meant. In other words, what a person conveys is what he means. For example, if a person declares "I am happy," and yet his facial expression appears depressed and he demonstrates otherwise, one would say that there is incongruence—lack of harmony between words and expressions. Rogers speculated that the greater the congruence of experience and awareness to communication, the more mutually satisfying would be the resulting interpersonal experience. For instance, the child learns the mother means business when she says "no" or learns that when the mother says "no" it may or may not mean no. Mixed messages with a lack of clarity lead to uncertainty. What is meant is open to speculation, as in the old song, "her lips say no, no; but there's yes, yes in her eyes." The implication of lack of congruence in personality development is that the child grows secure or insecure in message transmission. Clarity of communication promotes trust of others. If one cannot be certain what is being said, one becomes wary or lacks trust.

Another variation on the theory of interpersonal relationships is that of the transactional model, developed by Berne to explain and explore interactions.[14] Berne looked at the inner individual quite the way Freud had done in terms of the structure of the mind. But instead of calling these parts the id, ego, and superego, Berne called these aspects the child, the parent, and the adult. According to Berne, the child, which was analogous to the id, was seen as the part of the personality concerned with gratification of needs. Berne saw the child as rather shortsighted, primarily considering the now rather than looking to the future. The parent was in conflict with the child. The parent had incorporated the values of the society and reflected what is held in esteem by others. The adult, similar to Freud's ego, had as a major function the mediation between the child and

parent, as well as helping the individual adjust to reality.

Berne focused on how the individual functioned in society or in interpersonal situations. One major difference between the Freudian orientation and Berne's is that Freud specialized in using his framework to analyze psychopathology, such as his work on neurosis. Berne, however, chose to explore his theory of personality development with a backdrop of social situations. These social situations were called games by Berne. In games, people took roles in acting out scripts. For example, many overweight people respond differently to refusing food than do thin people. Overweight individuals may feel a need to explain why they aren't eating; the thin person says merely "no, thank you."

One major concept underlying interpersonal theory is that of **anxiety**. Anxiety can range from extreme discomfort to simply feeling ill at ease. The interpersonal theorist speculated that behavior is motivated by attempting to reduce anxiety, especially that which occurs because of difficulties in interpersonal interactions. Anxiety can be manifested by physical symptoms, such as sweaty palms or a fast pulse. It is an unpleasant, painful state. A little anxiety, say for instance about a forthcoming exam, causes the individual to spring into action, which is a positive aspect of anxiety. Huge amounts of anxiety, however, immobilize and prevent the individual from functioning. You have heard of people so overwhelmed with anxiety that they cannot speak. It does not matter what the cause of the anxiety is—a threat is real or perceived. The basic task of people is to learn effective methods to handle anxiety so that life becomes more pleasurable.

Existential-Humanistic Theory

Ideas of existential philosophers, such as Martin Heidegger and Rollo May, merged with the efforts of humanistic psychologists, including Carl Rogers and Sidney Jourard. Existential-humanistic theory is quite different from either the psychoanalytic or interpersonal, but they overlap. The major thrust of this theory is the holistic nature of human existence. Basic to all existential and humanistic theories is the belief that all human beings have potential for growth, and that it is up to the individual to decide and determine his fate. The goal of development is to achieve or move closer to potential, by means of "becoming." "Becoming" is a process rather than an outcome. The process consists of the individual attempting to liberate himself from the external world's view and gaining insight into his own nature. There is an emphasis on freedom to choose and the responsibility of the individual to achieve his goals.

Inherent in this theory is the aim to help people live more authentically. To live authentically means to stop misrepresenting oneself to others. One concept important in becoming more authentic is **self-disclosure.** Self-disclosure is a technique in which people share honest thoughts and feelings rather than "shoulds," "musts," and "oughts."[15] Jourard maintained that the greater the level of human potential reached, the higher the level of wellness. Jourard also stated the corollary—the more unauthentic the person, the greater the disorganization, and therefore, a lower resistance to stress and illness would result.[16]

Rogers focused on such tasks as the dropping of facades, discovery of unknown elements in oneself, freeing oneself in the discovery process, and gaining trust and confidence in one's perception, especially in regard to choices and decisions.[17] Both Jourard and Rogers acknowledge the unending nature of the process of "becoming."

Abraham Maslow, focusing on motivational aspects of becoming a whole, healthy person, brought forth a paradigm on the hierarchy of needs.[18] This hierarchy established an integrated, organized approach to consider human existence as related to needs. Maslow identified five broad categories of needs, starting with the basic ones of physiology and safety, and then moving to more sophisticated and advanced needs of belonging, esteem, and self-actualization.

The concepts inherent in the physiological needs were those of homeostasis and appetites. Examples of physiological needs are those for water, minerals, oxygen, food, an acid-base balance, and appropriate temperature. The need for safety brought concepts such as security, stability, protection, dependence, freedom from fear, anxiety, and chaos, and a need for structure, order, law, and limits. The need of belonging included concepts of love, affection, friendship, and affiliation. The esteem need involved attempts at self-respect, self-confidence, worth, and feelings of adequacy, prestige, appreciation, dignity, and having some status in the world. The most sophisticated of Maslow's hierarchy was the need for self-actualization, which included the individual's seeking self-fulfillment and achievement of potential. Maslow contended that until the basic needs were satisfied to some extent, more mature needs could not emerge. For example, it is difficult for a nurse to try to teach a client how to give insulin while the client is worried about being in a diabetic coma. First the nurse must deal with the needs presented by the client, in this case of fear.

Another existential-humanistic theorist was Erik Erikson.[19] Erikson, who began his career as a psychoanalytic thinker, devised a framework wherein the level of functioning was assessed by considering the tasks of the life-cycle. (For a detailed identification of the tasks that Erikson delineated, see Chapter 16).

Erikson felt that these tasks showed the conflicts, possible crises, and critical steps in becoming a highly functioning adult. Erikson, like the other theorists of this school, acknowledged that time was important in movement toward growth. But time alone was not the most important variable, as someone could be old in actual number of years but quite immature in terms of growth toward potential. As an example, one of the tasks Erikson wrote of was initiative in contrast to guilt. Imagine a person who, although 50 years old, is mainly motivated to action by guilt rather than because he wants to do something. This frequently underlies behavior of people who say "I should" or "I ought," rather than "I want to."

Erikson saw growth as somewhat painful. He felt that childhood was the time when the society systematically trained the individual to become a productive member.

Erich Fromm, another existential-humanistic theorist, took a slightly different point of view. He first analyzed the society and then decided what tasks of "social character" are developed. Fromm also stated that different classes in the same society will enforce or reinforce certain ideals based on what is or is not acceptable to certain groups.[20] Fromm thought that social character harnesses human energy primarily to meet the needs, economic or social, of a given system. This would affect what virtues are seen as important, depending on the developmental plan of the society. For instance, in a hunting and gathering society, traits such as artistic creativity or being articulate might be held in low esteem, while in a highly industrial society these same traits might be considered very worthwhile and rewarded with fame or money. Subgroups of society may have different values from the majority. Teen-agers may place a high value on a certain hairstyle, while their parents view it with less esteem. Fromm extended thinking about "becoming" as a societal and individual process.

The existential-humanistic scholars acknowledged needs, including individual and societal. They also speculated that people could go beyond basic needs and identified ideals. They offered explanations as to why people could become martyrs, giving up their lives, for an ideal. The theories of the existential-humanistic individuals paid heed to the society but advanced a position that individuals could be more mature than the culture in which they existed.

Learning Theory

This theory regarded personality development as a learning process, with learned responses as a major factor in dictating how a person reacts in specific situations. At one time this theory was considered to be antihumanistic and concerned mainly with putting human beings and the motivating forces of human behavior in the category of animals. But at present this theory is seen less negatively.

Much of the early work on which some aspects of this theory are based comes from the experimental method of study. The experimental method frequently studied laboratory animals to understand certain elements of the learning process.

B. F. Skinner's work looked at behavior in terms of the **stimulus-response** (S-R) interaction.[21] The stimulus is something that triggers a reaction. The response is the reaction. For example, a stimulus might be a brightly colored baby rattle; the response would be the baby reaching for the rattle. Another example is a hypodermic needle being the stimulus in a pediatrician's office. The response on the part of a 5-year-old child is crying. The S-R is a process. Skinner, expanding on the early work of Pavlov, added to the body of knowledge about how organisms learn. Using observation and carefully controlled studies, Skinner articulated relationships between two sets of variables. The variable of the stimulus was not merely one stimulus, such as an electric shock device or a push bar that gave out grain, but generally a class of variables that contained many things—the environment. The other variable, the response, was seen as a behavioral response that could and frequently did contain complex patterns of behavior. In addition to the concepts of stimulus and response, the terms **avoidance** and approach are used. Avoidance is the mechanism or process in which situations are seen as undesirable, and the person withdraws or moves away from the situation. Approach is the process of coming closer to or engaging in the activity.

The behaviorists were just one branch of learning theory scientists. Many others advocated learning as a theoretical framework for understanding personality. Piaget, working during the mid-portion of the twentieth century in Geneva, Switzerland, speculated that within the cognitive functions of the individual, a process took place that enabled and individual to adapt to new situations.[22] This process involved the person organizing past experiences and applying them to the present. Piaget's efforts were concentrated with the structure, the "hows" of learning, rather than looking at the content, or the "whats" of learning. Much of Piaget's work was done by observation of children. His method was to clinically observe the child, formulate a hypothesis, and then test the hypothesis by slightly altering the child's surroundings. Piaget identified a complex process, involving assessment of the stimulus, taking place within the individual. The present stimulus is viewed not merely on the perception of the current stimulus, but also on knowledge gained by the individual through previous situations.

According to Piaget the biological makeup of the child was not discounted, but the focus of his work was based on the ongoing interactions with the environment. Concepts important in Piaget's theory were **assimilation** and **accommodation**. Assimilation is the aspect of the mediating process where incoming sensory data interact with what has already gone on within the brain. It is a type of incorporating process. Accommodation is that other part of the mediating process that seeks to change the input. The goal of both these functions is to promote a general state of stability in the person. They both lead toward individual gain (or regain) of equilibrium. Piaget speculated that there is a better level of functioning if the person is in balance.

Piaget felt that language was the vehicle by which thought was socialized and rendered logical to the individual. People, by understanding structure and action, could transfer this understanding in the application of new knowledge. It should be noted that Piaget, like Erikson and Maslow, is frequently identified as a growth and development theorist.

One other aspect of learning theory work was done by Kurt Lewin on perceptional theory.[23] Lewin focused on how the individual perceives stimuli. One cannot examine stimulus apart from the environment. In other words, to understand one part of a situation, one must understand the broader field. One cannot look at a tree, for example, without realizing that the tree is just a part of the forest.

People, according to the learning theorists, think and act the way they do because, to a great extent, they have learned that they should do so. This theory does not negate the other theories, but adds another dimension to an understanding of the nature of personhood.

THE NURSING PROCESS

In carrying out the nursing process, the nurse uses knowledge of many different theories and concepts as she or he collects data, analyzes it, and plans care. The contributions of personality theorists may assist in the assessment phase, in planning and implementation, or in evaluation. Nurses who work in psychiatry or with clients who have significant personality or behavioral difficulties may base their entire practice on one or more theories of personality. Some of the concepts identified in this chapter might be used solely to better understand the motivation of

individuals or to decide on interventions to help the client adjust to illness or choose a more healthy life-style. Some concepts may seem more useful than others. Your use of this knowledge also will depend on the area of professional practice you are engaged in, how much experience you have had, and what your role is.

The following discussions on each of the phases of the nursing process will show, by example, how several of these theories can be clinically applied to nursing.

Assessment

How might the nurse use the concept of unconscious from the psychoanalytic theory in the assessment phase of the nursing process? It is not suggested that the nurse, unless quite sophisticated in both theory and practice, seek to undercover unconscious material. Unconscious material is hidden precisely because it is painful to the person.

Assume that a client who has been diagnosed as hypertensive is given a prescription for medication that will lower the blood pressure. While the nurse is visiting the home, giving prenatal instruction to the hypertensive client's wife, the nurse discovers that the client never had the prescition filled. Obviously, the client is not taking the medicine. The nurse should suspect that this noncompliance with the medical regimen is not merely a case of the client "not wanting" to take pills.

What might be the reason the client is not taking his blood pressure medicine? The nurse begins by asking questions. "Why" questions are more difficult to answer. Many times clients respond with "I don't know," and frequently they really do not recognize what motivates them to engage or to not engage in certain activities. One hidden reason for noncompliance might involve that client's perception that he feels he is not a "good provider," and therefore, his taking money to purchase the medicine might deprive his family. The nurse does not introduce this suspicion, but considers it as a possibility in speaking with the client. The goal is not to get the client to acknowledge unconscious thoughts but merely to help the nurse better understand the dynamics of the situation. In this case, the plan of the nurse might be to help the client identify the value of taking medicine. There should be reinforcement that medicine is important for several reasons. One reason might be that if the blood pressure is controlled, the client will be in better health to enjoy the baby and be better able to provide for his family. In this case, an appropriate nursing diagnosis might be noncompliance related to knowledge deficit.

Planning

Another example of theoretical application would be to consider the concept of anxiety for planning client care. Imagine the nurse trying to help plan care for a bedridden, arthritic client. Arthritis is a chronic condition that affects the client's joints, and frequently involves pain on movement.

In planning care, the nurse needs to consider clients' and their families' feelings and fears. For instance, in planning for the arthritic person, the nurse is attempting to enlist the aid of a client's elderly sister to do frequent turnings to prevent bedsores from forming. After a great deal of discussion, the nurse recognizes that the sister seems reluctant to do the turning for two reasons. She feels she might hurt the client, and she fears that by moving the client she might injure her own back. The nurse could use a straightforward approach to try to alleviate the anxiety. To deal with her fear about herself, the nurse might say, "I will teach you how to do it, and make certain that you are not putting yourself in danger of injury. I will make sure that you can do it correctly before you do it on your own." By providing an example, supervision, and suggestions, the nurse can help the sister reduce her anxiety. In regard to the expression about hurting the client, the nurse might say, "You may hurt your sister a bit, but is it far better for her to experience a bit of discomfort during turning than to suffer bedsores." Anxiety frequently can be diminished by confronting the issues that make the person anxious. When anxiety is reduced, the person is able to help in planning care.

Implementation

Use of the concept of stimulus-response from the learning theory might be considered in intervention or implementation. One example of using this concept might be in working with a mother who is trying to help her mentally retarded child stop biting his nails. The nurse would help the mother identify what situations (stimulus) seem to cause the child to chew on his nails (response). The mother then would be aware of those times that are especially stressful for the child. Together, the nurse and the mother might consider ways to see that the stimulus is diminished so that the response does not take place. This might be done by the mother offering a diversion, such as game playing at the stressful time, or maybe just holding the child, so that the response, the nail biting, does not happen.

Evaluation

Evaluation, which measures the effectiveness of nursing practice, including assessment, planning, and intervention, might be influenced by some of the concepts of needs theory, which is one aspect of existential-humanistic theory. One example might be to use Maslow's concept of self-actualization to determine the effectiveness of group therapy. Many psychiatric clients have problems with interpersonal relationships because they view their own self-worth unrealistically. In other words, because of their low self-esteem, their interactions with others may be disturbed. Treatment in psychiatric settings frequently is multifaceted, and group therapy is one common treatment mode.

One goal of a therapy group might be to increase self-esteem. In order to measure self-esteem, one would have to decide on behavioral aspects that could be noted and would be linked to self-esteem. The measure could be the frequency with which clients in a group speak disparagingly about themselves. It is assumed that as clients' self-esteem increases, the negative comments they make about themselves will decrease. The measure is behavioral change, which the nurse thinks is related to an affective change.

CONCLUSION

One of the major concepts that has been identified and appears in all these theories, is that of growth—the possibility of change. Growth is viewed as a positive movement toward a higher level of functioning and a healthier way of relating to the world and those in the world.

In terms of personhood, growth is a movement toward a greater feeling of worth and dignity and an increasingly positive view of oneself as a unique individual. No matter how seemingly disabled or distraught a client appears, the nurse can help the client becomes less so by capitalizing on his or her potential for personal and emotional growth.

The nurse might help clients grow in many situations. One opportunity may be leading a group of aged individuals with a focus on adjusting to moving into a retirement home. Giving parenting classes may help parents grow in their skills and self-confidence. Still another situation where a nurse can help clients grow is in health teaching in a junior high school. If the nurse works in a crisis intervention setting, growth may take place by helping the client learn from one situation to another.

One other important consideration is the nurse's own potential for growth. Within each of us, there exists a quality of striving, which involves doing better or becoming more mature. Growth includes being aware of our strengths and limitations. In order to grow, we must seek to capitalize on our strengths and work on our limitations. It is a constant process, but one with great rewards.

SUMMARY

This chapter presents several concepts that have emerged from various theories of personhood. The goal has been to identify concepts that are fundamental to the mental health, growth, and development aspects of people. The chapter gives a few examples of how the nurse might apply some of these concepts to nursing practice.

Personhood, as a state of being, depends on many things. Some of the factors that influence it are age, maturation, heredity, culture, state of health, and beliefs. These theories can improve our understanding of people. The more we understand about people, the more likely we are to be able to help them and care for them.

Nursing involves gaining knowledge in order to apply that knowledge to serve others more fully. Gaining an understanding of personhood is basic to treating people with respect and dignity. In your own nursing practice, you should try to apply some of the concepts discussed to help you address the needs of your patients.

Study Questions

1. Go to a playground and observe children. Are some introverted and others extroverted? How can you tell? List the behaviors.

2. Do you have a bad habit—maybe smoking, or handing in schoolwork late, or not hanging up your clothes? Make an effort for a week to try and break that habit. Notice how "breaking the habit" influences your feelings and thoughts. Keep a diary of what you think and feel about not following your usual behavior.

3. Try telling a friend a story. Say all the "right" words, but attempt "wrong" behavior (nonverbal clues). For instance, tell about a funny movie, but appear to be on the verge of tears. Does your friend notice? What does your friend say nonverbally? What does he say in words? Does the lack of congruence influence whether or not your friend thinks the movie is funny?

4. Keep a log for a week of when you feel anxious or uncomfortable. Try to determine the origin of these feelings. What do you do to become more comfortable? Does it work? If not, why not?

5. In what ways have you grown since you entered nursing?

References

1. G. Allport, "What units shall we employ?" in *Assessment of Human Motives* (New York: Rinehart, 1958), 48.
2. D. Orem, *Nursing: Concepts of Practice*, 3rd ed. (New York: McGraw-Hill Book Co., 1985).
3. C. Hall and G. Lindzey, *Theories of Personality*, 2nd ed. (New York: John Wiley & Sons, 1957).
4. Allport, *Assessment of Human Motives*, 48.

5. Hall and Lindzey, *Theories of Personlity.*

6. S. Freud, *The Basic Writings of Sigmund Freud* (New York: Random House, Modern Library Editions, 1938).

7. B. Bettelheim, "Reflections (Freud)," *The New Yorker* (March 1982):52–93.

8. C. Jung, "The symbols of the self," in *The Collected Works* (New York: Pantheon, 1960).

9. A. Adler, *Individual Psychology* (Worcester, Mass.: Clark University Press, 1930).

10. G. Mead, *Mind, Self and Society* (Chicago: Unviersity of Chicago Press, 1934).

11. E. Berne, *Games People Play.* (New York: Grove Press, 1964).

12. H. Sullivan, *The Interpersonal Theory of Psychiatry* (New York: W.W. Norton Co., 1953).

13. C. Rogers, *On Becoming a Person* (Boston: Houghton Mifflin, Co., 1961).

14. Berne, *Games People Play.*

15. S. Jourard, *Self-Disclosure: An Experimental Analysis of the Transparent Self* (New York: Wiley-Interscience, 1971).

16. *Ibid.*

17. C. Rogers, *On Becoming a Person.*

18. A. Maslow, *Motivation and Personality,* 2nd ed. (New York: Harper & Row, 1970).

19. E. Erikson, *Childhood and Society,* 2nd ed. (New York: W.W. Norton, 1963).

20. E. Fromm, Character and the social process, in *Appendix to Escape from Freedom* (New York: Rinehart, 1941).

21. B.F. Skinner, *The Behavior of Organisms: An Experimental Analysis* (New York: D. Appleton-Century, 1938).

22. J. Phillips, *The Origin of Intellect: Piaget's Theory* (San Francisco: W.H. Freeman & Co., 1969).

23. K. Lewin, *A Dynamic Theory of Personality: Selected Papers* (New York: McGraw-Hill, Book Co., 1935).

Annotated Bibliography

Fromm, E. 1956. *The Art of Loving.* New York: Harper & Row. (Available in paperback.) This classic book presents Fromm's ideas about the nature of love in terms of personality development. It is an excellent resource for assisting in self-development. Fromm emphasizes the importance of ongoing self-responsibility for reaching one's potential in life, particularly one's highest capacity for love relationships. It supports Fromm's personality theory.

Hymovich, D., and Chamberlain, R. 1980. *Child and Family Development: Implications for Health, Primary Health Care.* New York: McGraw-Hill. This is a family-oriented textbook that presents growth, development, and personality theories as they relate to nursing and health care. It is comprehensive and includes a section on theoretical frameworks.

Mussen, P., Conger, J., and Kagan, J. 1964. *Child Development and Personality,* 4th ed. New York: Harper & Row. This is a comprehensive, basic textbook on general growth and development with an emphasis on personality development through adolescence. It presents an excellent overview of all the possible factors that contribute to personality makeup.

Satir, V. 1972. *Peoplemaking.* Palo Alto, Calif.: Science and Behavior Books. This is primarily a book about the family process and parenting, but it gives tremendous insight into the complexities of personality development. It does not present personality theory per se but gives practical information and interesting viewpoints on interpersonal relationships within the family setting.

Skolnick, A. 1986. *The Psychology of Human Development.* San Diego, Calif.: Harcourt Brace Jovanovich. A coherent, comprehensive textbook formulated on a developmental schema. An excellent overview of traditional theories updated with current ideas, including a multicultural approach.

Chapter 19

Self-concept

Linda Manglass

Chapter Outline

- Objectives
- Glossary
- Introduction
- Definitions and Theory Development
- Theorists
- Self-concept Development
- The Nursing Process
  Assessment
  Planning
  Implementation
  Evaluation
- Summary
- Study Questions
- References
- Annotated Bibliography

Objectives

At the completion of this chapter, the reader will be able to:

▶ Identify self-concept as one way in which human beings adapt to biopsychosocial influences
▶ State a definition of self-concept congruent with theories of self-concept development
▶ Identify components of self-concept using an adaptation-approach model
▶ Identify factors useful in assessing self-concept in clients
▶ Describe nursing intervention strategies effective in the development of an adaptive self-concept and in promoting positive responses to influences on self-concept

Glossary

Body Image. An individual's concept of the shape, size, and appearance of his or her body and its parts.

Looking-glass Self. A person's view of self resulting from perception of others' responses.

Self-concept. An individual's self-definition; the composite of beliefs and feelings one holds about self.

Self-esteem. Evaluative attitudes toward self.

INTRODUCTION

Understanding of self-concept is important in nursing because an individual's self-concept affects and is affected by health and any deviation from health. How an individual functions in a given situation is dependent on how one perceives the self and how one perceives the situation. The self-concept is the point of orientation for all behavior.

Nurses are very concerned with individuals' physical, psychological, and social behaviors. Understanding the relationship between these and the self-concept will aid the nurse in promoting behaviors that are positive and adaptive.

Any time there is a change in an individual's state of wellness or illness, there must be adaptation as a total person. How well one is able to adapt, in part, depends on how one views oneself. This view of self is the self-concept.

Using a framework for assessing the client's self-concept enables the nurse to predict problems the person may have in adapting and promotes adaptation through identification and use of client strengths.

DEFINITIONS AND THEORY DEVELOPMENT

Self-concept is a composite of beliefs and feelings one holds about oneself. Self-concept is formed partly from perceptions or reflected appraisals of significant others, partly from environmental influences, and partly from inner resources. Self-concept is constantly evolving and directs one's behavior.[1]

This eclectic definition of self-concept is a composite of the major schools of thought regarding self-concept and reflects the what, how, and why of self-concept development.

THEORISTS

The term "reflected appraisals" and "significant others" are concepts originated by Harry Stack Sullivan, one of several social interaction theorists who wrote about self-concept development.[2] He used the term "reflected appraisals" to refer to the influences we get about ourselves as a result of ways we are treated and judged by significant others. "Significant others" are those people who provide rewards and punishments; most commonly, parents, spouses, helpmates, and best friends.

Another theory of self-concept development based on social interaction theory is the **looking-glass self** by Charles Horton Coolie.[3] This is seeing oneself through the eyes of others.

One imagines how one is perceived by another person, how the other person appraises one, and then makes a value judgment about that appraisal (i.e., one is proud of the perception or ashamed of it).

Both of these theories are based on the belief that interaction with others in a social world determines an individual's concept of self.

Perceptual psychology discusses self-concept in terms of individual perceptions. How a person behaves is determined largely by how the self is viewed. This self, referred to as the perceived self, is the point of reference for everything done. These concepts are the core of personality.[4] Raimy said of self-concept that it is more or less an organized perceptual object resulting from present and past observations. It is what a person believes about the self. The self-concept is a map that each person consults in order to understand the self, especially during moments of crisis or choice.[5] The self-concept is the self at all times and in all situations, and once established, has a high degree of stability.[6]

SELF-CONCEPT DEVELOPMENT

It is thought that an individual's concept of self actually begins at or soon after birth. This process begins in its earliest phases when the infant begins differentiation of self from others. The infant's differentiations are tactile, and the sense of who and what one is comes with exploration of the body and the discovery that one is separate from the surroundings. As the child matures, this process becomes less difficult and is greatly accelerated by the development of language. Initially, communication occurs on a nonverbal level with mother (or significant person). This nonverbal communication is the response the infant receives. Language, particularly the use of the child's own name, aids the clarification of self-concept. Using the child's own name helps identify the self and see the self as unique and special. The use of nonverbal language also allows approval and disapproval, affection and rejection. At this time, for example, it is particularly important for the difference between "bad boy" and "bad behavior" to be made clear.

Stanley Coopersmith has done significant research on development of self-concept in school-age boys. The results of his research, published in 1967, provided valuable information regarding the effect of the family on self-concept development.[7]

> No experience in the development of a child's concept of self is quite so important or far reaching as his earliest experiences in his family. It is the family which introduces a child to life which provides him with his earliest and most permanent self definitions. Here it is that he first discovers those basic concepts of life which will guide his behavior for the rest of his life.[8]

It is necessary, therefore, to understand what contributes to positive self-concept development and what does not.

Coopersmith used the term **self-esteem** to refer to evaluative attitudes toward self—the individual's perception of self-worth. He looked at many different areas in the family life of school-age boys in order to determine what kinds of parental characteristics and influencing familial factors had an effect on the feelings the boys developed about themselves and their resulting behavior. Some of the areas he studied and drew conclusions from are as follows:

- He found no clear or definite pattern of relationships between social class and positive or negative levels of self-esteem
- He found no difference between religion—Jewish, Protestant, or Catholic
- The prestige of the father's work had no bearing on levels of self-esteem. It was found that regular employment enhanced self-esteem, and that there was an exception with the children of police and members of the armed forces, who demonstrated lower levels of self-esteem
- Whether or not the mother was employed made no difference in levels of self-esteem
- Family size was unimportant, except that self-esteem was found to be higher in firstborns and only children

General characteristics of family life that were shown to contribute to the development of positive self-esteem were: *acceptance by parents, clearly defined and enforced limits,* and *respect for individual action that exists within those limits.*

Coopersmith summarized characteristics of children identified with low self-esteem and those with high self-esteem (Table 19–1). These factors are important in the process of assessing levels of self-esteem in clients.

As in any research study, Coopersmith reviewed the literature on self-concept and theoretical aspects of the development of self-concept. He found many of the same ideas in the existing writings. He summarized four factors inherent in any self-concept theory:

- The amount of respectful, accepting, and concerned treatment a person receives from significant others
- The individual's history of successes
- The person's experiences are interpreted and modified in accordance with aspirations and values (what is perceived as important)
- The individual's manner of responding to devaluation

Callista Roy, in her adaptation model, presents a similar summarization of stimuli affecting the individual's self-concept[9]:

- The individual's previous perceptions of feedback about self from significant others

TABLE 19–1. CHARACTERISTICS OF LOW AND HIGH SELF-ESTEEM

Low Self-esteem	High Self-esteem
Isolation	Maintains fairly constant image of self as a person
Inability to give or receive love	Capable of active expression
Decreased interactions	Can move realistically toward goals
Decreased socialization	
Fears and self-doubts	

- The individual's previous maturational and situational crises and how self-concept has been rearranged in response to the crises
- The person's self-expectations and experiences with success and failure
- Any experiences, such as interpersonal ones, that generate in the individual positive feelings and a sense of value or worth, or conversely, negative feelings
- The individual's physiological integrity

More recent studies have reconfirmed the importance of significant others' influence on self-concept. In studying the influences of employment and perception of the husband's appraisals on self-esteem in women, Meisenhelder found the perceived reflected appraisals of husbands was a remarkably strong prediction of self-esteem for all women and was especially influential for homemakers.[10]

THE NURSING PROCESS

Potential nursing problems related to self-concept are many and varied. The adaptation approach to nursing provides a useful framework for understanding self-concept and its relationship to individuals' behavior in health and illness.

Just as one adapts physiologically to one's environment (i.e., an increase in temperature causes sweating, which results in cooling), one also adapts through self-concept. Roy calls this the self-concept mode of adaptation.[11]

Individuals with positive self-concepts function effectively because they view themselves and their worlds positively. Negative self-concepts are associated with problems in many areas. For example, research has shown that clients with negative self-concepts believe their illnesses have a greater negative effect on their lives, have less hope and optimism about the future, and are more anxious about their illnesses.[12]

To understand and use the self-concept mode more easily, it is broken into components. These components are parts of the self that contribute to the overall concept of self that a person holds. The components provide a framework for assessing the individual's self-concept.

The following definitions with discussions on each mode and component are adapted from Roy and Buck.[13,14] There are two basic components: physical self and personal self. The physical self includes two components. The first component is body sensation, and the second is **body image**. The personal self is divided into self-consistency, self-ideal or self-expectancy, and moral-ethical-spirtual self (Fig. 19–1).

Assessment

In assessing self-concept, behaviors to look and listen for that indicate *adaptation* include general physical appearance reflecting a "cared for" look, appropriate height–weight proportions, good posture and gait, comfortable (for nurse and client) degree of eye contact, an energy level that reflects participation in and enjoyment of a reasonable number and variety of activities, an accurate view of reality, emotions within a range of normal, consistent verbal and nonverbal behavior, an ability to establish and maintain mutually satisfying interpersonal relationships, an ability to solve problems and make decisions, task achievement appropriate to developmental level, appetite and sleep patterns within normal limits, use of adaptive defense mechanisms, and what a person says about her- or himself.

Behaviors that may indicate less than positive adaptation are discussed next under problems commonly encountered in each component.

Physical self refers to one's appraisal of one's physical being. This includes body sensation—how one's body feels personally. The appraisal of body sensations as a component of self-concept enables one to experience self as a physical being. For example, "I feel pained," "I feel tense," "I hurt." Body image refers to how one's body looks to oneself and how one feels about how one looks. This includes physical attributes, functioning, sexuality, wellness, illness, and appearance. As with self-concept generally, a person's mental image of body (concept of physical self, or body image) may not correspond to actual body structure. In other words, the person may not see self as others do.

Problems encountered in nursing related to physical self often are caused by loss—real, imagined, or symbolic. Loss is defined as a sit-

The Physical Self

The Personal Self

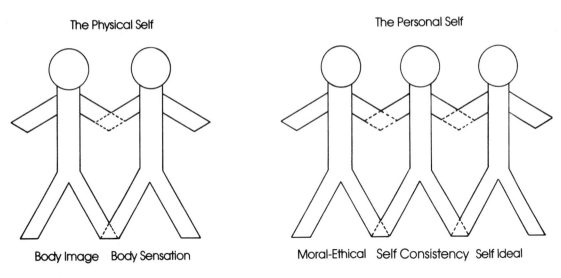

Body Image   Body Sensation

Moral-Ethical   Self Consistency   Self Ideal

Figure 19–1. The components of the self.

uation, either actual or potential, in which a valued object is rendered inaccessible to an individual or is altered in such a way that it no longer has qualities that render it valuable. The object, in its broadest sense, includes people, possessions, an individual's job, status, home, ideals, and parts and processes of the body (See Chapter 27 for a more thorough discussion of this important concept.)

Changes in physical body structure (e.g., amputation or mastectomy) commonly precipitate feelings of loss. Changes in physical functioning, loss of strength, central nervous system diseases, the aging process, pregnancy, a colostomy, obesity, and disfiguring surgery are losses that frequently are encountered in nursing situations.

The nurse can tell a great deal about how an individual feels about the self by looking at the client and listening to what the client has to say about his or her body and appearance. Areas to observe and listen for in assessing physical self include appearance, height–weight proportions, posture and gait, eye contact, and references made to body image and body sensation. Individuals who feel good about themselves tend to take care of themselves and look as though they care about themselves (Fig. 19–2). If an individual is unkempt, unable to make eye contact, and walks slumped over, for instance,

it may be an indication that the person has low self-esteem.

Physical changes, such as those described above, always demand adaptation, and the individual will experience concerns and possibly anxieties as a result of the changes. How well the person is able to adjust will be determined by numerous factors, such as previous perceptions of self, feedback from others including the nurse, suddenness and severity of change, previous experiences and growth and development level.

The first component of personal self is the moral-ethical-spiritual self, which refers to the aspect of self that functions as observer, standard setter, dreamer, comparer, and, most importantly, evaluator of who this person says he or she is. Moral-ethical-spiritual self judges desirability and undesirability of self-perceptions. Judgments a person makes about the self influence the value or esteem that is experienced. Examples of behaviors can include such statements as : "I believe in God"; "It is up to God"; or "it is up the doctor."

Since moral-ethical-spiritual self has a great deal to do with the values an individual holds, problems in moral-ethical-spiritual self commonly take the form of guilt. Areas to observe and listen for in assessing guilt include disparaging remarks about self, depression, apologies,

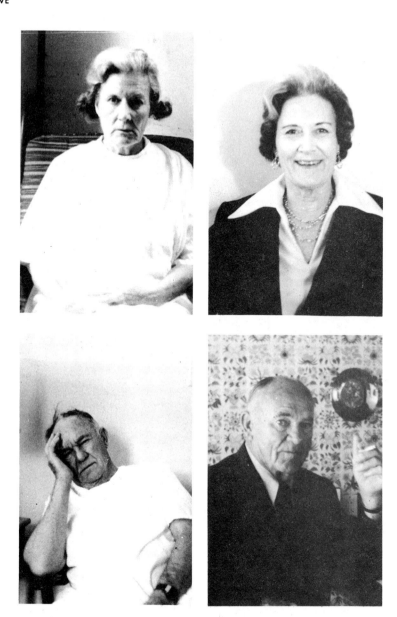

Figure 19–2. Physical appearance is an indicator of self-esteem. *(Courtesy of Nance Photo.)*

self-blaming statements, blushing, and stammering.

Self-consistency refers to a person's striving to maintain a consistent self-organization and thus avoid disequilibrium. People have a need to maintain a consistent or stable self-image; so, for example, a person who achieves a weight loss may still have an image of self as heavy. Only through consistent, repeated experiences of "thin" can this person change the concept of self from heavy to thin.

Problems in self-consistency produce anxiety. Anything that threatens who or what that person believes the self to be will result in anxiety. Problems in the self-consistency component of self-concept reflected as anxiety are encountered daily in all areas of nursing. Hospitalization alone is a threatening, anxiety-provoking experience. Addressing problems of anxiety in clients should be a part of every client's care plan. (See Chapter 26 for assessment factors and intervention strategies.)

Self-idea or self-expectancy is the aspect of the self that relates to what the person expects the self to be and do. It is also the ideal of what the person wants to become. These concepts guide the individual's behavior toward achieving identified goals.

Problems in achieving ideals and expectations often result in powerlessness. Feelings of powerlessness may be seen as a decrease in motivation and energy, depression, anger, passivity, or apathy. Illness and hospitalization may result in feelings of powerlessness, and nurses can intervene by ensuring that clients are given as much control over their experiences as possible. Control is enhanced by offering choices, giving information, and allowing time for questions and discussions.

This framework is one that can be used to organize data in assessing areas of self-concept that may be causes of concern or problems.

At the conclusion of the assessment phase, nursing diagnoses can be formulated from the data gathered. Some sample nursing diagnoses include:

- Disturbance in self-concept related to loss of role performance as bread winner
- Disturbance in body image related to pregnancy
- Anxiety related to perceived change in body image

Planning

In the planning phase of the nursing process goals and outcome criteria are established. Identifying precisely what the nurse is trying to achieve helps organize and direct nursing interventions. The plan should be in writing and placed either on the client's chart or on the Cardex.

Using the nursing diagnoses stated above, examples of goals might be:

- The client will be able to look at the amputation site within seven days and clean and care for site by discharge
- The client will state three positive aspects of self

In establishing goals to address problems in self-concept, keep in mind realistic time parameters. It is unlikely you will be able to raise a client's self-esteem and improve his or her body image during a short hospital stay, for example.

Implementation

The importance of helping individuals develop and maintain positive feelings about themselves cannot be overemphasized. Individuals function in any given situation according to how they perceive themselves and how they perceive the situation in which they are involved. The nurse's role in assisting clients to feel valuable and worthwhile and view themselves with confidence is paramount in the overall goal of working with clients to achieve maximum levels of adaptive functioning.

This is not an easy task. One characteristic of the self is stability. The self represents the fundamental frame of reference, the anchor to reality. Even an unsatisfactory self-organization is likely to prove highly stable and resistant to change.[15] For instance, it is difficult to change an individual's view of the self if that person doesn't like him- or herself much. He or she may be pleased by the praise, but continues to act in the same manner. Because of this characteristic stability, you can't "change" an individual's self-concept. That is not a goal. What you can influence is the individual's perception of the situation. How does this happen?

A change in the view of self occurs with repetition of experiences of adequacy and with much praise and encouragement. For example, a student who believes he or she is dumb will not change that view of self with one high grade. It will require many high grades. A client who feels unattractive and unlovable as a result of a physical alteration will only begin to be able to change that view of self with many positive interpersonal interactions and experiences.

Nurses are in unique and powerful positions with clients in influencing how they view themselves and the situations in which they find themselves. They often become, at least temporarily, a "significant other" to the client. For example, it is the nurse who usually works first and most closely with the client after surgery. How the nurse behaves with the client following her mastectomy, what kind of information she gives her, and how she treats her will have an impact on how the client incorporates this new aspect of self into her self-concept. If she is accepted, esteemed, and valued by the nurse, she will be more likely to accept, value, and esteem herself and incorporate her new self-image in a positive, adaptive manner. This relationship between the nurse and client is the primary tool of the nurse in intervening with clients experiencing problems related to self-concept.

Another important aspect of planning intervention strategies for clients is recognizing the client's strengths and looking for ways to focus on those strengths consistently and continuously. Focusing on strengths helps clients feel more confident and positive. If they can recognize worthwhile, positive qualities of self, then they will feel better able to cope with whatever situation comes along.

Evaluation

Evaluating your client's progress is necessary to determine whether your interventions are working. You are looking for the client to be able to view his or her situation in a different way that allows more positive, adaptive behavior. You will know your interventions are working if and when the client begins to talk about her- or himself in an accepting, positive way and with realistic self-confidence. The client's ability to interact with others and to identify with them is another area to evaluate. Remember that change takes time. Adapting to changes that occur in states of wellness and illness and that affect self-concept are difficult and challenging for both client and nurse.

SUMMARY

This chapter has introduced self-concept as an integral component of the total person. Self-concept influences and is influenced by an individual's state of wellness and illness and is, therefore, important for nurses to consider in providing total care to clients.

Social interaction theory and perceptual psychology were presented as two theories of self-concept development. Research was included on self-concept development in children,

which is also useful in assessment of self-concept.

Adaptation, as a framework, offers one approach to examining the self-concept of an individual. This approach allows for the steps of the nursing process to be carried out in assessing self-concept, planning and implementing nursing approaches, and evaluating the effectiveness of those nursing interventions.

Study Questions

1. List ten of your own strengths.

2. What is self-concept?

3. Relate two theories of self-concept development.

4. How does self-concept relate to self-esteem? body image?

5. Why is self-concept important in nursing?

6. What nursing strategies do you use to assess self-concept?

7. Indicate characteristics of positive self-concept and characteristics reflective of low self-concept.

8. Describe interventions appropriate in developing and promoting an adaptive self-concept.

References

1. Sr. Callista Roy, *Introduction to Nursing: An Adaptation Model*, 2nd ed. (Englewood Cliffs, N.J.: Prentice-Hall, 1983).
2. Harry Stack Sullivan, *The Interpersonal Theory of Psychiatry* (New York: W.W. Norton Co., 1953), 49–61, 158–71.
3. S. Epstein, "The self concept revisited or a theory of a theory," *Am Psychol* 28, (1973): 404–16.
4. Arthur Combs, Anne Richards, and Fred Richards, *Perceptual Psychology*. (New York: Harper & Row, 1976), 154.
5. V. Raimey, *The Self as a Factor in Counseling*

and *Personality Organization,* doctoral dissertation, Ohio State University, 1943. (Columbus, Ohio: Ohio State University Libraries, 1971).

6. Combs, Richards, and Richards, *Perceptual Psychology,* 160.
7. Stanley Coopersmith, *Antecedents of Self Esteem* (San Francisco: W.H. Freeman & Co., 1967).
8. Arthur Combs and Donald Snygg, *Individual Behavior: A Perceptual Approach* (New York: Harper & Row, 1959). 134–35.
9. Roy, *Introduction to Nursing,* 190.
10. J.B. Meisenhelder, "Self-esteem in women: The influence of employment and perception of husband's appraisal," *Image* 18, (Spring 1986): 8.
11. Roy, *Introduction to Nursing,* 171.
12. J. Schwab, R. Clemmons, and L. Morder, "The self concept: Psychosomatic implications," *Psychosomatics* 7, (January–February 1966): 1–5.
13. Roy, *Introduction to Nursing.*
14. M. Buck, Self-concept in: Roy *Introduction to Nursing,* 2nd ed. (Englewood Cliffs, N.J.: Prentice-Hall, 1984) p 259.
15. P. Lecky, *Self Consistency. A Theory of Personality,* F.C. Thorne, ed. (Hamden, Conn.: Shoe String, 1961), 162.

Annotated Bibliography

Chrzanowski, G. 1981. *The Genesis and Nature of Self Esteem. Am J Psychother* 35:38–46. This article discusses self-esteem as a foundation for understanding human behavior and in the psychotherapeutic situation.

Gruendemann, B. 1975. *The Impact of Surgery on Body Image. Nurs Clin North Am* 10:635. Discusses the impact of surgery on the individual's concept of self. Includes assessing, planning, and intervention.

Jourard, S. 1971. *The Transparent Self.* New York: Litton Educational Publishing. The concept of self-disclosure and its implications for the nurse-client relationship is discussed.

Maslow, A. 1962. *Toward a Psychology of Being.* Princeton, N.J.: D. Van Nostrand. Presents a theory of functioning based on needs, including self-esteem. It is particularly noted for the concept of self-actualization.

Money, J., and Ehrhardt, A. 1972. *Man and Woman, Boy and Girl.* Baltimore: Johns Hopkins University Press. Presents the results of the author's research on the development of sexual identity and sex-typed behavior.

Norris, C. 1970. *The Professional Nurse and Body Image.* In C. Carlson (ed.) *Behavioral Concepts and Nursing Interventions.* Philadelphia: J.B. Lippincott. Identifies problems related to physical self and discusses factors that influence the degree of threat to one's body image.

Otto, H.A. 1965. *The Human Potentialities of Nurses and Patients. Nurs Outlook* (August). This widely read and cited article discusses some of the findings of a human potentialities research project. Interesting and enlightening findings.

Satir, V. 1972. *Peoplemaking.* Palo Alto, Calif.: Science and Behavior Books. Highly readable, practical book that addresses the importance of self-concept in family relations.

Chapter 20

Human Sexuality

Carol N. Knowlton

Chapter Outline

- Objectives
- Glossary
- Introduction
- Components of Sexuality
- Human Sexual Response
- The Nursing Process
    Sexuality and Illness
    Effects of Hospitalization
    Overt Sexual Behavior
    Sexual Dysfunctions
    Assessment
    Planning
    Implementation
    Evaluation
- Summary
- Study Questions
- References
- Annotated Bibliography

Objectives

At the completion of this chapter, the reader will be able to:

▸ Describe human sexuality as a function of the total personality
▸ Differentiate between sex and sexuality
▸ Describe the influence of family and society on the child's psychosexual development
▸ Define gender identity, sex role, and sexual orientation
▸ Describe potential threats to an individual's sexual integrity
▸ Identify the effect of one's own feelings and value system on client care
▸ List some sexually related behaviors that may occur in the hospital setting
▸ Use a brief sexual assessment guide
▸ Describe nursing attitudes and interventions related to sexual health that will help clients maintain a positive sense of self

Glossary

Biological Sexuality. Anatomical and physiological "givens"—the sex organs, hormones, nerves, and brain centers.

Bisexuals. People sexually attracted to both males and females.

Celibacy. Abstention from sexual intercourse.

Chromosomes. The genetic material in the nucleus of every cell of the body.

Gender Identity. The inner persistent conviction that one is male or female.

Gender Role. Behavior that conveys to others that an individual is either male or female.

Genitals. Pertaining to the sex organs in the pelvic region; customarily refers to the penis, the testes, and the scrotum in the male; the vulva and the vagina in the female.

Gonads. Ovaries or testicles.

Heterosexual. Person with a sexual preference for partners of the opposite sex.

Homosexual. Person with a sexual preference for partners of the same sex.

Hormone. Chemical substance secreted by the endocrine system into the blood stream to be carried directly to the tissue on which it acts.

Masturbation. Self-stimulation of the sexual organs resulting in orgasm.

Ovaries. Paired structures located on each side of the uterus that contain and release eggs; female gonads.

Secondary Sex Characteristics. Those body characteristics that develop during puberty that distinguish the sexes.

Sex. Gender (male or female); sexual behavior; sexual anatomy; sexual intercourse.

Sex Identity. See gender identity.

Sex Role. See gender role.

Sexual Differentiation. The process that begins at the moment of conception to create a normal male or female.

Sexual Integrity. A comfortable, secure gender identity and sexual orientation; experiencing an increasingly satisfying sexual life, free of sexual dysfunction.

Sexual Orientation. Preference for sexual partner.

Sexuality. A pervasive life force that includes a person's total feelings, attitudes, behavior, and beliefs that relate to being a male or a female.

Testes. Paired male reproductive glands contained in the scrotum; the male gonads.

INTRODUCTION

Sexuality is a complex, unique human characteristic that pervades the whole of an individual's life. No other biological function is so personal and emotionally charged and yet so subject to legal and ethical regulation. The term *sexuality* is a broad concept, and it includes more than just biological sex. Sexuality encompasses the biological, psychological, social, cultural, and ethical aspects of sexual behavior. It designates the totality of being, one's experience of maleness or femaleness, and the way one expresses these attributes.

In contrast the word **sex** generally connotes genital sex, physical sex, or the sex act; thus, sex has a much narrower meaning than sexuality. Sexuality is a broad, integrating concept, synthesizing the varied aspects of an individual's expression of self and in many ways refers to what a person is. It does not exist only in the young and attractive or only between partners. It is a deep and pervasive aspect of the total human personality and of the total self from birth to death. It is observable in everyday life in endless variations conveyed by the way one dresses, moves, speaks, and relates to other human beings. Sexuality includes the need for attachment, sensuality, tenderness, intimacy, caring, and procreation. Attitudes toward relationships with people of the same and opposite sex and toward touching and being touched are also integral parts of sexuality.

As a significant concern throughout life, sexuality has the potential to enhance the quality of life, foster personal growth, and contribute to human fulfillment. Today, sexuality is seen as an important aspect of health for people of all ages.

Professional interest in sexuality as an integral part of human behavior has increased greatly in the past 40 years. Tremendous changes in openness about sexuality followed the publication in 1948 of Alfred Kinsey's first research in sexual behavior.[1] As a result sexual concerns are readily discussed today by both individuals and health professionals, and there has been a definite relaxation of societal norms pertaining to sexuality. Openness and candor about sexuality seem to be the norms of the 1980s, in contrast to a taboo about discussion of sexuality in previous decades. In addition, a larger knowledge base now exists in the area of human sexuality. Sex research is a legitimate area of scientific inquiry for researchers in fields such as biology, anthropology, sociology, psychology, nursing, and medicine. The basic facts about sexual functioning are now known, and the body of knowledge about human sexuality is continuing to grow at a rapid rate. Because of the marked expansion in knowledge and the increased availability of information on sexuality, our society has become more informed in sexual matters. Yet for many, sex myths still prevail or persist.

Myths, or beliefs with no foundations in truth, are by no means held only by the uneducated and unsophisticated. Health-care professionals can have a variety of misconceptions about sexuality. A few of the more common sexual myths and fallacies are listed in Table 20–1.

This increase in professional interest and knowledge in human sexuality has extended to the nursing profession as well. Before 1970, there were relatively few sexuality-related articles or texts in the nursing literature. The first nursing text dealing exclusively with sexuality was published in 1974.[2] At least a half dozen nursing texts on sexuality have since been published. Often health-care professionals are the primary source of information for people with sexual concerns, so it is essential that nurses be prepared and willing to manage sexually related health problems. Human sexuality content in nursing programs generally provides a framework of factual information about sexuality, modifies attitudes that block understanding of sexuality, and develops skills for assessment and management of sexually related concerns.

TABLE 20–1. COMMON SEXUAL MYTHS

1. Old people do not want or need sexual intimacy
2. Blacks have a greater sex drive than whites
3. A large penis is of great importance to a woman's sexual gratification
4. Menopause or hysterectomy terminates a woman's sex life
5. Homosexuals are usually identifiable by their appearance
6. Sexual intercourse should be avoided during pregnancy
7. Alcohol is a sexual stimulant
8. Emotional instability is caused by masturbation
9. A couple must have simultaneous orgasms for conception to occur
10. There is an absolutely "safe" period for sexual intercourse during which coitus cannot cause impregnation

All of the above statements are false

To comprehend how persons become the particular sexual being they are, certain fundamental principles must be understood. One's sexuality and sexual behavior result from the interplay of many influencing factors—a combination of inherited biological and physiological capabilities influenced by cultural factors—transmitted through the family and society. Human sexual feelings develop throughout the entire life cycle. One's sexual feelings, attitudes, and behavior are primarily learned, and the earliest sexual attachments are to one's parents.[3] Infantile sexuality begins as young children learn to enjoy the sexual pleasure of their own bodies and that of their mother. The physical and psychological closeness between parents and children that develops through holding, touching, and cuddling is essential to children's development of a belief that they are worthwhile and lovable. These early influences affect later behavior and attitudes in the area of sexuality. No aspect of human sexual expression can be fully understood without knowing how it is developed. The family's attitudes, feelings, and values about sexuality are influenced by the surrounding society and culture. Each society and culture determines what is sexual and what is not; what behavior is appropriate or acceptable and what is not. Each society and culture governs in what way each generation will learn the behavior of sex.

A sexual practice that is advocated in one society may be forbidden in another. For instance, sexual activity before marriage is encouraged by some societies and condemned by others. Premarital coitus is permitted by nearly half of the societies of which there is a record of sexual customs.[4] There are no predetermined, universally accepted sexual values or norms; in fact, it is virtually impossible to achieve consensus about sexual values. Individuals assimilate family and societal norms and develop their own religious belief systems regarding the purpose of sex (Figure 20–1).

COMPONENTS OF SEXUALITY

To understand sexuality, the interrelated components constituting the totality of the sexual self must be described. These components are

The concept of sexuality refers to the totality of being a person. It includes all those aspects of the human being that relate specifically to being a boy or girl, woman or man, and is an entity subject to life-long dynamic change. Sexuality reflects our human character, not solely our genital nature. As a function of the total personality it is concerned with the biological, psychological, sociological, spiritual, and cultural variables of life which, by their effects on personality development and interpersonal relations, can in turn affect social structure.

Figure 20–1. SIECUS Definition of Sexuality. *(From Sex Information and Education Council of the U.S., Inc. (SIECUS). "The SIECUS/Upsala Principles Basic to Education for Sexuality." SIECUS Report 8:3, (1980):8)*

biological, sexuality, gender identity, sex role or gender role, and sexual orientation.

Biological sexuality refers to the **chromosomes, hormones,** and primary and **secondary sex characteristics** that distinguish male from female. Before birth, in the prenatal period, sexual development is controlled mainly by biological forces. Normal sexual development or differentiation begins at the moment of conception. The chromosome pattern from each parent determines whether the **gonads** in the fetus will be **ovaries** or **testes.** Subsequent genital development of specific physical differences depends on hormones derived from the fetus and the mother. In the male fetus, growth of the testes begins about the sixth week after conception. For male sexual differentiation to occur, certain hormones (H-Y antigen and testosterone) must be present in adequate amounts at the right time of development.

Female **sexual differentiation** does not require hormonal stimulation. The ovaries develop by the twelfth week after conception. Prenatal sex differentiation in both sexes involves the **genitals,** the internal reproductive structures, and probably the brain.[5]

Current research is exploring the effects of fetal hormones on the brain. Some of this research theorizes that the brain is a bipotential structure; that is, it has the potential to differentiate differently in males under the influence of testosterone. (For detailed description of the differentiation processes, see the annotated bibliography for suggested readings.)

At puberty there are further physiological changes, as the secondary sex characteristics appear in response to increased hormone levels. Thus, the biological aspects of being male or female are determined by chromosomes, hormones, and internal and external sexual anatomy.

From the moment of birth, biological sex development is influenced by psychosocial factors. When a baby is born, it is declared to be either a boy or a girl. This gender assignment based on anatomy will greatly influence how the child is to be reared, because society prescribes different treatment for boys and girls.

Research has indicated that caretakers of babies, particularly parents, treat infant boys and girls differently. For example, during the first six months of life, boys receive more physical contact (being touched, held, nursed) and less nonphysical contact (being looked at and talked to) than girls. Girls are treated as though they were more fragile than boys.[6] The infant and older baby is receptive to and influenced by the input triggered by adult reactions to the baby's sexual anatomy.

As a result of these inputs, each child will develop a **sex** or **gender identity,** an internal sense of sexual self. Gender identity is a persistent conviction that one is either male or female, an awareness of one's masculinity or femininity. It encompasses much more than genital functioning. The child's gender identity, usually corresponding with his or her genetic makeup and anatomic sex, will be solidifed between the ages of 18 months and three years. Positive solid feelings about self are important foundation for the development of future healthy sexuality.

Gender role or **sex role** is an external or outward expression of one's maleness or femaleness and is a learned behavior. Every society ascribes different roles to males and females. For example, in American society, boys are often expected to be tough and action-oriented, whereas girls are expected to be domestic, quieter and refined. Gender roles permeate all human interactions. They affect how one perceives the other person, they allow one to know how to act, and what to expect from other people. Fulfilling gender role expectations can give a feeling of success and competence. Gender roles are learned in a variety of ways through the social and psychological mechanisms of reinforcement, role modeling, and socialization.

From the moment of birth when the infant is identified as a boy or a girl, reinforcement is given, by the parents or care givers, to behaviors that society sees as masculine or feminine traits. Through praise or discouragement, parents reinforce girls for what they believe to be feminine behaviors and discourage them from masculine behaviors. Likewise, parents and teachers give positive reinforcement to boys for masculine behaviors and negative reinforcement for feminine behaviors. In American society, it is much more acceptable for a girl to exhibit behaviors that are seen as masculine than is the reverse. Boys are strongly prohibited from exhibiting what are viewed as feminine behaviors.

A second way that children learn gender role behaviors is through imitation, or role modeling. Children choose the same sex parent as a role model and use these models to form their own behavior.

The third way a child learns role behaviors is through socialization. Children observe what goes on about them and then try to fit behavior into the norm for the social group. Socialization begins with the parents or care givers, then extends to toys, clothes, television, books, and a whole myriad of sources in society. In American society, the overlap between male and female role behaviors has greatly increased in the past ten years. Many previously considered male role behaviors are being assumed by women, such as head of family, assertiveness, and competitiveness.

In addition, contrary to older views that looked at masculinity and femininity as mutually exclusive opposites, it is now evident that masculine and feminine traits coexist in many people. Males and females are far more similar than different.[7]

Throughout the life cycle, various components of biological sexual function develop. For example, in infancy and childhood, the sexual reflexes for males and females are all present except for the ability of the male to ejaculate.[8] At puberty, with the increases in sex hormone levels and concomitant development of secondary sex characteristics, sexual orientation comes into full force. The term **sexual orientation** is used to describe an individual's prefer-

ence for one or several means of expression of sexual thoughts and feelings. Sexual behavior, like all human behavior, is varied, complex, and defies simple classification. Sexual feelings are most commonly expressed in a **heterosexual** relationship between males and females. In most societies, heterosexual behavior is the preferred pattern. Other forms of sexual expression include **homosexual** relationships, where sexual satisfaction is obtained in a relationship in which partners are of the same sex. **Bisexuals** choose both the same and opposite sexed partners. Some persons may choose **celibacy**, abstaining from sexual intimacy and intercourse, as a temporary or lifelong pattern. For some, solitary sexual behavior, such as **masturbation**, will be a source of sexual gratification. The factors determining sexual orientation are incompletely understood but include some combination of genetics, hormones, and environment. One's sexual orientation is probably established by the age of five to seven years but is thought to be a dynamic, lifelong process of growth.[9]

Homosexuality, or sexual attraction to the same sex, requires special mention. Within the context of both male and female homosexuality, it is a prevalent, controversial, and poorly understood form of sexual orientation. Attitudes toward homosexuality range from acceptance to condemnation. The causes of homosexuality may include genetic factors, hormonal imbalance, and faulty child–parent relations. There is no firm research evidence for any of these, possibly because there may be different types of homosexuality, each of which originates in a different way.[10] Some persons enter a homosexual relationship because they are strongly attracted to someone of the same sex. Others may enter a homosexual relationship because heterosexual partners are unavailable, or out of loneliness or rebellion. Transitory homosexual experiences during adolescence are not uncommon. (See the annotated bibliography for additional references on homosexuality.)

HUMAN SEXUAL RESPONSE

The human sexual response represents an integration of physiological responses with thoughts and feelings within an interpersonal relationship. Masters' and Johnson's work in the area of human sexual response greatly contributed to understanding of the physiological aspects of sexual expression.[11]

Sexual arousal is very individual and can occur in response to a wide variety of stimuli including touch, visual input, and fantasy. Masters and Johnson identified four basic phases of sexual response experienced by both men and women: excitement, plateau, orgasm, and resolution. The excitement phase begins with responses to sexual stimulation and is characterized primarily by vasocongestion of the genitals and breasts, vaginal lubrication, and erection of the penis.

The plateau is characterized by the maintenance of sexual arousal and the building of excitment toward orgasm.

The orgasmic phase is a highly pleasurable reflex characterized by muscle spasms and accompanied by ejaculation in the male.

The resolution phase is characterized by a gradual return to the preexcitement phase. A refractory period in males occurs immediately after orgasm during which ejaculation is impossible, but women have the capacity to be multiorgasmic.

THE NURSING PROCESS

As a basic human need, sexuality is one of the essential dimensions of holistic health care. Nurses are recognizing **sexual integrity** as an integral part of a client's health and well-being as well as recognizing the impact of illness on sexual functioning. Nurses encounter many clients whose sexuality is threatened by disease, trauma, surgical intervention, situational or maturational crises, or psychological problems. The resulting alterations in self-concept, changes in body image, and inability to meet role expectations are significant areas of concern. (Table 20–2).

Many nurses believe they have a responsibility for promoting sexual health in their professional practice. To be effective in helping people with sexual concerns, nurses must[12]:

- Confront feelings, values, and attitudes of sexuality in themselves and in those differing in sexual orientation and practices

TABLE 20–2. BASIC ASSUMPTIONS ABOUT SEXUALITY

Sex is a part of sexuality; a part of total personality

All people are sexual from birth to death

All people have the right to facts about sex and sexuality

Sexual behavior will vary greatly from one person to another and in the same person over time. A wide range of sexual behavior is normal

Because sex is a natural function, guilt need not be associated with sexual thoughts and feelings

Sexual feelings and fantasies are normal. All people experience them

Health professionals can help clients deal with sexual concerns if the professionals are comfortable with their own feelings and values about sexuality

- Develop a sound and comprehensive body of knowledge about sexuality
- Develop assessment, intervention, and communication skills in all aspects of health

Much personal and professional effort is necessary to develop these skills. However, it is appropriate for the beginning nurse to begin to develop sophistication in each of these areas.

A clinician who has achieved a healthy attitude toward her or his own sexuality can deal most effectively with the client's sexuality. Sexuality is an area to which many people attach strong emotions, religious ideas, and rigid opinions. Sexual attitudes, values, and behaviors that are acceptable to one person may be repulsive to another. There is no consensus about sexual values in our society. The nurse must be able to clarify and acknowledge her or his own feelings, attitudes, and opinions about sexual issues as well as develop a value-free attitude toward sexual practices. In identifying the effect of one's attitudes and values on one's nursing practice, one does not have to give up one's own moral standards. One's goal is to develop an atmosphere of acceptance and respect for the rights of individuals to self-determination.

For instance, attitudes of nurses and medical staff toward homosexuals may be negative (e.g., the focus of jokes). Negative staff feelings may compromise the health care they offer these individuals. These individuals are often struggling for acceptance as persons and deserve to be treated with the same dignity and respect as heterosexual individuals.

Assessment of one's own attitudes is a time-consuming but invaluable process. One can begin by listing topics related to sexuality (such as male and female anatomy, intercourse, masturbation, homosexuality) and then record how one feels about each topic. Discussing feelings about sexuality in small groups guided by an experienced professional can contribute not only to clearer identification of feelings, but to increased comfort in discussing emotionally laden topics. Courses in human sexuality often focus on desensitization to sexual topics. In helping people with sexual concerns and questions, the single most important factor is the ease and comfort of the professional in discussing sensitive and value-laden topics (Table 20–3).

Sexuality and Illness

There is increasingly widespread recognition that there is a reciprocal relationship between most medical illnesses and an individual's sexual functioning. Illness may cause changes in one's self-concept, role, sense of self as a man or woman, as well as physical ability to function. It is known that over 50 chronic illnesses and surgical conditions adversely affect sexuality,[13] and that the medication, plus the depression, stress, and fatigue that are often a part of chronic illness also can affect sexual functioning.[14] For instance, diabetes has a potentially destructive effect on sexual function. Some pros-

tatectomy procedures destroy or interfere with normal sexual response. Many medications used to treat hypertension interfere with sexual function.

Transient disinterest or lack of desire in sexual activity occurs in most persons when they are preoccupied with the symptoms of illness. Sexual problems often disappear when the illness improves. The fear that sexual behavior may cause or aggravate existing physical illness is common in clients. For example, although a myocardial infarct has no direct effect on sexual response, many male post-myocardial-infarction clients are unable to achieve an erection. The client fears that sexual activity will cause another attack or that sex will be "weakening." Fear may last long after recovery—and this fear may be experienced by both partners.

Effects of Hospitalization

Hogan states that admission to the hospital, physical exams, and diagnostic procedures may be more disturbing to the individual's sexual integrity than the disease itself. Hospitalized individuals are separated from significant others and stripped of their identity by removal of accustomed clothing, jewelry, and personal possessions.[15] Assessments and treatments such as rectal temperatures and pelvic exams may be perceived as intrusive. Questions focus on areas that have been considered private and that may be embarrassing to discuss. Invasion of one's privacy and violation of one's territory might surely be viewed as threats to one's sexual in-

TABLE 20–3. NURSING VARIABLES FOSTERING CLIENT SEXUAL INTEGRITY

Variables Affecting Nurse's Ability to Deal Effectively with Client's Sexual Concerns	Responsibilities of Health-care Team for Maintaining Sexual Integrity of the Client	Desired Client Outcomes
Comfort level in discussing sexual concerns	Anticipating potential sexual problems	Client feels free to verbalize sexual concerns
Knowledge level about concepts related to sexuality	Preventing problems from developing	Client understands effect of illness on sexual behavior
Awareness of own sexual value system	Validating normalcy	Client maintains a positive sense of self
Ability to perceive the underlying meaning and needs expressed by the client's behavior	Offering early treatment for problems that develop	Client functions sexually to the limits of his or her particular capacity
Interpersonal skills, such as communication, interviewing, and teaching techniques	Seeking consultation or offering referral for problems beyond the expertise of the health-care team	

tegrity. For instance, women often have feelings about a pelvic examination such as fear of the procedure, embarrassment, concerns about normalcy. Nurses can be a positive influence here. They can use knowledge and sensitivity to create an atmosphere of caring and consideration. Explaining the procedure, providing verbal support, and answering questions can contribute to maintaining the client's sense of self.

People react to illness and hospitalization in various ways—some with overt sexual behavior. Sexual behavior within the hospital setting may be the expression of a variety of needs, such as the need to reaffirm one's sexual identity, to express sexual feelings, to affirm one's ability to function sexually, or to control the situation.

Most people conduct sexual behavior privately, but there are times when staff members are confronted with a client's sexual behavior. This may be embarrassing and anxiety-producing for both nurses and clients. Health-care professionals sometimes respond by ignoring the behavior, humiliating and punishing the client, becoming angry, or avoiding further contact with the person. Instead, nurses need to look at the meaning of the behavior as a basis for choosing the most therapeutic response. The way nurses respond will be dependent on their knowledge of sexuality and comfort with sexual issues. They may see the client as asexual, or not having sexual needs because of age or illness. They may see the client as not having a right or need to express sexuality. For instance, it is sometimes assumed that sexuality is not a concern for older people, especially in nursing home settings. For an older person to exhibit interest in sex is often considered perverse or pathological. Interest in sex, despite age or illness, is a component of health throughout the life cycle and is a positive, vitalizing force.

In providing care, nurses have the responsibility to help the individual maintain a positive sense of self and sexual integrity within the limits of the client's particular capacity. Nurses can accomplish these objectives by avoiding practices that contribute to shame, by helping to ameliorate guilt related to sexuality, and by providing privacy.

Overt Sexual Behavior

There are several overt sexual behaviors that commonly occur to clients in health-care settings. Erections often occur spontaneously in men and are not under conscious control. An erection occurs when arterial blood rushes into the body of the penis. Erections are of two types—psychogenic and reflexogenic. Psychogenic erections can be triggered by fantasies, thoughts, and memories. Reflexogenic erections are stimulated by tactile stimulation of the penis or genital area or by a full bladder. By giving the individual a few minutes warning before any procedure involving exposure of the genital area, the nurse can usually avoid confronting erections. The nurse can respond to the presence of an erection by ignoring it or by acknowledging the client's sexuality by saying, "It must be frustrating to be in the hospital!"

Masturbation or self-stimulation is a normal part of sexual maturation and behavior. It can be a healthy outlet for sexual drives, an alternate method for experiencing sexual release. Masturbation is especially significant for the hospitalized individual who does not have access to a sexual partner. It can also serve to reduce anxiety. It is the responsibility of health-care personnel to provide privacy. Allowing predictable times during which the client can enjoy solitude, drawing curtains, closing doors, and knocking on doors before entering show respect for the individual and contribute to privacy.

Masturbation can also be used in a dysfunctional way if it is conducted publicly without respect for the rights of others. The possible meanings of this type of behavior are to draw attention, to express hostility, or to embarrass the staff. When nurses encounter this type of behavior, they should confront the behavior and request that the individual seek privacy for masturbation.

Although the need for sexual interaction is normal, the hospital setting is not conducive to intimacy. The nurse needs to be sensitive to clients' sexual needs, help them gain privacy, yet ensure that the rights of others are protected. If the nurse encounters a client and partner engaging in sex, the response might be, "Pardon me, I didn't realize you had company. I'll close the door."

Seductive or sexual acting-out, such as sexual overtures, compliments, sexual jokes, exhibition of genitals, provocative suggestions, attempts to touch the nurse, and bragging about sexual capabilities may be directed at the nurse. Nurses may become objects of seductive behavior by clients. The nurse must kindly but firmly set limits on the behavior. Reject the behavior, but not the person. Sometimes a sense of humor is helpful. The nurse must attempt to understand the meaning of the behavior as an expression of an underlying need. Clients may doubt their attractiveness and consider the nurse a safe person on whom they can test their desirability. It is possible that nurses may be provocative or give mixed messages about their own needs. Nurses are sexual people, too, but they must make their role clear without reacting negatively to the clients or humiliating them.

Promoting sexual integrity for clients is a complex task, especially for the beginning nurse. By discussing experiences one has had with individuals who were sexually acting out, one can master feelings and understand the needs underlying the behavior. In this way, the nurse can devise more effective strategies for future interactions.

Skills in assessing, interviewing, teaching, and counseling are needed if nurses are to become able to promote sexual health. Nurses must become sensitive in recognizing sexual concerns and problems in clients. Establishing a therapeutic atmosphere is a first step.

Despite increasing openness in American society about sexual matters, clients will seldom initiate discussion of a sexual concern. They may not wish to reveal their ignorance, feel guilty about having a problem, be uncertain how to state the concern, or fear being viewed by the staff as overinterested in sex. Sexuality is an area of self that needs to be treated with discretion, but the secrecy and taboos related to sexuality have often led to shame and guilt. Health-care professionals, through their own openness, help to change this atmosphere. It is the nurse's responsibility to provide a climate where clients feel comfortable expressing sexual concerns. The nurse needs to give the permission to discuss such concerns. This can be done indirectly in several ways. The nurse can bring up the topic of sex by saying, "Many people with your condition note changes in their sexual feelings. How about you?" Or the nurse can provide reading material that includes information on sexual activity. When the client has read the material, the nurse can discuss questions and concerns related to the situation. Once the nurse has sanctioned the topic of sexuality, the client will be much more likely to express sexual concerns. The nurse can assess whether the client has correct information or misconceptions about sexuality and especially about the effects of illness on sexual function. The nurse can listen for nonverbal cues of sexual problems. For example, telling sexual jokes, bragging about sexual prowess, or exhibiting genitals may be clues about underlying concerns the person may have.

Sexual Dysfunctions

Sexual dysfunctions are conditions in which the ordinary physical responses of sexual function are impaired. Women can experience problems in getting aroused and maintaining arousal as well as having difficulty in reaching orgasm. Men can have difficulty getting or maintaining an erection, ejaculating too quickly, or difficulty in ejaculating. Sexual dysfunctions may have psychological or relational causes (such as fear of failure or marital conflict), but many dysfunctions have an organic cause such as diabetes, neurological disease, alcohol, or prescription medications.[16] When confronted with a client's expressed anxieties and concerns, the nurse can gather data as the basis of a referral to a sex counselor or therapist. Because of the possibility of an organic cause of the dysfunction, it is imperative that the client have a thorough medical evaluation.

Assessment

Assessment of sexual health can be made as early as admission. The scope of sexual assessment will be dictated by the professional's preparation and experience as well as by the client's health situation. Sexual health assessment is a legitimate concern of the health professional and is the first step for the health-care team in meeting its responsibilities for maintaining the person's sexual integrity.

Sexual health assessment requires greater skill than any other interview. If the nurse is ill at ease, this discomfort will be conveyed to the client. A sexual health assessment should be part of every routine history. Including a sex history early in the nurse–client relationship communicates to the client the nurse's appreciation of the importance of sexual health and comfort in discussing these health needs. Whether or not the initial assessment elicits problem areas is insignificant. Perhaps none exists, or perhaps it will take time for the client to develop sufficient comfort and trust to confide a longstanding problem. When a problem does arise, the client will seek out the nurse as someone in whom to confide.

Several strategies can be used to facilitate obtaining a sexual health assessment:

- Provide privacy while conducting the assessment; ensure confidentiality
- Prepare client for the assessment with an introductory statement by briefly explaining the purpose of the interview. "To plan care for your health needs, I am going to ask you for information. You may find some of the questions personal, but these are issues about which clients often have questions or concerns"
- Ask questions in an open ended manner that helps the client to explain the situation rather than merely answer "yes" or "no." "Many people, after an operation (illness, accident) like yours, have concerns about their sexuality. What are your concerns?"
- Allow the client to refuse to answer. "You seem reluctant (anxious, embarrassed) about answering that question. Would you prefer I bring it up later?"
- Give the client a chance to ask questions. "What questions about sexual health would you like answered?"

Woods suggests three broad questions that can be asked to assess the effect or potential effect of illness or hospitalization on self as a sexual being, and on the individual's ability to function sexually:

- "What about your illness (surgery, accident, pregnancy) has interfered with your being a (mother, wife, father, husband)?"

- "Has anything (for example, heart attack) changed the way you feel about yourself as a man (woman)?"
- "What about your illness (surgery, accident, pregnancy) has changed your ability to function sexually?"[17]

By including questions related to sexuality on the health history, nurses convey the message that sexuality is a matter of legitimate concern and that sexuality is a topic they are comfortable discussing. It also provides an opportunity to provide education and to dispel myths and misinformation. Nursing diagnoses are formulated at the end of the assessment phase of the nursing process. Examples of these can be found in Table 20–4.

Planning

Once the assessment has been completed, the next phase in the nursing process, planning, can take place. Goals and mutual objectives are prepared, based on the assessment (Table 20–4).

Implementation

Education and counseling are the prime interventions that promote sexual integrity. The assessment process is, by its nature, a positive force toward health and can be considered to have the effect of an intervention. The nurse's comfort level in discussing sexual matters will encourage and facilitate clients' discussion of their own sexual problems and concerns, and this openness will contribute to self-understanding and enhancement of sexual integrity.

Secondly, clients frequently approach professionals to find out if what they are experiencing is acceptable or normal. By validating the normalcy of a particular practice, the nurse is contributing to problem prevention. Providing anticipatory guidance is another intervention useful in promoting sexual health. This involves providing the client with information about what to expect. For example, the nurse can provide a middle-aged woman with information about predictable physiological and emotional changes related to menopause or reassure a hospitalized client that loss of interest in sex after surgery is a normal but transient feeling.

TABLE 20–4. NURSING CARE PLANS

Assessment	Nursing Diagnosis	Goal	Plan and Intervention	Evaluation
Parental fear that sex education in the schools will cause promiscuity in their teenage children	Knowledge deficit related to misinterpretation of information	Client feels free to verbalize sexual concerns and values Client has accurate information and is able to discuss and list facts after reviewing materials	Provide opportunity for discussion of concerns about sex education Involve parents in planning of sex education program Validate normalcy of adolescents' interest in sexuality	Parents verbalize that increased knowledge of sexuality does not cause promiscuity Parents feel free to verbalize additional concerns about sexuality
Belief that hysterectomy (removal of the uterus) will cause loss of sexual desire	Knowledge deficit related to lack of information	Client verbalizes effect of hysterectomy on sexual desire Client can (prior to surgery): Describe the anatomy and physiology of the reproduction system Describe the surgical procedure Dicuss the human sexual response	Anticipatory guidance: Provide accurate information preoperatively Offer reading materials on hysterectomy Give permission to discuss sexual concerns	Client verbalizes that hysterectomy will have no effect on sexual desire Client verbalizes sources of accurate information on sexuality

Evaluation

Evaluation completes the nursing process. The nurse establishes whether or not interventions have been successful. In conclusion, nurses can provide accurate information and dispel myths and misconceptions. As members of the health-care team, nurses can anticipate potential sexual problems and, through education and counseling, prevent some problems from developing. Nurses need to have referral sources for interventions beyond their ability. As with any skill, practice is needed for proficiency in sexual history taking, education, and counseling.

SUMMARY

Sexuality is a function of the total personality. It is a lifelong process that has many variations.

The concept of sexuality, a function of the total personality, is concerned with the biolog-ical, psychological, sociological, spiritual, and cultural aspects of life. The interrelated components constituting the totality of the sexual self are biological sexuality, gender identity, sex role, sexual orientation and sexual response.

Sexual behavior is varied; each person has a right to his or her own values and beliefs about sexuality.

Sexuality is an essential dimension of health care, and nurses have a role in promoting sexual integrity in their clients. By becoming comfortable with their own feelings and values about sexuality, health professionals can more effectively help clients deal with sexual concerns. A sound and comprehensive body of knowledge about sexuality is essential for the care giver.

Nurses' ability to use the nursing process effectively in caring for clients with sexual concerns will depend on their preparation, level of self-awareness, and ability to communicate effectively through listening, eliciting feelings, acceptance, and problem solving. Mastery of these interpersonal skills will enable nurses to create a comfortable atmosphere in which the client can express concerns.

In providing care, nurses have the responsibility to help the individual maintain a positive sense of self and sexual integrity within the limits of the client's capacity.

Study Questions

1. What is the role of the family in determining the child's sexual identity and sex role?

2. Who was your most important role model when you were a child? When you were a teenager?

3. Differentiate between sex, sexuality, sexual identity, and sexual orientation.

4. For you, what is the meaning of touching? of companionship? of intimacy?

5. What is the relationship between human sexuality and nursing?

6. Whose responsibility is it to talk with clients about sexual concerns?

7. What are some of the reasons health professionals are reluctant to talk with clients about sexuality?

8. What are some nonverbal cues of sexually related problems clients may express?

References

1. Alfred Kinsey, Wardell Pomeroy, Clyde Martin, and Paul Gebhard, *Sexual Behavior in the Human Male* (Philadelphia: W.B. Saunders Co., 1948).
2. Nancy F. Woods, *Human Sexuality in Health and Illness*, 3rd ed. (St. Louis: C.V. Mosby Co., 1984).
3. Warren Gadpaille, *The Cycles of Sex* (New York: Charles Scribner's Sons, 1975), 3.
4. Frank A. Beach, ed., *Human Sexuality in Four Perspectives* (Baltimore: The Johns Hopkins University Press, 1977), 115–63.
5. William Masters, Viriginia Johnson, and Robert Kolodny, *Human Sexuality*, 2nd ed. (Boston: Little Brown & Co., 1985), 152–55.
6. Eleanor Maccoby and Carol Jacklin, *The Psychology of Sex Differences* (Stanford, Calif.: Stanford University Press, 1974), 309.
7. Masters, Johnson, and Kolodny, *Human Sexuality*, 224.
8. Ibid. 152–73.
9. Robert T. Francoeur, *Becoming a Sexual Person* (New York: John Wiley & Sons, 1982), 512–13.
10. Masters, Johnson, and Kolodny, 315–39.
11. William Masters and Virginia Johnson, *Human Sexual Response* (Boston: Little Brown & Co., 1966).
12. Fern H. Mims and Melinda Swenson, *Sexuality: A Nursing Perspective* (New York: McGraw-Hill Book Co., 1980), 4.
13. Helen S. Kaplan, *The New Sex Therapy*, (New York: Brunner/Mazel, 1975), 75–103.
14. Gadpaille, *The Cycles of Sex,* 427–33.
15. Rosemary Hogan, *Human Sexuality, A Nursing Perspective* (New York: Appleton-Century-Crofts, 1980), 297.
16. Masters, Johnson, and Kolodny, 399–404.
17. Woods, *Human Sexuality,* 79.

Annotated Bibliography

Boston Women's Health Collective. 1979. *Women, Our Bodies, Our Selves.* New York: Simon & Schuster. A book by and for women about how women feel about their sexuality.

Francoeur, R.T. 1982. *Becoming a Sexual Person.* New York: Wiley. A comprehensive textbook on human sexuality with a strong emphasis on self-health, cultural influences, and values. Extensive information on gender differentiation, contraception, sexually transmitted disease, and the quest for intimacy.

Gadpaille, W. 1975. *The Cycles of Sex.* New York: Scribner's. Detailed portrayal of each of the developmental phases of normal psycho-sexual development.

Hogan, R. 1980. *Human Sexuality, A Nursing Perspective.* New York: Appleton-Century-Crofts. Coverage of biological, psychological, and socio-cultural aspects of sexuality in health and illness with emphasis on the nurse's role in promoting and maintaining sexual health. Good chapters on effects of illness and hospitalization on sexuality, and sexual problems throughout the life cycle.

Kaplan, H.S. 1975. *The New Sex Therapy*. New York: Brunner/Mazel. A detailed handbook on sex therapy.

Masters, W.H., Johnson, V.E., and Kolodny, R.C. 1985. *Human Sexuality,* 2nd ed. Boston: Little, Brown. Comprehensive coverage of the field of human sexuality written in an interesting and lively manner. Striking artwork. Especially good coverage of gender identity, sex roles, homosexuality, bisexuality, fantasy, sexual assault, and contraception.

Mims, F.H., and Swenson, M. 1980. *Sexuality: A Nursing Perspective*. New York: McGraw-Hill. An excellent, concise text on promotion of sexual health with focus on prevention and health maintenance and care of individuals with acute, chronic, or terminal illnesses affecting sexual health. Es-

pecially good chapters on drugs affecting sexuality, sexuality and dying, and taking a sexual history.

Morison, E., and Price, M. 1974. *Values of Sexuality*. New York: Hart. A collection of group exercises, games, and role-playing suggestions useful in values clarification and in increasing the comfort level in discussing sexuality.

Moses, A.E., and Hawkins, R. 1982. *Counseling Gay Men and Women*. St. Louis: C.V. Mosby. Coverage of many of the aspects of being homosexual in American culture with specific information on counseling approaches.

Woods, N.F. 1984. *Human Sexuality in Health and Illness,* 3rd ed. St. Louis: C.V. Mosby. An excellent text with emphasis on sexual health, health care, and clinical aspects of human sexuality. Good chapters on assessment of sexual health, roles for professional nurses in sexual health-care delivery, fertility and infertility, and sexual assault.

Chapter 21

Perspectives on Aging

Sister Rose Therese Bahr

Chapter Outline

- Objectives
- Glossary
- Introduction
  Definition of Aging
  Demographics of Aging
  Importance of Studying Geriatrics,
  Gerontology, and Gerontological
  Nursing
- Attitudes Toward Aging
- Theories Related to Aging
  Biological Theories
  Psychological Theories
  Sociological Theories
  Summary of Current Status of Research in
  Aging
- Health Status and the Aging Process
  Life Expectancy, Mortality, and Morbidity
  Stress and Adaptation
  Primary Care Issues
  Social Welfare Needs
- Gerontological Nursing as a Specialty
- The Nursing Process
  Assessment
  Planning
  Implementation
  Evaluation
- Summary
- Study Questions
- References
- Annotated Bibliography

Objectives

At the completion of this chapter the reader will be able to:

- Define the terms in the glossary
- Define aging as a concept
- Describe the demographics of the aging population
- Explain the importance of studying geriatrics, gerontology, and gerontological nursing
- Discuss the societal attitudes toward aging and aging persons
- Explain the major ideas in three popular theories of aging
- Identify the status of research in aging
- Discuss health status and the aging process as related to morbidity and mortality, stress and adaptation, primary care issues, and the social welfare needs of the aged
- Discuss the specialty of gerontological nursing
- Discuss the nursing process in terms of assessment, planning, implementation, and evaluation of nursing care of aging individuals

Glossary

Aging The normal cycle of living from conception through death, in which changes in the function of organs and organ systems occur.

Agism. A process of systematic stereotyping of and discrimination against individuals because of the aging process.

Cohort. The peer group of any one age group, e.g., all persons who are living at age 65 at any one period of time.

Geriatrics. The study of diseases, primarily chronic, in the older age group.

Gerontology. The total process of studying the normal cycle of aging. It encompasses the biological, psychological, sociological, and spiritual dimensions of older adults.

Gerontological Nursing. That specialty in nursing concerned with assessing the health needs of the older person, planning and implementing nursing care to meet those needs, and evaluating the effectiveness of the care by measurement of outcomes beneficial to the older adult.

Frail Elderly. Elderly people in the population that are 85 years and older; this group is largely female and widowed.

Theories of Aging. The scientific explanations offered to understand the dynamics of aging and its causes in the human; the dimensions of biology, psychology, and sociology each provide theoretical input that assists in shaping such explanations.

INTRODUCTION

Human **aging** is a reality. It is part of the normal cycle of life.[1] When an individual is endowed with excellent (from a biological perspective) genetic material that provides for longevity, aging occurs and the person is benefited with a long life of 70, 80, 90, and even 100 years or more of life. All persons age. It is a universal concept that is inherent in the individual from the moment of conception. As each cell divides and matures within the human body, from the fibroblast stage throughout the life cycle, aging is taking place. The intent of this chapter is to present an overview of the concept of aging with application in the clinical nursing practice settings.

Definition of Aging

Aging as a phenomenon of society has been studied by various disciplines, primarily the bi-

ological, sociological, and psychological sciences. At the most fundamental level aging can be defined in terms of its biological characteristics.[2] There are, however, many different approaches to aging and its complexities, depending on the perspective identified by the various disciplines.[3]

Aging, according to Birren and Renner is "the regular behavioral changes that occur in mature genetically representative organisms living under representative environmental conditions as they advance in chronological age."[4] This definition suggests that not only does the organism or individual change biologically as it lives from year to year, but also that behaviors of that organism take on unique characteristics as adaptation to different situations and conditions in the environment evolve and are experienced. From a biological perspective, a projection or estimate of the present status and potential future of the organism or individual is termed biological age.[5] This approach to aging describes the functional capabilities of vital organ systems that allows an individual to continue to engage in activities of daily living, e.g., eating, bathing, walking or exercising. Using this approach, aging is defined in terms of the ability to live a life consisting of length or number of years lived, commonly called a life span. It also connotes the organismic structure biologically composed of molecule, cell, organ and the aging changes within the uniqueness of the individual.[6]

From a psychological perspective, aging—or the psychological age—is defined as the responses the person makes to an ever-changing environment and its demands, causing the person to continually adapt to new situations as they arise.[7] These responses are seen in terms of insights, feelings, and emotional reactions the person is continually called upon to produce by the aging process. These projected psychological behaviors help the older adult to cope with biological changes as they appear, and with the experienced nuances of living. The mental capacities of memory, concentration, and integration of information are also considered a vital part of the psychological aging dimension.[8]

Sociological age is defined as the social habits or roles an individual assumes within the context of a society.[9] Roles of an older adult refer to the ability to continue with activities begun in earlier years associated with being a parent, grandparent, worker, volunteer, teacher. In addition to social roles, social habits evolve within the individual from the environment in which that individual resides and from the effects of behaviors of family, friends, and associates of the older person. As one ages sociologically, losses are experienced in terms of job, occupational colleagues, friends, neighbors, and spouse.

Aging, then, is a phenomenon that is multifaceted and highly complex and requires many explanations to fully understand the process. A number of these explanations offered by scientists will be considered in the discussion of theories related to aging.

Demographics of Aging

Demography, the statistical study of populations of people in a nation, identifies size, distribution, density, and vital statistics as its major contribution.[10] Such study in the past has yielded interesting information about the elderly population in the United States. These factors include[11]:

- Older people are increasing in numbers
- An increasing proportion of the total population of the United States is constituted by the older members

- Life expectancy of people is on the increase
- The population of older people is itself aging (more **frail elderly**)
- An increase of chronic illness and disability in the aging population is a potential hazard to their health

The graying of America has been occurring since 1900 when approximately 3 million people were 65 years or older. In 1980 more than 22.5 million people were considered elderly, or an 8.3 percent increase over the number in 1900, when 3.8 percent of people were 65 years or older.[12] By 1984, one in five Americans was at least 55 years of age (55 million) and one in nine was at least 65 years of age (28 million).[13] The number of persons who will have celebrated their 65th birthday by 2020 is projected to be almost twice the number who have done so in 1985.[14]

Highlights of the growth in the older population at this writing can be viewed in Table 21–1.

The major factor for the presence of older adults in America is fertility. The number of individuals who become 65 in any given year is dependent upon the birthrate 65 years earlier. Large numbers of babies born around 1900 resulted in a large group of elderly in society 65 years later. With more births occurring during

TABLE 21–1. GROWTH OF AGING PERSONS IN THE UNITED STATES (1985–1986)

The older population grew twice as fast as the rest of the population in the last two decades

The median age of the U.S. population is projected to rise from 31 today to 36 by the year 2000

The 85-plus population is growing especially rapidly. This "very old" population is expected to increase seven times by the middle of the next century

The elderly population is growing older. By the year 2000, half of the elderly population is projected to be 75-plus. In 1984, 39 percent of the elderly population was age 75 and older

Elderly women now outnumber elderly men three to two. This disparity is even higher at age 85 and older; in this group there are only 40 men for every 100 women

The ratio of elderly persons to persons of working age has grown from 7 elderly per 100 persons age 18 to 64 in 1900 to 19 per 100 today. By 2010, there are expected to be 22 elderly persons per 100 of working age and by 2050, 38 per 100

Life expectancy at birth improved drastically over the last century. People born today have a life expectancy 26 years longer than those born in 1900

Improvement in life expectancy is particularly dramatic for women. In 1983 life expectancy at birth for women was 78.3 years, while for men it was 71.0 years

Aging is an international phenomenon. The number of persons 60-plus in the world is expected to increase from 376 million in 1980 to 1.1 billion in 2025

From U.S. Senate Special Committee on Aging in conjunction with the American Association of Retired Persons, the Federal Council on the Aging and the Administration on Aging, Aging America: Trends and Projections, 1985–86 Edition. (Washington, D.C.: U.S. Department of Health and Human Services).

World War II and the following years, a large increase in the aged in society is expected in the years 2010 to 2050.[15]

A decrease in mortality is another factor influencing the increased number of elderly in society. Death rates among children and infants have been reduced through technological advances in sanitation, medicine, and hospital care. Better economic conditions have also contributed through improved employment practices that have allowed for better health-care accessibility. Thus, many more persons survive to age 65 and beyond.[16]

Another major contributor to the increased gerontological population in America was the large influx of immigrants before World War II. This increase in the elderly population through immigration will continue as new immigrants from the Orient and Latin America arrive on American shores asking for asylum and a chance for a new life.[17]

An interesting fact uncovered by the 1980 census survey has been that many more individuals are living to be centenarians (100 years or more). In 1983, the number showed 32,000 Americans had reached the century mark and that the majority (three out of four) were women.[18] In 1985, 210 Americans celebrated their 100th birthday every week.[19] In addition, the group of elderly that is 85 years and older is the fastest growing group among the elderly, totaling 2.6 million, or 9.1 percent of the population that had increased between 1980 and 1984.[20] This group also is the group with the highest consumption of health and support services.

Women outlive, men as shown by the projections above. It is estimated that the ratio of women to men will be 154 to 100 by the year 2000 and 191 women to 100 men for those who reach 75 years.[21] Aging is and will continue to be a highly visible feature of the American societal scene for many years into the future. The nursing profession, and particularly, **gerontological nursing,** has a unique role to play in American society, to understand and broaden professional knowledge about this emerging population with unique needs and demands, and to take the lead in helping to meet those needs.

Importance of Studying Geriatrics, Gerontology, and Gerontological Nursing

Given the demographic evidence provided by statistical survey information, the need for studying the aging process and its unique presentation in each individual is imperative for nursing professionals.[22] The importance of understanding **geriatrics** or the chronic illnesses peculiar to the older population is demonstrated by the increased vulnerability of older adults to heart disease, cancer, and strokes that impair their health status. In **gerontology,** or the study of the normal aging process in older adults, it is important for the nurse to appreciate the well elderly and their many health-maintenance challenges. With assistance, older individuals may achieve projected life goals through improvement of functional ability, optimal living, and meaningful activities.

Nurses are especially urged to study the aging process and gerontological nursing so that high-quality care may be administered to elderly clients served in hospitals, nursing homes, long-term care facilities, community nursing service agencies, and the elderly person's own home. Gerontological nursing is an emerging specialty that is achieving its own recognition within the nursing professional circle.[23] Nurse gerontologists are being sought as highly specialized clinicians who can assess and evaluate the health status of the older adult, develop nursing interventions to overcome highly complex and challenging nursing problems, assist the older adult to a higher satisfaction with achievement of life goals, and study the complications of the aging process. The study of geriatrics, gerontology, and gerontological nursing is an essential facet of the holistic approach to scientific knowledge, which, applied to nursing practice, will benefit the elderly citizens in American society.

Discussion in the next section focuses on prevalent societal attitudes toward aging. Theoretical explanations of the phenomenon of aging are also presented. It is hoped that these explanations will dispel myths about aging, and that aging will be perceived as a benefit, not only for the individual who is aging but also for the society in which these older persons reside. Many of these aged individuals have contributed greatly to the major progressive movements that characterize the twentieth century. We owe much to these citizens who now, as elders, look to the nursing profession for meeting many of their health-care needs.

ATTITUDES TOWARD AGING

Society tends to hold negative images of and attitudes toward the aging process and aging persons.[24,25] DeBeauvoir notes this attitude in the following statement:

> The purified image of themselves that society offers the aged is that of a white-haired and venerable sage, rich in experience, planning high above the common state of mankind: if they vary from this, then they fall below it. The counterpart of the first image is that of the old fool in his dotage, a laughingstock for children. In any case, either by their virtue or by their degradation they stand outside humanity.[26]

This approach to the negative attitude toward the elderly is commonly called **agism.**

Agism described by Butler is "the process of systematic stereotyping of and discrimination against people because they are old."[27] Agism is a phenomenon that has occurred in America because our relatively young country and its youth-oriented society has produced an attitude that anyone not young is not productive to America's growth. Consequently, these older individuals tend to be ignored, abused, and pushed to the periphery of societal life. As this negative attitude prevails more and more, opportunities for older persons are denied them and their rights suppressed in favor of more youthful citizens.

Negative attitudes toward the aged have been noted by the myths commonly held about the aging process and the aging person. Myths about aging that have been promulgated in the past and have had detrimental effects include[28]:

- The majority of old persons are senile or demented
- The majority of old persons feel miserable most of the time
- Most older people cannot work as effectively as younger people
- Most old persons are unhealthy and need assistance with daily activities
- Most old people are set in their ways and unable to change
- In general most old persons are alike
- The majority of old persons are socially isolated and lonely

Each of these myths have been refuted through research findings or through clinical experiences. For example, only 2 to 3 percent of aging individuals are institutionalized with any diagnosis of mental illness[29]; and less than 20 percent of the total population over the age of 65 has any measurable memory impairment.[30] In addition, 80 percent of all elderly people are healthy enough to continue with activities of daily living in an independent manner. The National Council on the Aging sponsored a Harris poll in 1975, which found these myths without foundation when a sample of 4254 individuals over the age of 55 were surveyed.[31] Yet, these myths persist within the structure of society. The only basis for such untruths about aging and the aged is lack of current knowledge regarding elderly persons who live in the twentieth and will survive into the twenty-first century.

Within recent years, however, the elderly have increasingly joined organizations with heightened political activity. Organizations have been established by and for the elderly to promote a better image of aging and an improved understanding of the issues, such as society's negative attitudes toward older adults. Organizations such as the Gray Panthers, founded by Margaret Kuhn, a retired union organizer, the American Association of Retired Persons (AARP), and the Catholic Golden Age (CGA) in the last 10 years have been successful in retiring some of the myths about unproductive older citizens.[32] It is interesting to note that people may join AARP at age 50. This enables them to take advantage of excellent publications, services, and learning experiences at an age when they are just beginning to make the transition to an older age group. In consequence, strong lobbying efforts at the state and Federal level have resulted in laws promoting the welfare of the aging population. Such laws include the Discrimination Act, which provides that persons may not be barred from employment opportunities or denied their rights because of age, sex, or race; the Elder Abuse Law, making an abusive act toward an older adult a felony punishable by fine for the offender; an Ombudsman Act, in which each state must establish an office to receive complaints filed by institutionalized elderly, and assure that positive results are obtained through correction by administrators and nursing personnel at the institution; and, the upgrading of the retirement age from 65 to 70, a revision of the Mandatory Retirement Act that was a major breakthrough for older workers permitting continuity of income and better retirement pension payments for their later years.[33]

As a result of these political activities by older adults, society is slowly changing its attitude from a negative one to a more positive one. Cutler and Kaufman project that by the year 2020, older adults will have attained a high visibility in society as a result of political behavior and an age-consciousness within the citizenry.[34] They note further that age issues will be an increasingly essential dimension of the aged themselves and of political organizations. Since the aged of the twenty-first century will be more highly educated, there will be a more sophisticated approach to solving problems faced by the aged through their own efforts. Thus, their needs will be met through channels that will be more effective and efficient in producing the expected results. With this heightened awareness of older adults in America, the results will be a willingness to allow them to exercise their rights and assume responsibilities as citizens with respect and dignity. The division of the youth and the aged of society will move from separateness to a unified collaboration for the benefit of all.

Behaviors resulting from changed attitudes will have an impact on improved understanding of the aging process and the capabilities of older adults as suggested through scientific conceptualization of aging. Theories of aging have aided in this improved understanding and, as refinement occurs, greater depth of insight will be attained.

THEORIES RELATED TO AGING

Understanding of aging comes through scientific intellectual activity. Scientists project their insights or explanations drawn from their study of a subject, to formulate conceptual models, which may instruct others on the possible causes or reasons for the phenomenon under study. These explanations have been labeled as theories.

A theory is defined as an internally consistent set of concepts, propositions, and definitions that organizes a systematic perspective on phenomena by identifying relations among the concepts.[35] A theory has as its purpose to describe, explain, predict, and control phenomena. Because it organizes observations into logical relationships, scientists find a theory useful to guide their approach to the subject. With the theoretical guide, scientists can more easily plan the steps to be taken to investigate the subject in an organized, systematic fashion and derive from their findings greater insights into the phenomenon. In this testing of the theoretical concepts, more conclusive evidence is produced to allow other scientists to predict and even control the phenomenon in the future.[36]

Currently, there is no general theory of aging in existence.[37] There does exist a compilation of proposed hypotheses and concepts to explain limited aspects of people's behavior as they progress through the life span, which have been labeled as "theories of aging."[38] A more appropriate term would be conceptual framework(s), a set of statements that present descriptions and explanations of phenomena with the potential, through testing, for prediction and control.[39] The failure so far to develop **theories of aging** is due to the newness of the science of gerontology. Publications about aging began to appear in the literature in the 1930s.[40] Only as the numbers of aged persons have increased in society has the possibility existed to study the biological, psychological and sociological dimensions of aging.

Biological Theories
The biological theories of aging attempt to present explanations of the physiological processes and structural changes in people that determine

changes that affect longevity and death.[41] The process of aging in the biological realm is manifested by deterioration in the major organs and physiological systems of the body such as lungs, kidneys, heart, nervous system, liver, and digestive systems and the loss of ability to resist disease (immune system). Cellular changes have been the main focus of theories of aging to explain these phenomena. Many unanswered questions remain as to the ways the body begins to demonstrate aging changes and the complexities of causes for such changes.

Major biological theories of aging that appear to have a high degree of credence include the free radical theory, the cross-link theory, the immunological theory, the somatic mutation and error theory, and the programmed aging theory.[42] Each theory attempts to explain what scientists believe may be the cause for the aging process. A summary of the biological theories of aging is shown in Table 21–2. As a result of these explanations, the basic mechanisms of the aging process are better understood, but further research is needed for theory development.

Psychological Theories

Theories concerned with behavior changes within and between individuals are called psychological theories.[43] These behavior changes, based on personality development, have allowed scientists to probe the psyche of the older adult to describe emotional and psychological differences that may have an impact on the interactions of individuals. Feeling tones and emotional reactions to environmental conditions are important to the well-being of aging persons. Understanding behaviors promotes a more sensitive orientation to the individual who is becoming old—a new and sometimes frightening experience.

One of the major psychological theories providing explanation of aging from a developmental perspective comes from Erickson.[44] He described the life span in developmental stages and tasks for each stage of life. He viewed the last stage of life as the opportunity to review one's life with integrity, as a life of worth, or despair, as a life wasted and without satisfaction. His view of life stressed development in an orderly progression, with proper timing in each

stage for all tasks to be accomplished before progressing to another level of development. With the satisfactory accomplishment of tasks, normal development of the personality was possible, and appropriate adjustment to another stage of living readily achieved. As one aged, the satisfaction with one's life was evident in productivity and the meeting of all psychological needs. This appreciation for one's life, as lived, gave a person a sense of worth about his or her life, a life lived with integrity—all goals accomplished and all expectations met. On the other hand, if guilt was experienced by the aging individual for not meeting goals or for a life wasted, without evidence of accomplishment, the failures generated a sense of despair and a sense of bitterness.

Another theory was developed by Peck.[45] In this theory identification of specific tasks of old age promoted integrity. These tasks included[46]:

- Ego differentiation versus work preoccupation
- Body transcendence versus body preoccupation
- Ego transcendence versus body preoccupation

Many questions continue to be raised about the psychological orientation of the aging person and how changes in behavior are explained. A more thorough explanation is needed. Many of the conceptualizations are vague and incomplete at this time. More research is needed to understand fully the complexities of the psychological components of the aging process in the elderly.

Among the important psychological conceptualizations is the development of the spiritual life of the older adult. Hall identified spirituality as an important part of development in the later years and a means for developing wholeness and integrity as described by Erickson.[47] Spiritual needs of the older adult involve relationships with self, others, and a deity.

Sociological Theories

Sociological aging theories describe ways in which older adults adapt and the environmental

TABLE 21–2. SUMMARY OF BIOLOGICAL THEORIES OF AGING

Theory	Sources	Retardants
Damage Theory		
Free radical theory. Increase in unstable free radicals produces effects deleterious to the biological systems such as chromosome changes, accumulation of pigment, and alteration of macromolecules (collagen).	Environmental pollutants; oxidation of fat, protein, carbohydrate, and elements	Improve environmental monitoring; decrease intake of free-radical-stimulating foods; increase vitamin A and C intake (mercaptans); increase vitamin E intake
Cross-link theory. Strong chemical bonding between organic molecules in the body causes increased stiffness, chemical instability, and insolubility of connective tissue and DNA.	Lipid, protein, carbohydrate, and nucleic acids	Caloric restrictions; lathyrogens-antilink agents
Immunologic theory. Theorists have speculated on several erratic cellular mechanisms capable of precipitating attacks on various tissues through autoaggression or immunodeficiencies. This arises with greater frequency in the aged and may be an explanation for the adult onset of conditions such as diabetes mellitus, rheumatic heart disease, and arthritis.	Alteration of B and T cells of humoral and cellular systems	Immunoengineering—selective alteration and replenishment or rejuvenation of the immune system
Somatic mutation and error theories. DNA failure of replication, transcription, or translation between cells may be responsible for aging. Malfunction of RNA or related enzymes is also considered in the error theory.	Faulty synthesis of DNA (somatic mutation theory) or RNA, proteins, and enzymes (error theory); irradiation	
Program Theory		
Programmed aging theory. Organism is capable of a specific number of cell divisions. Diet and hypothermia can delay the rate of cell division, but the number of cell replications remains relatively constant.	Usually somatic cells	
Popular Theory		
Wear and tear theory. Body structures and functions wear out or are overused.	Repeated injury or overuse	
Stress-adaptation theory. Effects from the residual damage of stresses accumulate, and the body no longer is able to resist stress and thus dies.	Internal and external stressors (physical, psychological, social, and environmental)	Possibility of re-evaluation and adjustment of life-style

From P. Ebersole, and P. Hess, Toward Healthy Aging (St. Louis: C.V. Mosby Co., 1985), 125.

influences on this adaptive process. These theories have focused on the outcomes of adaptation and the status older persons hold in the group compared with other age groups in society.

Five major sociological theories of aging have been put forth. These include: the disengagement theory, the activity theory, the exchange theory, the continuity theory, and the phenomenological theory.

Disengagement theory is defined as the mutual and satisfactory withdrawal of the aging population from society and of society from the aged. This sense of withdrawal is projected as the completion of goals, with few future expectations in life, the idea of the "rocking chair" period for older adults.[48,49]

The activity theory describes the dynamic involvement in events and activities in which the older adult may pursue interests such as hobbies, social events, club and spa memberships, and volunteer activities. These activities are carried out to continue life in the mainstream, as experienced throughout the life span. The theory suggests that such activity continues to have a positive impact upon the older adult and life remains interesting and meaningful for the aged.[50]

The exchange theory offers explanations about the interactions between individuals and groups from which each profit. This exchange is demonstrated as being mutually beneficial and energizing for goal accomplishment.[51]

The continuity theory suggests stability of individual associations throughout adult and late life. This continuity orientation provides the opportunity for the individual to maintain an environment in which activities of interest in earlier years will be continued into late life. Consequently, little in the life of the individual changes because life-style, friends, acquaintances, and work opportunities continue beyond what is considered the retirement age.[52]

The phenomenological theory of aging identifies the impingement of all perceived events on human adaptation. It is the individual's perception of life that forms a gestalt from which the individual operates for living out his or her life in the later years.[53]

These sociological theories of aging are especially important for nursing practice. They teach appreciation for the position of the older adult in society and how the nurse may assist by becoming an advocate for older adults cared for within clinical health settings. Further study of societal issues may give greater insight into such phenomena as abandonment of the older person by family, friends, spouse, neighbors; liberation, the freedom of the older adult to pursue his or her own future without regard to stereotypes and myths projected to control aging behavior; and, solidarity, appreciating the rights of older adults to associate with other adults and citizens in society without being isolated into a segregated world for the aged only.[54]

Summary of Current Status of Research in Aging

Although research in the field of aging and gerontology has been carried on since the mid-1960s, many issues still need investigation to explain scientifically the process of aging and its implications for nursing practice. Recommendations for future research activities have been projected both for a national research program as well as a clinical protocol of research activities.

The national research program for gerontology and aging was projected in 1982 by a planning group as an update on the congressional mandate when the National Institute on Aging was established. The research recommendations were published and included the following highlights[55]:

Basic mechanisms of aging	Emphasis on genetic research including research on molecular genetics to explore possible structural and functional alterations in DNA that might play a role in determining longevity; develop a variety of markers of aging processes; establish centers of excellence to test methods, study populations, or develop animal models
Clinical manifestations of aging	Top priority to later life dementia disorders, particularly Alzheimer's disease, including determination of constitutional, genetic, and environmental factors (e.g., toxins or infections), diagnostic procedures, animal models of histopathological changes, significance of increased aluminum and other trace elements found in the brains of patients with Alzheimer's disease

| Interactions between older people and society | Emphasis on societal context of old age and the interactions of older people and social institutions, especially (1) longevity differences among population subgroups; (2) family and other institutions supporting older persons; and (3) work and retirement |
| Increasing productivity among older people | Conduct field trials to apply research findings on increasing productive activity of older persons, including paid work, unpaid mutual help, and self-care |

From a clinical nursing perspective, research recommendations based on a Delphi survey conducted in over 90 nursing homes and home health-care agencies in southeast Florida suggested areas for future research in gerontological nursing. These findings included[56]:

- Decubitus ulcers: prevention, formation, treatment
- Coping mechanisms used by clients and families to manage care after discharge
- Measures to increase physician interest in geriatrics
- Age differences in responses to medications
- Methods to improve gerontological preparation of nursing personnel (students and staff)
- Urinary tract infections: epidemiology and treatment
- Eating patterns and preferences of older adults
- Means to improve physician follow-up of clients
- Effective strategies to improve nurse–physician communications
- Strategies for attracting and retaining knowledgeable and interested staff.

The field of gerontological nursing research is growing but still needs much more money appropriated on the national level. In addition, there is a need for many more researchers willing to devote their time and skill to conducting sophisticated research projects that will produce scientifically valid findings for application to practice fields, especially that of nursing.

HEALTH STATUS AND THE AGING PROCESS

A healthy mind and body is a gift at any age, but it becomes especially appreciated as a person ages. Health maintenance and health promotion become more important than ever and need to be integrated within the nursing care plan for the older adult.

Health is defined in many ways, but basically it is "the state of optimum capacity of an individual for the effective performance of the roles and tasks for which he has become socialized."[57]

Wellness for the aged may be defined as "a balance between one's environment, internal and external, and one's emotional, spiritual, social, cultural and physical processes."[58] The aging process incorporates the changes experienced in these dimensions over a life span. When the stressors facing the aging adult are coped with so that functional ability continues, wellness is enhanced and the health of the individual can endure. The health status of this group is based on life expectancy, morbidity and mortality, stress and adaptation, primary care issues, and social welfare needs.

Life Expectancy, Mortality, and Morbidity

Life expectancy, according to the 1986 analysis of trends in the population in the United States by the Census Bureau, has increased overall to 74 years. Women continue to enjoy a longer life expectancy than men, with men having a life expectancy of 71 years and women 78.3 years. For whites, the average is 75.3 years and for blacks, 69.7 years. Mortality of aged individuals increased in 1985 to 2,083,000 or 8.7 deaths per 1,000 population, up from the 2,046,000 recorded in 1984.[59]

Aging itself does not cause specific diseases, but chronic illnesses are more prevalent among older adults. Health problems experienced in aging persons increase limitations for functional ability: seeing, hearing, walking, speaking, thinking clearly, and controlling elimination of bowel and bladder. The major chronic illnesses reported by aged people include: arthritis (44 percent), hypertension (39 percent), hearing impairment (28 percent), vision impairment (12 percent), and arteriosclerosis (12 percent).[60] Chronic illnesses are defined as those lasting three months or longer.[61]

Functional ability appears to become more impaired as the aged reach the age of 85 and above. It is the group of frail elderly, more than other age groups among the elderly, who are institutionalized because of increasingly prevalent chronic illnesses which become debilitating. Heart disease, cancer, and cerebrovascular accidents (strokes) lead the list of diseases that are most prevalent causes of mortality among the frail elderly.[62] Deaths from cancer increased 11 percent from 1965 to 1978, with 29 percent of deaths attributed to cancer by 1982.[63]

A recent report from the United States Census Bureau (1986) noted that there were more deaths of aged pesons in 1985 than ever before in the history of America. The report suggested that the death statistics reflected the continued aging of the population in our society.[64]

Stress and Adaptation

The factors of stress and adaptation in the older adult contribute significantly to the health status of this age group. Stress for the older adult, perhaps more than any time during the life span, may be a precursor of illness. Aging people, for example, have many of the same needs as when they were younger, but aging alters their roles and functions. This, in turn, heightens the struggle for adaptation and survival and, inevitably, produces stress. Also many of the losses commonly experienced by the aged (loss of family and friends through death, loss of physical capabilities, loss of control over finances, etc.) are highly stressful and produce varying numbers of stress-related symptoms, including depression and anxiety. When stressors in the physiological, psychosocial, and spiritual dimensions of life are reduced, older adults can more easily adapt to the environment and keep their life in a balance that promotes health and well-being. Stress reduction management is therefore a key factor in the health-maintenance program for the older person.[65]

Primary Care Issues

Primary care, in the broadest sense, encompasses all of the reasons and occasions that might lead an individual to seek initial health-care services. Primary care includes health prevention and health maintenance activities as well as the diagnosis and treatment of illnesses and injuries. The range of primary health-care needs of older persons is great. This is due, in part, to an increased vulnerability to episodes of chronic illness, disability, sensory losses (hearing, eyesight, smell, and taste alterations), cognitive and intellectual changes, and other physiological and biological changes caused by age. In addition, and sometimes of greater consequence when it comes to primary care needs, are psychosocial issues. Loneliness, isolation, and a lack of stimulation and motivation are particularly common situations for older people and can significantly interfere with health, directly or indirectly causing many signs and symptoms of illness and lead to disease.

Everyday living patterns and the health choices older persons make are of prime importance in determining their level of wellness and their needs for primary health-care services. Activities that individuals engage in to prevent illness and promote and maintain their health are called health behaviors. Health behaviors that are particularly crucial for the older adult include maintaining proper diet and nutrition, exercising, controlling weight appropriate for size, height, and age, responding to stress in a healthy manner and reducing it as quickly as possible, and maintaining habits of reduced or moderate intake of alcohol, drugs, and tobacco. When unhealthy habits or patterns of living are detected early, through primary-care services, correction can be initiated with positive results for good health. If poor living patterns are allowed to continue, the consequences could be deteriorating health.[66]

Social Welfare Needs

The social welfare needs are those needs the aging person has in terms of financial security, adequate living arrangements, and a social support system that provides assistance, friendship, and sense of belongingness. Older people experience may losses in their lives as they advance in age—loss of job, spouse, friends, neighborhood, home, church, physician, dentist. These losses can be devastating to the individual's sense of well-being and good mental health. Retirement, for example, is often a time of confusion and crisis rather than the long anticipated "life of leisure." It is important for the aging person to maintain good interactions and interpersonal contacts both with individuals in their **cohort** group and with younger adults and children. The circle of friends must always be strengthened by broadening contacts through involvement in activities such as senior citizen centers, church functions, civic organizations, and other volunteer activities where new friends may be found and maintained. To have several confidantes and intimate friends with whom one's life circumstances can be shared is both productive and essential for maintenance of physical, psychological, sociological, and spiritual health.[67]

Financial security is a concern of many older people, especially in times of inflation and the spiraling costs of health care. Being caught between escalating costs and a low, relatively fixed income, for example, can lead not only to extreme worry and anxiety but to a tendency *not* to seek needed health-care services.

The fast-growing population of older adults in the United States and their diverse health-care needs hve generated the need for a nursing specialty that promotes the well-being and general welfare of the elderly. This nursing specialty has been named gerontological nursing by the American Nurses' Association.

GERONTOLOGICAL NURSING AS A SPECIALTY

Gerontological nursing, the newest specialty area in the profession of nursing,[68] and gerontological nursing practice are coming of age.[69] The specialty received national recognition in 1966 with the establishment of its own division of nursing within the professional organization of nursing, the American Nurses' Association.[70] In 1966 the name of this organizational unit was Division of Geriatric Nursing; in 1976 the name was changed to Division of Gerontological Nursing, and in 1984 it became known as the Council of Gerontological Nursing, to reflect the newly restructured organization of the parent group, the American Nurses' Association. The goal of gerontological nursing is to assist elderly clients to function fully and as much as their potential allows.[71]

In 1973 the American Nurses' Association published Standards of Geriatric Nursing, which were revised and refined in 1976 and titled Standards of Gerontological Nursing Practice to reflect the divisional title change within the organization (Table 21–3). These standards set the criteria for quality nursing care to older adults and reflect the nursing

---

TABLE 21–3. ANA STANDARDS OF GERONTOLOGICAL NURSING PRACTICE

Standard I	Data are systematically and continuously collected about the health status of the older adult. The data are accessible, communicated, and recorded
Standard II	Nursing diagnoses are derived from the identified normal responses of the individual to aging and the data collected about the health status of the older adult
Standard III	A plan of nursing care is developed in conjunction with the older adult and/or significant others that includes goals derived from the nursing diagnosis
Standard IV	The plan of nursing care includes priorities and prescribed nursing approaches and measures to achieve the goals derived from the nursing diagnosis
Standard V	The plan of care is implemented, using appropriate nursing actions
Standard VI	The older adult and/or significant other(s) participate in determining the progress attained in the achievement of establishing goals
Standard VIII	The older adult and/or significant other(s) participate in the ongoing process of assessment, the setting of new goals, the reordering of priorities, the revision of plans for nursing care, and the initiation of new nursing actions

From Council on Gerontological Nursing, American Nurses' Association Standards of Gerontological Nursing Practice. (Kansas City, Mo.: American Nurses' Association, 1976).

process as it includes the older-adult client and the significant others in the determination of goals of care.[72]

The following factors specific to nursing of older adults formed the basis for the development of the Standards of Gerontological Nursing[73]:

- The aging process and its ramifications
- The different rates at which aging occurs in individuals
- The multiple losses that aging persons experience as the collectivity of these losses
- The grieving process for acceptance of those losses
- The interrelatedness of economic, social, biological and psychological factors
- The unique response of the aging individual to disease and its treatment
- The accumulating effects of multiple chronic illness and degenerative processes
- The societal attitudes and cultural values associated with aging

In 1981 a statement on the scope of gerontological nursing practice was developed by the American Nurses' Association Division on Gerontological Nursing. The scope includes health promotion, health maintenance, self-help, disease prevention, and self-care of the older adults with the goals of restoration and maintenance of optimum physical and psychosocial functioning and spiritual health. Further stated goals are the prevention and control of disease and provision of comfort and dignity for the older adult throughout the life span, even to the point of death.[74]

Numerous roles are projected for the gerontological nurse who is prepared for the specialty of gerontological nursing through undergraduate education initially and through advanced graduate educational programs. With advanced education, the nurse with a baccalaureate degree in nursing is prepared to be a geriatric nurse practitioner or gerontological nurse specialist. Each program is housed within a Master of Science program in a school of nursing accredited by the National League for Nursing. The program of each educational institution has its unique philosophy, curriculum design, and clinical practicum sites that develop skills

and competencies for the practice of this specialty.*

Roles assumed by nurses in gerontological nursing incorporate the expectations of society and the needs of the aging client. These roles, identified by Bower and Bevis and Eliopoulos include[75,76]:

Communicator	Listening, initiating, developing and maintaining relationships that effectively assist in health maintenance of the individual, family, and community
Planner	Individual or collaborative efforts in directing or attaining desired outcomes or change; potential problems are to be anticipated
Protector	Arranging the environment by removing barriers for maintenance of homeostatic balance or resolving difficulties for health purposes
Healer	Facilitation of normal regulatory or recuperative processes of the individual through use of specific techniques that allow and promote restoration of function
Comforter	Release of social, physical, psychological and spiritual distress; restore pleasure and sense of well-being and preserve respect and dignity of the individual; this role may be accomplished by direct intervention of medication or therapeutic touch
Teacher	Promotion of information sharing, analyzing, and

*Information about various gerontological nursing programs may be obtained from the National League for Nursing, Ten Columbus Circle, New York, N.Y. 10091 or from the Council of Gerontological Nursing, ANA, 2420 Pershing Road, Kansas City, Mo. 64108.

	synthesizing content and validation of material for learners
Rehabilitator	Assistance in promotion of the optimal potential of the individual so that maximization of capabilities is reached through patient and resourceful approaches
Coordinator	Provision for the actualization of activities through promotion of a team approach
Implementor	Projection of knowledge, skills, and practice components to allow the older adult to advance in meeting individual needs
Advocate	Assertion of rightful positions in attainment of unique needs or wants of older adults in all clinical settings

These roles of the gerontological nurse are executed jointly with the older client in whatever unique ways the older adult dictates to the nurse. It is in cooperation with the aging person that the various roles are undertaken. It is through role projections that the nurse may systematically help the older adult meet the challenges arising in clinical settings. This systematic problem solving is termed the nursing process.[77] As it relates to gerontological nursing practice, the nursing process can furnish a guide to complete, comprehensive practice of nursing to promote a holistic health orientation for the older adult. The nursing process is now discussed in relation to its separate and distinct, integrated components of assessment, plan, implementation, and evaluation.

THE NURSING PROCESS

The nursing process is systematically applied when nursing care is given to the older adult and in determining his or her unique needs. An understanding of aging and the older adult helps nurses to use this process by permitting accurate assessment and determination of individual needs. Priorities for resolution of health chal-

lenges are established and optimal levels of functioning are promoted.

The following discussion of the four components of the nursing process focuses primarily on the individual aging person. These components are discussed as a step-by-step progression of activities but are to be viewed as integrated into the total systemic approach to client care.

Assessment

The nurse's initial step in the application of the nursing process is the assessment of the individual health needs of the older person. Assessment is the act of "reviewing a human situation from a data base in order to affirm the wellness state and diagnose potential client problems; to affirm an illness state, diagnosing the client's prevailing problems; determining the potential for problems; and identifying the wellness aspects of the ill client."[78] The initial part of the assessment is to obtain historical data from the elderly adult about life-style practices, food preferences, activities of daily living, goals in life, and a determination of the health status on the health continuum. After the history interview, the nurse proceeds with the assessment by reviewing each system with the client to gather pertinent information, and by performing the physical examination.

The history section of the assessment provides information about past health status and the unique experience of living for this individual. A planned interview obtains data in a systematic manner for completeness and comprehension. In certain circumstances, depending on the condition of the client and the setting of the services being provided, the nurse may choose to rely partially on past health records of the individual or on a family member. Taking down the life history of an 85-year-old client who is frail and ill, for example, may be difficult and tiring for the client. If past records are available and accurate, the nurse may wish to go over them briefly verbally and obtain acknowledgment of past health history, family, social, and personal history in this way.

The review of systems (ROS) is generally done on each occasion the client is seeking care. The ROS is completed by asking the individual to state if any problems have been experienced within the last year or from the last time a physical examination was conducted by a health professional. The ROS gives the client the opportunity to tell in his or her own words what complaints have been experienced. As each system is reviewed, the nurse should keep in mind some of the common problems affecting elderly persons and age-specific signs and symptoms that might be brought up. In this way, pertinent questions can be asked to clarify and identify all avenues of concern. These comments are recorded by the nurse for future analysis.

After the ROS, or along with it, the nurse focuses more specifically on the physical health status of the person. In this step, the nurse uses the five assessment skills which are reviewed in Table 21–4. With these skills the nurse determines the levels of wellness or illness based on the normal changes of aging exhibited by the older client. The normal changes of aging are presented in Table 21–5. Assessment tools for performing physical, psychosocial, and spiritual assessments are available through various media, e.g., textbooks, commercial publishing establishments, or the institutions and agencies responsible for providing health-care services. These tools are useful to nurses as guides in obtaining complete data necessary for accomplishing the next step, the nursing diagnosis.

When data regarding the aging individual has been obtained and organized, the nurse completes a thorough analysis of the information, sets priorities for those needs that appear to be most urgent, and formulates nursing diagnostic statements.[79] The nursing diagnosis statements should be clear and concise, using language that conveys the client's problems and their amenability to nursing intervention. These statements are then validated with the client or family member as to priority and classification, using the ANA Standards of Gerontological Nursing Practice as a procedural guide.[80] Validation of the nursing diagnosis with the client is a very important part of the assessment phase of the nursing process. It is well worth making an extra effort with clients, especially the frail elderly, who might require additional time to process the information or might have alternative ideas based on many years of experience. Only after the older adult has agreed that the prioritized listing of nursing diagnoses are those that project urgent health needs *from his or her perspective* does the nurse initiate—with the client's assistance, if possible—the plan for goals of care with expected outcomes. An example of this approach is the case of Mrs. B.J.

TABLE 21–4. PHYSICAL ASSESSMENT SKILLS

Observation	An overview of the general appearance of the individual to determine overall physical and mental well-being
Inspection	Validation of observed and reported data through actual investigation and view of the areas of the body
Palpation	Examination of areas of the body through touching, such as taking measurements of pulse, respiration, blood pressure, temperature, and feeling for any surface abnormalities such as bumps, lumps, moles, etc.
Percussion	Tapping or striking a portion of the body to evaluate the deeper organs for signs of tenderness, pain, or enlargement
Auscultation	Use of instruments, such as a stethoscope, to determine sounds of bodily organs, e.g., heart sounds, bowel sounds, air conduction of ears, etc.

From M. Mezey, L. Rauckhorst, and S.A. Stokes, Health Assessment of the Older Individual (New York: Springer Publishing Co. 1980).

Mrs. B.J., a 74-year-old unmarried female, fell on an icy sidewalk while walking home from a grocery shopping trip in the late afternoon of a winter day. As she fell she struck her right ankle on the curb of the sidewalk. A young man walking behind her came to her assistance immediately and helped her to her feet. She tested the foot by putting full weight on it, feeling little pain at the time. She continued to walk to her home approximately two blocks away. Living on the second floor, she climbed several flights of stairs to her room. That night her foot became edematous and extremely painful. She soaked the foot in witch hazel, a favorite home remedy, which eased the pain somewhat. The next morning the foot was so swollen she could not wear her shoe. She called a nurse friend who worked for the Visiting Nurse Association and asked for her assistance. When the nurse stopped by to assess the situation, she began by observing Mrs. B.J.'s overall status. Mrs. B.J. was sitting in a rocking chair with her foot resting on a footstool. She appeared alert,

TABLE 21–5. NORMAL PHYSICAL ASSESSMENT FINDINGS IN OLDER PERSONS

Cardiovascular Changes

Cardiac output	Heart loses elasticity; therefore heart contractility decreases in response to increased demands
Arterial circulation	Decreased vessel compliance with increased peripheral resistance to blood flow occurs with general or localized arteriosclerosis
Venous circulation	Does not exhibit change with aging in the absence of disease
Blood pressure	Significant increase in the systolic, slight increase in the diastolic, increase in peripheral resistance and pulse pressure
Heart	Dislocation of the apex is due to kyphoscoliosis; therefore diagnostic significance of location is lost
Murmurs	Over half the aged have diastolic murmurs; the most common are heard at the base of the heart due to sclerotic changes on the aortic valves
Peripheral pulses	Easily palpated because of increased arterial wall narrowing and loss of connective tissue; vessels feel more tortuous and rigid
	Pedal pulses may be weaker due to arteriosclerotic changes; lower extremities are colder, especially at night; feet and hands may be cold and have mottled color
Heart rate	No changes with age at normal rest

Respiratory Changes

Pulmonary blood flow and diffusion	Decreased blood flow to the pulmonary circulation; decreased diffusion
Anatomic structure	Increased anterior-posterior diameter
Respiratory accessory muscles	Degeneration and decreased strength; increased rigidity of chest wall
	Muscle atrophy of pharynx and larynx
Internal pulmonic structure	Decreased pulmonary elasticity creates senile emphysema
	Shorter breaths taken with decreased maximum breathing capacity, vital capacity, residual volume, and functional capacity
	Airway resistance increases; there is less ventilation at the bases of the lung and more at the apex

Integumentary Changes

Texture	Skin loses elasticity; wrinkles, folding, sagging, dryness
Color	Spotty pigmentation in areas exposed to sun; face paler, even in the absence of anemia
Temperature	Extremities cooler; perspiration decreases
Fat distribution	Less on extremities; more on trunk
Hair color	Dull gray, white, yellow, or yellow-green
Hair distribution	Thins on scalp, axilla, pubic area, upper and lower extremities; facial hair decreases in men; women may develop chin and upper lip hair
Nails	Decreased growth rate

Genitourinary and Reproductive Changes

Renal blood flow	Due to decreased cardiac output, reduction in filtration rate and renal efficiency; subsequent loss of protein from kidneys may occur
Micturition	In men frequency may increase due to prostatic enlargement
	In women decrease in perineal muscle tone leads to urgency and stress incontinence
	Nocturia increases for both men and women
	Polyuria may be diabetes-related
	Decreased volume of urine may relate to decrease in intake, but evaluation is needed
Incontinence	Occurrence increases with age, specifically in those with organic brain disease
Male Reproduction	
Testosterone production	Decreases; phases of intercourse slower, refractory time lengthens
Frequency of intercourse	Changes in libido and sexual satisfaction should not occur, but frequency may decline to one or two times weekly

TABLE 21–5. (Continued)

Testes	Decreased size; sperm count decreases, and the viscosity of seminal fluid diminishes
Female Reproduction	
Estrogen	Production decreases with menopause
Breasts	Diminished breast tissue
Uterus	Decreased size; mucous secretions cease; uterine prolapse may occur because of muscle weakness
Vagina	Epithelial lining atrophies; canal narrows and shortens
Vaginal secretions	Become more alkaline as glycogen content increases and acidity declines
Gastrointestinal Changes	
Mastication	Impaired due to partial or total loss of teeth, malocclusive bite, and ill-fitting dentures
Swallowing and carbohydrate digestion	Swallowing more difficult as salivary secretions diminish Reduced ptyalin production impairs starch digestion
Esophagus	Decreased esophageal peristalsis Increased incidence of hiatus hernia with accompanying gaseous distention
Digestive enzymes	Decreased production of hydrochloric acid, pepsin, and pancreatic enzymes
Intestinal peristalsis	Reduced gastrointestinal motility Constipation caused by decreased motility and roughage
Musculoskeletal Changes	
Muscle strength and function	Decrease with loss of muscle mass; bony prominences normal in aged, since muscle mass decreased
Bone structure	Normal demineralization, more porous Shortening of the trunk due to intervertebral space narrowing
Joints	Become less mobile; tightening and fixation occur Activity may maintain function longer Posture changes are normal; some kyphosis Range of motion limited
Anatomic size and height	Total decrease in size as loss of body protein and body water occur in proportion to decrease in basal metabolic rate Body fat increases; diminishes in arms and legs, increases in trunk Height may decrease to 1 to 4 inches from young adulthood
Nervous System Changes	
Response to stimuli	All voluntary or automatic reflexes are slowed Decreased ability to respond to multiple stimuli
Sleep patterns	Stage IV sleep reduced in comparison to younger adulthood; frequency of spontaneous awakening increases The elderly stay in bed longer but get less sleep; insomnia is a problem, which should be evaluated
Reflexes	Deep tendon reflexes remain responsive in the healthy aged
Ambulation	Kinesthetic sense less efficient; may demonstrate an extrapyramidal Parkinson-like gait Basal ganglions of the nervous system are affected by the vascular changes and decreased oxygen supply
Voice	Range, duration, and intensity of voice diminish; may become higher-pitched and monotonous
Sensory Changes	
Vision	
Peripheral vision	Decreases
Lens accommodation	Decreases, requires corrective lenses
Ciliary body	Atrophy in accommodation of lens focus
Iris	Development of arcus senilis
Choroid	Structure shows atrophy around disk

(continued)

TABLE 21–5. (Continued)

Vision (cont.)	
Lens	May develop opacity, cataract formation; more light is needed to see
Color	Fades or disappears
Macula	Degeneration occurs
Conjunctiva	Thins and looks yellow
Tearing	Decreases; increased irritation and infection
Pupil	May be different in size
Cornea	Presence of arcus senilis
Retina	Vascular changes can be observed
Stimuli threshold	Threshold for light touch and pain increases Ischemic paresthesias in the extremities are common
Hearing	High-frequency tones are less perceptible, hence language understanding is greatly impaired; promotes confusion and seems to create increased rigidity in thought processes
Taste	Acuity decreases as taste buds atrophy; may increase the amount of seasoning on food

From L. Gress and R.T. Bahr. The Aging Person: A Holistic Perspective (C.V. Mosby Co., 1984).

but frustrated, and was wincing in pain whenever she tried to move her injured foot. Upon physical examination the foot was found to be red, painful, and swollen. Mrs. B.J. did not have any immediate plans for seeking medical attention, i.e., to have her foot checked for internal injuries. The nurse briefly asked her about any present or chronic illnesses and if she was currently taking any medications. She inquired about Mrs. B.J.'s regular source of medical care but did not dwell on getting a complete medical history or doing a review of systems. She did examine her carefully to ascertain there were no additional injuries that might have resulted from the fall.

From this data she concluded there were three main areas in which she could help Mrs. B.J. with and formulated three nursing diagnoses:

- Comfort, alteration in, pain
- Health maintenance, potential for injury
- Mobility, impaired physical

In reviewing the three problem areas with the client, they decided together that comfort was the most immediate priority, then mobility, followed by referral to a health-care facility for medical diagnosis. The nurse was very concerned about the possibility of a fracture, given Mrs. B.J.'s age. "The risk of attaining serious fractures rises

steeply after age 40. Unless treatment is prompt and aggressive, the temporary loss of function caused by the fracture may progress to permanent disability and dependency in the elderly."[81] She also realized the client needed relief from pain as soon as possible and, at a minimum, to be able to get around her apartment safely until the extent of injury could be determined.

After the formulation of the nursing diagnoses, the nurse is ready to plan the care based on the data obtained and the nursing interventions required for this individual person's welfare.

Planning

When the nursing diagnosis has been established by the client and the nurse, the next step is to plan care by establishing nursing goals and the steps to be accomplished in achieving the goals. This action is important so that necessary resources are available for the health maintenance of the individual.

In the case of Mrs. B.J., the nursing goals established in the planning phase of the nursing process based on the nursing diagnoses cited above included[82]:

- Prevent further injury by protecting injured part

- Relieve or prevent pain
- Minimize complications and maintain maximum function of the limb

To achieve these goals it is helpful to decide with Mrs. B.J. how she can function within her living space with an injured foot. Questions to be asked may include:

- How far must she move to reach the bathroom? Living room? Dining room? The outdoors?
- Are there railings on the staircase leading to the first floor and to the street for safety purposes?
- Is there a support person available who could assist Mrs. B.J. to the physician's office? To store for grocery shopping? To pharmacy for medications?
- What financial status does she enjoy—health insurance to cover doctor's expenses? Medicare?
- Is there transportation available—bus? Medicab? Taxi? Relative or friend who could provide transportation as required?

As the nurse seeks information from the client regarding the situation and potential resources available to achieve the nursing goals, the nurse's awareness of the aging person's personal resources for dealing with this problem is also a consideration. Such concerns include:

- What is the threshold of pain tolerance of the individual?
- Is the nutritional status adequate?
- What nutritional deficits might be present? Calcium intake? Mineral intake on daily basis?
- Is the person in good mental health? Any depression? Confusion?
- Is the person able to take care of self? Any self-care deficits?

Responses to these questions help the nurse choose the best means for meeting the nursing goals through implementation of the nursing care plan, in compliance with the client's wishes. Any plan of care is only as good as the motivation exhibited by the client. It is thus essential that the nurse work with the client and take into account the client's unique approach to the health problem if the goals are to be achieved successfully.

Implementation

Implementation is the third part of the nursing process. In this step the nurse, with the aging person, proceeds to execute the nursing care plan based on the priority nursing diagnoses and projected outcomes. In the example of Mrs. B.J., the nurse and the client initiate the implementation of the care plan with the following interventions[83]:

- Continue immobilization of the injured part as much as possible
- Elevate injured part
- Investigate and document any pain or pressure noted by the client and relieve as quickly as possible
- Explain to the client how pain can be prevented or minimized by gently moving the part, not hitting the part on any hard surfaces, keeping the bedclothes off the injured part
- Maintaining sufficient level of analgesia to control pain from becoming severe
- Soak foot as required to reduce edema
- If swelling or pain not relieved within 24 hours, seek medical consultation regarding potential fracture

Roles the gerontological nurse demonstrates during this phase of nursing process include:

Surveillance	Observe for any complications such as infection, redness of area, pressure areas near the injured site
Teaching	Instruct the client and significant others about potential complications and care measures that assist them to remain independent and assume self-responsibility until a joint decision (the client and nurse) regarding medical referral if needed
Collaboration	Facilitate cooperation between the client, significant others, and other interdisciplinary team members as needed, which makes care a team effort with the older adult retaining control

Direct care	Give nursing care as required to alleviate pain and to maintain comfort
Referral	Use community resources as required by the client such as homemaker services, visiting nurse association, home health aid, physician referral, and physical therapy

Throughout the implementation phase the nursing goals are used as the guide for providing quality nursing care. Ongoing evaluation is required to ensure that proper care is administered to meet the presenting needs of the individual. Evaluation of the nursing care is the last but essential component of the nursing process.

Evaluation

In the evaluation phase the nurse and the aging person assess the progress made in meeting the projected nursing goals and outcomes of care. This phase is considered the feedback phase from client to nurse. The evaluation should be conducted at least once a week or daily as the need presents itself to maintain adequate and quality nursing care. The nurse uses the Standards of Gerontological Nursing Practice as the guidelines for evaluation of nursing care. When such an evaluation is accomplished, additional health problems may surface and require attention through revision of the original nursing goals and outcomes, including the planned interventions. Evaluative questions that would be appropriate in the case of Mrs. B.J. might include:

I. Has the client perceived changes in the health status?
   A. To what degree has the ankle and foot pain subsided?
   B. In what ways does she have greater ability to move about without pain?
   C. Which activities of daily living is she capable of achieving more successfully?
   D. Can she state she feels less worried about the accident?
II. Have there been satisfactory contacts with the family physician and community re-

sources if needed by the older adult and her family?
III. Have there been satisfactory arrangements made to meet financial needs at this time? What, specifically, are they?

Evaluation is an essential and integral part of the total nursing process in caring for the older adult. The primary nurse contact with the older adult and the family has the responsibility to assure that the care provided is comprehensive, thorough, and complete in meeting all needs of the aging person. If the care is lacking in some way, the evaluation process provides a chance to reassess and make needed changes.

The interdisciplinary approach to caring for the elderly is gaining recognition as a valid alternative to traditional methods of health-care delivery and is worthy of mention here as an adjunct to the use of the nursing process. An interdisciplinary team is a group of health-care professionals, e.g., psychologists, nurses, physicians, dentists, social workers, dietitians, and occupational therapists, who collaborate toward a common goal involving an individualized plan of patient care or specific patient outcome. In geriatric settings where such teamwork is supported, the nurse collaborates with other team members and *together* an assessment is made and a plan of care implemented. As in the nursing process, evaluation is also an important function of the interdisciplinary team approach. Because geriatric clients often have chronic, multiple problems requiring continuing care, the interdisciplinary team can offer a valuable service in efficiently assessing problems and developing treatment plans without going through lengthy consultation and referral processes. When working as a member of an interdisciplinary team, the nurse uses her knowledge of the nursing process.

SUMMARY

Aging is a normal phenomenon of society. It is a complex process, characteristic of all living things as they complete the life cycle from birth to death.

The population of America is growing

older and it is projected that by the year 2030 persons over 65 will constitute 17 to 20 percent of our total population. This rise in percentage of older people will have profound consequences for nurses and other health-care workers. With this statistical picture it is essential that nurses who are being educated to practice professional nursing in the remaining years of the twentieth century and into the twenty-first century possess sophisticated knowledge about gerontology and its application in the area of gerontological nursing.

Society tends to view aging and the aging process in a negative and stereotyped way. Myths that are common about older people include beliefs that most elderly are senile, cannot work as effectively as younger persons, and are unable to change their ways. Images such as "little white-haired lady in a rocking chair" and "bent old man with a cane" are all too often initial associations with the older population. Within recent years, however, efforts among elderly people and advocate organizations have done much to debunk these myths and promote the positive aspects of aging. Political activism, fitness programs, and special employment plans are among the activities currently popular with the elderly and are helping to change the old stereotypes.

Theories related to aging can be found in biology, psychology, and sociology. There is no one comprehensive theory of aging, but combined information from all of these theories allow us to describe aging and predict some of its consequences. Ongoing research in aging is carried out on the Federal level through the National Institute on Aging and various other agencies such as the Veterans Administration. A number of professional and private organizations also fund and promote research in aging. Although gerontological research is a growing field, the preparation of geriatric researchers and the funds allocated need to be increased.

Older persons are susceptible to numerous chronic illnesses and their functional abilities tend to deteriorate with age. Stress is a concern in all dimensions of older people's lives as they experience the loss of close friends and family through death. Many have to adjust to reduced finances, disabilities, and other life changes. Primary care becomes especially important in the areas of health prevention and health maintenance. Social welfare needs such as financial security, adequate living arrangements, and a social support system are paramount. All of these needs impact on the health status and general well-being of the older person. Nurses and other health-care providers are challenged to deliver holistically oriented primary-care services that reflect a knowledge of gerontology and sensitivity to the uniqueness and individuality of each person.

Gerontological nursing, as a specialty, is gaining national recognition as a respected and worthwhile professional practice area. Gerontological nurses are prepared to give comprehensive health care to older adults in nursing homes, long-term care facilities, hospitals, the community, and the home. Gerontological nurse specialists are prepared as clinical nurse specialists or geriatric nurse practitioners at the master's level, and are competent to provide independent primary health care to aging individuals.

An understanding of the normal aging process helps nurses to use the nursing process accurately when caring for the elderly. Nursing diagnoses must reflect judgments based on differentiation of normal health and disease processes from those manifested as a result of aging factors. When the steps of the nursing process are skillfully and thoughtfully carried out within this framework of knowledge, successful nursing care of the older person can take place.

Gerontological nursing challenges nurses to provide health care for older persons in an atmosphere that promotes feelings of dignity, self-worth, and respect. The gerontological nurse is an advocate in upholding the rights of health, liberty, and the pursuit of happiness, rights that the elderly are often at risk of losing. All persons are unique in terms of how they respond to the aging process. The experience of discovering this uniqueness and developing a caring and therapeutic relationship with an older person can be most rewarding. An optimistic perspective of aging and knowledge of gerontological nursing will greatly assist the beginning nurse in meeting the challenges of future nursing care practice.

Study Questions

1. Give several examples of how the nurse benefits from the study of gerontology and geriatrics in terms of providing nursing care to aging individuals.

2. Why is a theory of aging needed?

3. Explain the theories of aging as they relate to the biological, psychological and sociological dimensions of the older adult.

4. Give three examples of how stress may affect the health of the older adult.

5. Discuss the importance of meeting the primary care needs of the older adult.

6. List at least four statements that are found in the ANA Standards of Gerontological Nursing Practice.

7. Give an example of how the nurse carries out the nursing process and its five steps in providing care for the older adult.

8. Formulate nursing diagnoses using the care-plan example.

References

1. E. Palmore, E. Busse, G. Maddox, et al., *Normal Aging III: Report from the Duke Longitudinal Studies, 1975–1984* (Durham, N.C.: Duke University Press, 1985), viii.
2. C.M. Gaitz and T. Samorajski, eds., *Aging 2000: Our Health Care Destiny, Vol. 1: Biomedical Issues* (New York: Springer-Verlag, 1985), 29.
3. P. Selby and M. Schecter eds., *Aging 2000: A Challenge for Society* (Boston: MTP Press, 1982), 11–12.
4. J.E. Birren and V.J. Renner, "Research on the psychology of aging: Principles and experimentation," in J.E. Birren and K.W. Schaie, eds., *Handbook of the Pscyhology of Aging* (New York: Van Nostrand Reinhold, 1977), 4.
5. Ibid.
6. S. Robb, "Theory in aging and theory-related

issues," in A.G. Yurick, B.E. Spier, S.E. Robb, and N.J. Ebert, eds., *The Aged Person and the Nursing Process,* 2nd ed. (Norwalk, Conn.: Appleton-Century-Crofts, 1984), 67.
7. Birren and Renner, "Research on the psychology of aging, 5.
8. Ibid.
9. Ibid., 4.
10. S. Robb, "The elderly in the United States: numbers, proportions, health status and use of health sciences," in Yurick, Spier, Robb, and Ebert (eds.), *The Aged Person,* 33.
11. Ibid.
12. Ibid., 35.
13. U.S. Senate Special Committee on Aging in conjunction with the American Association of Retired Persons, The Federal Council on the Aging, and the Administration on Aging, *Aging America: Trends and Projections, 1985-86 Edition* (Washington, D.C.: U.S. Department of Health and Human Services), 8.
14. Social Security Administration, 1985.
15. Robb, "The aged person", 35.
16. Ibid.
17. Ibid., 36.
18. If you live to be 100, it won't be unusual. *U.S. News and World Report* 94, (August 10, 1983): 18.
19. *Aging America,* 8.
20. Ibid., 15.
21. H.B. Brotnan, Analytic and summary reference tables, *The older population estimates for 1975 projecting through 2000* (Baltimore: National Institute on Aging, 1976).
22. R.T. Bahr, "An overview of gerontological nursing," in M.O. Hogstel, ed., *Nursing Care of the Older Adult* (New York: John Wiley & Sons, 1981), 27.
23. Ibid., 18.
24. Ibid., 15.
25. P. Ebersole, and P. Hess, *Toward Healthy Aging: Human Needs and Nursing Response* (St. Louis: C.V. Mosby Co., 1985), 106.
26. S. deBeauvoir, *The Coming of Age* (New York: C.P. Putnam's Sons, 1973), 11.
27. R. Butler, "Successful aging and the role of the life review," *J Geriatr Soc* 22(1974): 553.
28. Ebersole and Hess, *Toward Healthy Aging,* 108–109.
29. E. Busse and E. Pfeiffer, *Behavior and Adaptation in Late Life* (Boston: Little, Brown & Co., 1977).
30. Ebersole and Hess, *Toward Healthy Aging,* 108.
31. Ibid., 109.
32. Bahr, "An overview of gerontological nursing," 6.

33. Ebersole and Hess, *Toward Healthy Aging*, 455–459.

34. S. Cutler and R. Kaufman, "Cohort changes in political attitudes," *Public Opinion Q* 39, (1975): 69.

35. F.N. Kerlinger, *Foundations of Behavioral Research* (New York: Holt, Rinehart & Winston, 1973).

36. P.L. Chinn, and M.K. Jacobs, "A model for theory development in nursing," *Adv Nurs Sci* 1(1), (1978): 1–11.

37. Robb, "The aged person," 67.

38. Ibid.

39. Chinn and Jacobs, "A model for theory development," 2.

40. K.F. Reigel, History of pscyhological gerontology, in J.E. Birren and K.W. Schaie, eds., *Handbook of the Pscyhology of Aging*, 93.

41. Robb, "The aged person," 68.

42. Ebersole and Hess, *Toward Healthy Aging*, 17.

43. P.B. Baltes, and S.L. Willis, Toward psychological theories of aging and development," in J.E. Birren and K.W. Schaie, eds., *Handbook of the Pscyhology of Aging*, 148.

44. E. Erikson, *Childhood and Society*, 2nd ed. (New York: W.W. Norton & Co., 1963).

45. R. Peck, Psychological developments in the second half of life," in B. Neugarten, ed. *Middle Age and Aging* (Chicago: University of Chicago Press, 1968).

46. Ibid.

47. E.G. Hall, "Spirituality and aging" (abstract), *Gerontologist* 23, (1983, special issue): 210.

48. W.E. Henry, "The theory of intrinsic disengagement," in P.F. Hansen, ed., *Age With a Future* (Philadelphia: F.A. Davis Co., 1964).

49. E. Cumming and W.E. Henry, *Growing Old* (New York: Basic Books, 1961).

50. B.W. Lemon, V.L. Bengston, and J.A. Peterson, "An exploration of the activity theory of aging: Activity types and life satisfaction among in-movers to a retirement community," *J Gerontol* 27, (1972): 511–23.

51. Ebersole and Hess, *Toward Healthy Aging*, 129.

52. R.C. Atchley, *The Social Forces in Later Life* (Belmont, Calif.: Wadsworth, 1977).

53. K. Reigel, "Adult life crises: A dialectic interpretation," in N. Futon and L. Ginsberg, eds., *Life Span Developmental Psychology, Normative Life Crises* (New York: Academic Press, 1975).

54. Robb, "The aged person," 86.

55. I. Schecter, ed., "NIA plan for development of aging research and training completed," *Aging Research and Training News* 51, (1982): 3–6.

56. H.T. Brower and M.A. Christ, A Delphi Study of Research Priorities for Long-Term Care Nursing. Paper presented at the 55th Annual Scientific Meeting of the Gerontological Society of America, Boston, Mass.: November, 1982.

57. A.C. Twaddle and R.M. Hessler, *A Sociology of Health* (St. Louis: C.V. Mosby Co., 1977).

58. Ebersole and Hess, *Toward Healthy Aging*, 146.

59. "'85 deaths show aging of America," *St. Louis Globe-Democrat* (August 20, 1986): 7A.

60. Robb, "The aged person," 44.

61. H.B. Brotman, *Every Ninth American, 1982 Edition: An Analysis for the Chairman of the U.S. House of Representatives Select Committee on Aging* (Washington, D.C.: U.S. Government Printing Office, 1982), 12.

62. Ibid., 14–15.

63. Ibid., 15.

64. *St. Louis Globe-Democrat*.

65. Ebersole and Hess, *Toward Healthy Aging*, 155.

66. Ibid., 150–58.

67. L. Gress and R.T. Bahr, *The Aging Person: A Holistic Perspective* (St. Louis: C.V. Mosby Co., 1984), 230–258.

68. M. Schwab, "Professional nursing and the care of the aged", in W. Reichel, ed., Clinical Aspects of Aging (Baltimore: Williams & Wilkins Co., 1978), 470.

69. Bahr, "An overview," 3.

70. C. Eliopoulos, "Services for the aged," in C. Eliopoulos, ed., *Gerontological Nursing* (New York: Harper & Row, 1979), 350–51.

71. Council on Gerontological Nursing, *American Nurses' Association Standards of Gerontological Nursing Practice* (Kansas City, Mo.: American Nurses' Association, 1976).

72. Ebersole and Hess, *Toward Healthy Aging*, 5.

73. *American Nurses' Association Standards of Gerontological Nursing Practice*, 3.

74. Ebersole and Hess, *Toward Healthy Aging*.

75. F.L. Bower and E.O. Bevis, *Fundamentals of Nursing Practice: Concepts, Roles and Functions* (St. Louis: C.V. Mosby Co., 1980).

76. Eliopoulos, "Services for the aged."

77. H. Yura and M. Walsh, *The Nursing Process: Assessing, Planning, Implementing, Evaluating*, 4th ed. (East Norwalk, Conn.: Appleton-Century-Crofts, 1983), 1.

78. Ibid., 135.

79. M. Gordon, "Nursing diagnosis and the diagnostic process," *Am J Nurs* 76 (1976): 1298–1300.

80. *American Nurses' Association Standards of Gerontological Practice*.

81. E.C. Gioiella and C.W. Bevil, *Nursing Care of the Aging Client* (Norwalk, Conn.: Appleton-Century-Crofts, 1985), 461.

82. M.E. Doenges and M.F. Jeffries, *Nursing Care Plans: Nursing Diagnoses in Planning Patient Care* (Philadelphia: F.A. Davis Co., 1984), 518.

83. Ibid.

Annotated Bibliography

Carnevali, D.L., and Patrick, M. 1986. *Nursing Management for the Elderly*, 2nd ed. Philadelphia: Lippincott. This excellent text provides a comprehensive presentation of care of the older adult in various settings, with a strong focus on the nursing process and its application to older adults and their health needs. Features include an excellent discussion of normal aging, characteristics of the aged population, chronic diseases common to the aging population, and the nursing management of these disorders.

Dychtwald, K. 1986. *Wellness and Health Promotion for the Elderly*. Rockville, Md.: Aspen Systems Corp. This compendium of material is excellent for prevention of health problems and the promotion of the health status of aging individuals.

Ebersole, P., and Hess, P. 1985. *Toward Healthy Aging: Human Needs and Human Response*. St. Louis: C.V. Mosby. An excellent text for nurses to gain an appreciation of the application of nursing principles within the context of Maslow's Theory of Human Needs and the responses made by individuals to those needs in the biological, psychological, sociological, and spiritual dimensions. A very comprehensive text.

Gress, L., and Bahr, R.T. 1984. *The Aging Person: A Holistic Perspective*. St. Louis: C.V. Mosby. An excellent text describing the holistic orientation of the person who is aging. Descriptions of the biological, psychological, sociological, and spiritual dimensions within the context of gerontological nursing are presented as are the need for the older adult to have a support system and motivation to meet demands of aging, and a futuristic orientation to trends facing elderly in society.

Hall, B.A., ed. 1984. *Mental Health and the Elderly*. Orlando, Fla.: Grune & Stratton. This is a text that all nursing students should read to appreciate the mental health status and needs of older adults. Special features of this text include pyschosocial aspects of aging, approaches to nursing care of the elderly emphasizing the psychosocial and spiritual needs of older adults, with models for delivery of care to the aged.

Hogstel, M.O. ed. 1981. *Nursing Care of the Older Adult*. New York: Wiley. This is an excellent text on nursing care of aged individuals in the hospital, nursing home, and community. It features information about changes in aging, essential components of nursing care of the older adult, and special problems and concerns in gerontological nursing.

Part V

Concepts Related to the Care of Individuals

This section discusses selected concepts that relate specifically to various pathophysiological or behavioral responses in individuals. The concepts are broad in scope and were selected because they are universal and affect many individuals of all ages in any health-care setting.

In most instances nurses relate to these concepts every day and an understanding of their theoretical principles can enhance nursing practice. The chapter on sensory perception, for example, discusses how various health and illness states affect a client's basic ability to receive and understand information from the environment and how nursing intervention can improve sensory perception. Likewise, the concept of sleep as a basic human response is discussed in terms of how it can be affected by various health and illness states and how nursing intervention can alleviate or improve sleep disturbances.

Subsequent chapters in this section introduce the reader to other concepts that have an impact on the lives of individuals and, in some instances, the lives of other family members. These concepts include immobility, pain, stress, loss, and crisis intervention.

The chapters included in this section build on the concepts introduced in the previous sections. Each reviews the theoretical basis for the concept and then discusses the relevance of the concept to nursing. A nursing process approach is used throughout these chapters, with examples when appropriate.

Chapter 22

Sensory Alterations

Janet-Beth McCann Flynn

Chapter Outline

- Objectives
- Glossary
- Introduction
- The Sensory Process
- Sensory Alterations
  Sensory Deprivation
  Sensory Overload
- Alterations of Consciousness
- Sensory Deficits
  Alterations in Vision
  Alterations in Hearing
  Alterations in Smell and Taste
  Alterations in Touch
- The Nursing Process
  Assessment
  Planning
  Implementation
  Evaluation
- Summary
- Study Questions
- References
- Annotated Bibliography

Objectives

At the completion of this chapter, the reader will be able to:

▸ Define the terms in the glossary
▸ Discuss the sensory process
▸ Compare and contrast sensory deprivation and sensory overload
▸ Assess key factors contributing to sensory deprivation

▸ List the levels of consciousness
▸ Discuss sensory deficits and list examples from each of the senses

Glossary

Levels of Consciousness
- **Alert:** conscious, alert, and oriented
- **Lethargic:** sleepy, oriented when aroused
- **Semicomatose:** unconscious but may respond to pain
- **Comatose:** unconscious and may not respond to pain

Reticular Activating System (RAS). The portion of the brain that activates the cerebral cortex and prepares it for incoming information.

Reticular Formation. A complex area of the nerve fibers in the brainstem that controls wakefulness.

Sensory Alterations. Changes in the ability to correctly use the sensory organs to receive information from the environment.

Sensory Deficit. An alteration in one of the five senses.

Sensory Deprivation. A reduction in the number of meaningful stimuli from the environment.

Sensory Overload. Too many unpatterned stimuli in the environment.

Sensory Perception. The ability to process data gathered by the senses into meaningful information.

459

Sensory Process. The ability to receive information through the senses and then translate it into meaningful information.

Sensory Reception. The ability to receive information from the environment through the senses.

INTRODUCTION

Individuals are dependent on their sensory systems in order to interact with the environment. Environmental stimuli are collected through the five senses and processed by the brain into meaningful information. It is by use of these processes that people are able to adapt to the environment. Changes in the ability to accurately receive and perceive sensory stimuli can seriously affect one's ability to adapt to the environment and to maintain health.

Changes in the ability to correctly use the sensory process can be caused by a wide variety of physiological, psychological, and environmental factors. For example, one individual may become blind because of increasing opacity of the lens of the eye; another may have a stroke. Severe depression can limit an individual's contact with the outside world, thereby narrowing sensory experiences. Environmental factors, such as meaningless sounds or blinding lights, also can contribute to altered perception.

Alterations in sensory input can cause individuals to become confused or disoriented. Many hospitalized individuals, for example, are exposed to stimuli that are unfamiliar. They may be overwhelmed by a wide variety of machines, noises, light, and medical language that is not understood.

Persons experiencing sensory alterations may demonstrate behavior that is not directed toward achieving a higher health state. An elderly person, for example, may attempt to get out of bed by climbing over the side rail and may fall and break a hip, adding further health problems.

In order for individuals to be able to function in their environment, they must be able to interpret incoming stimuli so that they become meaningful information. Too many or too few stimuli may lead to thought disorganization and confusion.

When individuals enter the health-care system, they must adapt to a variety of changes in environmental stimuli. Many times, because of the unfamiliarity of the new environment, persons find it difficult to make necessary adaptations. Individuals in an intensive care unit (ICU) are bombarded with a variety of incoming stimuli from the environment, but because they do not understand them, they become meaningless (Fig. 22–1). There has been a great deal of research on why people become confused by alterations in the environment. The findings of these studies have shown that confused and disorganized behavior can be caused by **sensory deprivation, sensory overload,** altered **levels of consciousness,** and **sensory deficit.**

THE SENSORY PROCESS

Before nurses can work with people experiencing **sensory alterations,** they first must understand the sensory process, which consists of an individual's ability to *receive* stimuli through the sensory organs and the ability to *perceive* or interpret the stimuli received.

Sensory reception is the collection of data through the five senses. **Sensory perception** refers to the ability to organize and translate environmental stimuli into meaningful information. The nervous system controls and directs the **sensory process.**

The human nervous system is a complex and wonderful organ system consisting of the brain, the spinal cord, the cranial nerves, and the peripheral nerves. The peripheral nerves act as gatherers of sensory information and transport it along nerve fibers. The brain acts as a control tower receiving stimuli from the senses. By using highly developed mechanisms, it processes the information gathered and responds by signaling the motor nerves to act.

Thousands of pieces of information are gathered by the peripheral nerves and the sensory organs and are transmitted by the peripheral and automatic nerves through the spinal cord to higher brain centers. The spinal cord segregates incoming information into tracks and transmits it to the various appropriate sites in the brain.[1]

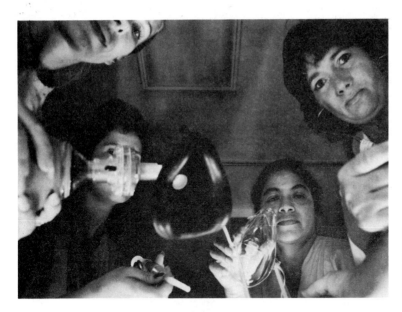

Figure **22–1.** Environmental stimuli can be meaningless and overwhelming to the client. *(Photo courtesy of the Methodist Hospital, Texas Medical Center, Houston, Texas.)*

After reception and transmission, some information is integrated in the brainstem, which regulates many of the vital body functions and contains the **reticular formation.** The reticular formation is a diffuse network of neurons that extend throughout the brainstem boundaries.[2,3]

The output of the reticular formation can be divided into ascending and descending systems. The descending system influences the function of the somatic and autonomic efferent neurons, and the ascending system affects wakefulness and the direction of attention to specific stimuli.[4] This portion of the reticular formation, which coordinates input and modifies levels of awareness, is called the **reticular activating system (RAS).**[5]

The RAS begins in the lower brainstem and extends upward through the mesencephalon, thalamus, and the cerebral cortex.[6] The RAS activates the cerebral cortex and prepares it for incoming information. It is the RAS that coordinates input from the senses and modifies the level of awareness necessary to interpret incoming stimuli (Fig. 22–2).[7]

The cortex is the highest level of the nervous system, and its role is to process, interpret, use, and store incoming sensory data in an organized and systematic manner.

Just how much stimulus is needed from the environment is highly individual. Some people thrive on high amounts of sensory input, while others require much less.

The nervous system would not be at all effective if all sensory information caused a reaction. Only about 1 percent of incoming information is processed and used. When we put on cologne, for example, we can smell it as we apply it, but shortly thereafter we become adapted to the fragrance. We can perceive it if we focus our attention on it, but if we do not, we simply do not smell it. What would happen if we attended to all of our incoming stimuli? Attention would be heightened to the world around us, but so much information would be coming into the system that the brain would be unable to sort it all and, consequently, unable to function. There is an optimal level of cortical arousal for adaptation to occur. Too high a level, for example, interferes with organizing and processing, and the RAS is unable to adapt. Too low a level does not provide enough stimuli for the RAS, and again, it may be temporarily unable to adapt.

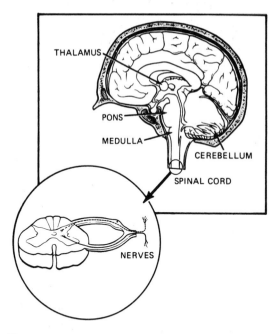

THALAMUS

PONS

MEDULLA

CEREBELLUM

SPINAL CORD

NERVES

Figure 22–2. A portion of the sensory system that transmits stimuli from the receptors to higher centers.

SENSORY ALTERATIONS

Alterations in reception and perception of sensory information can lead to disorganized behaviors and can limit the ability to adapt. The most common of these alterations are sensory deprivation and sensory overload.

Sensory Deprivation

Any major change in a person's environment may produce an alteration in sensory input, in turn upsetting the balance in the RAS. Sensory deprivation results when the sensory input is lower than the person requires to function.[8] Under conditions of decreased sensory input, the RAS is not able to maintain a normal level of activation to the cerebral cortex. The client, experiencing less stimulation than normal, becomes more attuned to the remaining sensory stimuli and consequently receives a distorted view of reality.

Studies have investigated the effects of sensory deprivation of persons in the hospital or subjects in a simulated hospital environment.[9–11] In one study researchers observed the effects of prolonged exposure to environments with extremely limited sensory experiences.[12] They used 22 healthy college students as subjects. The subjects were placed in beds in single sound proof cubicles for 24 hours a day. They wore translucent goggles that admitted light but prevented normal vision, and gloves and cardboard sleeves to reduce tactile stimulation. Sound was limited to the monotonous drone from the air-conditioner. They were not told the time of day, but were permitted two to three hours of breaks for meals and personal needs.

Subjects found the experiment extremely difficult to endure. The researchers found that they could not keep their subjects for more than two to three days. Subjects reported that they could not stand the experience because it was too stressful and reported that after sleeping for most of the first day, they were very bored and eager for any type of stimulus. They reported experiencing hallucinations and other types of perceptual distortions. Furthermore, they demonstrated the inability to concentrate, and their decision-making capacities were limited. If healthy experimental subjects report sensory changes within 24 hours after limited sensory input, one must wonder what happens to ill individuals who are exposed to a totally new sensory environment and altered sensory input.

Hospitalized persons are exposed to an environment that may have limited sensory input. Meaningless and unpatterned stimuli are present in the hospital in the form of medical equipment, sounds, lighting, and meaningless medical jargon. Limited mobility further reduces the amount of variation of stimuli and contact with significant others and medical personnel. Technical language, which the client does not understand, is frequently used and reduces the possibility of meaningful communication. Segregation of individuals to prevent spread of infection is common and increases the chance for sensory deprivation. Dying, belligerent, or confused clients often are isolated physically from others, so as not to disturb them.

There are numerous occasions in which clients can suffer from sensory deprivation. It is the nurse's responsibility to identify these situations and to manipulate the environment in order to control some of the meaningless stimuli and to provide meaningful stimuli.

Certain people are at risk for developing the maladaptive behaviors caused by sensory deprivation. These persons include those who have diminished sensory capacities because of a physical condition or have limited interactions with others because of psychosocial conditions (Table 22–1).

Decrease of meaningful stimuli in the environment has been observed to lead to boredom, irritability, inability to concentrate, confusion, and inaccurate perception of information gathered by the senses. For example, people relate seeing dots, colors, and shapes, and hearing distorted sounds, such as wind rushing, water running, and whispers. More complex perceptual distortions include seeing people, animals, or scenes; hearing voices or music; sensations of floating or falling; and experiencing strange odors and tastes. Clients may have vague somatic complaints or demonstrate maladaptive, noncompliant behaviors that may be harmful to them.

It is important for nurses to recognize these behaviors as they occur in order to provide the client with the best possible care and support.

Sensory Overload

Sensory overload is the opposite of sensory deprivation and can be described as a condition in which individuals receive more sensory stimuli than they can tolerate. The physiological mechanism is unclear. It is believed, however, that the effects on the RAS and on behavior is similar to that of sensory deprivation.

TABLE 22–1. INDIVIDUALS AT RISK FOR DEVELOPING SENSORY DEPRIVATION

Persons at risk include those who are:
Isolated
Restricted to bedrest
Elderly
Very young
Terminally ill
Critically ill
Visually impaired
Deaf or hard of hearing
Dysphasic
Confused
From a different culture
Socially isolated
Paralyzed

In the hospital, individuals are exposed to many sensory stimuli—bright lights, noise, odors, pain, machinery, visits from health-care staff, phone calls, visitors, TV, and so on. When individuals have trouble processing all of the stimuli, they become fatigued, irritable, and may exhibit agitation. Clients also show some of the more severe signs of sensory deprivation, such as confusion and hallucination. Think of an amusement park with all of its glaring lights, rides, noise, music, smells, and confusion. Quite a nice place to have fun for a few hours, but think of what it would be like to live there. No doubt this would quickly lead to fatigue and irritability. There would be too many random sounds and sights to attend to, and perceptions could become distorted. Almost everyone has experienced sensory overload at one time or another—students during course orientation, or nurses when caring for a large number of clients.

ALTERATIONS OF CONSCIOUSNESS

Occasionally, the nervous system has difficulty receiving or processing stimuli from the environment because of an altered level of consciousness (LOC). Levels of consciousness can be affected by metabolic or nutritional disturbances, neural or renal dysfunction, psychiatric conditions, circulatory failure, stroke, trauma, substance abuse, or fever.

In most instances, clients experiencing an altered level of consciousness cannot make their needs known. Every need must be anticipated by the nurses caring for these persons. Nursing interventions must be planned carefully and carried out to meet these needs.

Unconscious and semiconscious clients need total care and need to be protected from hazards in the environment. Caring for unconscious or semiconscious clients is one of the most challenging nursing experiences.

SENSORY DEFICITS

Individuals depend on all of their senses to adapt to the environment and actively participate in the world. When one of these senses is altered, ability to adapt may be temporarily reduced.

When one or more of the five senses is limited, a sensory deficit is said to exist. For example, the blind or visually impaired individual is unable to receive clear visual stimuli, the deaf or hearing impaired individual is unable to receive auditory stimuli, and so forth. With the loss of one or more of the senses, the entire life-style of an individual may be threatened; even if the alteration is temporary, a sense of disequilibrium can occur. Nurses are in a key position to assist individuals as they adapt to sensory deficits.

Alterations in Vision

Vision is considered by most people to be the most crucial of all the senses in terms of autonomy and independence. Loss or impairment of vision is a threat to the individual's self-concept and self-image. Vision can be affected by a variety of disease processes or conditions, for example, high blood pressure, diabetes mellitus, glaucoma, cataracts, and trauma. Through careful use of the nursing process, nurses are able to facilitate adaptation and perhaps prevent further damage to the eyes.

Alterations in Hearing

Hearing is probably the second most important of our senses because it enables us to interact with other people and the environment. Alterations in hearing can lead to social isolation and decreased self-esteem. Hearing-impaired individuals sometimes conceal the fact that they are hard of hearing or deaf. It is important to identify individuals who have impaired hearing, so that health care can be most efficient.

Alterations in Smell and Taste

Olfaction, the sense of smell, is the least developed of human senses. Research has demonstrated that the sense of smell arises from a small area of mucous membrane deep within the nose. Because of its location and lack of refinement, it is the hardest of the senses to study, and consequently, it is the least well understood. The sense of smell is important because it contributes to our relationship with others, protects us by detecting smells such as gas and fire, and aids in appetite stimulation.

Gustation, the sense of taste, is the function of taste buds in the mouth and on the tongue.

The exact physiological mechanism of the perception of taste is not known, but it is known that there are four distinct taste sensation areas. These areas detect the tastes of salt, sweetness, sourness, and bitterness.

Although smell and taste are two distinct senses, they complement each other. They are important senses, because they allow people to select their nutritional needs. If individuals are not able to smell and taste their food, they may lose all interest in eating and become malnourished and ill.

Most alterations in smell and taste result from illness or trauma. Sense of smell can be altered by nerve damage or dry nasal mucosa. Sense of taste can be altered by nerve damage, salivary gland disorders, or zinc deficiencies. Many times, a loss of sense of smell or taste is not sufficiently serious to bring individuals into the health-care system. Usually, individuals will seek care because of pain or weight loss.

Alterations in Touch

The sense of touch is most closely associated with the skin and is the earliest sense to develop in the human embryo.[13] The skin is the largest of the sensory organs.[14,15] It covers the entire body. The sense of touch comes from millions of nerve fibers located all over the skin and covers a wide spectrum of sensations, including pressure, pain, itching, and temperature.

There are two temperature receptors in the skin: cold and hot. If these are damaged, individuals may have difficulty in receiving environmental stimuli, and may be prone to frostbite or burns.

Pain receptors serve to prevent adverse effects of the environment. By this mechanism, individuals are able to prevent trauma to the body. When pain is perceived, individuals are able to withdraw and, if injured, seek help. If this mechanism is not working appropriately, injury can be sustained and left untreated, causing further injury.

There are three types of maladaptive skin (or touch) responses. Anesthesia is the absence or loss of feeling, hyperesthesia is an increase in the skin's sensitivity, and paresthesia is a tingling sensation.

Alterations in touch generally are caused by impaired sensory nerve function or central nervous dysfunctions because of disease or trauma. Alteration in the ability to perceive touch or feeling can be both physically and emotionally traumatic. There are many causes for alterations in touch—some temporary and some permanent—that may have an effect on how well an individual will adapt.

THE NURSING PROCESS

Nurses need a systematic approach to nursing care of persons experiencing sensory deprivation. The nursing process is an excellent framework for this. The nursing process has four phases: assessment, planning, implementation, and evaluation.

Assessment

The assessment phase is the data-gathering phase. Information about the client and the environment is gathered by observation, interviewing, and history taking, examination, and record review.

The following case study provides an example of *sensory deprivation.*

Mrs. Kathryn Jones, an 80-year-old woman, lived alone in an apartment. She fell when walking to the store, broke her hip, and lost her glasses. She was rushed to the hospital in an ambulance and underwent hip-pinning surgery the following day. After the surgery, she was placed in the intensive care unit because she developed a cardiac dysrhythmia during surgery.

Lights were left on at all times, and her room was opposite the nurses' station.

Mrs. Jones began to spend a great deal of time sleeping and was becoming more and more irritable. She became confused and couldn't remember where she was. She attempted to climb over the side rails on several occasions and had to be placed in a posey jacket restraint. She thought that the nurses were discussing her at the desk and she treated them with suspicion.

Mrs. Jones was demonstrating many of the symptoms of sensory deprivation. A careful assessment of the situation discovered many stressors in the environment that contributed to Mrs. Jones' disorientation. Mrs. Jones was attached to a cardiac mon-

itor, which emitted monotonous sounds and had twinkling lights. There were no windows, clock, or calendar in her room. Mrs. Jones had lost track of time, and this was reinforced by the environment because the lights were only slightly dimmed at night. Being near the nurses station also added to the noise and disruption she was experiencing.

In addition to these factors, contact with her family was restricted to a few minutes an hour. The staff were quite busy with Mrs. Jones, since she required a great deal of care and monitoring. Her vital signs were checked at least every hour around the clock, disturbing her ability to rest. Interactions with the staff were limited and not interactive on a personal level.

Her glasses were lost; therefore, her ability to see was altered. She was unable to read or watch TV.

After the data are gathered, nursing diagnoses are formulated. Nursing diagnoses related to sensory deprivation for Mrs. Jones might include:

- Sensory perceptual alterations (visual) related to sensory deprivation
- Anxiety related to sensory overload
- Sleep pattern disturbance related to sensory overload
- Thought process, alterations in, related to sensory overload

Once the assessment is complete and the nursing diagnoses written, the planning phase of the nursing process can be started.

Many of the symptoms of *sensory overload* are the same as sensory deprivation but instead of boredom, individuals exhibit irritability and agitation. Visits from friends and family tend to increase these behaviors. Additional stimuli in the environment also adds to the clients irritation.

The environment should be assessed. Are the lights too bright? Do they shine in the client's eyes? Are they ever dimmed or turned off? What is the noise level? Do staff make excessive noise? Is the housekeeping department always buffing the floor? How many health-care workers and support staff are in the environment at any given time? Telephones and intercom systems contribute to the noise level and confusion on a busy unit. There are many strange smells in the hospital, adding more stimuli for the sensory system to interpret.

After the assessment of sensory overload, the nursing diagnosis can be prepared. Examples of nursing diagnoses related to sensory overload might include:

- Anxiety related to sensory overload
- Sensory perceptual alterations related to sensory overload

Any changes in a client's *level of consciousness* may indicate underlying life-threatening pathologies, all clients must be carefully assessed as to their level of consciousness. Initial LOC assessment should be made and recorded for all clients when they are admitted to the health-care system. Subsequent changes should be reported and recorded immediately.

There is a series of stages of consciousness ranging from alert to comatose (Table 22–2). Nurses need to be aware of these stages in order to distinguish among them. Distinguishing between stages is at times difficult and tends to be subjective, so many hospitals have begun to use flow sheets to standardize observations of LOC. These flow sheets provide space for nurses to record data regarding LOC. A good example of a standardized LOC flow sheet is the Glasgow Coma Scale (GCS).[16] The value of the GCS lies in its ability to help health-care providers objectively document clients' LOC by focusing on measurable responses to verbal commands and painful stimuli. The GCS eliminates the more subjective descriptions of LOC mentioned above and focuses on more concrete, observable data (Table 22–3).

Factors to be considered in an LOC assessment cover a wide range of parameters. The most obvious is the client's level of awareness, mentation, and orientation. The most important is the respiratory status, because without an adequate airway, the client will not survive. Further assessment of vital signs includes pulse, temperature, and blood pressure. Pupil size and response to light is measured for constriction, consensuality, and convergence construction.[17] Assessment includes size, rate of constriction (brisk or sluggish), and equality of the pupils and their equal response to light.

Motor response is also a part of the LOC exam. Can the client move body parts on command? Against gravity or resistance? Are the movements and strength equal on both sides? Does the client respond to pain? What other reflexes are present (cough, swallow, blink)?

In addition to the LOC assessment, nurses should assess the client's hygiene needs. Many clients require total care, including bathing, skin, mouth, and eye care. Careful positioning is essential and turning side-to-side every two hours or more frequently is helpful in reducing aspiration and pressure damage. Bowel and bladder functioning is important to assess, too. Examples of nursing diagnoses include:

- Alteration in thought processes related to altered LOC
- Impaired mobility related to altered LOC

Taking a careful *visual history* of clients is important. Particular attention should be given to any visual changes, trauma, previous eye conditions, and present eye diseases. Nurses should determine if the visual changes were sudden or gradual. Clients with eye conditions may use eye drops. Noting other conditions that might

TABLE 22–2. LEVELS OF CONSCIOUSNESS

Level of Consciousness	Client Behaviors
Alert	Conscious, alert, fully oriented to person, place, and time. Answers questions appropriately
Drowsy (lethargy)	Sleepy. Oriented when aroused but may appear confused. May answer questions appropriately. May be oriented to person and place
Stuporous (semicomatose)	Loss of consciousness. May be aroused but with great difficulty. Generally not oriented to place or time. May respond to painful stimuli
Comatose	Unconscious. Cannot be aroused. May not move spontaneously. Reflexes may not be present. May not respond to painful stimuli

TABLE 22–3. THE GLASGOW COMA SCALE

Eyes	Open	Spontaneously	4
		To verbal command	3
		To pain	2
	No response		1
Best motor response	To verbal command	Obeys	6
	To painful stimulus[a]	Localizes pain	5
		Flexion—withdrawal	4
		Flexion—abnormal (decorticate rigidity)	3
		Extension (decerebrate rigidity)	2
	No response		1
Best verbal response[b]		Oriented and converses	5
		Disoriented and converses	4
		Inappropriate words	3
		Incomprehensible sounds	2
	No response		1
Total			3–15

[a]Apply knuckles to sternum; observe arms.
[b]Arouse patient with painful stimulus if necessary.
Adapted from Upjohn, January 1980, based on G, Teasdale, and B. Jennett, "Glasgow Coma Scale," Lancet, No. 7872, p 81.

contribute to visual impairment, such as diabetes, provides additional data. Inspection of the eye and surrounding tissue and structures is another step in the process, and any abnormalities, such as edema, crusting, or redness, should be noted.

Pertinent data regarding visual acuity can be gathered easily during the initial eye exam by asking the client to read from the newspaper or a menu for near vision. A Snellen eye chart is used for assessing distance vision. If the client wears glasses or contact lenses, he or she should be assessed with and without these devices. If the client is blind, the nurse must assess if the client can determine light, dark, shapes, and forms.

Seven danger signals indicate the possibility of eye disease, and these should be assessed.

- Persistent redness of the eyes
- Persistent pain in the eye or around the eye
- Visual disturbance, e.g., blurred vision
- Crossing of the eyes
- Growths on the eyes or lids
- Persistent discharge, crusting, or tearing
- Unequal pupils

If these signs are caught at an early stage, more severe complications may be prevented.

If the client does have an uncorrectable alteration in vision, then assessment of the client's degree of acceptance is essential. If the client denies that the impairment is permanent, planning and implementing care will be difficult. Examples of nursing diagnoses with an alteration in vision include:

- Anxiety related to altered vision
- Mobility, impaired related to altered vision
- Potential for injury related to blindness

The key to working with a person with an *alteration in hearing* is accurate assessment of hearing ability. Once this ability has been established, planning can begin. As with the blind or visually impaired person, it is necessary to know how long the hearing loss has been present, if there is a way of reversing it, and how the person has adapted to the loss. The person who has lost his hearing gradually is more likely to be adapting successfully. The person experiencing a sudden loss of hearing resulting from trauma will experience feelings of loss, fear, and anxiety.

Clients with a minimal or gradual loss of hearing may be the hardest to assess, because they might not be aware of the loss, or they may be too embarrassed to admit to it. Does the client turn one ear toward the person speaking? Does the client answer questions appropriately? Does he or she have trouble following orders?

Does the client start if touched? Is his or her voice abnormally loud? Does he or she respond to loud noises? If several of these behaviors exist, the nurse will be able to formulate a nursing diagnosis relating to an alteration in hearing.

Communicating with hearing-impaired clients can be difficult at times. There is no set way of establishing communication, because needs vary with the severity of the impairment and at what age the impairment developed. Any aids that a client uses must be observed, as well. Does the client lip-read, use a hearing aid, or an interpreter? Ways in which clients communicate and their assistive devices must be noted and incorporated into the nursing plan. Sample nursing diagnoses include:

- Sensory perceptual alteration related to impaired hearing
- Potential impaired verbal communication related to hearing deficit

Generally, the senses of smell and taste are assessed in the examination of the head and the neurological system (see Chapter 9). The senses of smell and taste are easy to assess by asking the client to close the eyes and presenting objects to smell and taste. Responses are noted on the chart. Any changes or distortions in these senses should be measured and reported, because it may imply accelerating physiological or psychological health problems. In addition to a routine assessment, appetite and food preferences should be noted and any recent weight loss recorded.

- Potential alteration in nutrition: less than body requirements related to altered sense of smell

Assessment of sense of *touch* is based on history, observation, and other data-collection methods. Superficial touch, pain, and temperature should be assessed as well.

Anesthesias, hyperesthesias, or paresthesias should be noted. The color and condition of the client's skin should be observed and noted. At the conclusion of the assessment phase, the nursing diagnoses are prepared. Nursing diagnoses for a person with impaired touch might include:

- Potential injury related to inability to perceive sensation

- Alteration in sense of touch related to lack of circulation

Planning

The written plan should be placed on the chart or the cardex. Goals and objectives are written to direct the nursing plan and are derived from the assessment. If possible they should be agreed on by both the client and the nurse. In some instances clients may be too disoriented or confused to assist in setting the goals, but they should be encouraged to participate as much as possible. Examples of goals with outcome criteria for the client with *sensory deprivation* might be: The client will be able to state name and location within 24 hours. The client will not climb over side rails and will state safety reasons within 24 hours.

When planning care, nurses should consider the potential problem of sensory deprivation and employ methods to prevent it. Prevention of a problem is always the best form of nursing care. Clients who are at risk for developing sensory deprivation need to be identified and meaningless stimuli minimized.

Meaningful stimuli should be provided in the form of clocks and calendars. Clocks that distinguish night from day by using two colors on a 24-hour face also are helpful. These persons also need access to windows to add more meaningful stimuli.

Newspapers, television, and radios are another means of providing additional stimuli. If clients wear glasses or hearing aids, they should be encouraged to wear them in the hospital.

Persons at risk for developing sensory deprivation should not be placed in single rooms unless absolutely necessary (or by their own request). Assignment of staff should be adequate, so that time can be spent with these clients. Time can be spent talking with clients and letting them ask questions.

Team or staff conferences can be scheduled to discuss approaches for controlling sensory deprivation. It is important that everyone on the health-care team assist in reducing the effects of sensory deprivation. Many times, the fast pace of an intensive care or other hospital unit does not give the staff time to reflect on these effects.

An example of a goal related to *sensory overload* might be: To rest in a quiet room for

1 hour every day as evidenced by sleeping or resting in the quiet, darkened room. Planning nursing interventions for persons experiencing sensory overload would include control of the environment, so that clients are exposed to fewer stimuli. This can be done by minimizing noise and light and by planning rest periods so that the client can integrate sensory input.

Because of the comprehensive care that clients with altered *LOC* require, adequate time must be given to perform the needed interventions. Additional support for family members is essential, because they usually are extremely concerned about their loved ones.

Goals and outcome criteria can involve the client and the family. For example: The client will be free of skin breakdown as evidenced by clear skin at all times. The family will assist in care as evidenced by turning client with assistance at least once during visit.

In the planning phase, the family should be encouraged to participate in the physical care of the client and touch and talk to the client as well. Many persons who have recovered from a comatose state have related daily incidents, identified nurses by their voices, and thanked family for sitting with them and talking. Family members can be encouraged to bring tape recorders and recordings of favorite music to play for the client, too. If they are able to hear, these actions keep the client in contact with familiar things.

Control of the environment also should be incorporated into the plan of care. Methods are similar to those mentioned earlier in this chapter. Safety features should be incorporated into the care plan to decrease the chance of complications. Anticipating emergencies before they occur is an important step in planning the care of a semiconscious or unconscious client. Complications can be reversed before they become harmful.

Mutual goals may not be possible for unconscious clients, but family members can be encouraged to participate in preparing goals and objectives.

The Visually Impaired Client. A care plan is essential to ensure comprehensive care of the *visually impaired client.* A note should be placed on the cardex and the intercom system to alert the staff to the client's impairment.

Mutual goals should be derived. For example: Client demonstrates safe mobility in room after orientation. If unsure of environment client asks for assistance when getting out of bed.

In addition to assistance with the activities of daily living, the nurse will have to plan an orientation to the unit for the client. If clients are aware of the surroundings, they will be less anxious and better able to function. Environment must be controlled to prevent injury. Precautions must be taken to eliminate electric cords, small stools, and trash baskets that might be a safety hazard to the visually impaired patient. Other safety features include keeping side rails up, attaching the call bell within easy reach and telling the client where it is and how to use it, and placing the bedside cabinet and telephone close to the bed so that it is within easy reach. Also, if clients smoke, they should be assisted to the lounge and supervised to prevent burns and fires.

Rehabilitative measures should be incorporated in the plan. Supportive measures and encouragement assist the client in gaining independence. Family members need support and encouragement, too. Visits from other blind persons or representatives from organizations for the blind can be incorporated into the rehabilitation plan. Referral to other agencies can be planned.

The Hearing Impaired Client. The nursing plan for the *hearing impaired* person incorporates the client's special needs. Planning to meet these needs revolves around the amount of the loss of acuity and the client's present state of adaptation. Family members should be encouraged to participate in the plan. If the client is totally deaf, the nurse may need to arrange for an interpreter. One of the national service agencies for the deaf (Table 22–4) can refer a skilled interpreter. Additional information can be obtained by contacting local agencies and organizations.

Once the plan has been determined, the implementation phase of the nursing process can begin. Goals might include:

- Client wears hearing aid while awake.

The Client with Altered Sense of Smell and Taste. The nursing care plan should incorporate all of the client's needs including the specific

TABLE 22–4. NATIONAL AGENCIES LISTING INTERPRETERS FOR THE HEARING IMPAIRED

Information regarding skilled interpreters in local areas can be obtained by contacting:

The Registry of Interpreters for the Deaf
Box 1339
Washington, D.C. 20013

or

The National Association of the Deaf
814 Thayer Avenue
Silver Spring, Maryland 20910

If the client is deaf and blind, information about assisting these clients can be obtained by contacting:

Helen Keller National Center for Deaf–Blind Youths and Adults
111 Middle Neck Road
Sands Point, New York 11050

---

needs caused by alterations in smell and taste. Since altered appetite may be a problem, the dietician should be consulted in the planning phase of the nursing process. Any food preferences should be emphasized. Family can be encouraged to bring favorite foods from home, if these are unavailable in the health-care setting. Smells that can be distorted should be removed from the unit, because these will be disturbing. Foods that are found disagreeable should be removed from the tray before it is taken into the room. All staff should be aware of the care plan, so that care is consistent. Preferences and dislikes should be noted on the cardex and on the client's door.

The Client with an Altered Sense of Touch. A written care plan for the client with an altered sense of *touch* will include mutual goals and objectives that are derived by both the nurse and the client. Goals might include:

- Client will use bath thermometer to determine water temperature prior to bathing
- Client states reason for testing water temperature

Implementation

Implementation of the plan is the next phase of the nursing process and is extremely important in reducing the effects of *sensory deprivation*. The environment can be manipulated to in-crease meaningful sensory stimuli. This can be accomplished in a variety of ways. Large clocks can be placed where the bedfast client can see them, or clients can be encouraged to wear their own watch, if possible. A large calendar can be placed in view. When entering the room, nurses on each shift can tell the client the day, the date, and the time. Discussion of the weather is highly appropriate, too, as it helps orient to the season.

Small children do not understand time and climate changes, so it would add meaningless stimuli to the environment to discuss it. Orienting stimuli for children might include reading stories, especially ones from home that the child already knows. Mobiles can be hung from the ceiling to add additional stimuli, and familiar toys can be placed in their beds, in most instances.

Nurses should address adult clients by their title (Mr., Dr., Mrs., Ms., Miss) and surname and identify themselves by what they wish clients to call them. This reinforces the client's name and reminds him or her of the nurse's name.

The morning bath is a good time for the nurse to spend some extra time with the client. Problems encountered during the hospital stay and possible solutions can be discussed. They can be allowed some control in this activity. For example, "Would you like to bathe before or after breakfast? Do you want to start with your teeth? Do you use mouthwash?" These may seem like small items but they can be quite meaningful to a person who has had all control of the situation removed.

Environmental lighting can be controlled by opening drapes during the day and turning on lights if needed. Lights should be turned off at night to permit patients to maintain their normal biorhythms and assist them in distinguishing night from day.

Clients may distort what they hear, so talking in a whisper is not good practice. Moving the client out of the room for a period of time every day increases the variety of stimuli. If at all possible, clients can be moved to the sunroom or visiting area. Clients can meet and talk, and this provides them with a very important change of environment. Children can be taken to the playroom to play with their parents and other children.

Encouraging exercise is another important intervention. Clients can be taught range of motion (ROM). If they are able to transfer to a wheelchair, they can assist with its propulsion in the halls. Clients restricted to bed for intravenous (IV) therapy can be mobilized by placing their IV bag on a pole on wheels, and they can be taught to push the pole safely.

Exercise is an excellent diversion and relieves some of the boredom of sensory deprivation.

Interaction with family members is important for hospitalized clients. Family and friends provide meaningful stimuli for clients, and should be encouraged to visit. Clients should be encouraged to call family and friends from the room and receive calls there as well. Photographs can be displayed in the client's room to provide additional visual stimuli. Cards from friends and family can be arranged within view.

Clients in acute-care settings can be encouraged to have articles brought from home to brighten their rooms. Such things as a favorite afghan, pillow, and photographs of loved ones can mean a great deal. Large, breakable, or irreplaceable, expensive items should be discouraged, however. Also, if possible, individuals should be encouraged to wear their own pajamas, robes, and slippers, and bring their own toilet articles.

Persons demonstrating confused or disoriented behavior should have reality reinforced constantly and consistently. All members on the staff must be consistent. Reports on what the client has believed to be true should be discussed, as well as what the staff has done to reinforce reality.

Clients experiencing *sensory overload* need to have a controlled environment where extreme stimuli are kept to a minimum.

The same nurses should care for clients experiencing sensory overload in order to provide consistent care and to minimize the number of health professionals involved. Establishing a routine each day is a way of providing consistency for the client and reducing the aspect of surprise. Visitors can be limited to close friends and family and the visits kept short to control some of the stimuli.

Lights may be dimmed during the day and rest periods provided. Lights should be turned off at night. Reducing noise also reduces the number of stimuli in the environment.

Odors should be kept to a minimum. Soiled linen should be changed immediately, removed from the room, and the client bathed.

The person experiencing sensory overload may need to stay in the familiar environment of the room. Trips to the sunroom may not be needed. The client can be ambulated in the room minimizing contact with stimuli from the hospital unit. In controlling the number of stimuli clients receive, caution should be taken so that the client does not begin to experience sensory deprivation.

Implementation of the nursing care plan is quite challenging and may vary as the client's LOC changes. Basically, nursing interventions meet all of those needs that the client cannot meet. The key to intervention is prevention of complications. The airway must be kept clear, hygiene measures met, range of motion exercises performed, position changed frequently, nutritional status and elimination needs maintained. Emotional support is necessary, as is providing sensory stimulation. The client's privacy must be maintained and worth and dignity respected. Addressing the client by title (Mr., Mrs., etc) and surname is one way of demonstrating this. The nurse should always tell the semiconscious or unconscious client who he or she is and what he or she is going to do.

Side rails should be kept up at all times and they should be padded with bath blankets in case of seizures. Padded tongue blades and plastic airways should be in reach in case of emergency.

The Visually Impaired Client. A strong nurse–client relationship is essential in caring for the *blind*. There are specific ways of fostering this relationship. When the blind individual enters the health-care system, the nurse should be introduced by name and tell the client what nursing services will be provided. Once these amenities have been concluded, the client should be oriented to the environment. It is important to indicate where the furniture is placed and where the bathroom is located. Introductions to roommates and other members of the health-care team are necessary.

Helping the client unpack may be helpful, but permission should be obtained first. Once unpacking has started, the client should assist in the placement of belongings, so that they can be found. Arranging the food on the blind person's tray is another way of assisting the client. An effective way is to describe the tray as the face of a clock. For example, juice is at one o'clock, coffee at 4 o'clock, plate at 6 o'clock, and so on. Blind individuals need help in selecting their meals from the menu.

When performing treatments on blind clients, the nurse should call the client by name, introduce her- or himself, and carefully explain the treatment and equipment.

Forms of sensory stimulation are needed when providing assistance for the blind client. Frequent visits should be made by the nurse, and visits by family and friends should be encouraged. Radios and TVs can be used to reduce sensory deprivation. Braille readings can be obtained from local agencies that provide services for the blind. Interventions appropriate for the client with sensory deprivation can be applied to the blind client, as well. Providing a meaningful environment, rich in experiences that a blind person can appreciate, is an essential part of caring for the blind.

The Hearing Impaired Client. The key to working with the *hearing impaired* is the establishment of a trusting relationship. Assistive devices, such as glasses or hearing aids, should be used. Verbal means of communication have to be altered to maximize interaction. The nurse should face the client at eye level when speaking and stand fairly close especially if the client is lipreading.

Lip movements should not be exaggerated as this tends to make speaking more difficult to interpret. Nurses also should make every effort to keep their hands away from their lips, so that clients can easily see them.

When speaking, a normal voice level should be used, because when shouting, the voice becomes higher in pitch, and most hearing impaired clients have lost the ability to hear high-pitched tones. Eliminate competing noises from the environment, so that the client is able to concentrate on what is being said.

Nonverbal cues can be used to support verbal communication, but should not be distracting. If the person communicates by notes, several things should be kept in mind. The first, of

course, is supplying the client with enough paper and pencils. Flash cards may be prepared for commonly used words and phrases. After the nurse and client have communicated by note writing, the notes should be destroyed to maintain confidentiality.

Be calm when working with a hearing-impaired person. If both nurse and client are anxious, the communication system can break down quickly. Interpreters are very helpful and arrangements should be made for one especially when the hearing impaired client will be exposed to stressful situations.

Finally, for consistency and safe care, a note should be placed on the chart and on the cardex to advise everyone on the staff that the client is hearing impaired. Another small sign should be placed on the intercom system. When the client puts on the call light, the nurse should respond in person.

The Client with an Altered Sense of Smell and Taste. Smells and tastes that are enjoyed should be increased. Emotional support should be given to the client and family. Family members can learn from the dietician how to maintain a nutritious diet at home. Offending smells can be removed (where possible), and room fresheners can be used.

The Client with an Altered Sense of Touch. When the ability to perceive touch is diminished, the nurse should teach health-care practices to prevent accidents, such as measuring the temperature of water before getting into the tub or shower, wearing shoes or slippers, inspecting the feet daily, and having a podiatrist cut toenails. Clients also should be cautioned about using cold applications, as they can lead to tissue damage.

Heating pads, hot water bottles, hot packs, etc., should be used with caution, if at all, and clients should be taught about their potential danger.

Clients should be positioned carefully and skin assessed frequently for breakdown. Back massage may be comforting, therapeutic, and prevent skin breakdown.

Evaluation

Evaluation is the fourth phase of the nursing process. This is the phase in which the client's present behavior is measured and compared with the goals and objectives written during the planning phase. Has the client met these goals? Behavior before the plan was instituted should be compared with behavior demonstrated afterwards. There should be substantial evidence, if the desired outcomes were reached.

The evaluative process will identify omissions that occurred during the assessment phase of the nursing process. In pinpointing the omissions, the evaluation then guides reassessment, future planning, and interventions.

Nurses frequently encounter clients who are at risk for developing sensory alterations or who have sensory deficiencies. Through careful use of the nursing process, nurses can minimize sensory alterations and effectively communicate with individuals experiencing sensory deficits.

SUMMARY

Individuals are dependent on their sensory system to interact with the environment. Stimuli from the environment are collected from the senses—vision, hearing, touch, taste, and smell. The brain translates the sensory stimuli into meaningful information. By receiving and perceiving environmental information, human beings are able to adapt to a dynamic environment.

Changes in ability to receive or perceive information from the environment can be caused by physiological, psychological, or environmental changes. Alterations in sensory input may lead to confused or disoriented behavior that may cause individuals to exhibit symptoms that are not healthful.

When people enter the health-care system, they are exposed to a different kind of environment, and it is confusing and frightening. The stimuli may be overwhelming and meaningless. Clients may be unable to adapt under these circumstances and may demonstrate confused behavior.

Sensory deprivation results when the sensory input is lower than people require to function. Under these conditions, the RAS is unable to maintain normal levels of activation to the cerebral cortex, and individuals receive a distorted view of reality.

Research on healthy people has shown that the effects of sensory deprivation can have a rapid onset. Symptoms of boredom and irritability begin almost at once, and hallucinations appear between 24 and 48 hours. The findings of these studies are staggering. If well subjects respond to sensory deprivation so quickly, sick individuals may be affected at an even faster rate. Clients who are immobilized for any reason are particularly at risk.

Sensory overload is the opposite of sensory deprivation and generally is caused by too many stimuli in the environment. Behaviors demonstrated by clients experiencing sensory overload may be like those exhibited by persons experiencing sensory deprivation.

Occasionally, because of disease or trauma, individuals may experience an altered level of consciousness (LOC). Changes in LOC are extremely serious and should be monitored and reported immediately. There are four LOCs and these include: alertness, lethargy, semicoma, and coma. Recently, methods such as Glasgow Coma Scale have been developed to measure LOCs. These focus on measurable responses and eliminate more subjective descriptions of LOCs.

Sensory deficits exist when a sensory organ is not functioning at its optimum level. With the loss of one or more of the senses, an individual may not be able to adapt to the environment and may not be able to function adequately.

Nurses play a key role in assisting clients with sensory alterations and deficits. The nursing process provides a framework for providing systematic, comprehensive nursing care.

Study Questions

1. Describe an environment that might lead to sensory deprivation.

2. Put on gloves, a blindfold, put cotton in your ears, and lie down for as long as you can in a quiet place. Describe your feelings during and after this activity.

3. What types of clients are most likely to develop sensory deprivation?

4. What is sensory overload? Have you ever experienced it? What was it like?

5. Why was the Glasgow Coma Scale devised? How is it used?

6. Observe a friend's pupillary response to light.

7. Put on a blindfold. Walk around. Eat lunch or a snack. Describe your feelings.

8. Wear gloves and attempt to perform normal activities such as taking coins from a purse or pocket to buy a cup of coffee.

References

1. Laura K. Hart, Jean L. Reese, and Margery O. Fearing, *Concepts Common to Acute Illness, Identification and Management* (St. Louis: C.V. Mosby Co. 1981), 152.
2. J. Hole, *Human Anatomy and Physiology* 3rd ed. (Dubuque, Iowa: Wm C. Brown, 1984) 359–60.
3. Arthur J. Vander, James H. Sherman, and Dorothy S. Luciano, *Human Physiology: The Mechanisms of Body and Function,* 2nd ed. (New York: McGraw-Hill Book Co, 1976).
4. Vander, Sherman, and Luciano, *Human Physiology,* 168.
5. Barbara L. Conway, *Carini and Owens' Neurological and Neurosurgical Nursing* (St. Louis: C.V. Mosby Co., 1978), 152.
6. Arthur C. Guyton, *Textbook of Medical Physiology,* 6th ed. (Philadelphia: W.B. Saunders Co., 1981).
7. Conway, *Neurological Neurosurgical Nursing,* 81.
8. J.P. Shelby, "Sensory deprivation," *Image* 10:2, (1978):49–55.
9. Leo Madow and Lawrence Snow, *The Psychodynamic Implications of Physiological Studies on Sensory Deprivation* (Springfield, Ill.: Charles Thomas Co. 1970), 6.
10. Philip Solomon, *Sensory Deprivation* (Boston: Harvard University Press, 1961), 73.
11. F.S. Downs, "Bed rest and sensory disturbances," *Am J Nurs* 74, (1974) 3:435–38.
12. W.H. Bexton, W. Herron, and T.H. Scott, "Effects of decreased variation in sensory environment," *Can J Psychiatry* 8:6 (1954):70–76.
13. Ashley Montagu, *Touching, The Significance of the Skin* (New York: Harper & Row, 1971), 1.
14. J.R. Dunn, "Regulation of the senses," in Callista Roy, *Introduction to Nursing: An Adaptation Model* (Englewood Cliffs, N.J.: Prentice-Hall, 1976), 133–50.
15. Ashley Montagu, *Touching,* 3.
16. C. Jones, "Glasgow coma scale," *Am J Nurs* 79 (1979):1551–53.
17. N. Mauss-Clum, "Bringing the unconscious patient back safely. Nursing makes the critical difference," *Nursing 82,* 12(1982):34–42.

Annotated Bibliography

Bolin, R.H. 1974. Sensory deprivation: An overview. *Nurs Forum* 8(3):240–58. A concise description of sensory deprivation, citing the major concepts and interesting research findings.

Buisseret, P. 1978. The six senses. Part 3: The peripheral sensation. *Nurs Mirror Suppl* 146(4):iii–vi. This article provides basic information and enlightening drawings of the peripheral nervous system.

Chodel, J., and Williams, B. 1970. The concept of sensory deprivation. *Nurs Clin North Am* 5(3):453–65. This classic article describes the sensory process and aspects of sensory deprivation.

Downs, F.S. 1974. Bedrest and sensory disturbances. *Am J Nurs* 74(3):434–38. This classic article cites research on sensory deprivation and the hazards of bedrest.

Jones, C. 1979. Glasgow Coma Scale. *Am J Nurs* 79(9):1551–53. This article describes the use of the GCS and provides an example of a completed assessment scale.

Lindenmuth, J.E., Brew, C.S., Malooley, J.A. 1980. Sensory Overload. *Am J Nurs* 80(8):1456–58. A description of sensory overload is outlined in this brief article.

Mauss-Clum, N. 1982. Bringing the unconscious patient back safely. Nursing makes the difference. *Nurs 82* 12(8):34–42. This important article describes the physical attributes of unconscious clients and discusses four crucial responsibilities for nursing care.

McNamee, C. 1976. Communicating with the hard-of-hearing. *Can Nurse* 74(3):27–29. This short article provides very good pointers for establishing a good nurse–client relationship with hard-of-hearing clients.

Norman, S. 1982. The Pupil Check. *Am J Nurs* 82(4):588–91. This article describes the process of pupil checks and provides an illustration of pupil sizes.

Stewart, L.M., and Dawson, D.F. 1979. Blind client—sighted therapist: The interface. *J Psych Nurs Ment Health Serv* November: 31–35. This unique article describes some of the difficulties in establishing relationships with blind clients and gives some interesting suggestions for nurses.

Wolf, E.M. 1977. Communication with deaf surgical patients. *AORN J* 26(1):39–47. This article provides an assessment tool for determining the communication profile of the deaf client.

Chapter 23

Sleep

Janet-Beth McCann Flynn

Chapter Outline

- Objectives
- Glossary
- Introduction
- Stages of Sleep
- Alterations in Sleep Patterns
- The Nursing Process
  Assessment
  Planning
  Implementation
  Evaluation
- Summary
- Study Questions
- References
- Annotated Bibliography

Objectives

At the completion of this chapter, the reader will be able to:

▶ Define sleep
▶ Compare and contrast REM and NREM sleep
▶ Describe the five stages of sleep
▶ Discuss alterations in sleep
▶ Discuss nursing interventions to facilitate sleep

Glossary

Circadian Cycle. The human 24-hour biological clock.

Electroencephalogram (EEG). A painless study in which EEG machines convert the electrical impulses of the brain into a visual graph.

Enuresis. Bed-wetting beyond the age when bladder control should have been reached.

Hypersomnia. Periods of prolonged sleep.

Insomnia. The inability to fall asleep or to stay asleep.

Narcolepsy. Uncontrollable sleep.

Nightmares. Vivid dreams occurring during REM sleep and remembered upon awakening.

Night Terrors. Feelings of fear that occur when a person, usually a child, is awakened from NREM sleep.

Parasomnias. Sleep disorders in which events occur during sleep that generally occur during the waking state.

Reticular Activating System (RAS). A neural system, located in the reticular formation, which is responsible for the wakeful state.

Reticular Formation. A complex area in nerve fibers in the brainstem that controls wakefulness.

Sleep. An adaptive recurrent state of unresponsiveness that occurs clinically every 24 hours and has five stages.

Sleep Apnea. Self-limiting cessation of respiration during sleep.

Somnambulism. Sleepwalking.

INTRODUCTION

Sleep is a normal process important in the maintenance of physical and mental health. Human beings spend one-third of their lives asleep or approximately eight hours a day.

Almost a century ago, sleep was considered essential to human well-being. Pierce wrote in 1895,

> It is a well-established physiological fact, that during the wakeful hours the vital energies are being expended, the powers of life diminished, and, if wakefulness is continued beyond a certain limit, the system becomes enfeebled and death is the result.[1]

The amount of sleep that individuals need to feel rested and refreshed varies with age, activity, health, and emotional state. Whereas young children need a great deal of sleep, the need for sleep decreases with age. The normal adult needs 5 to 10 hours of sleep per night, with the average being around 7 to 8. A large amount of physical activity might increase the amount of sleep needed. Altered physical and emotional states might cause individuals to sleep more. Nutritional states also may influence the amount of sleep that individuals need.

An adequate definition of sleep does not exist. Definitions of sleep are present in the literature of anthropology, biology, physiology, philosophy, and many other disciplines. Definitions of sleep can be traced back thousands of years, but there has never been one definition that has been accepted by all schools of thought.

A historical definition described **sleep** as a period of profound relaxation, much like a comatose state. Current researchers have modified this definition through clinical research by demonstrating that sleep is a state of consciousness, not unconsciousness, in which the individual's state of perception of the environment is decreased but not absent.[2] Sleeping persons are able to attend to certain noises while sleeping. Some noises will awaken the sleeper, such as a smoke detector alarm, an alarm clock, or a crying baby, while other noises—traffic and birds singing—will not. This appears to occur because stimuli that are relevant to individuals will awaken them, while less essential stimuli will not.

Sleep can be considered as a recurrent healthy state of unresponsiveness that occurs cyclically and has stages within the sleep state. The 24-hour day–night or awake–sleep cycle has been referred to by scientists as the **Circadian cycle** and is a part of the human biological clock. The nature of the Circadian cycle or biological clock is still a mystery, but it appears that it is related to the light and dark cycles. It is our biological clock that causes us to fall asleep at one time and awaken at another.[3]

The Circadian cycle develops around the third month of life and appears to be inherited from the mother.[4] The site of this clock has not been determined, but several theories have been suggested.[5] The pineal gland is one of these anatomical sites, located deep in the brain between the two hemispheres. It is light-sensitive, and this may be how it regulates the body clock. The adrenal glands also appear to have some effect on the body clock. The hypothalamus has been considered as a location for the body clock as well. These are just a few of the body clock locations hypothesized, and there is no universally acceptable theory to date.[6]

The **reticular formation** in the brain has been shown to control wakefulness.[7] It consists of neurons distributed in the medulla, the pons, mesencephalon, and portions of the diencephalon (Fig. 23–1). Within the reticular formation there is a neural structure known as the **reticular activating system (RAS)**, which is believed to be responsible for normal wakefulness. The brainstem portion of the RAS transmits signals to the cortex to produce the awake state.

When people sleep, the RAS is mainly dormant.[8] It is inhibited by two neuronal systems that oppose its stimulating effect. These neuronal clusters are located in the central core of the brainstem and in the pons. The brainstem core neurons secrete serotonin (5-hydroxytryptamine), and when this level becomes high enough, the RAS is inhibited. When this inhibition occurs, the individual loses consciousness and is asleep.[9]

Dreams are associated with sleep, and it appears that brainstem core neurons facilitate sleep centers in the pons, where paradoxical or dream sleep originates (Fig. 23–2). Pathways

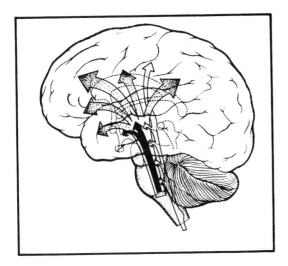

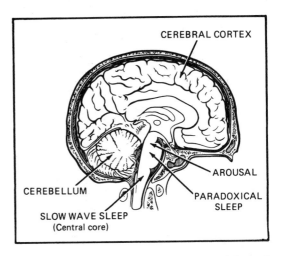

Figure 23–2. Paradoxical or dream sleep originates in the pons.

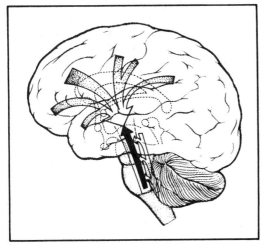

Figure 23–1. The reticular formation.

ascending from the paradoxical sleep centers produce brain waves like those of the awake stage and also produce eye movement.

Many studies have been done concerning wakefulness and sleep. Data in these studies have been gathered through use of an **electroencephalogram** (EEG) that measures the electrical activity of the brain. Researchers now have empirical, objective, and scientific data, as opposed to the highly subjective data obtained in the past.

The EEG is a painless study in which probes are placed on the scalp to measure electric po-

tential between two points on the scalp, and a mechanical printout results.[10] The wave-like pattern of the EEG changes as a person goes from an awake state, through a drowsy state, to a sleep state. An individual who is awake and resting produces a slow wave known as the alpha wave (Fig. 23–3A). When these waves are being generated, a person, when questioned, will verbalize feelings of contentment and relaxation. In the awake state, the alpha waves become smaller but are still alpha waves.

STAGES OF SLEEP

The EEG pattern changes during the sleep state. As the individual becomes drowsy, the rhythmic alpha wave is replaced by an irregular pattern, the beta wave (Fig. 23–3B). As sleep deepens, the waves become slower, larger, and more irregular—delta waves (Fig. 23–3C). These sleeping waves are interrupted through the sleep cycle by other waves that resemble the wakeful waves (Fig. 23–3D) and are generated during paradoxical sleep. In this stage, the individual still appears to be asleep, but the EEG is like the alert, wakeful pattern.

Based on sleep research, two types of sleep have been identified: rapid eye movement (REM) sleep and non-REM (NREM) sleep, or

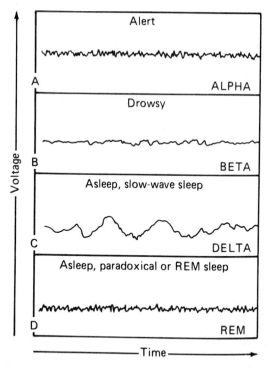

Figure 23–3. An electroencephalogram measures the changes in electrical activity in the brain. REM = rapid eye movement.

slow-wave deep sleep. REM sleep, also known as active or paradoxical sleep, is characterized by rapid eye movements of the sleeping person, and the EEG pattern is much like the pattern of a wakeful person. NREM sleep occurs in four stages, from light, drowsy sleep to heavy, deep sleep, and it occurs in cycles, each lasting about 90 minutes.[11] Sleep is a dynamic process during which individuals move through five sleep stages.

Stage I is the drowsy state. The person still knows where he is but is relaxed. It is that pleasant transition state just before dropping to a deeper stage of sleep. Alpha waves are demonstrated on EEG tracings at this stage. Frequently, as one begins to drift into a deeper stage, the legs may jerk, causing the person to jerk awake.

Stage II is a light sleep. The alpha rhythm is lost completely. Beta brain waves are shown on EEGs in stage II sleep. Stage II sleep has been called the door stage, because it precedes and

follows REM sleep. Of total sleep time, 40 to 45 percent is spent in stage II. External stimulation at this stage may awaken the sleeper.

Stage III is a medium depth sleep. This stage is characterized by delta waves on EEG. Occasional bursts of "spindle" activity may be seen on the EEG.

Stage IV is a stage of deep, profound sleep during which individuals are difficult to arouse. There is little body movement in this stage, and vital signs and metabolic rates decrease. These EEG waves reveal slow delta patterns. This is the sleep that restores, builds, relaxes, and rests the body physically. After a day of heavy physical exercise or work, the need for stage IV sleep increases. Research has found that somatotropin or growth hormone is released during this stage of sleep.[12] It appears that some dreaming occurs during stage IV sleep. The eye movements associated with this NREM sleep are slow and rolling. NREM dreams are more realistic and thought-like than vivid REM dreams. NREM sleep, especially those stages that produce delta waves, is most prevalent in the first third of the sleeping time and decreases in each subsequent sleep cycle.

Stage V sleep is called REM sleep and is the stage most identified with dreams that are described as vivid and unrealistic. REM dreams are more often recalled than NREM dreams, and dreams that are threatening to an individual's psyche usually are repressed on or before waking. Research has lead to simple explanation of this phenomenon of paradoxical sleep.[13] Certain factors suggest that catecholaminergic neurons are responsible for the cortical arousal seen both in the wakeful state and in paradoxical sleep.

There are four to five periods of REM sleep per night, and approximately 20 percent of the sleeping time is spent in REM sleep. As the sleep cycle progresses through the sleeping time, the REM phases become longer and occur closer together. The dreams that occur toward the end of the sleep cycle tend also to be more vivid and to be remembered on awakening (Fig. 23–4).

This stage of sleep is characterized by rapid eye movements that can be observed through the closed eyelids, and the EEG pattern resembles the wakeful pattern. Other observable behaviors include muscular twitching, and irreg-

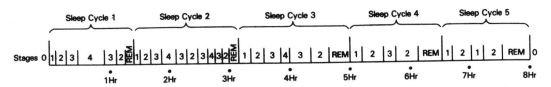

Figure 23–4. The sleep cycle schema. *(From Helen Yura, "The need for sleep," in Helen Yura and Mary Walsh,* Human Needs and the Nursing Process, *(New York: Appleton-Century-Crofts, 1978), 265.)*

ular breathing and pulse rates. Breathing can stop (sleep apnea) at the onset of REM sleep and the period of apnea lasts up to 30 seconds.[14] This phenomenon appears to be more common in men than in women.

The purpose of REM sleep is to catalog and process the day's events, to integrate thoughts, and add to the memory storehouse. Because infants and young children have a great deal to process and store they spend a great deal of their sleep time in REM sleep. As people grow older, they spend much less time in REM sleep (Table 23–1).

REM sleep can be suppressed by use of drugs and alcohol. When this occurs, individuals lose the ability to integrate new information and process stressful events. They may begin to exhibit disorganized behavior or the inability to cope with stressful situations.[15]

ALTERATIONS IN SLEEP PATTERNS

Alterations in normal sleep patterns are frequently seen in ill persons and occasionally in those individuals who are healthy. There are a variety of reasons for sleep disturbances. Some are caused by physical discomfort, some by psychological factors, and others are environmental in origin.

The most common alteration in sleep is **insomnia**. Insomnia is the inability to obtain an adequate amount of sleep because of problems falling asleep or difficulty remaining asleep. Statistics reveal that one in three Americans suffers from a form of insomnia,[16] and Americans spend millions of dollars on over-the-counter sleep preparations. Just the thought of another sleepless night can create enough anxiety to produce the very state that the individual wishes to avoid.

Insomnia affects all of us at times, but it is not a problem unless it is chronic. Chronic insomnia deprives individuals of the needed rest and restorative functions of sleep. Research has demonstrated that NREM stages III and IV are decreased in the insomniac, so not only does the insomniac suffer from decreased amounts of sleep but also from altered sleep patterns.[17] Insomnia is related to physical discomfort, anxiety, depression, environmental conditions, and drug or alcohol abuse. Because the causes are various, treatment is diverse, ranging from exercise to sleeping medications. Treatment should be based on a thorough physical, history, and proper use of a client-kept sleep log or diary.

Hypersomnia is the opposite of insomnia, in that periods of sleep are quite long, lasting to several days. Waking, for individuals suffering from this condition, can be difficult, and they may be confused when awakened. Hypersomnia has been reported in individuals with anorexia nervosa or obesity, causing researchers to hypothesize that hypersomnia is related to a central nervous system disorder involving the hunger–satiety center in the hypothalamus.

TABLE 23–1. CHANGE OF SLEEP AND DREAM PATTERNS WITH AGE

Age	Sleep (hr/day)	Dreams (REM %)
Birth–30 days	16–20	50–80[a]
1 month–1 year	12–16	30–40
1–3	12–14	25
3–5	10	20
6–16	8–10	18–20
18–40	8	22
40–60	6–8	19
65	5–7	20–23

[a]Higher for premature infants

Other conditions causing hypersomnia may include head injury, cerebrovascular accidents, brain tumors, depression, and high stress levels.

EEG tracings of individuals suffering from hypersomnia follow the normal pattern except for the long duration of the sleep period. Treatment of this condition involves limiting the amount of time spent sleeping and possibly the use of physician-prescribed stimulants.

Narcolepsy is similar to hypersomnia in that individuals tend to sleep more, but the urge to sleep cannot be controlled. Sleep patterns of a narcoleptic are characterized by frequent uncontrollable periods of sleep of short duration. After these brief periods, narcoleptics report feeling refreshed. Attacks usually follow meals, are toward the end of the day, or occur in boring situations. This condition can be quite hazardous and incapacitating for individuals driving or using machinery.

EEGs performed during the daytime narcoleptic attack show REM sleep patterns. This disorder is usually treated with physician ordered drugs such as Ritalin (methylphenidate hydrochloride) or amphetamines.

Sleep apnea syndrome is a cessation of respiration during sleep. It is a potentially lethal condition characterized by multiple obstructive or mixed apneas. This condition is fairly common in infants up to three months of age, in obese males, post-menopausal females, and in all individuals during REM sleep.[18-20] Sleep apnea occurs during NREM sleep, too, and is associated with heavy snoring, snorting, extreme restlessness, sleepwalking, enuresis, morning headache, personality changes, daytime drowsiness, anxiety, depression, and sexual dysfunction.

Guilleminault et al. have proposed that a sleep apnea syndrome can be diagnosed if during a 7-hour nocturnal sleep period at least 30 apneic episodes are documented.[21] In most instances the etiology is unknown.

Treatment includes weight reduction,[22] abstention from alcohol and smoking, and more invasive procedures, such as tracheostomy, or removal of tissue from the oropharynx.

Extreme care needs to be taken when administering sedatives to individuals who have sleep apnea. Death can occur from this additional stress on an already strained respiratory system. If these clients are sedated, they must be closely monitored.

Parasomnias are sleep disorders in which events occur during sleep that usually occur during the waking state. Types of parasomnias include somnambulism, or sleepwalking, and enuresis, or bed-wetting.

Somnambulism is seen primarily in male children and adolescents. There is usually a strong family history of sleepwalking. EEG reports show that this state occurs during NREM sleep, in stages III and IV. The child is able to get out of bed, though totally asleep, and walk around. Children have been known to get lost or into rather tricky locations, such as window ledges or behind large appliances, but do not generally hurt themselves. Eyes are generally open, but the child is unresponsive when questioned or answers briefly in a monotone. If left alone, the child generally returns to bed and sleep. Characteristically, the child has no recall of the sleepwalking process. There may be an underlying emotional problem or anxiety, and the child may act this out during the sleepwalking activity. Most children outgrow sleepwalking. Only 1 to 5 percent of the adult population sleepwalk, and this is usually only during periods of extreme tension and anxiety.

Treatment involves providing a safe environment for the sleepwalker and includes using side rails both at home and in the hospital.

If sleepwalking continues, treatment might include administration of physician-ordered medication and psychotherapy.

Enuresis is the involuntary release of urine beyond the age when bladder control should have been acquired, at around four years of age. Enuresis is the most common of parasomnias and appears to run in families. The majority of bed-wetting episodes occur during NREM sleep. Children generally outgrow this condition by the time they are 12, but it can have embarrassing effects on them until then. Causes of enuresis include psychological problems, pathology such as diabetes mellitus, and organic lesions. Treatment depends on the cause and might include exercises to enlarge the bladder capacity, psychological support for both child and parents, and limiting fluids after the evening meal. Psychological problems are treated with psychotherapy for the child and the family.

Other sleep disorders include nightmares and night terrors. **Nightmares** occur during REM sleep and can be remembered upon awaking. They are common in children but less so in adults. Adults tend to have nightmares during time of stress. **Night terrors** are most common in preschoolers. The child wakes from sleep screaming and may be difficult to console. The cause of the terror as well as the attack generally are not remembered in the morning. Night terrors occur when the child is awakened from NREM sleep, and the attacks occur infrequently. If they become more frequent, help should be sought.

Alcohol abuse and drug use also can produce alterations in sleep patterns. Alcohol abuse decreases REM sleep and appears to disturb normal progression through the sleep cycle. The alcoholic awakens unrefreshed due to this disturbance. With the withdrawal of alcohol the alcoholic will spend much sleeping time in the REM stage. Drug use and abuse also can produce a decrease in the amount of REM sleep. Individuals experiencing the lack of REM sleep may not be integrated emotionally and physically. They may complain of fatigue, jitters, and a "hangover" in the morning. When drugs or alcohol are withdrawn, individuals may experience vivid dreams and night terrors. In addition to this, they may become anxious about not being able to take sleeping medications or alcohol. They also suffer from insomnia and fitful sleep.

Many hospitalized persons suffer from sleep deprivation caused by frequent disturbances during the sleeping hours. Lack of sleep can delay the healing and recuperation processes. Persons who are awakened often, such as the critically ill or postoperative clients, lose NREM sleep that is needed for restoration and may become irritable, anxious, and have difficulty concentrating. Total sleep deprivation can lead to hallucinations and confusion. Another interesting phenomenon can also occur in cases of sleep deprivation. Individuals who need both REM and NREM sleep may drop into REM sleep during the bath and begin talking in their sleep or may appear confused until the proper nursing diagnosis is made and they are permitted to sleep undisturbed.

Physiological conditions, such as hypothy-roidism, hyperthyroidism, coronary artery disease, and nocturnal dyspnea can produce alterations in sleep patterns. Pain and discomfort can contribute to alterations in sleep, too, and need to be monitored.

The nurse can provide an environment conducive to sleeping and adequate sleeping time. Providing clients with adequate and restful sleep is probably one of the most useful services that the nurse can perform in helping clients to adapt.

THE NURSING PROCESS

Adequate, restful sleep is essential for proper healing and emotional well-being. In order to meet clients' sleep requirements, the nurse should base nursing interventions on a careful sleep and rest assessment.

Assessment

A careful assessment of previous sleep habits is essential for determining general patterns. Important data to be gathered are age, number of hours slept nightly, naps or rest periods taken daily, aids to facilitate sleep (reading, baths, alcohol, medications—both prescribed and over-the-counter), number of awakenings and cause, sleeping arrangements (furniture, lighting, bed linens, light, noise, etc.), whether the person sleeps alone or with someone, amount of daily exercise, prayers or religious readings, and how much sleep the client needs (Figure 23–5). Other data to be gathered include the nutritional status, presence of stress in the environment, and the presence of noise and light in the hospital environment. Once the sleep history has been taken and observations of the environment completed, the nurse can observe the sleeping client in the hospital over a period of several days to assess the client's present sleep behaviors.

Nursing diagnoses are drawn from the findings of the assessment. Examples of nursing diagnoses related to sleep might include:

- Alteration in sleep patterns related to pain
- Alteration in REM sleep related to alcoholism
- Potential alteration in sleep related to impending surgery

Sleep Assessment

Sleep Habits

Hours slept per night _____ Number of awakenings _____
Why? _____
Hour of retiring _____ Awakening _____ Naps _____ Time _____
Awaken refreshed _____ Fatigued _____ Alteration in pattern _____
How much sleep is generally required _____ hrs.

Sleep Environment

Type of bed _____ Number of blankets _____ Number of pillows _____
Any special devices _____ TV _____ Radio _____
Sleeping companion _____
Ventilation _____ Temperature _____ Light _____ Noise _____
Music _____ Other _____

Aids

Reading, TV, radio _____ Exercise _____
Foods and beverages _____
Behaviors (baths, showers, tooth brushing, etc.) _____
For children: bedtime rituals _____
Medications taken: _____
Alcohol _____ type _____ amount _____

Figure 23–5. Sleep assessment tool.

Planning

Planning should be based on the assessment phase and should incorporate data gathered from the client's sleep history. Planning also should include client and family teaching when appropriate. The purpose of a sleep plan is to provide for maximum periods of sleep and to relieve sleeplessness.

Treatments, vital signs, and medications should be scheduled in such a way as to maximize the amount of time between them, so that the client can have several hours of uninterrupted sleep. It is possible to have medications ordered for 10 P.M., 2 A.M., and 6 A.M. and treatments at 12 A.M. and 4 A.M. In most instances, these times can be rearranged so that medications and treatments occur simultaneously and the client is allowed to sleep between interruptions.

The nurse also should schedule time so that time can be spent at bedtime assisting clients to meet their bedtime needs. Careful planning leads to an organized and consistent approach to facilitating sleep.

Implementation

A great many nursing interventions can be used to facilitate rest and sleep. Some are rather sim-

ple and take only a few minutes, while others are more complex and may take more time.

The simplest are the comfort measures, which involve straightening the bed linens, providing more blankets, fluffing and turning pillows so the cool side is against the client's body. Back rubs and sponge baths are relaxing, too. Placing the client in a comfortable position or a favorite sleeping position will facilitate sleep.

Another simple care measure is assessing the client's physical discomfort and administering prescribed pain medication before the client's pain tolerance is surpassed. Employing other comfort measures will aid the client, as well.

Helping the client maintain normal routines promotes sleep. Providing reading materials and snacks may help, if these are practices usually carried out at bedtime when at home.

The environment should be manipulated to provide a restful atmosphere. Phones can be turned down or off, lights dimmed, and noise reduced. The room door can be closed as a buffer from hall lighting and noise. When checking sleeping clients, the nurse should be as quiet as possible, so they are not disturbed.

Some clients are under a great deal of stress and are unable to sleep because of this. Talking with them and providing support is essential. If they can discuss their problems, they may feel better and be able to get to sleep.

If the clients are not sleeping at night or are sleeping fitfully, other nursing measures can be taken. Care can be planned to leave periods of time for naps. Naps should be encouraged during the morning hours, because it has been found that individuals continue to have REM sleep during these hours. Naps should be discouraged during the afternoon, because individuals tend to drop into stage IV sleep and awake feeling more fatigued than they did prior to their nap. Elderly persons may stay awake at night and sleep all day. Efforts should be made to keep these individuals awake during the day. They can be placed at the nurse's desk and walked in the corridors frequently. They may become noisy at night and disturb others and have to be placed in a room alone. This adds to their sensory deprivation.

Teaching relaxation technique is a good method to promote sleep. One method is to assist the client into a comfortable position and have him or her concentrate on various body parts and relax them. The individual is taught to begin with the feet and work up through the calves, thighs, hips, abdomen, chest, arms, and neck while stating "Feet go to sleep," "calves go to sleep." This is a type of meditation and works for many people.

A dependent nursing action for promoting sleep is administration of physician-ordered drugs. These should be administered with care, usually at the client's request. The client should be monitored frequently throughout the night. Great care should be taken when administering sleeping medications to individuals with medical histories of respiratory problems or sleep apnea. It should be remembered that these persons will have reduced periods of REM sleep and may awaken with a drug hangover. It should be kept in mind that if sleeping medications are not administered to clients who have been taking them for a long time, they may experience vivid dreams or even night terrors caused by withdrawal of the drug.

Evaluation

Evaluating the quality of the client's sleep should be based on what the client verbalizes.

Many nurses have observed clients sleeping all night only to be told in the morning that the client had a terrible night's sleep. Sleep, like pain, is a subjective experience. If the client says that he or she did not rest well, then he or she did not. Evaluation of sleep can focus on the client's subjective description of the activity, the nurse's objective observation, and on the waking behavior of the client, such as irritability or dropping off to sleep at odd times.

Once careful assessment planning and intervention has brought about restful sleep, the client is well on his way to regaining the optimal health level.

SUMMARY

Sleep is a natural, recurring process important in maintaining physical and mental health. The amount of sleep individuals need to feel rested depends on age, activity, health, and mental state. Most normal adults need between 5 and 10 hours sleep per night, and children need from 10 to 12.

At this time, no completely acceptable definition of sleep has been advanced, but it seems safe to say that sleep is a recurrent healthy state of unresponsiveness that occurs cyclically and has several stages. The day–night cycle that humans adhere to is referred to as the Circadian cycle, and it is a part of the biological clock. The Circadian cycle appears to be controlled in part by the pineal gland and the reticular formation.

Within the reticular formation is an area known as the reticular activating system (RAS) that appears to control sleep and wakefulness. Brainstem core neurons facilitate sleep centers in the pons, where paradoxical or dream, sleep originates.

Researchers have used electroencephalograms (EEG), which measure the brain's electrical activity, to obtain empirical data on sleep. This research has shown that an individual's EEG changes with passage from an awake state to a sleep state. Based on this research, two types of sleep have been identified: rapid eye movement (REM) sleep and nonrapid eye movement sleep (NREM).

Sleep has five stages. Stage I is the drowsy

state. Stages II and III are progressively deeper stages of sleep. Stage IV is a stage of deep profound sleep, which individuals need for physical restoration. Stage V is REM sleep and is associated with dreaming, and its EEG pattern resembles the wakeful pattern. The purpose of REM sleep is to catalog and process the day's events, to integrate thoughts, and to add to the memory storehouse. Infants and young children have a great deal of information to store and process, and they spend a great deal of time in the REM sleep, while older people need less REM sleep. Lack of REM sleep can produce disorganized behavior and mental confusion.

Alterations in normal sleep patterns are common and can be caused by a wide variety of factors, including physical discomfort, emotional disturbances, and environmental factors. The most common sleep disorder is insomnia. Other disorders include hypersomnia, narcolepsy, sleep apnea, parasomnias, nightmares and night terrors, REM deprivation, and sleep deprivation.

Adequate sleep and rest are essential for adaptation, and by using the nursing process, the nurse can facilitate sleep. Careful sleep assessments are necessary in order to determine the problem. Then the plan can be determined, implemented, and evaluated.

Study Questions

1. What is sleep?

2. What is NREM sleep? Why is it necessary?

3. What is REM sleep? Why is it necessary?

4. What stage of sleep is essential for psychological well-being?

5. How can the nursing process be used to help individuals with alterations in sleep patterns?

6. How can the nursing process be used to promote sleep?

References

1. R.V. Pierce, *The People's Common Sense Medical Adviser in Plain English: or Medicine Simplified,* 50th ed. (Buffalo, N.Y.: World's Dispensary Printing Office and Bindery, 1895), 278.
2. Karen C. Sorenson and Joan Luckmann, *Basic Nursing. A Physiologic Approach* (Philadelphia: W.B. Saunders Co., 1979), 540.
3. K. Adams, "A time for rest and a time for play," *Nurs Mirror* (1980), 150.
4. M. Walsh, "Prologue: Biologic rhythms and human needs," in Helen Yura and Mary Walsh, *Human Needs and the Nursing Process* (New York: Appleton-Century-Crofts, 1978), 1–33.
5. Arthur L. Guyton, *Textbook of Medical Physiology,* 6th ed. (Philadelphia: W.B. Saunders Co., 1981), 705.
6. M. Walsh, "Prologue," 8.
7. A. Guyton, *Textbook of Medical Physiology,* 705.
8. Ibid.
9. A. Vander, *Human Physiology,* 2nd ed. (New York: McGraw-Hill Book Co, 1976).
10. Ibid., 553.
11. J. Hayter, "The rhythm of sleep," *Am J Nurs* 80 (1980): 457–61.
12. J.A. Horne, "Human sleep and tissue restitution: Some qualifications, some doubts," *Clin Sci* 65, (1983):569–78.
13. T. Canavan, "The psychobiology of sleep," *Med Educ* (1984): 682–83.
14. C. Guilleminault, "State of the art sleep and control of breathing," *Chest* 73, (1978) 293–96.
15. H. Yura, "The need for sleep," in Helen Yura and Mary Walsh, *Human Needs and the Nursing Process.* (New York: Appleton-Century-Crofts, 1978), 259–318.
16. Pamela H. Mitchell and Anne Loustaw, *Concepts Basic to Nursing,* 3rd ed. (New York: McGraw Hill Book Co. 1981), 612.
17. I. Oswald, "Drug research and human sleep," *Ann Rev Pharmacol* 13 (1973), 213.
18. A. Kales and J. Kales, "Sleep disorders," *N Engl J Med* 290 (1974) 9:478.
19. J. Washburn, "Sleep disorders," *Am J Nurs* 82 (1982): 936–40.
20. Sorenson and Luckmann, *Basic Nursing. A Physiologic Approach,* 548.
21. C. Guilleminault et al., "Clinical overview of sleep apnea syndromes," in C. Guilleminault and W. Dement eds., *Sleep Apnea Syndromes* (New York: Alan R. Liss, 1978), 1–12.
22. Ibid.

Annotated Bibliography

Bahr, S.T. 1983. "Sleep–wake patterns," *J Gerontol Nurs* 9 (4): 534–41. This excellent article provides guidelines for assessing sleep patterns in the elderly.

Bassler, S.F. 1976. The origins and development of biological rhythms. *Nurs Clin North Am* 11(4):575–82. In this article, the body rhythms of sleep, wakefulness, and physiological rhythms are discussed.

Grant, D.A. and Klell, C. 1974. For Goodness Sake—Let Your Patients Sleep! *Nurs 74* (11):54–57. This article discusses the Circadian cycle and the need for all stages of sleep. It offers suggestions for nursing interventions based on day, evening, and night hours.

Hayter, J. 1980. The Rhythm of Sleep. *Am J Nurs* 80(3):457–61. This excellent article discusses the stages of sleep and implications for nursing practice.

Long, B. 1969. Sleep. *Am J Nurs* 69(9):1896–99. The author of this article discusses how knowledge of sleep can help nurses assess the sleep needs of hospitalized clients.

Orem, J., and Barnes, C.D., 1980. *Physiology of Sleep*. New York: Academic Press. Excellent discussions of physiology and technology of sleep are provided.

Tom, C.K. 1976. Nursing Assessment of Biological Rhythms. *Nurs Clin North Am* 11:621–30. This interesting article proposes an assessment tool for assessing Circadian cycles.

Yura, H. 1978. The Need for Sleep. In H. Yura and M. Walsh. *Human Needs and the Nursing Process*. New York: Appleton-Century-Crofts. This comprehensive chapter discusses all aspects of sleep and cites current sleep research. In addition, it uses the nursing process as a framework for client care.

Zelchowski, G.P. 1977. Helping Your Patients Sleep: Planning Instead of Pills. *Nurs 77* 7:63–65. Alternative methods for assisting clients to sleep without medications is outlined in this brief article.

Chapter 24

Immobility

Nancie H. Pardue

Chapter Outline

- Objectives
- Glossary
- Alterations in Mobility
- Physical Problems of Immobility
  Respiratory System
  Cardiovascular System
  Skin
  Musculoskeletal and Peripheral Nervous Systems
  Elimination
- Metabolism and Nutrition
- Psychosocial Aspects of Immobility
- The Nursing Process
  Assessment
  Nursing Diagnosis
  Planning
  Implementation
  Evaluation
- Summary
- Study Questions
- References
- Annotated Bibliography

Objectives

After completing this chapter, the reader will be able to:

▶ Define the terms listed in the glossary
▶ Discuss the concepts of mobility, immobility, and therapeutic bedrest
▶ Describe the effects of immobility and extended bedrest on the client's respiratory, cardiovascular, musculoskeletal, and peripheral nervous systems, and on skin, elimination, metabolic, nutritional, and psychosocial status
▶ List the nursing diagnoses appropriate to a client on extended bedrest based on the assessment of his or her problems and needs
▶ Specify client outcomes necessary for evaluating the client on extended bedrest
▶ Discuss nursing interventions that will assist the client and family to adapt to physiological and psychosocial changes induced by immobility and prolonged bedrest

Glossary

Anorexia. Loss of appetite.

Aspiration. The drawing in of foreign bodies or fluids into the lungs on inspiration.

Atelectasis. Collapsing of the alveoli of the lung caused by mucus plugs, excessive secretions, or obstruction by foreign bodies.

Constipation. Infrequent passage of stool.

Contractures. Shortening and atrophy of muscles or joints resulting in resistance to passive stretch caused by disuse and prolonged maintenance of a flexed position.

Decubitus Ulcers. Pressure sores or ulcers that are breaks in the surface skin or mucous membrane, characterized by disintegration or death of the tissue.

Defecation. Evacuation of the bowels.

Edema. The swelling of tissues when fluid is held intercellularly.

Embolus. A mass of undissolved matter, such as a blood clot or air, traveling through a blood vessel.

Fecal Impaction. A collection of hardened stool in the rectum or sigmoid colon.

Hypostatic Pneumonia. An inflammation of the alveoli and buildup of secretions within the alveoli because of lack of expansion and contraction of the lung tissue.

Immobility. An intentional or involuntary limitation of activity in any sphere of a person's physical, emotional, intellectual, social, or cultural experience.

Lateral Position. Sidelying.

Mobility. The ability to move freely and easily without restrictions in one's own environment.

Orthostatic Hypotension. The occurrence of a marked fall in the blood pressure occurring when a person rises from the recumbent to the erect position.

Osteoporosis. Loss of the protein matrix of the bone.

Prone. Lying flat with the face downward.

Reactive Hyperemia. A temporary increase in blood flow to an area of the skin that occurs just after blood flow to the area has been blocked and then released.

Recumbent. Lying down.

Shearing Forces. Forces that pull tissues and move one layer of tissue over another as a client changes position in bed.

Supine. Lying on the back with the face up.

Therapeutic Bedrest. The confinement of a person to bed to aid in the healing process and in the treatment of disease.

Thrombophlebitis. Inflammation of a vein developing before the formation of a blood clot.

Thrombus. A blood clot loosely attached to the wall of a vein, caused by stasis of the blood, injury to the vessel, or hypercoagulability.

Urinary Incontinence. An involuntary release of urine from the bladder.

Urinary Retention. Accumulation of urine within the bladder due to the inability to urinate.

Urinary Stasis. The pooling of urine in the urinary tract.

Valsalva Maneuver. The attempt to forcibly exhale with the nose and mouth closed, resulting in increased intrathoracic pressure and a decreased return of blood to the heart.

Venous Stasis. Pooling of blood in the veins.

ALTERATIONS IN MOBILITY

Mobility is the ability to move freely and easily without restrictions in one's own environment. An individual defines health and physical fitness through the ability to be mobile. Not only does mental well-being depend on one's ability to be mobile, but the body functions best with the ability to change positions. The body organs and systems perform their functions much more easily when the person is standing. The kidneys are able to drain completely in the standing position; the lungs expand more easily; and peristaltic movements of the bowel are more effective in the upright position. The functioning and repair of joints, muscles, tendons, and bones are dependent upon the forces of motion.

Immobility may be defined as an intentional or involuntary limitation of activity in any sphere of a person's physical, emotional, intellectual, social, or cultural experience. Throughout the life span, individuals experience various types of immobility. Certain occupations, for example, are sedentary, requiring the body to be held in one position for long periods of time. People who practice meditation or other forms of relaxation exercises also are engaging in a limited type of immobility. Extremes of immobility are seen in nursing and medicine, and range from the unconscious or totally paralyzed client to the person with a temporary arm sling or finger splint.

Immobility, as seen in nursing situations, is often imposed for beneficial reasons. **Therapeutic bedrest** is the confinement of a client to bed in order to aid in the healing process and in the treatment of disease. Rest in bed *immobilizes fractures and wound edges,* enabling them to heal together more easily. *Relief of pain* is also provided by bedrest and immobility, especially in clients with operations, trauma, wounds, and arthritis. Bedrest is frequently prescribed to *limit exercise,* such as in those individuals suffering from a myocardial infarction.

Rest reduces the metabolic needs, oxygen requirements, and body system demands of various injured and diseased organs. Certainly the heart and lungs have a reduced workload during bedrest. Armchair rest is frequently just as effective as bedrest for clients who need cardiac rest.

To remove the local effects of gravity is another use of bedrest because gravity causes a strain on the lower circulation. Ankle edema and venous congestion improve with elevation. Also, clients with **orthostatic hypotension** are generally kept on bedrest until they can be gradually introduced to standing. Another indication for bedrest is the need for *support* for clients who are too weak or ill to remain upright and active; for example, cancer clients and those with neurological diseases who need bedrest to aid them in physiological adaptation to various bodily changes and stressors. Through rest, energy is freed, making it possible for the injured or diseased body systems to repair themselves.

It is often the nurse's function to assess, with the physician, a person's basic needs and adaptability, and then to determine if some form of immobility will help the client to cope with the situation. It is important to look carefully at the decision to immobilize a client because bedrest has definite hazards. Disabilities caused by immobility can affect every system and major organ of the body. Malnourished clients, the elderly, the critically ill, quadraplegics, and comatose clients, for example, are especially susceptible to the hazards of bedrest. For many years, the problems and severe disabilities associated with bedrest have been documented and warned against, yet one still sees these complications in hospitals and nursing homes. By the completion of this chapter, the following quote from 1947 will take on new meaning.

> Look at a patient lying long in bed. What a pathetic picture he makes! The blood clotting in his veins, the lime draining from his bones, the scybala staking up in his colon, the flesh rotting from his seat, the urine leaking from his distended bladder, and the spirit evaporating from his soul.[1]

A person experiences *physical immobility* when there is a restriction of physical movement or bodily processes. The limitation of movement within the environment may be due to bedrest, a body cast, isolation, or an intensive care unit. A client may be unable to walk due to severe emphysema or congestive heart failure.

When overstressed, a person's usual ability to adapt may be ineffective and *psychological immobilization* may occur. When a client experiences a terminal illness, for example, or is faced with paralysis or loss, the responses may consist of withdrawal, depression, crying, or denial, all of which are demonstrations of psychological immobility.

Certain persons do not adapt well to threats within their environments or injuries to their bodies, due to a lack of knowledge of how to act effectively. This is called *intellectual immobility*. This lack of knowledge may occur for several reasons. Physiological reasons include an impaired intellect caused by drugs, trauma, cerebrovascular accidents, and arteriosclerosis. Clients after surgery may be so exhausted and in pain that they are physically drained and have no mental energy left. Cultural barriers, such as language, may prevent clients from understanding their problems and how they will be treated. The nurse needs to assess a client carefully for possible ineffective adaptation and determine if the level of knowledge or potential to learn is interfering with the ability to adapt.

Social immobility can occur when there are restrictions placed on normal patterns of social interaction. A quadriplegic person, for example, will experience social immobility when returned home, since he or she is no longer able to participate in certain activities. Elderly people who gradually lose their families and friends can become socially immobile as they spend increasingly more time alone and become afraid to go out by themselves. Hospital clients with extended illnesses begin to lose touch with their friends and the community and find that their social contacts are limited to hospital personnel.

PHYSICAL PROBLEMS OF IMMOBILITY

Immobility affects many of the body's physiological subsystems (Fig. 24–1). This section will

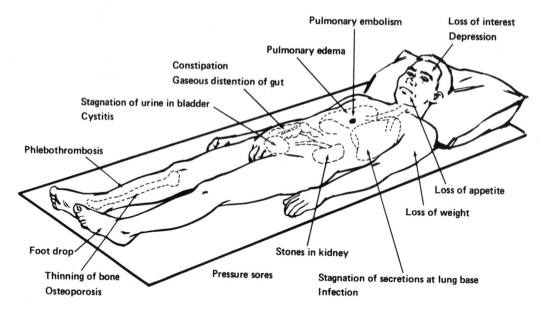

Figure 24–1. The hazards of prolonged bedrest on various body systems.

present a review of the effects of immobility on these various systems.

Respiratory System

The respiratory system is perhaps most dangerously affected by immobility, since adequate functioning of the lungs is critical to life. People who are immobile or confined to bed have decreases in all of the lung volumes except for the tidal volume.[2] As the client uses the respiratory muscles less, they become weaker and less efficient. If there are pressures against the chest caused by bedding, restraints, or clothing, the client may not be able to take adequate deep breaths. A person in the **supine** position has an elevated diaphragm, a constricted chest, and a redistribution of blood flow from the legs to the chest. Abdominal distention, fear of incisional pain, and the use of drugs, such as morphine, are all causes of restricted respirations and can prevent clients from taking periodic deep breaths. Absence of periodic lung expansion results in decreased surfactant activity, contributing to early airway closure. Also, when a client is left lying on one side for an extended period of time, the airways tend to close. There is less traction on the airway due to the reduced size

of alveoli, which in turn results from the decreased negative intrapleural pressures and increased blood volumes that are present in dependent lung zones. If a client continues in a pattern of minimal lung expansion, **atelectasis,** a collapse of the alveoli, may develop. Atelectasis is characterized by crackles and tubular breath sounds in dependent zones of the lung. Decreased transmission of breath sounds occurs when the airways are occluded.

Many clients on bedrest tend to develop **hypostatic pneumonia,** in which the alveoli and bronchioles of the lungs become inflamed and plugged with a fibrous exudate. When a client lies down and remains still for a long period of time, normal mucous secretions of the bronchial goblet cells tend to pool on the dependent side (Fig. 24–2). Bacterial organisms have a chance to proliferate in the pools of mucus. The cough reflex, important for mobilization of secretions, may be decreased by abdominal muscle weakness, abdominal surgery, narcotics, and anesthetics. When clients are placed lying on the side of the lung with atelectasis or pneumonia, gravity will cause an increase in blood flow to the dependent lung, and the client's blood arterial oxygen level will drop.

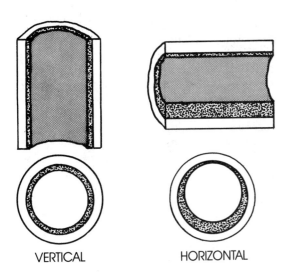

VERTICAL   HORIZONTAL

Figure 24–2. The effect of body positions on mucous secretions in the bronchioles.

The immobilized individual may also be susceptible to problems of **aspiration.** This problem occurs especially among clients receiving nasogastric tube feedings and in those who have had strokes or seizures, are unconscious, or have inadequate cough reflexes. Paralysis or selected medications may slow the reflex actions of the epiglottis, thus permitting aspiration of secretions from the nasopharynx. When gastric contents are aspirated into the lungs, an inflammatory reaction may occur, leading to complications.

Cardiovascular System

Changes in the cardiovascular system occur rapidly when a person is placed on bedrest. Studies have shown that the shift of fluid from the lower to the upper half of the body produces more deleterious effects on the cardiovascular system than the lack of physical activity during bedrest. Thus, getting the client out of bed for a walk or into an armchair is very important. **Venous stasis** can occur as a result of vasodilation and impairment of venous return to the heart. During muscular inactivity, the veins in the legs and other dependent parts tend to dilate. With normal activity, pressure changes on the venous bed aid venous blood to return to the right side of the heart. Changes in thoracic and abdominal

pressures from movement of the diaphragm promote blood return to the heart. Pressure changes in the veins of the legs are provided by the contraction and relaxation of leg muscle, referred to as the muscle pump.

Gravity can be a factor in the impairment of venous return. When an individual is supine and inactive, the veins in the legs are dependent, resulting in slow emptying of these vessels. Pressure also impedes venous return. The sitting position puts pressure on the vessels at the back of the knee, resulting in pooling of venous blood. When the body is horizontal and supine, external pressure from the bed causes impairment of venous return. If a client is placed on the side in the **lateral recumbent position** without a pillow between the legs, damage to leg veins may occur. **Edema** can occur as a result of circulatory stasis. As the venous backup and pressure increases, fluid is forced into the tissues, and edema occurs most commonly in the legs and sacrum. This edema may cause pain, impairment of mobility, and skin breakdown.

Some immobilized clients develop signs of a **thrombus** formation. In addition, clients on bedrest often become dehydrated and have higher than normal calcium levels, which contributes to increased blood viscosity and hypercoagulability. Clients susceptible are those who have conditions that increase the coagulability of the blood and those who have had previous thrombi or recent trauma.

Calf pain may indicate **thrombophlebitis,** which is inflammation of a vein. A tender, red, swollen cord may be palpable over the affected superficial vein. There will be an increased warmth of the affected extremity and a bluish mottling of the skin, particularly in the dependent position. The longer a client is immobilized, the greater the risk of a blood clot. Factors contributing to blood clot formation begin after immobilization. If a thrombus breaks loose from a vein and enters the circulation it becomes an **embolus.** This can occur when a client is allowed to sit or stand after prolonged inactivity. An embolus can travel to the heart and into the lung. Damage to the lung can cause a pulmonary infarct. Of those clients who develop a pulmonary embolus, nearly 40 percent die within two hours of onset. An embolus may lodge in a peripheral artery of the leg and cause symptoms such as pain, pallor, coolness, and tingling.

Clients on bedrest can inflict damage to their cardiovascular systems through the increased use of the **Valsalva maneuver.** This occurs when a bedridden client performs a pushing, pulling, or straining movement, such as using the upper trunk muscles to turn in bed or lift with an overhead trapeze. Straining during bowel movements also results in the Valsalva maneuver. After holding the breath, the person releases it and the drop in intrathoracic pressure causes the blood to rush to the heart. This surge of blood causes a corresponding increase in heart rate. For individuals with heart problems, continual use of the Valsalva maneuver can have detrimental effects.

Orthostatic hypotension is the inability of the autonomic nervous system to adapt to a sudden change from a lying-down to an upright position. As a result, there is a rapid fall in blood pressure and increase in heart rate accompanied by dizziness, weakness, and fainting. The client is considered to have orthostatic hypotension if the blood pressure drops over 20 mm Hg and pulse rate increases 20 beats per minute or more from the lying to the sitting or standing position. Nearly all clients, including healthy, active people, find that they may become light-headed when they get up too quickly after lying down, even after as little as 6 hours of bedrest. Orthostatic hypotension occurs for several reasons. Prolonged immobilization causes a decrease in blood volume because of changes in blood pressure and the redistribution of blood. Also, if a client remains in bed for a long time, many arterioles of the muscles and splanchnic circulation lose their ability to constrict. When the person changes position, the peripheral vessels fail to constrict and blood pools in the legs. There is a decreased return of blood to the heart and a subsequent decrease in blood pressure. The pressure of leg muscles against the veins is very important in helping to pump the blood back to the heart.

Prolonged immobility can also cause an *increased workload for the heart.* The recumbent position does not rest the heart. The work of the heart is at its lowest when the client is in a sitting position. In a supine position, blood volume is redistributed from the legs toward the head and some enters the pulmonary circulation. With this increase of blood to the heart, the cardiac output and heart rate increase, so that the heart works 30 percent harder.[3] Bedrest does not harm the heart, however, and damaged or enlarged hearts do improve with a reduction in stress and muscular work. Prolonged bedrest increases the resting heart rate 4 to 15 beats per minute and decreases the pulse pressure.[4] This is due to the redistribution of the fluid components of the body and the unfitness of the entire cardiovascular system. Without exercise, the heart does not function as well, however, and its efficiency deteriorates. A muscle that is well exercised is able to use oxygen from the blood more efficiently. Continual use of muscles also results in greater mechanical efficiency.

When clients begin to get out of the bed, they will experience a *decreased exercise tolerance.* The cardiovascular system will not be able to deliver adequate oxygen to perform activities that could be performed easily before bedrest, and clients will tire easily. It may take from days to months of gradual reconditioning before the cardiac and skeletal muscles perform as in the preimmobile state.

Skin

Immobility can have an especially rapid and visible effect on the skin. Nurses, because of their close association with bedside care, assume a primary responsibility for inspecting and caring for the client's skin. In addition most of the interventions relating to the prevention of skin breakdown are carried out by the nurse. Since nurses are responsible for skin care, it is especially important for them to understand the effects that immobility can have on the skin.

The pressure that occurs when clients remain in the same position for too long can result in a **decubitus ulcer.** These pressure sores or bedsores are breaks in the surface skin or mucous membrane characterized by disintegration of or death of the tissue. Pressure sores form when the external pressure on the skin exceeds capillary hydrostatic pressure (32 mm Hg). The first stage in the development of a decubitus ulcer is called blanching hyperemia.[5] At this stage when pressure is removed from the sore the areas remains red, a condition called **reactive hyperemia.** Light finger pressure will cause blanching, indicating that the microcirculation is intact. During the next stage, nonblanching hyperemia occurs, where the redness remains when light finger pressure is applied. At this point one can begin to classify the ulcer according to a grading system (Fig. 24–3).[6]

A *grade I* pressure sore is an acute inflammatory response within the epidermis with areas of irregular edema and induration. The epidermis remains warm and intact and the condition is reversible if pressure is relieved. A *grade II* pressure sore is a break in or blistering of the epidermis and dermis and extends into subcutaneous fat. A necrotic base in the subcutaneous tissue must be removed before healing can take place. A grade II pressure sore will heal after several weeks or months. A *grade III* pressure ulcer extends deeply into subcutaneous fat. There is distortion of muscle by swelling and inflammation. In a *grade IV* pressure ulcer, epithelial, adipose, and muscle tissue have necrosed; underlying bone or joint structures are involved. Grades III and IV ulcers require surgical closure after dead tissue has been removed and infections resolved. One of the severest complications that can result from the latter two ulcers is septicemia. What is seen at the skin surface is only the top of the ulcer, since 70 percent of the ulcer is below the skin. Pressure is transmitted in a cone-shaped manner from the skin through each layer of tissue to the body prominence so that a cone of tissue destruction is created (Fig. 24–4).

Many factors contribute to decubitus ulcer formation, and it is the nurse's responsibility to be fully aware of these factors. When clients move in bed they are exposed to **shearing**

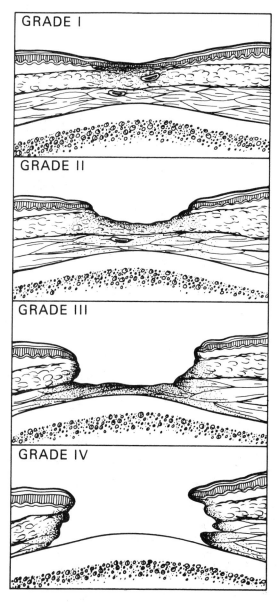

Figure 24–3. The development of a decubitus ulcer.

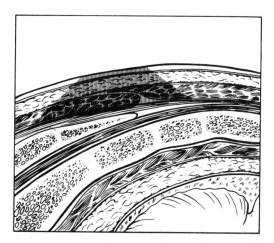

Figure 24–4. Cone of tissue destruction. The decubitus ulcer is almost always larger than its surface would suggest.

forces, where bone and underlying tissues move one way while the skin is held in place (Fig. 24–5). Shearing forces pull tissues rather than press on them. They move one layer of tissue over another. When the shearing forces are strong, the subcutaneous blood vessels can be kinked or stretched, and the soft tissues can be torn. When clients slip down in the bed in the inclined position (Fig. 24–5), and are pulled up or down in bed instead of being lifted properly, or if they dig their heels and elbows into the mattress, they are exposed to shearing forces. *Friction* injuries can be caused by rubbing against wrinkled sheets and overvigorous massage with towels. The danger sites include the front of the knees, the elbows, and the inner sides of the knees and ankles. *Moisture* from perspiration, draining wounds, or incontinence can cause skin to become swollen, soft, and easily damaged. Skin creases in fatty skin can develop moisture and friction resulting in sores around the genitals, between the thighs, and under pendulous breasts. *Edema* causes tissue pressure, so that cells have a reduced rate of oxygen and nutrient exchange. Edematous tissues also are more fragile and more liable to be injured.

Drugs injected into subcutaneous tissue in the same areas, instead of rotating sites, can cause skin breakdown. *Injuries* of the skin resulting in cracks or abrasions caused by long fingernails, poor equipment, and careless handling of clients may lead to ulcers. *Poor hygiene* can allow bacterial invasion of ischemic tissues, increasing the likelihood of development of an ulcer. *Fever* causes a client's metabolic rate to increase, increasing the demand for oxygen in an already compromised tissue area. *Anemia,* resulting in decreased hemoglobin, causes the oxygen supply to the skin to be reduced and can lead to skin breakdown or slow healing.

Several groups of clients are particularly susceptible to the development of sores. Most pressure sores occur in the elderly. Changes in the elderly brought about by the aging process include depression of resistance to infection and healing processes, hypertension, arteriosclerosis, tissue atrophy, and skin and muscle wasting. In general, the elderly have a loss of adaptability and are unable to respond to threats to their skin integrity with sufficient speed and flexibility. Other susceptible persons include thin, bony persons, and people who have peripheral edema, loss of peripheral sensation, loss of bowel and bladder control, motor paralysis, or complete immobilization. Anemia, cancer, obesity, and diabetes are examples of other precipitating factors.

Instruments are available to place under clients for measuring the surface pressure of weight against their skin. When a person is on a bed in the supine position, it has been found that the highest surface pressures are recorded under six locations, in order of highest to lowest: heel, occiput, buttocks, calves, scapulae, and elbows. The majority of decubitus ulcers have been found to occur over the sacrum, trochanter, heel, ischium, and ankle. The remainder of them occur on the lower leg, lateral edge of the foot, thigh, ear, scapula, iliac crest, anterior superior spine, knee, spinous process, achilles tendon, sole of the foot, shoulder, elbow, and big toe (Fig. 24–6).

Musculoskeletal and Peripheral Nervous Systems

Prolonged bedrest without protective measures can lead to much damage within the musculoskeletal and peripheral nervous systems. Changes occur that are not visible to the nurse

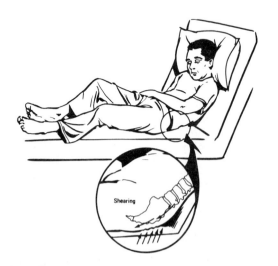

Figure 24–5. When a client assumes a poor position in bed, shearing forces occur where the bone and underlying tissues move one way while the skin is held in place.

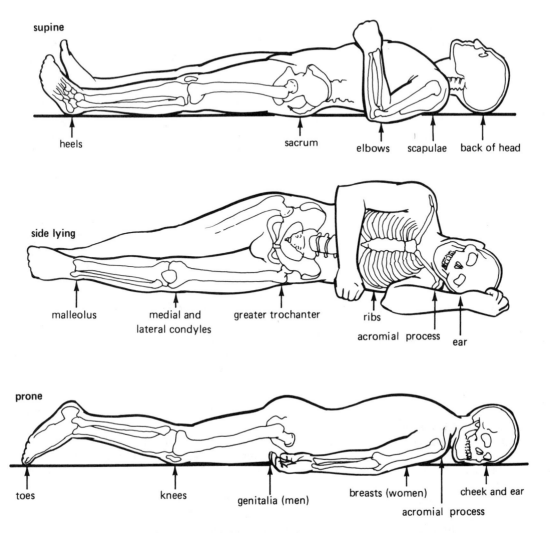

Figure 24–6. Pressure points in various positions.

until it is too late to prevent them. One of the problems that can occur is disuse **osteoporosis.** In a healthy person, bone is continually being built (osteoblastic activity) and at the same time being broken down (osteoclastic activity) at similar rates. These processes occur because of the normal stresses created by the pull of muscle on the bone. When a person becomes inactive, stress on the bones is decreased secondary to a decrease in muscle tension and resulting decreased stress on the long bones of the upper and lower legs. The osteoblastic and osteoclastic activities become imbalanced, and the osteo-

clasts break down the bone at a faster rate. The matrix of the bone becomes thinned and porous, and calcium and phosphorus are dissolved into the bloodstream and excreted. A high blood level of calcium can result in kidney stones and the deposition of calcium in the muscles and joints, causing pain. When bones become porous and spongy, they break under weight bearing, so that a client can develop a *pathological fracture.* This type of fracture occurs with slight or no trauma. The long bones of the lower extremities, the bodies of the vertebrae, and the heel bone are most involved in osteporosis.

Studies have shown that the loss of calcium can be reversed by weight bearing, such as standing for a few hours a day, which results in compression forces acting on the bone. Supine or sitting exercises or quiet sitting will not prevent calcium loss.[7]

Immobility results in a *decreased muscle mass and strength,* especially pronounced during the initial period of immobilization. A muscle maintains and increases strength through frequent contractions of muscle fibers. Without activity, there is a loss of strength and mass. Muscle mass is also lost in bedrest because of the concurrent protein breakdown. The muscles that are affected the most by immobility are those that the client uses for walking and the maintenance of an upright position.

Joints are also affected by immobility, because the flow of the synovial fluid ceases and its diffusion in and out of the cartilage stops. Absence of pressure fluctuations causes a stagnation of the intercellular fluid of the cartilage and decreases its nutrition. After prolonged immobilization, contractures of the joint capsule and periarticular muscles cause restriction of motion. Within the joint cavity connective tissue grows and causes adhesions. Clients who experience trauma, edema, and insufficient arterial circulation are prone to develop periarticular **contractures.** Their joints become contracted rapidly because of the formation of dense connective tissue once they stop walking unless range of motion exercises are performed regularly.

A *muscle contracture* is an abnormal shortening of muscle tissue resulting from decreased range of motion or immobilization in a shortened position. When a joint is poorly positioned, a dynamic imbalance of muscle power can occur as a stronger, unopposed muscle shortens and is never lengthened by its weak opponent. If not allowed to persist long, this condition is reversible. Eventually much of the muscle substance is replaced by fibrous tissue, and normal length and function cannot be restored.

If the foot is allowed to rest in an unsupported position, the muscles in the anterior portion of the leg become stretched. Also the tendon of the calf muscle tends to shorten. This results in a *foot-drop* deformity. When the client is ready to get out of bed and ambulate, the client's heel will not rest on the floor and the client has difficulty walking. When clients sit for long periods of time with their knees flexed and supported by pillows, they can develop knee-flexion contractures. At the posterior aspect of the thigh, the hamstring group of muscles, whose tendons pass under the knee, tends to contract quickly during immobility.

Clients on bedrest who are allowed to remain in the sitting position for prolonged periods of time have a danger of a prolonged outward rotation at the hips. Also, since the hips are flexed, such a client may develop a *hip-flexion contracture.* If there is a depression of the mattress at hip level, a contracture of the hip flexor muscles may occur, which will prevent the client from being able to fully extend (straighten) the hips when in the upright position. Clients who are continuously turned from side to side with their legs adducted (moved toward the body) and their hips and knees flexed will also develop contractures. If pillows are not placed between the thighs for alignment of the extremities, the person may develop a dislocation of the hip that was unsupported and adducted for too long.

Clients on bedrest with very little energy frequently lie with their arms held closely to the sides of the body, their wrists crossed and dropped, and their elbows flexed at right angles. The muscles at the axillary (armpit) level, especially the pectoral group, can develop contractures. Also, clients wearing a sling who do not perform range of motion exercises may get tight pectoral muscles and an adduction contracture.

Clients confined to bedrest frequently experience backaches. When the complaint is investigated, it is usually found that the client sits in a slumped position on the sacrum or lumbar spine with the chest caved in and shoulders sagging forward, pulled down by the weight of the arms. Pain and spasms then occur in the muscles of the back. Hips may not be back as far as possible in the angle of the bed so that body weight can be correctly borne on the ischia and the thighs. Pillows are sometimes found bunched up under the shoulders and head, leaving the spine out of its normal alignment. A soft mattress can also contribute to poor support for the client's back.

Immobility can cause damage to the nervous system. *Peripheral nerve damage* may occur from the improper use of tight restraints and poor body positioning, which cause compression and ischemia of superficial nerves that course around body prominences. Prolonged pressure on the peroneal nerve as it courses around the head of the fibula can occur from a tight plaster cast. Foot drop, or the inability to flex the foot and toes, can result. Characteristics of the ulnar nerve make it especially vulnerable to compression injury during bedrest.[8] Ulnar nerve compression results in altered sensory and motor function of the hand and occurs in the elbow area where the nerve crosses a joint and is close to the skin surface. With the forearm pronated (Fig. 24–7) the cubital tunnel is in contact with a surface so that *cubital tunnel compression syndrome* may occur. When the forearm is supinated, the ulnar nerve is free of external pressure at the cubital tunnel.

Elimination

Because of restriction of activity and changes in body positioning from upright to lying down, clients on bedrest frequently develop problems eliminating body wastes. When not adequately treated or controlled, elimination problems can become one of the immobile client's most trying problems.

When clients on bedrest are in a strange environment with a changed daily routine and lack of privacy, they may suppress the desire to defecate. If a person continues to avoid defecating when the urge is felt, gradually the **defecation** urge will become weaker. Also, as food enters the stomach and upper small intestine, the gastric reflexes normally cause fecal material to be emptied into the colon. Recumbency and inactivity alter the effect of meals, and the passage of fecal material is delayed. Physical activity and gravity both normally contribute to the propulsive movements of the colon.

Some immobilized people do not have the muscle strength to pass stool, especially if it is hard. Abdominal and perineal muscles used for defecating become weakened by bedrest. Also it is very difficult to bear down on a bedpan while in the sitting position in bed. Many clients do not have the physical strength to position themselves and lean forward on a bedpan. The changes in intrathoracic pressure caused by the Valsalva maneuver and the stimulation of the vagus nerve can cause complications such as heart block or cardiac arrest. Also, hemorrhoids, anal fissures, ulcers, and rectal prolapse can result from excessive straining at stool. Straining can increase intracranial pressure, which can cause serious damage to neurosurgical and eye surgery clients.

If the stool is allowed to become hard and dry, **constipation** can occur. When constipation continues, **fecal impaction** may result. With prolonged retention of feces in the colon, more water is absorbed and the stool becomes hard and dry. Liquid stool may begin oozing out around the impaction and mistakenly identified

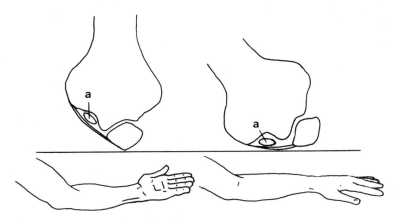

Figure 24–7. The ulnar nerve (a) is held in the cubital tunnel. In the supine client, with the forearm supinated (left), the cubital tunnel is free of external pressure. With the forearm pronated (right) in the supine client, the ulnar nerve is susceptible to injury by external compression at the cubital tunnel.

as diarrheal stool. A fecal impaction may result in a *mechanical bowel obstruction,* which interrupts the normal intestinal propulsions and movement of digested food and feces. This is a very serious situation and must be treated immediately.

Supine immobility has relatively little direct effect on the kidneys; however, when a client is first immobilized there is an increase in renal blood flow with a subsequent increase in urine volume. Immobility also causes an increase in the volume of tissue fluid being reabsorbed into the plasma, which in turn creates a temporary increase in urinary excretion. When a person is lying immobile on his or her back, the kidney pelvis does not completely drain. The opening of the kidney leading to the ureter is anatomically positioned to provide constant drainage of urine in the upright position. This prevents stasis of the urine. After just a few days in the supine position **urinary stasis** occurs in the kidney pelvis, and can result in infection and damage (Fig. 24–8).

Complete emptying of the bladder occurs more easily in the upright position. Many men find it very difficult to void while lying or sitting in bed. Once they are able to stand, they find that they can urinate quite easily. When voluntary actions are not adequately carried out due to awkward positioning or embarrassment, the urination cannot be initiated. The client may either wait too long to empty the bladder or only partially empty it. **Urinary retention** can cause bladder distention, which can result in a loss of bladder muscle tone, so that the client has no desire to void even though the bladder is full. The bladder becomes distended and urine may back up into the kidney pelvis, causing damage. The client may have to be catheterized in order to determine if there is residual urine in the bladder. Additional problems include severe discomfort, sensitivity to palpation, and restlessness.

During immobility, calcium is mobilized from the bone in the process of bone resorption and is excreted in the urine. When a client is in the supine position, as the urine sits in the renal calices there is more time for the calcium to precipitate. As tiny particles settle out of the urine, they are the beginning of *kidney or bladder stones.* Alkaline urine, dehydration, infection, and a decreased citric acid concentration also contribute to the formation of renal stones. Less calcium is held in solution as the urine becomes more alkaline, while dehydration produces less urine for washout of particulate matter. Infection can provide bacterial nuclei around which stones can form. Bacterial activity may decrease citric acid levels that normally help to maintain an acid pH. Fifteen to thirty percent of clients who have been on prolonged bedrest have kidney stones.

METABOLISM AND NUTRITION

At present little is known about what happens to a person's metabolism, fluid and electrolyte balance, and endocrine system, once the person is subjected to prolonged bedrest. It is well known, though, that proper nutrition plays a large role in maintaining crucial metabolic balances. Immobility induces a *decrease in the basal metabolic rate* and oxygen consumption of the body. The body requires less energy to function while on bedrest because there is less activity. Also, during bedrest the process of building new tissue from nutrients is slowed, whereas the processes that break down tissues are increased.

Normally the body tissues break down nitrogen, which is excreted through the urine and stool. On about the fifth to sixth day of im-

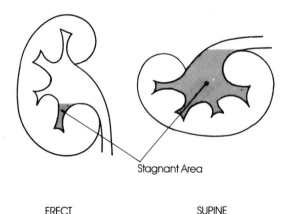

ERECT   SUPINE

Figure 24–8. The effect of body positions on the drainage of the pelvicaliceal system of the kidney.

mobilization, more nitrogen is excreted than is taken in, and a condition known as *negative nitrogen balance* develops. If people are immobilized after surgery or accidental trauma, excretion of nitrogen occurs earlier. By the second week of bedrest the negative nitrogen balance reaches its peak and gradually returns to a normal state. With negative nitrogen balance there is a depletion of stores for protein synthesis essential to healing skin ulcers and surgical or traumatic wounds. It is assumed that muscle tissue is the source of the excreted nitrogen. Clients on bedrest have *muscle mass decreases*, although their body weight tends to remain stable. With reduced muscular activity there is atrophy of skeletal muscle and the smooth muscles associated with gastrointestinal functioning. A client's protein status can be determined by subtracting nitrogen intake from output after a 24-hour collection has been analyzed. Protein status can also be assessed by evaluating lymphocyte production and the liver's production of transport proteins (albumin, transferrin, and prealbumin).[9]

Fluid and electrolyte imbalances can occur as a result of immobility. The kidneys' response to the changes in tissue metabolism induced by prolonged bedrest is excessive excretion of potassium and calcium. Another change that occurs during immobility is loss of appetite, or **anorexia.** A client who is inactive or immobile uses less energy and has a decreased rate of metabolism, and as an adaptive mechanism, appetite soon decreases. The client may also develop constipation and gas pains. Medications or other therapies may affect the client's ability to digest, absorb, or use nutrients in the food eaten. Boredom, depression, uninteresting unpalatable institutional food, and limited chewing abilities are other causes of anorexia. When a client does not eat enough, the body adapts to its lack of needed caloric intake by breaking down its own fat and protein supply. The client then goes into a negative nitrogen balance.

PSYCHOSOCIAL ASPECTS OF IMMOBILITY

When an individual experiences immobility, some of the ability to be independent within the environment is lost. This can be a confusing and sometimes threatening situation. Frequently, the nurse tends to focus so heavily on the client's physical problems that the psychosocial aspects of care are neglected.

Throughout the life span, each person has developed needs, a self-concept, and values that are essential for satisfaction, security, and comfort as a human being. A person may be feeling unwell and must be confined to bed but still needs safety and security, love and belongingness, self-esteem, privacy, and respect from others. Needs and values relating to prestige, status, and expectations of the self do not suddenly disappear when a person becomes physically ill.

A person who experiences immobility will begin to notice many changes—physical, internal, interpersonal, environmental, social, and cultural—all of which can cause a great deal of stress. Changes that can occur include sensory, perceptual, and tactile deprivation (see Chapter 22). Immobility, sensory deprivation, illness, and injury also cause changes in one's body image. Clients who are immobile in some way or who are on bedrest experience a variety of feelings, perceptions, and information about their bodies. They bring with them to the hospital previously formed, culturally determined values of how their bodies should look and feel. Clients with artificial limbs, for example, experience emotional stages of loss of the body part they once took for granted. Physical changes related to immobility present a significant threat to the identity.

The social isolation and depersonalization of a health-care institution also present problems. Immobility can cause a deprivation of interpersonal relationships and other self-actualizing activities. Clients can lie in bed for days, for example, without having a meaningful conversation with anyone. Unfortunately, nurses rarely have enough time to spend talking to clients. The client is likely to sleep or doze for longer periods of time. Sleep becomes an escape; however, it reduces all body functions such as respiratory rate and gastrointestinal motility. Sleep is a dangerous vicious cycle for the immobilized hospitalized client.[10]

Clients who are hospitalized and on bedrest also can experience isolation from loved ones. They are removed from close contact with family and close friends. People in the outside world may find it very inconvenient to visit. They may gradually come less frequently, as they find that they have increasingly less in common with the client. Elderly people who live alone and have problems with mobility also may find that they are deprived of close personal relationships.

Immobility can bring about temporary or permanent interpersonal and social role changes, too. Clients are suddenly unable to fulfill their basic self-care needs and become dependent upon others. They may lose their roles in the family as breadwinner, homemaker, decision maker, or parent. Financial, job, and community status changes occur. The client may have been making a large contribution to meeting the family's economic needs and providing valuable services to an employer. Clients may be painfully aware of their lowered community status and worry that their families are suffering financially. Time spent on bedrest also interferes with developmental tasks and valued goals. A client may be losing a large block of time out of his or her life. Children miss school and learning of developmental tasks. Adults must delay achieving various goals in life.

There is, inevitably, a cultural dimension to clients' and families' experiences of and reactions to immobility. The American culture places great emphasis on youth, vigor, strength, beauty, and activity. A client may feel an acute need to appear attractive and presentable for visitors. This need may not be recognized by a nurse who fails to look beyond the person's physical needs. The hospital environment can be very threatening to people who have lived in a society and culture different from that represented by institutionalized care. Men tend to have more difficulty than women in expressing their emotions, and some fare poorly in the dependent, sick role. Hospitalized men feel unproductive, for example, having been raised in a society with a strong work ethic. Foreign clients may be totally unaccustomed to being in a different cultural environment and require special foods, rituals, and religious services. Families in various cultures also react differently to the idea of caring for an immobile client at home.

As clients experience these many threatening changes, they can develop initial emotional responses of loneliness, depression, anger, frustration, anxiety, lowered self-esteem, inferiority, worthlessness, powerlessness, and a sense of boredom and monotony. These signs and symptoms of psychological stress may range in severity, and their significance is related to the client's coping patterns and support systems.

After experiencing initial psychological stress, the person goes through a phase of adaptation to psychological stress. A client uses adaptive measures to cope with and seek immediate relief from the discomfort of initial emotional responses. Behaviors may not involve conscious problem solving or be effective unless help is received. Ineffective adaptation behaviors exhibited by clients attempting to cope with their emotional responses to immobility include: extreme denial, dependency, disorientation, confusion, auditory and visual hallucinations, exaggerated emotional reactions, demanding and manipulative behaviors, aggressiveness, regression, withdrawal, apathy, and lessened motivation to learn and solve problems.

The psychological and physical stress of immobility also causes changes in certain mental functions and abilities. Changes include:

- Inability to sleep
- Decreased abilities to learn and solve problems
- Diminished drives and expectations
- Inability to cooperate with treatment programs
- Decreased speed of perception
- Deteriorated perception of time and place
- Decrease in the perceptions of pattern and form, weight discrimination, and pressure
- Decrease in temperature sensitivity

Many clients adapt well to psycological stress. They are able to direct their energies to accomplish important goals rather than to waste their time in ineffective, regressive activities. Those who adapt poorly and are unable to resolve their problems through defensive measures or problem solving tend to lose control until a state of crisis occurs. A client experiences a crisis situation when he or she is no longer able to respond with adequate coping mechanisms (see Chapter 26). Studies indicate that coping mechanisms determine adaptation to problems of life. A study of Harvard men over a 30-year period found that the coping mechanisms that most facilitate adaptation to life events and a changing environment are altruism, anticipation of events and actions, sublimation, humor, and suppression.[11] Social isolation is also a factor to consider when examining a client's abilities to cope. Loneliness, lack of social integration, and living alone are all somewhat detrimental to a client's motivation and functional improvement. Studies have shown that patients need to be in close contact with a significant other. They need a sense of social support and encouragement in order to enhance their motivation, which, in turn, contributes to their ability to respond to treatment.[12]

THE NURSING PROCESS

The main steps in the nursing process include assessment, nursing diagnosis, planning, implementation, and evaluation. Once the nurse assesses the client, using data collected in a systematic fashion, nursing diagnoses can be formulated. The nursing diagnoses communicate the client's problems and form the basis for the plan of care. When writing nursing diagnoses for a client the nurse is concerned with correcting and preventing problems and providing for maintenance, restorative, and rehabilitative needs and concerns of the client. All of the client's more basic needs are aimed at the ultimate goal of becoming a self-actualized, self-sufficient member of society. During the planning phase of the nursing process the nurse establishes priorities for the nursing diagnoses and establishes client outcomes. The outcomes consist of observable behaviors that the nurse would like for the client to demonstrate. Then nursing orders are written that will help the client to achieve the proposed outcomes. The implementation phase consists of performing the nursing orders and documenting the client's care. The evaluation phase of the nursing process consists of documenting whether or not the client outcomes were met and continual reassessment of all steps of the nursing process.

Assessment

During the assessment phase, the nurse performs an orderly collection of data relating to the client's physical, emotional, family, social, and environmental needs and problems. An assessment tool may be designed specifically for the purpose of assessing the client's responses to immobility. Refer to Figure 24–9 for an example of key components to include in such a tool. It is very important for nurses to make their assessments carefully and in sufficient detail to formulate accurate nursing diagnoses related to the client's independent nursing care. Because immobility can evoke such a broad range of responses, some of which develop slowly, it is important to include as much of this information as possible at the early stages of immobility. This initial baseline assessment usually is done at the time of admission or on the first home visit. In the case of hospitalized clients (or nursing home residents, etc.), a shorter version of this same type of assessment can be devised in a checklist format. Figure 24–9 can be used as a guide for either type of assessment.

The data for the psychosocial assessment of the client can be collected gradually as the nurse provides bedside care. Of particular importance is knowledge about how a client handles stress, what the support systems are, and how the client feels about him- or herself in general. Nonverbal behaviors, such as gestures, movements, and facial expressions, often give additional important information. A slumped body posture, for example, may indicate depression or withdrawal.

As nurses complete their assessments, they begin to identify problem areas and client needs that will lead to nursing diagnoses and form the basis of the nursing care plan. In addition to the information found in Figure 24–9, the following data categories are presented as guidelines in the assessment of responses to immobility:

Data Categories/Physical Components
- Oxygenation adequacy
- Acid-base balance
- Sensory functions
- Hormonal/metabolic functions
- Body temperature regulation
- Fluid and electrolyte balance
- Nutrition of body cells

Nursing Assessment for Problems of Immobility
Flow Sheet Checklist

Date						
Time						
Respirations regular/lungs clear						
Irregular respirations						
Shortness of breath						
Ashen/pallor/cyanosis						
Rales/rhonchi/wheezing						
Cough/sputum production						
Alert, awake, oriented						
Confused						
Restless/combative						
Drowsy/lethargic						
Comatose						
Heart sounds regular						
Peripheral pulses present						
Heart sounds irregular						
Peripheral pulse/pulses absent						
Legs unequal size/color/temp.						
Ankle edema						
Orthostatic B.P. changes						
Skin clear, warm, and dry						
Skin cool/moist						
Pressure sores/redness/edema						
Abrasions/burns/wounds						
Dry, scaly skin						
Good range of motion in joints						
Contractures						
Joint swelling						
Decreased muscle strength						
Fractures/casts/splints						
Daily stool						
Urine clear/adequate amount						
Bowel sounds absent						
Constipation						
Cloudy urine						
Burning/frequency of urination						
Incontinence						
Appetite good						
Good response to illness						
Taking nourishment poorly						
Complaints/poor coping patterns						
Sleeping poorly						
Presence of pain						
Family visited						

Figure 24–9. This assessment tool can be used each day as a guide and as a method of documenting that an assessment of the client was done. The nurse should mark the date and time the assessment was performed and then place a check mark by the appropriate signs, symptoms, and observations.

- Level of consciousness
- Elimination of body wastes
- Sleep, rest, and relaxation
- Hygiene and physical comfort
- Exercise, general mobility

Psychosocial Categories
- Protection from psychological threat and physical harm
- Privacy and a feeling of integrity
- Dependence and stability
- A predictable, orderly environment
- Love, affection, and sexual expression
- Acceptance, approval, and companionship
- A sense of value and usefulness
- Adequacy, self-reliance, and independence
- Goal achievement and mastery of skills
- Dignity, recognition and appreciation from others
- Attention, status, and importance
- Personal growth and maturity
- Increased learning and development of potential
- Religious and philosophical satisfaction
- Increased reality perception and problem-solving abilities

Nursing Diagnosis

Nursing diagnosis is the second phase of the nursing process. A nursing diagnosis statement consists of two parts joined by the phrase "related to" and begins with a determination of the problem of the client or client response (part I) and the *etiology* or associated contributing factors (part II). Occasionally the second part of the nursing diagnosis, or the etiology, may need to be extended into two parts, using the words "secondary to" or the abbreviation "2°." There are several guidelines for writing a nursing diagnosis. The diagnosis should be written in legally advisable terms without value judgments, using the term "related to" rather than "due to" or "caused by." Nurses should write the diagnosis in terms of the client's response to the health state rather than as a need. One should include only problems in the first part of the diagnosis, avoiding signs and symptoms of illness. The medical diagnosis should not be included in either of the two parts of the nursing diagnosis, and the two parts should not mean the same thing.[13] The following list of nursing diagnoses represent some typical examples appropriate for a client on prolonged bedrest[14]:

- Ineffective airway clearance related to pooling of tracheobronchial secretions secondary to immobility or ineffective cough
- Alteration in urine and bowel elimination related to decreased activity, lack of privacy, supine position, medications
- Potential fluid volume deficit related to altered intake secondary to immobility
- Potential for infection related to urinary stasis, pressure sores, pooling of lung secretions, dehydration, thrombus formation secondary to bedrest
- Impaired physical mobility related to contractures, muscle weakness, orthostatic intolerance secondary to bedrest and immobility
- Alteration in nutrition: Less than body requirements related to inability to ingest foods secondary to immobility
- Sleep pattern disturbance related to extended bedrest
- Social isolation related to extended hospitalization
- Spiritual distress related to removal from cultural and religious ties, challenged belief and value system
- Alteration in tissue perfusion related to venous stasis, dependent edema, thrombi, emboli secondary to immobility

Planning

During the planning stage the nurse determines what can be done to assist the client. This is when priorities are decided, *client outcomes* are written, and methods are designed to resolve problems and meet the client's needs. Client outcomes should be written so that they are observable and measurable. They are positive, realistic behaviors and signs that the nurse expects the client to exhibit. In many hospitals the written care plan is a legal document and is considered part of the client's chart. The evaluations of client outcomes are used in chart audits for quality assurance determinations. Therefore outcomes must be carefully written and time-limited so that they can be easily evaluated. The nurse should not use words such as absence of, lack of, or free from, since such outcomes are difficult to prove and measure and the list could become very lengthy. Instead of documenting the lack of a symptom, one should document exactly what one hopes to observe by a specific time. The following client outcomes are selected examples of objectives for the immobile client on extended bedrest[15]:

Client Outcomes, Example

- *Client evidences:*
  Clear lungs with bilateral equal breath sounds on auscultation
  Spontaneous, unlabored respirations, of normal pattern, 12 to 18 times per minute
  Pink or normal skin color for client
  Thin, clear or white sputum
  Negative sputum cultures
  Arterial blood gases within desired limits for client, usually Pao_2 60 to 100 mm Hg and $Paco_2$ 35 to 45 mm Hg
  Normal chest x-ray
  Extremities of equal size and color, temperature, and skin turgor
  Palpable peripheral pulses
  Stable blood pressure between 90/60 and 140/90 or within client's normal limits (may vary with age)
  Hemoglobin, hematocrit, and red blood cell levels within normal limits for client
  Clear, well-hydrated skin of normal coloration, turgor, and temperature
- Client exhibits freely movable joints with normal range of motion for client
- Client manifests normal equal muscle strength in all extremities
- Client performs active range of motion and breathing exercises independently
- Client increases amount of ambulation
- Client easily passes soft, formed, guaiac-negative stool of normal color every one to two days
- Client voids clear urine in reasonable amounts and intervals to a total of over 30 ml/hr
- Client displays alertness and orientation to person, place, time, and recent and remote memory
- Client displays calm, relaxed facial expressions and body posture
- Client participates in diversion and recreation
- Client communicates questions, needs, and problems to staff
- Client discusses own effective and ineffective coping patterns
- Client expresses preferences regarding his own plan of care
- Client makes contact with socially significant others

Implementation

After the planning stage the nurse is ready to implement the nursing plan. In the implementation phase the actual nursing care is provided, based on defined goals and outcomes. Nurses use technical, intellectual, and interpersonal skills to implement their objectives. Other members of the health-care team, such as dieticians, physical therapists, and respiratory therapists help the nurse to meet goals set for the client. Family members and the client should participate during the implementation phase. Many clients are able to live at home and be cared for comfortably by family members because of equipment available to assist persons who are immobile, such as portable lifters, multipurpose wheelchairs, and well-designed walking aids (Figure 24–10). Mechanical prostheses have been designed for useless limbs, and wheelchairs are even motorized now. Even with the best intentions, it is not always possible for the nurse to implement all of the goals set for the client and to prevent all of the hazards of bedrest and immobility. It is important to know, however, those nursing actions that are most likely to meet the needs of immobilized clients. The following discussion summarizes some of the most important nursing actions.

Proper positioning and body alignment are very important concepts to understand in the care of immobilized clients. A straight, hard bed supporting the body cannot match the normal curves of a person. Therefore, when a person is supine, the body parts that protrude posteriorly (occiput, sacrum, heels) must share most of the body weight. The segments in between them have no support and, therefore, tend to sag until the base of support is reached. These natural hollows need to be filled in or supported in order to maintain the axes of the hips and shoulders in relation to the spine. It is important to avoid the *hammock,* or *sling, effect,* which can occur when a client sits on a wheelchair cushion or lies on a bed with a tight cover (Figure 24–11A).

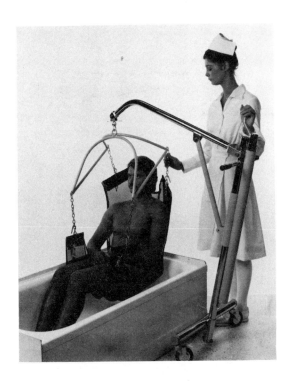

Figure 24–10. This portable lifter is for lifting people from supine to sitting and for transfer to wheelchair, commode, bath, and auto during home care. Such home aids can enable a severely immobilized person to live at home. *(Courtesy of Trans-Aid Corportion)*

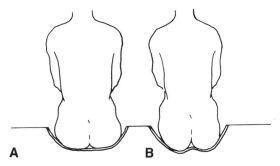

Figure 24–11. The hammock, or sling, effect can occur when draw sheets are tucked in too tightly over mattresses or wheelchair cushion covers are too tight.

A cushion cover must be loose and able to conform to the body's curves in order to prevent the effects of pressure (Fig. 24–11B).[16]

An important concept is that a good posture for a client on bedrest to assume is the same alignment of body segments that would be assumed to provide good posture in the vertical position (Fig. 24–12). Much equipment is available to help in positioning clients in bed, including pillows, footboards, special boots, splints, and palm grips (Fig. 24–13). Joints may occasionally have to be immobilized to treat a trauma or burn wound. The joint should be *optimally* positioned so that its stiffness will least interfere with the overall function of the extremity. If the joint surfaces are not under pressure, and the immobilization does not extend past four weeks, no permanent damage may result. Positioning a client properly in a wheelchair is also very important. The size of

the wheelchair should be prescribed by an occupational therapist to prevent pressure from the chair seat in the popliteal space and to allow free movement of the arms when propelling the chair.

A client should be given a role in maintaining proper positioning and promoting adequate circulation. When a client is on extended bedrest or in a chair, blood tends to pool in the legs. *The legs may be elevated* and elastic compression of the veins can be provided by using elastic bandage wraps or elastic stockings. *Elastic bandages* should terminate below the knee because those that are wrapped across the knee tend to act as tourniquets. The nurse can also discuss with the physician the possibility of using inflatable leggings that provide intermittent compression of the lower legs. Clients should be taught to exercise their lower extremity muscles to get the blood to flow more rapidly, preventing clotting. Certain positions cause impairment of venous return. *Positions to avoid* are flexion of the knees with the knee gatch or pillows, flexion of the hip with elevation of the head, leg compression from the bed, and the lateral recumbent (sidelying) position without support for the upper leg. Clients should be cautioned against crossing their legs at the knees, and they should be checked for garters, tight dressings, or constrictive clothing above the knees. Leg massages must be avoided so as to prevent turbulence and dislodged emboli. *Abdominal distention* should be relieved as soon as possible, because it causes compression of the great veins. For those clients with cardiac prob-

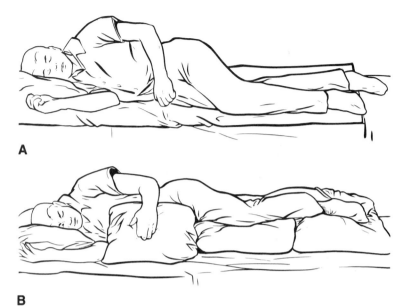

A

Figure 24–12. A. Poor body alignment. The arm rests on the chest and the calf of the upper leg compresses the tibia of the lower leg. **B.** Pillows are placed between the legs in order to align the lower extremities. A flat pillow should be provided so that the neck is not hyperextended.

B

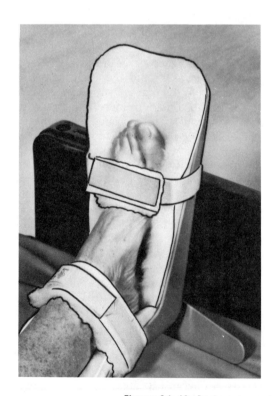

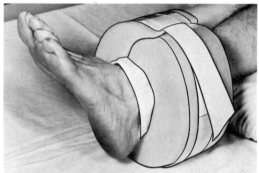

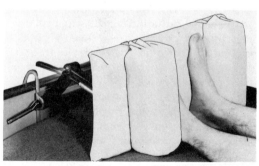

Figure 24–13. Bed equipment. *(Courtesy of the J.T. Posey Co.)*

lems, the head of the bed should be slightly elevated. This results in a decreased blood volume returning from the legs to the heart, thereby reducing the work of the heart. Clients should not be allowed to assume a *"slumped," half-lying position* in bed. This position causes backaches and compression of the abdominal viscera with restriction of the descent of the diaphragm. The pulmonary capacity becomes restricted.[17]

Turning a client to various positions, such as the side, back, other side, a sitting position, and possibly the **prone** position is very important for every body system. Clients who are able to move themselves will usually shift their positions automatically when they feel discomfort from pressure, but often they lie in one position in bed because of heavy sedation and fear of pain. Turning clients and having them shift their weight frequently prevents the blockage of blood flow caused by external pressure on the veins in the legs and promotes gravity drainage. The body's position should be altered frequently in relation to gravity, stimulating the postural neural reflex and *preventing orthostatic intolerance*. The client should periodically ambulate, have the head of the bed elevated, and sit on the side of the bed or in a chair. One should investigate the need for a bed that allows for position changes (Fig. 24–14). Also, nurses should avoid placing clients on fluid-filled beds for too long. A client resting on a fluid-filled bed tends to sag at the hips, resulting in slight but continuous flexion at the hip joints. This can lead to hip contractures and the pooling of blood in the pelvic area.[18] The nurse can instruct the client to breathe through an open mouth when moving in bed and straining at bowel movements, so as to *prevent the Valsalva maneuver*. An overbed frame and trapeze can be provided to help prevent the client from straining. To protect the skin, when clients are moved in bed they should not be pushed or pulled along the bed surface, to avoid strong shearing forces.

Because infrequent repositioning permits the same lung regions to remain dependent and at low lung volumes, it is necessary for a client to *change positions* at least every two hours to allow for decreased arteriovenous shunting and full expansion of all parts of the lung. Turns from side to side (120 degrees) help secretions to drain by gravity from the outer segments of each lung into the major bronchi, where they can be removed by coughing or suctioning. *Postural drainage,* or "tipping," can be used to drain pulmonary secretions by gravity. To aid in dislodging the secretions, the physician may order the physiotherapy techniques of manual percussion and vibration. After a thoracotomy or in unilateral lung disease, gas exchange is better when the client is sidelying with the "good lung" dependent and the affected lung uppermost. This allows increased perfusion to the healthy lung, which has better ventilation.[19] The client should be rolled well forward when being treated in the side-lying position to release the diaphragm from the pressure of the viscera.

Providing exercise for one's client is important in the prevention of contractures and muscle wasting and helps to empty the veins via the muscle pump. In-bed exercise also minimizes symptoms during recovery such as unsteady gait, backache, and leg pain. There is some evidence to suggest that during exercise a biochemical reaction is induced within the body that leads to mood elevation and enhanced mental functioning.[20] The various types of exercises available include an *active assistive* exercise carried out by the client with the assistance of the nurse or therapist, a *resistive* exercise in which the muscle contracts in pushing or pulling against a stationary object, an *active range of motion* exercise in which the client moves a joint through its full range of motion, and a *passive range of motion* exercise in which the therapist moves the client's joints through their complete range of motion. If joints are inflamed, exercises should be preceded by heat application, which relieves pain and muscle spasms. Occasionally *stretching* of a muscle contracture is performed by a physical therapist. The objective of stretching is to lengthen the fibrous connective tissue of the periarticular structures.

A client should be encouraged to perform *self-care activities* that encourage the use of the arms in abduction and outward rotation, including combing hair and fastening the gown. Using a footstrap or pushing against a footboard are also helpful. An overhead trapeze should always be available when the client is able to use it. Handblocks can serve the same purpose, and a rope ladder tied to the foot of the bed allows the client to maintain an upright

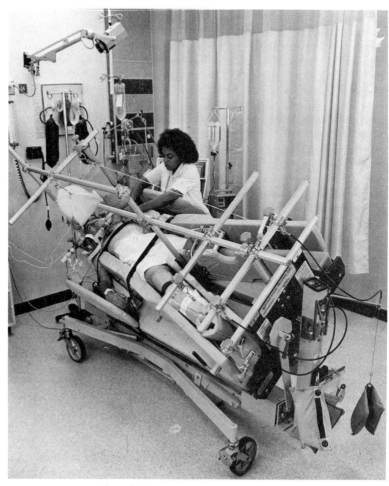

Figure 24–14. Roto-Rest Kinetic Treatment Table. For kinetic care of trauma clients. The Roto-Rest's silent motor slowly turns in a relaxing, continuous motion over 300 times a day. For therapeutic reasons, the immobile client is rotated automatically in an arc of 124 degrees every 3.5 minutes. The rotation is so slow it will not cause nausea or alarm, and the gentle vibration promotes sleep all night long without waking for turning. When properly positioned there is no head or neck movement that can cause further irreversible injury. Constant traction can be applied, and the weight does not vary. The constant motion of the bed prevents stasis of urine and respiratory secretions and the occurrence of thrombosis and embolism. *(Courtesy of Kinetic Concepts, Inc. San Antonio, Texas)*

position (Fig. 24–15). The client should also perform exercises that transmit forces lengthwise along the bone shaft of the lower extremities. This slows the demineralization process and prevents immobilization osteoporosis. The nurse should provide an opportunity for the client to *stand and bear weight* as soon as possible. When a client is moved from the bed to a wheelchair, the client should perform a standing pivot transfer. Standing whenever possible is one of the more effective means of lowering elevated serum calcium levels. Clients who are paralyzed need to have their movable beds locked into a standing position occasionally in order to prevent disuse osteoporosis. For ambulatory clients with problems walking or

standing there are many walking and sitting aids available.

Treatments commonly used for the prevention or treatment of pulmonary complications include: voluntary coughing and deep breathing, incentive spirometry, intermittent positive pressure breathing (IPPB), bronchoscopy, aerosol therapy, chest physical therapy, and more recently, intermittent continuous positive airway pressure (CPAP) by mask.[21] *Incentive spirometry* has become very popular in the prevention and treatment of atelectasis. The benefits include an improved coughing mechanism because of improved inspiratory capacity and a strengthening of the diaphragm. The best type of spirometer to use is the one with the

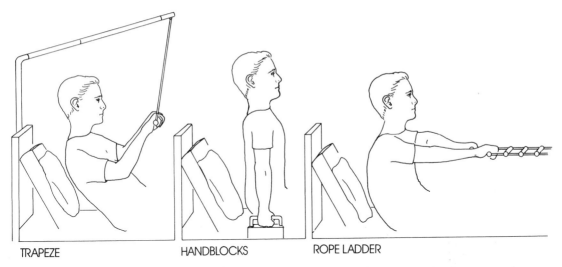

TRAPEZE   HANDBLOCKS   ROPE LADDER

Figure 24–15. Simple aids to help a client pull her- or himself up in bed.

breath-hold component. Research studies recommend that clients be asked to take ten maximal inspirations every hour while they are awake and that they incorporate the breath-hold if that option is available on the spirometer chosen.[22]

Coughing is the most important natural mechanism for the removal of secretions. Clients should be encouraged periodically to take a deep breath, hold it, and forciby cough two times. When possible, those with abdominal or chest surgery may be given pain medication 30 minutes before they are to be encouraged to cough. *Splinting* the abdominal muscles with a pillow is also helpful in providing support. A daily fluid intake of 2000 ml will help to prevent mucus secretions from becoming thick and viscous. Humidifiers or vaporizers are also useful to prevent irritation and drying of membranes and respiratory secretions. The promotion of self-care activities will increase a client's energy level, causing natural lung expansion and changes in position.

The prevention of *skin breakdown* is dependent on the provision of an ideal skin environment. A humidifier should be used to keep room relative humidity at about 40 percent. During the winter months room temperature should be as low as is reasonably comfortable (65°F or below). Nurses should *avoid excessive*

bathing of clients. It has been demonstrated that water—not lipid—governs the pliability of the epidermis. The most effective moisturizers reduce evaporation by forming occlusive or semiocclusive films that coat the skin surface.[23] They should be applied when the skin is moist after bathing or showering. A warm-water bath every 2 to 3 days is sufficient for most clients.

The nurse should teach the client and family about skin care and *skin inspection*. A paraplegic client who cannot shift position can be taught to use a mirror for inspecting posterior areas. Skin should be protected from abrasions and a wet environment. The need for absorbent bedpads or diapers should be investigated for incontinent clients. When plastic incontinent pads are used, they should always be covered with a soft drawsheet. Casts, braces, splints, and compression bandages should be inspected, adjusted, and padded. For clients who are highly susceptible to pressure sores, the nurse should investigate the possibility of obtaining devices designed to support either specific pressure areas or the entire body surface (Fig. 24–16). *Artificial sheepskins* help bring more of the client's body surface into contact with the supporting surface. They also help reduce friction, drain urine, and absorb moisture from the skin.

Decubitus ulcer care may become necessary for the immobilized clients who develop pres-

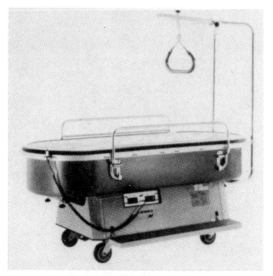

Figure 24–16. Clinitron therapy features an air-fluid-ized system of silicone-coated glass beads covered with a polyester sheet. This system reduces contact pressure to well below capillary closing levels and vir-tually eliminates friction, shear, and maceration. The unit also allows liquids and exudates to drain away from the client. *(Courtesy of Support Systems International, Charleston, South Carolina.)*

sure sores. There are many methods available. During the early stages of pressure sore devel-opment when a reddened area does not fade within the normal time, massaging the area should be avoided. Massaging will only cause greater damage. When *heat lamp therapy* is pre-scribed, the heat provides drying of skin and an increase in circulation to the area. Once skin is swollen and red or a small ulcer forms, often the physician will order a *protective dressing* or ointment to be applied. Desitin Ointment, tinc-ture of benzoin, and plastic sprays provide pro-tection against bedclothes and support fragile tissues (Fig. 24–17). The dressings should be porous, allowing hydration, and help to en-courage optimal regrowth of the external cel-lular layer.

Once a pressure ulcer with a moist exudate forms, research has shown that a moist, rather than a dry, environment may be more effective in promoting healing. Epidermal cells migrate across the wound bed about three times faster in a *moist exudate* than under a dehydrated ex-posed dermis.[24] Dressings such as Op-Site, when

left on for up to seven days, provide this desired moist environment. The exudate under the dressing contains leukocytes, which have a phagocytic action on bacteria and necrotic de-bris.

A deeper sore involving the tissue may ne-cessitate the *debridement* of necrotic tissue. The best method of reducing bacteria in pressure ulcers is to remove the dead tissue on which they thrive. Enzymatic agents, such as Elase Ointment, are used to remove this devitalized tissue. In some institutions Debrisan wound cleaning beads are used in large wet ulcers to absorb fluid and cleanse a wound area (Fig. 24–18). When a large decubitus ulcer is healing very slowly, the client may be susceptible to infection and loses serum and protein through the sore. Surgical intervention may be necessary. Preop-eratively the ulcer is debrided with irrigations and *wet-to-dry dressings* until a clean, healthy granulating bed of tissue is obtained. Surgery includes excision of the ulcer and scar tissue with skin grafting.

The prevention of *problems of elimination* is a major responsibility of the nurse. Clients need as much privacy as possible during elimi-nation, and unpleasant or foul odors should be removed from the environment. A client should be encouraged to respond to the urge to defecate in an unrushed manner and to perform exercises in bed that strengthen abdominal and pelvic floor muscles. Increasing activity and ambula-tion will help to stimulate gut motility. A plan of care can be developed to help the client stay on his or her *own schedule* of regular bowel movements. As soon as possible, the client should be permitted to get out of bed and use the bedside commode or bathroom so that he or she strains less and decreases energy expen-diture and anxiety. The best time for the client to attempt a bowel movement is after breakfast when the gastrocolic reflex causes the urge to defecate.

To avoid constipation in bedridden clients, they should be provided a *high-fiber diet* of be-tween 25 and 30 g.[25] Increased fiber in the in-testinal tract speeds a slow transit time, since fiber enlarges and softens stool. Foods high in dietary fiber include whole-grain breads and ce-reals, fresh fruit, root vegetables, and legumes. The cereal fibers seem to have maximum effect

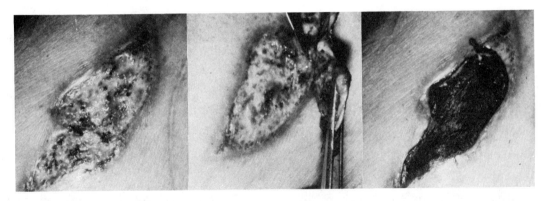

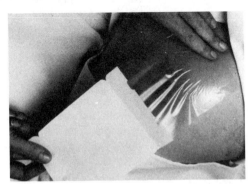

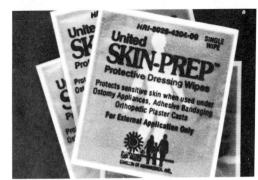

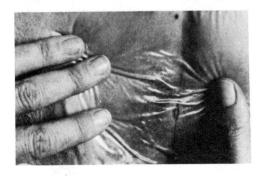

Figure 24–17. Various ointments and dressings are available to debride decubitus ulcers, support fragile tissues, and provide protection against bedclothes.

on bowel physiology.[26] When necessary a supplement of prune juice and apple pulp can be added. A minimum of *fluid intake* of 1500 to 2000 ml/day will help prevent stools from becoming hard, dry, and more difficult to evacuate. This excludes coffee, tea, or grapefruit juice, which are diuretics and tend to decrease body fluids. It is also important to check with the physician about weaning clients off constipating narcotics and other constipating drugs, such as some antacids.

To aid in emptying urine from the kidney,

a client should be placed in an *upright position* for at least part of the day (if permitted). A client with **urinary incontinence** may be encouraged to void every 2 hours. Then the interval can be lengthened as control is gained. Urine output should not be allowed to drop to less than 30 ml/hr. To help prevent urinary tract infections, the urinary pH can be kept *acid* by means of an acid-ash diet that includes cranberry juice, vitamin C, cereals, poultry, meat, and fish.

Ensuring adequate nutrition, fluid intake, and enough calories to meet the energy require-

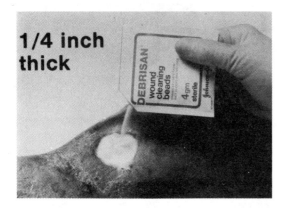

Figure 24–18. Debrisan wound cleaning beads are tiny hydrophilic beads of a dextranomer (sugar). As the beads swell with fluid, the spaces between them form a capillary system that draws bacteria and debris up and into the bead matrix. *(Courtesy of Johnson & Johnson Products, Inc., New Brunswick, New Jersey.)*

ments of the client is an important nursing intervention. The recommended daily caloric allowance for the average person in the resting state is 1500 calories for males and 1000 calories for females. Fever, stress, certain drugs, trauma, and wound healing can elevate a client's basal caloric requirements significantly. The immediately postoperative client requires between 2500 and 4000 calories per day. A daily calorie count can be kept with a record of exactly what the client eats. Clients should be encouraged to eat high-protein foods and supplements such as Ensure Plus, Magnacal, or Osmolite HN.

Vitamins A, C, and K are essential for wound repair. Trace elements such as zinc, copper, and iron play an important role in collagen synthesis and scar formation.[27] Monitoring for iron-deficiency anemia or anemia caused by blood loss and hypoalbuminemia is also recommended. An adequate fluid intake of at least 1500 ml/day is necessary to provide hydration to the skin and to provide dilute, free-flowing urine. Loose clothes, a comfortable room temperature, and position changes help to prevent fluid loss through perspiration. A low-calcium diet and sufficient fluids help to reduce kidney stones and blood viscosity, keeping blood clots from forming so easily.

A client's fluid intake, vomitus, stools, urine, and wound drainage should be carefully measured. One of the best ways to monitor progress is through *daily weights.* An environment conducive to eating, with a more sociable or variable setting may help the client to finish meals. Unpleasant procedures and the administration of sedatives before a meal can prevent the client from being alert and comfortable while eating. Good *oral hygiene* will help a client to retain the full range of chewing abilities. Self-help aids that include special cups and eating utensils are available for clients who lack the ability or energy to feed themselves (Fig. 24–19).

Meeting *psychosocial needs* is another important nursing intervention. After the nurse has assessed the threatening changes a client is experiencing and the emotional responses to them, the client must be helped to adapt to the new situation. The client will have to learn to adjust to negative events and realities. The client will need help in learning more about his or her emotional reactions to problems and how to use *effective coping mechanisms.* The nurse must always be alert for ineffectual adaptation behaviors. For the client who is adapting well, the nurse may serve simply as a good listener.

While clients are in bed they may need to be provided with *diversional activities* and *sensory stimulation.* The nurse should ensure that they wear their eyeglasses and hearing aids. Tactile stimulation like back massage is important, and a sense of caring and understanding can be conveyed when a nurse touches a client, holds a hand or arm, or gives a hug. Clients should continue satisfying relationships with others. Opportunities for them to *socialize* can be provided. A communication board can be used for the client who is severely physically disabled.[28] A client should be constantly *reoriented* to the environment and encouraged to maintain normal sleep patterns. He or she can help to make decisions about self-care. When possible, alternatives should be provided and he or she should be informed of what can be expected and what is expected of him or her. Families also need support and encouragement to participate in the client's care and to continue with their own lives.

Evaluation

The last phase of the nursing process is evaluation, which is an on-going process. The nurse collects specific evidence about the client's

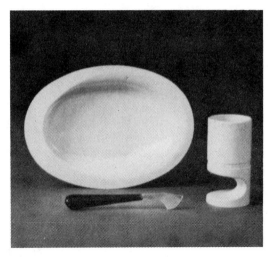

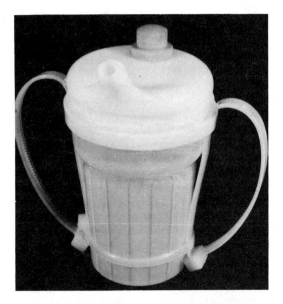

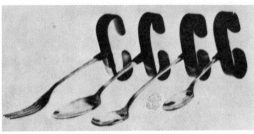

Figure 24–19. Self-help feeding aids can enable the immobilized client to become more independent.

health status to determine if the client's progress matches the outcome criteria set for him or her. If the client is not meeting the outcomes by the specified time limit, reassessment should occur, and the nursing care plan should be updated. The nurse documents the date of the evaluation of the outcomes on the client's written care plan. The evaluation of the client should be documented using specific observations or client statements. The care plan can then be used as a legal record for quality assurance purposes.

SUMMARY

The problems and disabilities associated with bedrest and immobility represent one of the nation's major health problems. Nurses must work toward maintaining and maximizing physiological and psychosocial mobility to avoid the in-evitable disabilities of immobilization. When immobility and bedrest are unavoidable, the nurse is responsible for helping the client to adapt. After a thorough assessment, nurses should determine the client's needs and problems and specify nursing diagnoses and client outcomes to provide for the preventative, maintenance, therapeutic, and restorative needs of the client. The nurse, client, family, and health-care team should all contribute to the planning phase of the client's care. Nurses should hold themselves accountable for using the most effective client care therapies and commercial products available for the client who is susceptible to immobilization disabilities. They must take the responsibility to ensure that the care is evaluated, outcomes are met, and corrective action is taken.

Immobility is an intentional or involuntary limitation of activity in any sphere of a person's physical, emotional, intellectual, social, or cultural experience. Mobility is the ability to move freely and easily without restrictions in one's chosen environment. A person can be rendered immobile in many ways. Types of immobility include physical, psychological, intellectual, and social. Bedrest and immobility do have some beneficial effects, but to immobilize a person for an excessive length of time can be damaging.

Problems with the respiratory system that may occur with prolonged bedrest include atelectasis, hypostatic pneumonia, aspiration, and pulmonary embolus. Hazards for the cardiovascular system can include circulatory stasis, edema, thrombus formation, thrombophlebitis, emboli, orthostatic hypotension, increased workload of the heart, and decreased exercise tolerance. Nursing interventions in the care of the cardiovascular and respiratory systems include elevation of extremities, in-bed exercises, use of elastic stockings, avoidance of supine position and Valsalva maneuver, early ambulation, frequent changes in position, postural drainage, chest physiotherapy, incentive spirometry, coughing and removal of secretions, hydration and humidification, and promotion of self-care and health teaching.

When a person remains too long in one position, decubitus ulcers may form, especially over bony prominences. Factors contributing to decubitus ulcer formation include shearing forces, friction, moisture, edema, anemia, poor hygiene and nutrition, skin creases, and injuries. Principles in the prevention and treatment of pressure sores include good hygiene and nutrition, hydration, protective dressings, topical therapy, surgical debridement, and frequent changes in body positioning. Immobility can also lead to problems in the musculoskeletal system, such as osteoporosis, loss of muscle mass and strength, muscle and joint contractures, backaches, and nerve damage. Preventative measures include range of motion exercises and good body alignment and positioning.

When a client on bedrest is in a strange environment with a changed daily routine and lack of privacy, bowel problems such as constipation, leading to fecal impaction and mechanical bowel obstruction may develop. Other elimination problems include those of the urinary tract—renal stones, difficulty in urination, and urinary stasis, retention, and incontinence. Measures that help to prevent elimination problems include a high-fiber diet, a good bowel regimen, exercise, and intake of sufficient fluids. Immobility also induces changes in the basal metabolic rate, a negative nitrogen balance, muscle mass decrease, fluid and electrolyte imbalances, and nutritional changes such as anorexia.

Internal, interpersonal, environmental, social, and cultural changes can also be caused by bedrest and immobility. These include sensory deprivation, sensory overload, distortion, and monotony; changes in body image; social isolation and depersonalization; significant-other deprivation; interpersonal and social role changes; changes in financial, job, and community status; interference with developmental tasks and valued goals; and exposure to different cultural expectations. As clients realize that their goals of security and need-satisfaction are not being met, they respond with various emotions. While attempting to adapt to unexpected changes, clients sometimes use ineffective coping styles. It is the responsibility of the nurse to assess the client's adaptation to immobility, to help him or her learn more about the emotional reactions to problems, and to teach him or her how to use effective coping mechanisms.

Study Questions

1. What are the various ways in which a person may be rendered immobile?

2. What are the stages in the development of a decubitus ulcer, and what factors can contribute to decubitus ulcer formation?

3. What is a contracture, where do contractures most commonly occur in the body, and how can they be prevented?

4. What are some of the problems that can occur within the cardiovascular system if a client remains on extended bedrest?

5. Why should a client avoid performing a Valsalva maneuver?

6. Why can anorexia occur in an inactive or immobile person, and what are some nursing interventions you might recommend for a patient who is malnourished?

7. How might a client develop respiratory problems while on bedrest?

8. What are four main problems that can occur within the urinary tract due to immobility? How do these problems occur?

9. What nursing diagnoses might be pertinent to describe ineffective psychosocial adaptation of a client on prolonged bedrest?

10. How might a nurse help a client to cope more effectively with feelings and reactions to immobility?

References

1. R. Asher, "The dangers of going to bed," *Br Med J* 2, (1947):967–69.
2. J. J. Marini, "Postoperative atelectasis: Pathophysiology, clinical importance, and principles of management," *Respir Care* 29, (May 1984): 516–21.
3. N.L. Browse, *The Physiology and Pathology of Bed Rest* (London: Thomas Books, 1965), 151.
4. E.H. Winslow, "Cardiovascular consequences of bed rest," *Heart and Lung* 14, (May 1985):236–45.
5. C. Torrance, *Pressure Sores. Aetiology, Treatment, and Prevention* (London: Croom Helm Ltd., 1983), 18.
6. M. Phipps, B. Bauman, D. Berner, et al., "Staging care for pressure sores," *Am J Nurs* 84, (1984):999–1003.
7. E.H. Winslow "Cardiovascular consequences of bed rest," 236–45.
8. M.A. Chuman, "Risk factors associated with ulnar nerve compression in bedridden patients," *J Neurosurg Nurs* 17,(December 1985):338–42.
9. C.R. Kneisl and S.W. Ames, ed., *Adult Health Nursing. A Biopsychosocial Approach* (Menlo Park, Calif.: Addison-Wesley, 1986), 200.
10. V.M. Fitzsimons, "Maintaining a positive environment for the older adult," *Orthop Nurs* 4, (May/June 1985):48–51.
11. M. Friedman-Campbell and C.A. Hart, "Theoretical strategies and nursing interventions to promote psychosocial adaptation to spinal cord injuries and disability," *J Neurosurg Nurs* 16, (December 1984):335–41.
12. F.U. Steinberg, *The Immobilized Patient. Functional Pathology and Management* (New York: Plenum Medical Book Co., 1980).
13. P.W. Iyer, B.J. Taptich, and D. Bernochhi-Losey, *Nursing Process and Nursing Diagnosis* (Philadelphia: W.B. Saunders Co., 1986), 98–102.
14. T.A. Duespohl, *Nursing Diagnosis Manual for the Well and Ill Client* (Philadelphia: W.B. Saunders Co., 1986).
15. J.R. Lederer, G.L. Marculescu, J. Gallagher, and P. Mills, *Care Planning Pocket Guide. A Nursing Diagnosis Approach* (Menlo Park, Calif.: Addison-Wesley, 1986).
16. Torrance, *Pressure Sores,* 1–29.
17. W.J. Crosbie and S. Myles "An investigation into the effect of postural modification on some aspects of normal pulmonary function," *Physiotherapy* 71, (July 1985):311–14.
18. M.L. Shannon, "Famous fallacies about pressure sores," *Nursing 84,* 14, (October 1984):34–41.
19. A. Hough, "The effect of posture on lung function," *Physiotherapy* 70, (March 1984):101–103.
20. C.J. Parent and A.L. Whall, "Are physical activity, self-esteem and depression related? *J Gerontol Nurs* 10(9),(1985).
21. R.K. Albert, "Prevention and treatment of postoperative atelectasis." *Chest* 87, (January 1985): 1–3.
22. L. Grant-Paterson and N.B. Moodie, "Incentive spirometry: An adjunct to chest physiotherapy," *Physiotherapy Can* 37, (November/December 1985):388–93.
23. W.I. Dotz and B. Berman, "Dry skin. Aids that preserve hydration and mitigate its loss," *Consultant* 24, (August 1984):46–62.
24. G. Kurzuk-Howard, L. Simpson, and A. Palmieri, "Decubitus ulcer care: A comparative study," *West J Nurs Res* 7, (February 1985): 58–79.
25. M. Burr and M. Alton, "Constipation in immobile patients," *Med J Aust* 14, (March 1984):446–47.
26. B. Resnick, "Constipation. Common but preventable," *Geriatric Nurs* 6, (July/August 1985):213–15.
27. C.G. Skiar, "Pressure ulcer management in the neurologically impaired patient," *J Neurosurg Nurs* 17, (February 1985):30–35.
28. Y. Wu and J.A. Voda, "User-friendly communication board for nonverbal, severely physically disabled individuals," *Arch Phys Med Rehabil* 66, (December 1985):827–28.

Annotated Bibliography

Christian, B.J. 1982. *Immobilization: Psychosocial aspects.* In C.M. Norris, Concept Clarification in Nursing. Rockville. Md.: Aspen Systems Corp. A comprehensive, fairly advanced-level discussion that classifies immobility into eight types of limitation of movement. Models for the sequential assessment of immobilization are developed.

Gardner, S.S., and Johnston-Whisman, L. 1985. Aids to Independence. *J Pract Nurs* 3:31–35. This article describes how to assess rehabilitative home-care needs. Various products and devices are depicted that are useful for the client with immobility handicaps.

Jackson, S. 1985. The Touching Process in Rehabilitation. *Aust Nurs J* 14(11):43–45. This sensitive, well-written article discusses the need for touch and task-oriented touch in the elderly institutionalized, the terminally ill, and in clients with confusion or inappropriate behavior.

Lucke, K., and Jarlsberg, C. 1985. How is the Air-Fluidized Bed Best Used? *Am J Nurs* 85:1338–40. This journal article summarizes the advantages, limitations, and complications of the air-fluidized bed, based on recent research.

Porecca, R.C., and Chagares, R.C. 1983. Op-Site: A treatment for pressure sores in the orthopaedic patient population. *Orthop Nurs* 2(5):30–35. This research article presents a study that demonstrated the benefits of Op-Site in producing significant wound healing of pressure sores in the orthopedic client population.

Shefts, D.L., Topping, R., and Zieman, L.K. 1984. Bowel Management Protocol. *Home Healthcare Nurs* 2(5):17–20. This article presents a very good assessment of a client's bowel history with a flow sheet and questionnaire. Bowel management steps and a fiber content food list are very helpful.

Tyler, M.L. 1984. The Respiratory Effects of Body Positioning and Immobilization. *Resp Care* 29(5):472–80. This is an excellent article which is a review of the research literature on the effects of the lateral decubitus, upright, prone, and head-dependent positions on arterial blood gas values.

Urosevick, P.R., ed. 1980. *Nursing Photobook. Providing Early Mobility.* Horsham, Penn.: Nursing 80 Books, Intermed Communications, Inc. This book has excellent illustrations that demonstrate in detail the technical care of the immobile client. Topics of the chapters include body mechanics, turning and positioning, strengthening exercises, performing transfers, special equipment, and environmental considerations.

Chapter 25

Pain

Marion R. Johnson
Joann M. Eland

Chapter Outline

- Objectives
- Glossary
- Introduction
- Pain Theories
- Characteristics and Classification of Pain
- Intervening Variables
- Persons at Risk
- Response to Pain
- The Nursing Process
    Assessment
    Planning
    Implementation
    Evaluation
- Summary
- Study Questions
- References
- Annotated Bibliography

Objectives

After reading this chapter, the reader will be able to:

- Discuss the concept of pain and relate it to the gate-control theory of pain
- Describe differences in types of pain: acute, chronic, and progressive
- Identify variables that may alter the perception of and resonse to pain
- Describe physiological and psychological re-
sponses to pain and relate them to types of pain
- Apply pain assessment techniques in a clinical situation
- Discuss factors to be considered in selecting a nursing intervention for the person experiencing pain
- Describe a process that may be used in relaxation and in distraction of persons who are experiencing pain
- Identify how various types of analgesics may be used most effectively in pain control
- Discuss the use of placebos in pain control
- Identify behavioral outcomes that may be used to evaluate pain control

Glossary

Analgesic. Medication used for the purpose of pain relief.

Endorphins. Endogenous opioid peptides. Chemical regulators that probably modulate pain by binding with opiate receptor sites throughout the nervous system, inhibiting release of neurotransmitters, and may alter pain perception.

Pain Reaction. Multiplicity of events or responses set up by a pain sensation.

Pain Sensation. Recognition of perception of pain.

519

Pain Threshold. The lowest stimulus value at which pain sensation is reported.

Pain Tolerance. Maximum level of pain sensation tolerated.

Placebo. An inactive substance used as an analgesic.

T-cells. A group of ascending neurons in the spinal cord that are influenced by the "gating mechanism"

INTRODUCTION

Pain is a symptom commonly encountered in individuals seeking health care, and it is, therefore, an important concept for nursing. The person with pain may be encountered in any clinical area and in any health-care setting. Nurses are often responsible for pain assessment and alleviation on a continuous basis. Because of the frequency with which the nurse encounters persons with pain, it is necessary to develop skills to assist the person experiencing pain.

What is pain? A warning, a sensation, a perception? Despite intensive study and research during the last decades, a concrete definition of pain, acceptable to all disciplines, has not been formulated. Richard Sternbach has defined pain as an "abstract concept which refers to (1) a personal, private sensation of hurt; (2) a harmful stimulus which signals current or impending tissue damage; (3) a pattern of responses which operate to protect the organism from harm."[1] Although this definition separates components of pain for the purpose of clarification and research, it must be recognized that these components overlap or occur simultaneously in the pain experience. Margo McCaffery's definition of pain is perhaps the most useful to the practicing nurse; she defines pain as "whatever the person says it is, existing whenever he says it does."[2] This definition of pain requires nurses to approach the pain experience from the perspective of the suffering individual.

PAIN THEORIES

In spite of the efforts of countless researchers, the exact mechanism of pain remains unknown.

Various theories have evolved over the years including specificity, pattern, and gate-control theory. The developers of each of the theories have attempted to improve previous theories to explain the complex phenomenon known as pain.

The *specificity theory* is perhaps the most traditional of the three, dating back at least 200 years (Fig. 25–1). It proposes that pain travels from specific pain receptors to a pain center in the brain. Furthermore, specificity theory assumes that the relationship between a pain stimulus and pain response is direct, uniform, and invariable. The impulses are picked up by undifferentiated free nerve endings and carried by peripheral nerves to the spinal cord and then transmitted to the pain center in the thalamus. Those opposing this theory have taken issue with its failure to explain why the same stimulus presented to two different people is not always felt as pain.[3]

Pattern theory evolved from specificity theory and includes several slightly different theories. Peripheral pattern theory, central summation theory, and sensory interaction theory are all examples of what has been classified as pattern theory. Proponents of peripheral pattern theory believe that peripheral nerve fibers are essentially the same and a given pattern of fiber stimulation is interpreted centrally as pain. Central summation theory is especially useful in explaining phenomena such as phantom limb pain, causalgia, and the neuralgias. It proposes that peripheral nerve input stimulates specific areas in the dorsal horn of the spinal cord; stimulations in these areas are interpreted as pain. The focus of this theory is within the dorsal horn of the spinal cord where input creates abnormal reverberatory activity in closed, self-exciting neuron loops. The prolonged activity stimulates the **T-cells,** which in turn project to brain mechanisms, and the result is interpreted as pain. Sensory interaction theory proposes that there are peripherally small- and large-diameter pain fibers. The small fibers carry the nerve impulse patterns that produce pain and the large fibers inhibit pain. Pain is perceived when the number of small fiber volleys outnumber the large-diameter volleys.[4]

In 1965, Melzack and Wall proposed what is now the most commonly accepted theory of the pain mechanism, the *gate-control theory.*[5]

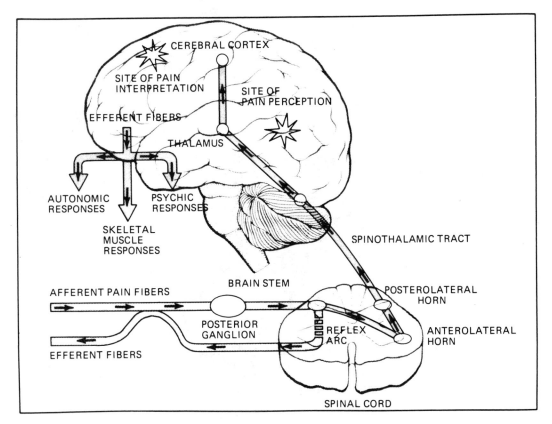

Figure 25–1. Specificity theory of pain.

The gate-control theory suggests that there is a gating mechanism (Fig. 25–2) in the dorsal horn of the spinal cord that can increase or decrease the flow of nerve impulses from peripheral fibers to the central nervous system. This gating mechanism is influenced by the activities of the larger-diameter A-Beta, smaller-diameter A-Delta and C fibers, and by descending influences from the brain. The small-diameter afferent fibers (A-Delta and C) conduct excitatory pain signals. Stimulation of the large-diameter cutaneous afferent fibers (A-Beta) inhibits the transmission of pain impulses. Both the small- and large-diameter fibers terminate in the dorsal horn of the spinal cord in an area known as the substantia gelatinosa (the gate and T-cell). The spinal gating mechanism also is influenced by nerve impulses that descend from the brain.

A specialized system of large-diameter fibers rapidly conducts impulses directly to the brain, activating selective cognitive processes that can influence the gating mechanisms by the descending fibers. This specialized system explains how an individual's past and present experiences influence current pain responses. The T-cell within the substantia gelatinosa acts as a calculator to sum information from the small fibers, the large fibers (A-Beta), and the descending fibers. When the excitatory input from the small fibers outnumbers input from the inhibitory (A-Beta) and descending fibers, the T-cell "opens" the gate and allows information about pain to be transmitted to the brain. Several ascending pathways are important contributors to pain transmission. The most prominently involved in pain transmission is the lateral spinothalamic tract, which has two parallel divisions: the *neospinothalamic tract* and the *paleospinothalamic tract*. (For further information consult a physiology text.)

These tracts enter the thalamus, which is a major relay system. Within the context of pain,

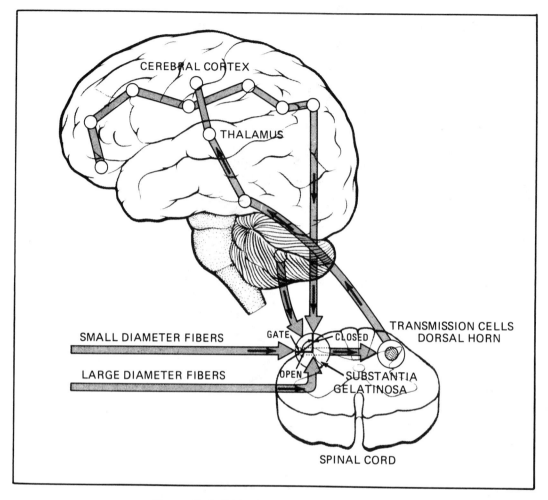

Figure 25–2. The gate-control theory of pain.

its function can be compared to a major telephone switchboard where thousands of messages are routed to specific destinations. Messages from paleospinothalamic ascending fibers are routed to reticular and limbic structures and then processed by the cerebrum. The retricular and limbic structures produce the *unpleasant affective quality* associated with pain, activate the stress response, and motivate the organism to stop pain. Sensory discriminatory messages are routed directly to the cerebrum. The cerebrum and thalamus together are called the *central control* center by Melzack and Wall.

Central control processes information from three sources: sensory discrimination information, motivational affective information, the body's fight or flight response; and cognitive information including such things as past experiences and response alternatives.[6]

In 1983 Melzack and Wall added to the gate-control theory of pain. The new model includes excitatory and inhibitory links from the substantia gelatinosa to the T-cell as well as descending inhibitory control from the brainstem systems. The specialization of the substantia gelatinosa has been the subject of much research and the additions of the information about the stimuli to the substantia are an attempt to incorporate new knowledge about this physiologically complex area within the spinal cord.[7]

Each person has cataloged, in central control, a variety of previous experiences involving pain as well as a number of intervening variables in the pain response, such as age, sex, socioeconomic status, race, and ethnic group expectations. Because pain stimuli are processed within each individual's own context, a wide variety of pain responses is seen.

CHARACTERISTICS AND CLASSIFICATION OF PAIN

Although agreement on definitions and theories of pain is not at present available in the literature, some attributes of the pain experience are more consistently described than others. **Pain threshold** identifies the lowest stimulus value at which the sensation of pain is reported, whereas **pain tolerance** identifies the maximum level of sensory stimulus one is willing to tolerate.[8] The difference between pain threshold and pain tolerance may be referred to as the pain *sensitivity range*.[9] Researchers have shown the pain threshold to be relatively constant, providing the central nervous system is intact, whereas significant variations in pain tolerance occur. Pain threshold depends on physiological factors, whereas pain tolerance depends on psychological and social factors.[10] It is also important to note that pain tolerance may vary in the same individual in differing circumstances. For example an individual may be less aware of, or more willing to tolerate, muscle spasm while involved in competitive sports than while recovering from an appendectomy. Studies of pain tolerance have significance to the nurse, since efforts to alter the pain experience will often be directed at altering the pain tolerance level rather than the pain threshold level.

Researchers usually distinguish between the pain sensation and pain reaction. **Pain sensation** could be equated with the pain threshold. **Pain reaction** may be used to include only the mental processing. The typical pain response seems designed to protect the individual from further harm and may consist of automatic behaviors and responses learned as methods of coping with pain. The pain response will be affected by[11]:

- The integrity of the central nervous system
- The level of consciousness
- Previous experience with pain
- Learned coping mechanisms
- Attention and distraction
- Fatigue
- Emotions

The pain sensation cannot be observed but must be reported by the subject; the reaction will be observable as the behaviors elicited by the pain stimulation. Both sensation and reaction are evaluated during a clinical assessment of pain.

A very simplified example of the components in a common pain experience may clarify the concepts. Slamming a finger in a door causes two distinct sensations in most individuals—a sharp, quick pain followed by a throbbing or dull ache. This is the basic sensory component and will be quite consistent with most people. What the individual does—the verbal expression of pain as well as motor behaviors, such as squeezing the finger—can be considered indicative of the reaction component. Even with such a simple pain, we might observe different verbal motor responses; this helps us appreciate the variety of responses that can occur with more complex pain experiences. What the individual feels and the degree of hurt experienced is the personal, subjective aspect of pain that can be shared only through verbal communication and only imperfectly, because of the constraints imposed by language.

Pain is classified using more than one typology. Common parameters used to classify types of pain include:

- Physiological versus psychological factors as sources of pain
- The physiological source of pain
- The duration of the pain

Pain is often labeled as psychogenic or organic, depending on whether a physiological cause for the pain can be determined. There is a tendency to treat organic pain as "real" pain and psychogenic pain as "imaginary" pain; this dichotomy carries the implication that suffering does not occur without demonstrable pathology. A more accurate and fruitful approach is to view pain as a continuum in which physiological and psychological factors play greater or lesser roles depending on whether the pain is triggered by a mental or physical stimulus. Psychological factors may cause pain or augment its severity. Three psychological mechanisms that may precipitate or increase pain are[12]:

- The occurrence of pain as a hallucination in conjunction which schizophrenia or endogenous depression
- Pain caused by muscle tension, vascular distention, or other physical changes caused by psychological factors
- Pain associated with conversion hysteria

Anxiety may intensify pain, therefore anxiety may need to be controlled if pain relief is to be obtained. Determining the degree to which psychological factors are important is a necessary requisite for determining the method of treatment that will prove most successful.

The type of tissue or organ that is the *source of pain* may determine aspects of the sensory characteristics of pain. Three distinctive sources of pain are cutaneous, deep somatic, and visceral. *Cutaneous* or *superficial pain* generally is well localized and may occur along dermal segments. The intensity of the pain correlates with stimulus intensity. It may be described as sharp, tingling or stinging. Cutaneous pain may take on a throbbing quality with tissue inflammation. *Deep somatic pain* may be more diffuse, may be felt as three-dimensional, and may be referred to other deep tissues. Somatic pain may be correlated with both stimulus intensity and movement of the involved area. It is often described as aching, dull, or piercing. *Visceral pain* tends to be diffuse but may localize if pain continues. It may be accompanied by symptoms of autonomic stimulation and by pain and tenderness referred to the body surface in locations adjacent to or removed from the affected organ (Fig. 25–3). The quality and chronology of the pain also may be determined to some extent by the source of the pain. It may be described as dull, aching, burning, or sharp. Visceral pain may be constant or occur in cycles. Characteristics of pain that may be related to the pain source can be identified.

Pain of neurological origin is not well understood, and acceptable models for such pain are not available. The term *central pain* traditionally has been used to describe pain arising from the brain and spinal cord; however, it more recently has been enlarged by some authors, to include pain arising from within the central nervous system regardless of the location. Central pain may be described as episodic or constant.[13] Central pain is usually experienced as intense pain and may be accompanied by a variety of sensations, such as cold, burning, itching, and tingling. All central pain problems have several commonalities: (1) the intensity of the pain cannot be explained by any known pain theory, (2) the resulting pain is usually worse than the pain of the original pathology, and (3) from a clinical perspective, they are extremely difficult to treat. Syndromes that are now commonly included under the category of central pain include: phantom pain, causalgia, neuralgias (including tic douloureux and postherpetic neuralgias), and thalamic syndrome. Gentle touch, warmth, barometric changes, and other non-noxious stimuli cause severe, excruciating pain in people with any of these syndromes. Pain from these conditions can last as long as 30 years, far beyond what would be considered normal healing. All are resistant to surgical control and there appears to be multiple input into the pain itself, including cutaneous, sympathetic, auditory and visual systems, and anxiety.[14] Although much is known about these various conditions, pain relief has been difficult. Some of the most promising results have come from interventions such as nerve blocks to the sympathetic nervous system and transcutaneous electrical nerve stimulation (TENS). Table 25–1 compares the characteristics of pain in relation to source.

The nature of pain cannot be adequately described without considering a model of pain as related to pain chronology and duration (Table 25–2). A model helpful in describing acute and chronic pain differentiates chronic pain as progressive or long-term. *Progressive pain* is frequently found in pathological conditions that progress over time and ultimately end in the client's death. Long-term pain occurs in pathological conditions that may remain stable or progress but are not of themselves terminal. Long-term pain also may occur when no known

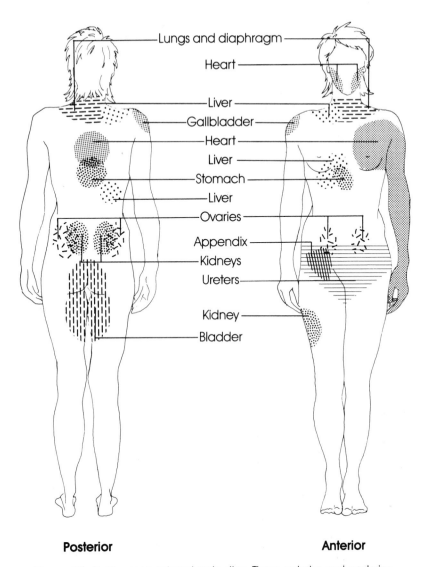

Lungs and diaphragm

Heart

Liver

Gallbladder

Heart

Liver

Stomach

Liver

Ovaries

Appendix

Kidneys

Ureters

Kidney

Bladder

Posterior   **Anterior**

Figure 25–3. Common referred pain sites. These anterior and posterior views of the body show where a client might feel pain referred from various visceral organs.

pathological cause can be identified, for example, some cases of low back pain. The model relied on most frequently in health-care settings is that of *acute pain,* and certainly many of the pain experiences encountered in a hospital setting fall into this category—incisional pain, renal colic, labor pains. Individuals experiencing chronic pain are not immune from hospi-

talization, and the characteristics that differentiate acute and chronic pain must be recognized.

Physiological signs that result from autonomic stimulation in acute pain do not occur with chronic pain. The body cannot sustain changes in blood pressure, pulse, and other physical symptoms that may occur with acute

TABLE 25–1. CHARACTERISTICS OF PAIN IN RELATION TO SOURCE

Source	Location	Intensity	Quality	Associated Factors
Superficial	Surface; well localized	Correlates with intensity of the stimulus; sharp, cutting, piercing	Described in terms of familiar surface injuries; sharp, cutting	May be intensified by contact; may protect area
Somatic	Deep; poorly localized. May radiate or be segmental; may be referred to body surface	May be mild to severe; correlates with stimulus. May be increased by muscle spasm	Vague, aching, piercing, pounding, sharp, or cutting	Intensified by movement; client may move awkwardly to prevent pain
Visceral	Deep; poorly localized. May radiate or be referred	Varies; may be mild to severe. Intensity may not remain stable	Gripping, cramping, aching, burning, stabbing. May be vague; an ache or soreness	May be intensified by motor activity or by compression of involved organ. Client may have found factors that relieve pain
Neurogenic	Follows neural distribution; may be on surface or deep; may radiate	Usually intense; does not necessarily correlate with stimulus	May be combination of painful sensations; difficult to describe. Burning, stinging, stabbing	Provoked by stimulation; client's guarding and protection of area is prominent behavior

Adapted from G.G. Engel, Pain, in C.M. MacBryde and R.S. Backlow eds., *Signs and Symptoms* (Philadelphia: J.B. Lippincott Co., 1970).

pain over prolonged periods without resulting in physical harm to the body. Thus, physical symptoms are absent or sharply modified in chronic pain. Many persons also adapt to chronic pain by eliminating behaviors normally associated with pain. One of the goals of a pain treatment center may be to decrease pain behaviors while increasing participation in daily activities. Individuals may learn coping mechanisms that allow them to increase their control over pain behaviors. These mechanisms may vary from increased activity as a method of distraction to sustained periods of quiet and meditation. An awareness of the potential differences in expression of acute and chronic pain is of importance to the nurse in assessing and evaluating pain; it emphasizes the need to rely upon the individual's report of pain.

Chronic pain may wear many faces, but whatever else, it becomes a constant companion, to be controlled if possible but always to be lived with. It imposes stress on the individual and can become the most debilitating and potentially destructive force in a person's life. Mental and physical resources of the individual

may be drained as energy is focused on the pain. In his classical description of the world of the patient in chronic pain, Le Shan compares chronic pain with a nightmare.[15] Terrible things are occurring to the individual with the possibility of worse to come, there is a lack of control in what the individual can do to provide relief, and there is no time limit, no known end to the nightmare. Chronic pain becomes a state of existence and, perhaps most tragic, this suffering no longer serves a useful purpose in warning the individual of potential harm. Chronic pain may, however, serve to enforce rest as an aid to healing.[16]

Fordyce suggests that a component of learned behavior may exist in chronic pain.[17] Reinforcement of pain behaviors may occur when the health-care worker provides attention only when pain is experienced and withdraws this attention when the person is comfortable. If this theory proves to be correct, we may unwittingly increase the learning of pain behaviors by activities such as medicating on an as needed (prn) basis for severe pain and increasing activity until painful.

TABLE 25–2. PAIN MODEL RELATING CHARACTERISTICS TO DURATION

| | Type of Pain | | |
Factors	*Acute*	*Chronic*	*Progressive*
Duration	Minutes→weeks	Weeks→lifetime	Until death, remissions may occur
Cause and treatment	Known and treatable	May be unknown or untreatable or both	Usually known but may be difficult to treat
Intensity	Moderate→severe	Low→moderate Severe episodes may occur	Low→moderate Severe episodes may occur
Function	Warning	No useful function	May warn of change
Related emotional component	Anxiety	Depression	May vary
Interference with activities	Temporary	Indefinite	Varies with remissions
Social acceptance of pain behaviors	Acceptable, no stigma	Not acceptable, stigma attached	Acceptable
Adaptation	No change, temporary	May lead to decreased self-esteem, requires behavior modification	May be associated with fear of greater pain Requires some behavior modification

INTERVENING VARIABLES

Age becomes a factor in both the young and old, particularly in the area of pain communication. Young people are in the process of learning a pain vocabulary, the names of body parts, and attempting to understand sensations coming from their body. They may be unable to communicate pain in adult terms. The geriatric client at one time had the capability of communicating pain but may have lost it through various deteriorations associated with age and sensory alterations.

The meaning pain has for an individual flows from *cultural, religious, and social expectations* and from *past experiences* and *future expectations.*[18] Zborowski pioneered the systematic study of pain responses of ethnic groups. He found wide variations in overt pain behaviors that had evolved from ethnic expectations. These variations held constant through second- and even third-generation immigrant groups. As a result of his work, four major cultural groups and their sociocultural attributes with respect to pain have been identified. Specifically, they are Old American, Jewish, Irish, and Italian. The "Old American" group were identified as individuals whose values and attitudes dominate in the United States. Members of this group were defined as white, native born, Protestant, and whose grandparents, at the least, were born in the United States. Zborowski's work provides a general framework for understanding various groups' responses to pain. Members of the Old American group will usually deny the existence of pain so that they may stay productive. Pain is described in an efficient, unemotional manner, and behaviors such as crying, moaning, or groaning are not seen with this group. Jewish people are very demonstrative with respect to pain and may use many affective descriptors, such as intolerable and agonizing, to describe pain. They expect family members to become involved in their suffering and are very concerned about the significance of their current pain on the future. Italian people are also very demonstrative about their pain and also expect family members to become involved in their suffering. Unlike the Jewish client, however, pain is viewed in the context of the current sensation and not future expectations. The Irish are similar to the Old American group in their calm, unemotional response to pain. Irish clients often will not complain about their pain and frequently will withdraw from other people when in severe pain. As a group, the Irish are also very proud of their ability to fight and endure severe pain. Zborowski's work provides a framework for understanding cultural variations in pain response, but care must be taken not to expect all clients of a given cultural group to behave in exactly the same manner.

Religious beliefs may also influence current responses to pain. Members of some religious groups believe that pain is punishment for wrongdoing and may not actively seek relief from the pain until penance has been performed.[19]

Children, in the magic-thinking years of four to seven, often view pain as punishment. They believe that they are hospitalized because of some bad deed they have done. Unfortunately, this view is frequently reinforced by parents during illness episodes. An example of this is the parent who threatens a child by saying, "If you don't behave, I'll have the nurse give you a shot."

Children are in the process of developing a cognitive background on which to base their interpretations of pain and do not have, as most adults have had, friends who have described pain experiences. The significance of an injection to a child is not fully appreciated by most adults. In a study by Eland, 186 hospitalized children were asked the question, "Of all the things that have ever hurt you, what's hurt you the worst?"[20] Of those children who were hospitalized in a large Midwestern university hospital, 49.7 percent answered "shot" or "needle." Interestingly, six of those children, between the ages of 4 and 10, had undergone 25 surgical experiences each, and every one of them answered "shot" or "needle" as being the most painful event. Children lack the cognitive understanding that momentary pain of an injection will alleviate the overall hurt that they are experiencing. Younger children around the ages of four and five lack a time concept and do not associate the painful event of an injection with pain relief at a later time.

Past experiences and responses to pain can be either positive or negative. A person who has had repeated painful experiences may have developed successful ways of coping. On the other hand, if frequent painful procedures and attempts at coping have been unsuccessful, the heightened fear and anxiety over having to endure them again may elicit an entirely different response. Anticipated pain can become an overwhelming threat to this individual.

The following is the protocol developed by Eland to assess pain in children 4 through 10 years of age. Eland used crayons and body outlines (Fig. 25–4).[21] The originator of the idea for the use of a chromatic array of colors to represent pain was Stewart, who designed a sensory matching device consisting of colored boxes ranging from yellow (no pain) through orange, red, and black (severe pain).[22] Eland adapted the idea for this use with young children and uses a felt board for this particular protocol. Body outlines and crayons also have been used to color pain.[23–25]

In an attempt to establish rapport, children were asked about pets, school, if they like to color, and play activities. Each child was asked what his or her favorite color was. The child was asked the question, "What kinds of things have hurt you before?" If the child did not reply, the researcher asked the child, "Has anyone ever stuck your finger to get blood? What did that feel like?" After discussing several things that have hurt the child in the past the researcher asked the child, "Of all the things that have ever hurt you, what hurt the most?" In this study the following protocol was followed:

1. Present eight felt squares in a row in the exact same order to every child—yellow, orange, red, green, blue, purple, brown, black—across the bottom of the felt board.
2. Ask the child, "Of these colors, which color is like (the event identified by the child as hurting the most)?"
3. Place the color square at the top of the felt board away from the other colors. (Represents severe pain.)
4. Ask the child, "Which color is like a hurt but not quite as much as (event identified by child as hurting the most)?"
5. Place the color that represents moderate pain below the square chosen representing severe pain.
6. Ask the child, "Which color is like something that hurts just a little?"
7. Place the color square below the colors representing severe and moderate pain.

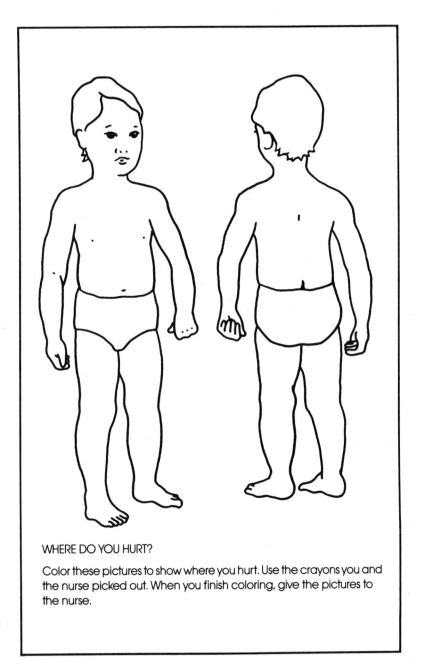

WHERE DO YOU HURT?

Color these pictures to show where you hurt. Use the crayons you and the nurse picked out. When you finish coloring, give the pictures to the nurse.

Figure 25–4. Assessment of pain in children.

8. Ask the child, "Which color is like not hurting at all?"
9. Place the color at the bottom of the column of color squares.
10. Ask the child to show on the color scale "What color is like a shot?"

PERSONS AT RISK

Antecedent conditions of pain—physiological, psychological, and sociocultural—determine the occurrence and magnitude of pain experienced in any individual. Many of these factors have been discussed previously. The influence that age and sex have on pain is not well documented. Traditionally it has been assumed that children and older individuals experience less pain because of lack of development or changes in the central nervous system. Research is not available to support these assumptions, however. Studies of children's pain done by Eland do not support the hypothesis that children experience less pain; when provided with a means to identify and describe pain they are able to do so quite accurately.

Cummings identified characteristics that have been found to signal a high potential for chronic pain in clients treated at the Veterans Administration pain clinic in Seattle.[26] Characteristics that have been identified include:

- Drug or alcohol abuse
- Several previous hospitalizations or other health problems
- Inappropriate affect
- Depression, hopelessness, anger
- Threatening or demanding behavior
- Rejection of self-help measures
- Negative feelings about job, marriage, family
- Litigation or compensation pending

These characteristics are not identified as causal factors of chronic pain but do suggest factors that can be considered in the initial evaluation of pain and that may influence responses to treatment.

RESPONSE TO PAIN

The potential range of individual responses to pain is both varied and complex. The labeling of pain responses or behaviors as adaptive or maladaptive is determined partially by the health-care system and the culture. For example, a culture may require stoicism as an appropriate pain response. These responses become most significant when considering chronic pain, although some behaviors, such as seeking assistance and complying with treatment, are expected of clients with acute as well as chronic pain.

Lipowski has identified mechanisms that are used in coping with illness, and defines *coping styles* as the relatively enduring dispositions in dealing with stress, while *coping strategies* are those techniques used to deal with a particular stress, such as illness.[27] The strategies used will be influenced by the individual's coping style, the situational factors, and the meaning the illness has for the individual. He identified eight common meanings of illness (Table 25–3) that are very similar to those identified by Copp as meanings that clients use to describe pain.[28] Lipowski's conclusions about coping strategies in illness can be applied to coping strategies used with pain. The way individuals perceive pain will influence the way in which they cope or respond to pain. He states that "coping may be evaluated as either adaptive or maladaptive depending on its appropriateness to the client's age and situation, as well as its effectiveness in achieving maximum possible function and recovery or compensation."[29]

Response mechanisms, such as addiction, manipulation of the sick role for secondary gain, and withdrawal, are usually culturally unacceptable to health-care workers as well as being ineffective for the client. Within the wide range

TABLE 25–3. COMPARISON OF LIPOWSKI'S CONCEPT OF ILLNESS WITH COPP'S MEANING OF PAIN

Lipowski: Illness	Copp: Pain
1. Challenge	Challenge
2. Enemy	Struggle or fight
3. Punishment	Punishment
4. Weakness	Weakness
5. Relief	Relief (restoration of health)
6. Strategy	Self-testing (fear, anxiety, strength to cope)
7. Loss or damage	Loss or grieving
8. Value	Value

of culturally acceptable responses, more information is needed to identify those responses that will prove most effective for the client. A study focusing on the relationships between individual differences in coping and the course of recovery in surgical clients found that clients using avoidance modes of coping did better than those using vigilant modes of coping.[30] Avoidance modes included behaviors that showed avoidance or denial of the emotional or threatening aspects of the surgery and were demonstrated by an unwillingness to discuss thoughts about the operation. Vigilance included those responses that indicated the client was overly alert to threatening aspects of the surgery, as demonstrated by a readiness to discuss thoughts about the operation. These findings are only suggestive of trends relating recovery and coping methods; additional recovery and coping methods; additional research of this type is necessary to determine causal relationships.

THE NURSING PROCESS

The nurse will assess pain to provide information that will assist in making a nursing diagnosis, formulating a plan, intervening, and evaluating the effectiveness of the intervention. The nursing diagnoses will be of most value in planning interventions if the factors that contribute to the pain are identified; for example, "pain related to tension on the abdominal incision."[31] These factors will be identified as part of the assessment. Interventions may be *independent* or *dependent nursing functions* and are identified as such. The use of **analgesics** is a dependent function requiring nursing judgments and collaboration with the client and physician; knowledge that will be helpful to the nurse is specifically addressed in a later section of this chapter on analgesics. Evaluation of the effectiveness of interventions may use the same protocol used for pain assessment, although general behavioral outcomes that may prove helpful are identified at the end of this chapter.

Assessment
Problems often arise with pain assessment because of the subjectivity of the pain experience. Individuals should be encouraged to describe pain in their own words; however, the evaluator

must recognize that pain may be difficult to report accurately without assistance. Judgment must be exercised by the nurse in determining when clients need help to describe their pain. Physiological indicators of pain, e.g., redness and swelling, and behavioral responses, e.g., crying, should be evaluated in conjunction with verbal reports of pain; if the client does not report pain, such cues may be the only indicators that the individual is experiencing pain or discomfort. In evaluating chronic pain, it must be kept in mind that the responses normally present with acute pain may be modified or absent.

A pain history should be modified to fit the needs of the usual population or of the individual client; questions posed to the postoperative client may differ from those asked of a person with chronic pain. The pain history should include the client's reports of pain (subjective) and physiological and behavioral responses (objective).

The report of pain includes an evaluation of location, intensity, quality, and chronology of pain. *Location* of pain is best described by having the person describe or trace the area of pain; the description should include the extent and spread of the pain as well as the location of pain-free areas. An anatomical diagram may be of assistance if the individual cannot describe or locate the pain or if multiple areas of pain are interspersed with pain-free areas. The use of such a tool with an individual experiencing multiple sites of joint pain is illustrated in Figure 25–5. Medical terms used to describe location include:

Localized	Confined to the area of primary focus
Radiating	Extending outward from the area of primary focus
Projected	Transmitted along a pathway; usually the distribution of a nerve
Referred	Occurs in an area other than the source

Location of the pain also should include whether the pain is deep or superficial and whether the location remains the same or changes. If the location of the pain changes, determine whether these changes are related to any factors that clients can identify.

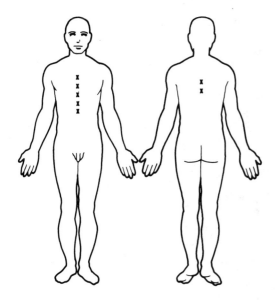

Figure 25–5. Anatomical diagrams can be used to identify pain locations.

Perceived intensity of the pain may reflect the intensity of the stimulus, the degree of tissue damage, the amount of psychological distress caused, or a combination of these factors. More precise assessments may be made by having clients rank the pain on some type of scale (Fig. 25–6). The most common method is one in which the individual ranks pain on a scale of 0 to 10; 0 represents no pain and 10 the worst pain. A 5-point ranking scale may also be used in conjunction with words commonly used to indicate pain intensity. Having the individual compare the intensity of this pain experience with that of previous pain experiences may help the person describe the pain, if other measures are not available.

The *quality* of the pain may be the most difficult aspect for the individual to describe. You can assist by asking, "How does your pain feel?" The McGill–Melzack Pain Questionnaire contains groupings of words frequently used to describe pain and may be given to the client if specifics about the quality of pain are desired.[32] The words describe sensory qualities (such as throbbing, burning, dull, tearing) and affective qualities (such as sickening, suffocating, nauseating). The presence of related sensations, such as tingling, fullness, or itching, also should be determined. The evaluator needs to determine if the quality of the pain remains constant or if changes occur; again, if the quality changes, is this related to factors the client can identify?

Chronology of the pain should be described by the client, but he or she may need to respond to questions in order to provide the required information. Information needed includes:

- Mode of onset (sudden or gradual) and what the client was doing at the time, if related to the onset of pain
- Pattern of the pain (steady or intermittent). If intermittent, does it follow a cycle or pattern?
- The duration of the pain, if intermittent or cyclic
- Whether this type of pain has occurred before and under what circumstances

Associated information to be considered includes the identification of factors that precipitate or intensify the pain, as well as factors that provide relief. Does the pain awaken the client from sleep? The amount of distress caused by the pain may be evaluated on a scale similar to the one used to rank intensity. The distress level will not necessarily be the same as the intensity level and may be anticipatory in situations that clients know will be painful, such as dressing changes. If the distress level is higher than the pain level, interventions to decrease anxiety may be of most benefit in controlling the pain.

Physiological responses may accompany acute pain and generally reflect stimulation of the autonomic nervous system. Assessing these responses is most important in situations where clients may not be reporting pain (e.g., a new postoperative client, a person with a depressed level of awareness). Responses to be evaluated include:

- Changes in skin color such as pallor, flushing
- Diaphoresis
- Alterations in blood pressure and pulse rate, increases being most common
- Increase in respiration
- Nausea, vomiting

Physiological symptoms most common with chronic pain include fatigue and inability to rest, weakness, anorexia, and in some cases, faint-

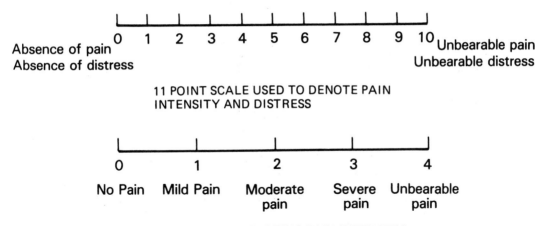

Figure 25–6. Pain scales.

ness or syncope. Many of these symptoms are most likely to occur when the individual becomes exhausted by the pain; providing pain relief and rest may alleviate many of these symptoms.

Behavioral responses associated with pain are diverse and frequently difficult to evaluate. Body movement may be decreased, and some persons state they lie quietly as a method of controlling pain.

A complete pain history requires that sufficient time be allowed so that the client does not feel rushed. If the cause of the pain is easily identified, the pain is acute, and temporary relief can be achieved with relative ease, the pain history can be shortened and completed quite rapidly; however, if the pain situation is complex, the time taken to do a thorough history will prove of value in planning interventions. Meinhart and McCaffery recommend a flow sheet providing a 24-hour summary of the client's pain and serving as a tool for communication with other health-care professionals.[33] The flow sheet includes time, pain rating, analgesics, vital signs, and other pertinent information.

Planning

The next phase of the nursing process entails the preparation of a written nursing care plan that includes the nursing diagnoses, client ob-

jectives, and the outcome criteria. Nursing diagnoses used by the North American Nursing Diagnosis Association include:

- Comfort, alterations in: Pain
- Altered comfort: Chronic pain

Since the diagnoses are broad, a statement that includes the diagnosis and the contributing factors can best guide practice. Examples of such statements could be:

- Acute pain related to decreased oxygenation of tissues
- Chronic pain related to neoplastic infiltration of tissues

Objectives are developed in conjunction with the client and the family. The client should be asked only for that information to be used in planning care; persons with chronic pain may be reluctant to share information unless they believe it will be used to plan appropriate interventions. The development of realistic objectives, especially in the presence of chronic pain, may require that the nurse explore the client's and family's perception of the pain problem as well as share information concerning the pain experience. A client goal related to the absence of pain in a situation in which pain cannot be totally alleviated will limit the choice of interventions. Client objectives will be specific for the individual situation. Goals useful in the development of more specific objectives can include:

- Absence of pain
- Lessening of pain
- Maintaining adequate rest and sleep patterns
- Maintaining adequate nutrition and elimination
- Decreasing muscle tension
- Maintaining activities of daily living
- Maintaining mobility
- Maintaining a productive life-style
- Maintaining desired interactions with others
- Decreasing occurrence of factors that trigger pain episodes
- Lessening anxiety and depression
- Increasing client control over pain management
- Increasing client self-sufficiency
- Decreasing or eliminating pain behaviors

Specific objectives can be derived from these goals. A more specific goal for a postoperative client might be: Can participate in required activities such as coughing and ambulation.

Outcome criteria will be related to the specific objective. The criteria may be based on the client's verbal statements, observations of physiological parameters, physical activities, and other client behaviors. More than one criterion may be used to evaluate an objective. Maintaining adequate rest and sleep patterns may be evaluated by the following criteria:

- Client states he or she feels rested
- Client is able to rest or sleep at night for a 6-hour period
- Client is not wakened by pain
- Client requires only one rest period during the day

Outcome criteria can vary and may be dependent upon such factors as the physical condition of the client, the source of the pain, the client objectives, and the degree of pain.

Once the plan has been completed, the selection, implementation, and evaluation of interventions can follow.

Implementation

The third phase of the nursing process is implementation of the plan. Numerous articles on nursing management of pain can be found in the nursing literature. Many of the interventions recommended are based on the experience of practitioners rather than on research, but they reflect a variety of creative techniques for assisting the client with pain. Some of the approaches are based on the gate-control theory of pain and are methods of altering pain sensation or pain reaction by "closing the gate." Other methods focus on increasing body response mechanisms, such as **endorphin** production. A number of physical approaches can be used for pain control. Heat and cold affect the vascular and muscular systems, but just as important are their effects on hormone production. Warmth and warm weather stimulates the production of serotonin, and cold and cold weather stimulates the production of norephinephrine.[34] Moist heat can be applied with warm soaks, compresses, or heating pads. Dry heat is applied with heating pads or as radiant heat. Cold can be applied by using ice bags, cold towels, gel packs, or as an ice massage. Cold and heat usually are most effective if applied directly to the painful area. The client may have a preference for heat or cold and should be encouraged to try both, if appropriate, to determine which method is most effective. Heat and cold are most frequently used with somatic pain but may provide relief with cutaneous pain.

Chinese medicine has relied on acupuncture for 2000 years for pain relief, and with increased interest in pain it was only appropriate for Western medicine to evaluate its effectiveness. An acupuncturist places solid core needles (gauge 27 to 31) into specific points on the body—some of which are near the painful part and others that are remote from the pain itself. Acupressure is practiced by applying finger pressure on the same points. After research by many anatomists and physiologists, it was found that many of the acupuncture points correspond to the superficial aspects of peripheral nerves, whereas others correspond to neurovascular or lymphatic elements. Regardless of the physiological explanation, for some clients stimulation of these points provides pain relief. They can be stimulated by heat, cold, TENS electrodes, finger pressure, or an acupuncture needle. The identification of specific points is far beyond the scope of this chapter and the reader is referred to Mannheimer and Lampe,[35] and Travell and Simone[36] for more information on stimulation and location of specific points.

Massage, range of motion exercises, and positioning can be used to relieve pain of muscle tension or spasm. Massage should not, however, be used for calf pain or in any instance in which a thrombus may be present. The use of a menthol ointment may be included with massage. It is not known how menthol ointments relieve pain, but many persons find them effective with muscular pain.[37] Range of motion and positioning can be effective if muscle tension or spasm is reduced. The initial movement may increase the pain temporarily but this may be partially controlled with smooth, continuous motion and avoidance of sudden jerky motions. Relaxation techniques, which are discussed later, may be appropriate to relieve muscle tension. Exercise and movement may need to be planned for in conjunction with periods of decreased activity or rest. Rest may be used alone as an effective method of pain control, particularly when pain is being aggravated by fatigue or when injured tissue can heal if rest is provided. Control of environmental factors, such as noise, temperature, and light, are important considerations when providing periods of rest.

Cognitive approaches aimed at assisting the client to gain control over the symptom or alleviating the affective distress associated with pain are recommended by practitioners. These approaches include relaxation, distraction, information distribution, and alleviation of pain apprehension. The use of relaxation in pain control is based on its effects in decreasing anxiety and decreasing muscle tension, both of which may increase the perception of pain. General relaxation techniques that are focused on total body relaxation require cooperation of the client and adequate time to learn the technique. It is necessary to evaluate the mental and physical capability of the client to participate. The client must be alert and physically capable of doing the exercises. The procedures used for progressive relaxation include the following sequence.[38] The client:

- Focuses attention on a muscle group
- Tenses the muscle group when a predetermined signal is given by the nurse
- Maintains tension at a level that does not cause discomfort or pain for five to seven seconds

- Releases tension at a predetermined signal
- Focuses on the muscle group and the sensation while relaxing as completely as possible

Relaxation also may be promoted by the use of breathing exercises, which do not require much effort or time on the part of the client. Breathing techniques are frequently used for childbirth. The techniques require abdominal breathing to be done at a specified rate and depth. The client assumes a comfortable position and concentrates on relaxing. A deep cleansing breath is taken, followed by slow, deep, rhythmic abdominal breathing for about 60 seconds. Relaxation is most effective if taught prior to anticipated pain or during periods of less acute pain to allow the individual to focus on learning the technique. Breathing techniques may be used without previous practice during acute pain if the nurse coaches the client through the technique.

Distraction can be provided by any method that will successfully focus attention away from the pain. Relief will last only as long as the distraction and may be followed by increased awareness of the pain. Techniques that will provide distraction vary from person to person. Some commonly used distractors include:

- Physical activities, such as pacing, visiting with others, talking on the phone
- Listening to music; this is most beneficial if the client uses a headset to allow concentration on the music and prevent distraction from other stimuli
- Relating events or happenings. The nurse has the client relate an exciting or pleasant experience. Items such as family pictures or scrapbooks can be used to tell about the people or activities involved
- Counting in a rhythmic manner, such as with a metronome, while concentrating on the activity of counting

The distraction selected must serve as a focus of concentration strong enough to overcome concentration on the pain. The client should be actively encouraged to use distraction and be assisted in finding those methods that will be most effective. In general, distraction will work best with brief periods and milder forms of pain.

It is not as effective with chronic pain but may be used intermittently in these cases.

Discussion of pain and provision of information may reduce pain, particularly if a lack of information is increasing anxiety, or if the client does not know how to assist in pain control. Provision of information is focused on the needs of the client. It can include information about the source of the pain, expected course of the pain, methods that can decrease the pain, and how the individual can control the pain. Providing information about sensations that occur in situations associated with pain has been shown to decrease the amount of pain experienced.[39] Suggesting that an intervention will provide pain relief was shown to be effective in relieving pain in postoperative clients.[40] Conscious suggestion can be used to dispel anxiety and increase relaxation. The voice and attitude of the helper are crucial to the effectiveness of this technique.

General nursing care measures that decrease discomfort and distress associated with pain can be used alone or in conjunction with other interventions. These comfort measures can include touch, listening, and just "staying" with the client. Reassurance and support can be provided by diminishing the client's feeling of being alone with pain.[41] Others, of the client's choosing, also may serve the function of "staying" with the person in pain. Care must be exercised to determine the client's wishes as well as the needs of those staying with the client.

Nurses can administer medications as ordered by the physician to relieve the client's pain. Some analgesics alter central control's perception of pain; some work at small-diameter (A-Delta and C fibers) or large-diameter (A-Beta) fibers. Administration of pharmacological agents with differing action sites, when combined with other nursing comfort measures, such as back rubs and position changes, maximize the potential for pain relief. The action sites of some common medications that provide a framework for combining them are as follows:

Aspirin	Small-diameter fibers[42]
Morphine sulfate	Large-diameter fibers and central control[43]
Barbiturates	Central control and T-cell[44]
Codeine phosphate	Small-diameter fibers and central control[45]
Meperidine hydrochloride	Central control[46]
Tylenol (acetaminophen), Butazolidin (phenylbutazone), Motrin (ibuprofin)	Small-diameter fibers[47]

Aspirin remains one of the best anti-inflammatory agents and analgesics available today. It works by inhibiting prostaglandin production at the level of the small fiber. For aspirin to be most effective, a blood level must be maintained in the body, and it needs to be administered every four hours.[48] Many clients have difficulty believing aspirin will work, for several reasons. It is readily available to all and does not require a prescription or special handling to acquire it. It is relatively inexpensive and side effects associated with administration are low. Many individuals believe that if a drug has these qualities, it must not be strong, and if it is not strong, it will not work. If someone believes this, the drug probably will not work.

Barbiturates have long had a recognized role in providing adequate sleep and rest for clients, but they also have a role in pain management. There is growing evidence to show that barbiturates alter the small fibers (A-Delta, C) input to the T-cell.[49,50] In addition, barbiturates diminish the electrical activity in the midbrain reticular area, which in turn alters the pain-transmitting capabilities of the substantia gelatinosa.[51]

If pain becomes extremely intense, normal doses of analgesics will not successfully alleviate it. This frequently happens when clients attempt to endure pain for a long period of time, or a nurse has not initiated pain management. As a result, the pain is excruciating before a nurse can administer an appropriate analgesic. If the usual dose of an analgesic will not eliminate the client's pain, the client needs to be told why, and the nurse must make attempts to secure additional medication.[52] Nurses occasionally withhold the client's pain medication for fear of the client's becoming addicted. In most instances, this will not occur. If the client is promptly and adequately medicated for pain, less medication may be needed over the course of treatment. Unfortunately, the fear of creating addiction is one of the most common reasons that nurses withhold narcotics. In a study by Porter and Jick, only four out of 11,882 hospitalized patients became addicted to their narcotics, and all four had previous histories of drug abuse.[53] Having some basic information regarding addiction will be helpful for nurses.

There is no one, recognized definition of addiction. A generally recognized definition states that addiction is an overwhelming involvement with obtaining and using drugs for their *psychic* effects rather than for medically or socially approved reason.[54] Therefore, by definition, relief or prevention of pain is a reason to use narcotics. Another reason given by nurses for not administering narcotic analgesia is the fear of respiratory depression. Narcotics can cause respiratory depression, just as antibiotics can cause anaphylaxis and insulin can cause hypoglycemia. However, the risk of anaphylaxis and hypoglycemia do not prevent nurses from giving antibiotics and insulin respectively and neither should the risk of respiratory depression prevent nurses from administering narcotics for pain relief. When the topic was studied, Miller and Jick found only three cases of respiratory depression in 3263 hospitalized patients.[55]

Nurses also need to anticipate painful experiences and medicate clients prior to these occurrences. For example, on a postoperative surgical unit, when it is necessary for a client to deep-breathe and ambulate, a nurse needs to enter the client's room at least one hour prior to the required activity, administer the appropriate analgesic, and allow the medication to take effect. Adequate pain control in these situations allows the client to move more easily, to participate in care activities, and to maximize recovery.

A **placebo** is an inactive substance that resembles a medication. Previously it was thought that placebos worked because of the power of positive suggestion and of the brain's power over pain.[56–59] Beecher found that 35 percent of all clients could receive benefit from chemically inert substances. Therefore, physicians occasionally order placebos (such as normal saline for an intramuscular injection, or a flavored syrup or a pill of inert substance for oral administration) instead of a narcotic. Placebos frequently are chosen for clients whose pain has been resistant to ordinary therapeutic modalities and when health-care professionals can think of nothing else to do. A nurse, when administering a placebo, tells clients everything they want to hear: that the medication is a new medication when the old ones have not worked and conveys that someone is paying attention to their pain and suffering. The client wants the medication to work; pain is very real to him or her. New research by Halpern has shown that placebos activate the descending system, leading to release of endorphins, and at least 40 percent of all clients should be able to mobilize their own endorphins when given a placebo.[60] This raises more ethical questions on placebo administration. The nurse who refuses to give a placebo when ordered may be denying pain relief to at least 40 percent of clients. If all members of the nursing staff are not part of a team effort in giving placebos and clients discover they are receiving an inert substance, the nurse–client relationship may be permanently altered. The client may feel that his or her credibility is being questioned and responses to other potentially successful treatment modalities during that hospitalization will be less successful and cooperative because of the deception. The use of placebos raises many ethical issues, because clients have the right (see Chapter 12) to know what treatments are being used, and dishonesty is considered unethical.

Nurses need to consider this ethical issue before they are confronted with it in the clinical area. Then, when the issue becomes a reality, the nurse can make a decision based on conscience and the individual situation. If nurses feel that they do not wish to participate in that particular part of the client's care, they should make their stand clear to the other members on the health-care team. Regardless of one's ethical stand, the ethical stand of another may be different, and it is within the other's right as a professional to choose.

Some health-care disciplines provide measures for pain relief that may require coordination with nursing functions. Surgical measures, for example, may include a variety of techniques designed to interrupt the pain stimulus through destruction of part of the sensory pathway. These procedures were originally performed through open exposure of the cerebrum or spinal cord under general anesthesia. More recently, surgery has provided a means of performing these techniques under local anesthesia. Interruption of the lateral spinothalamic tract in the spinal cord (cordotomy) is the surgical procedure most commonly preferred; however, procedures that interrupt tracts at another point in the central nervous system are frequently performed. Because of the ability of the central nervous system to protect itself, suspended function may recover, and pain may recur.[61] Sympathetic blocks and sympathectomy may be of benefit in posttraumatic injuries or causalgia. A temporary block usually will be done prior to a surgical procedure to determine if relief will be obtained with interruption of these fibers.

Other forms of treatment that may be used include acupuncture, hypnosis, operant conditioning, and biofeedback. The responsibility of the nurse may range from teaching the technique, especially biofeedback, to support and positive reinforcement. Acupuncture, which is being more widely used and researched in this country, involves the insertion and rotation of metal needles in the body at specific, designated points. These acupuncture points also have been used in massage techniques that substitute hand pressure and massage for the needle.

Hypnosis can be used in the management of pain problems. Removal of pain by hypnosis should be done by one skilled in the practice of hypnosis and aware of the diagnostic and treatment problems of the disease.[62] Pain is generally reduced rather than blocked completely, so as to leave sufficient pain perception to note changes in the course of the illness. Not all persons are responsive to hypnosis, but among those who are, repeated hypnosis may provide periods of pain relief for several weeks before reinforcment becomes necessary.[63] Operant conditioning is aimed at reducing learned pain behaviors.[64] The objectives are to: reduce pain behavior by withdrawing positive reinforcement, increase activity with positive reinforcement, retrain the family to enforce well behaviors and to avoid enforcing pain behaviors, and modify deficiencies other than pain that may

limit activity. Operant conditioning is most effectively provided in a controlled setting such as a pain clinic. Biofeedback is used to alter and bring under control physiological responses and may be used in conjunction with other treatment techniques. At the present time, one of the most common uses of biofeedback in pain control is for the individual with tension or migraine headaches.[65]

Electrical stimulation, although not a new concept, is another method used by physicians to control pain. The ancient Egyptians in 600 B.C. placed their gout-affected feet in buckets of water with specific electrical fish for pain relief. Recent technological advances have brought about new electrical devices for pain relief, and an increased number of physicians, nurses, physical therapists, and auxiliary personnel are finding themselves involved with them.

TNS or TENS units work by sending impulses along large-diameter fibers (A-Beta). There is also recent evidence to suggest that stimulation from TENS units can result in the exogenous release of endorphins. Tens units are used for acute postoperative pain, chronic pain, and as a screening device for determination of the plausibility of surgically implanting a more sophisticated unit, such as a dorsal column or a peripheral nerve stimulator. TENS units consist of two electrodes (one positive, one negative) that are attached by flexible wires to a battery pack. On the battery pack there are two or three controls that control the voltage, frequency, and pulse width of the electrical current. In an acute-care setting, postoperative clients have electrodes placed along their incision lines for pain relief. In chronic pain situations, electrodes are located where large fibers become superficial over acupuncture points or sometimes geographically near the source of pain.

Nurses working with clients with nerve stimulators need to know electrode placement and taping, conductive jellies, battery changing, and adjustment of the voltage, pulse width, and frequency controls. For clients to receive maximum benefit, a program of nurse education needs to be undertaken. If the nurse doesn't know about the device, the placebo effect will not be operant, existing pain can be made worse, and maximum benefits will not be attained. The reader is referred to Mannheimer and Lampe for the specific management of patients with TENS.[35]

Evaluation

Whatever form of treatment is used to alleviate pain, the *evaluation* of its effectiveness is a necessary nursing function. Behavioral outcomes can be used to assist in this evaluation. Outcomes that can be observed and can be positive cues that some degree of pain control has been achieved include:

- Relaxation of skeletal muscles
- Increase in normal, daily activities
- Increased ability to rest or sleep
- Elimination of pain postures
- Decreased use of affective descriptors in describing pain
- Decreased report of pain, soreness, or tenderness
- Increased attention span
- Focus of attention on topics other than pain
- Verbalization that pain sensations are absent

Once the evaluative phase of the nursing process has been completed, the cycle can begin again with a reassessment. If the established plan proved to be partially or totally ineffective, the plan has to be redesigned. If the plan was effective, then the successful outcomes need to be supported.

Through careful use of the nursing process and a firm knowledge base about pain, nurses are able to anticipate client's needs and provide meaningful client care.

SUMMARY

Pain is a symptom frequently encountered in the health-care setting, but it is not easily defined, and there is no agreement about the mechanisms leading to pain. The gate-control theory is the most widely accepted theory at present, although it is being modified by new research. Pain may be identified as acute, long-term, or progressive. Physiological and psychological responses vary with the type of pain and may require differing emthods of pain treatment. A number of variables may modify the pain experience and include such things as age, cultural background, and general coping mechanisms. Pain assessment should be thorough and include the characteristics of the pain, responses to pain, and pain history. Nursing interventions include both independent and dependent activities. The use of physical and general comfort measures as well as the use of analgesics are recognized nursing interventions. The role of interventions, such as teaching, suggestion, relaxation, and biofeedback, are newer and being developed at a rapid rate. The role that the nurse chooses to assume in relation to the person experiencing pain will be a vital factor in the effectiveness of pain evaluation and alleviation. The nurse can facilitate the accurate reporting of pain, the use of independent control measures, and the effectiveness of other forms of treatment. The responsibility is great, but the rewards of helping the client with pain are even greater.

Study Questions

Case Study I

Mr. McCloskey is a 21-year-old, 120-pound male who was involved in a motor vehicle accident three years ago. At the time of the accident he sustained L-2-3-4 compression fractures. He has undergone two spinal fusions and three lumbar laminectomies to relieve his pain, but is still in pain. He is currently hospitalized for reevaluation of his pain problem.

At the time of the accident, Mr. McCloskey was employed as a steelworker. Since the accident, he has been totally disabled. (His fiancée was killed in the accident.) Mr. McCloskey now lives in his parents' home. He was forced to give up his apartment for economic reasons.

The lumbar spine x-rays, myelogram, and electromyogram (EMG) all indicate what will most likely be permanent damage bilaterally to the nerve roots at the L-2-3-4 levels. Medical orders include:

- Regular diet
- Bedrest with bathroom privileges
- Laxative of choice
- Client may straight cath self prn
- Intake and output
- Bedboards
- Overbed trapeze

- Codeine 15 mg q 4 hr prn pain PO or IM
- ASA gr X q 3–4 prn pain PO
- Valium 2 mg qid PO
- 2 ccs Bacteriostatic water IM q 3–4 hr if codeine does not relieve pain

1. Identify the data you need to assess Mr. McCloskey's pain. List the data in order of priority.

2. A new pain relief device that you have never seen before is given to the client. What effect can your attitude toward the device have on its success?

3. List the advantages and disadvantages of using the placebo.

4. Under what circumstances would you give the placebo?

Case Study II

Mr. Wesley is a 55-year-old, admitted to a unit with intractable pain secondary to advanced heart disease. He has undergone heart surgery twice in the past two years. One surgery was for a mitral valve replacement and the other removed approximately one-third of his heart muscle because of ischemia. He is in severe congestive heart failure and will not live long. Mr. Wesley is as accepting as he could possibly be of his own death but wants to be more comfortable than he is. During your initial interview, he admits to being suicidal over the pain.

His pain is in several locations and is present at all times. The areas of his pain include: heart, left arm, right shoulder, entire rib cage, and leg (from intermittant claudication).

Mr. Wesley has not had a good night's sleep in as long as he can remember. He lives with his two sisters in a large house he built himself. He was the head of a large university department until forced into total disability two years ago.

1. What assessment information do you need from Mr. Wesley?

2. What nursing comfort measures could you institute that would most likely make him more comfortable?

3. You have the complete resources of a large medical center at your disposal and unlimited power to take over Mr. Wesley's care. What would you do for him? What areas of the gate-control mechanism would be affected by your interventions?

4. What is the nursing plan of care regarding pain for Mr. Wesley (for all 3 shifts)?

References

1. Richard Sternbach, *Pain: A Psychophysiological Analysis* (New York: Academic Press, 1968), 12.
2. Margo McCaffery, *Nursing Management of the Patient with Pain* (Philadelphia: J.B. Lippincott, 1972), 32.
3. Ibid., 32.
4. Ronald Melzack and P.D. Wall, *The Challenge of Pain* (New York: Basic Books, 1983), 208–15.
5. Ronald Melzack and P.D. Wall, "Pain mechanisms: A new theory," *Science* 150 (1965): 971.
6. Ronald Melzack, *The Puzzle of Pain* (New York: Basic Books, 1972).
7. Melzack and Wall, *The Challenge of Pain*, 235.
8. S. Kim, "Theory, research and nursing practice," *Adv Nurs Sci* 2, (1980):43–54.
9. B.B. Wolff, "Factor analysis of human pain responses: Pain endurance as a specific pain factor," *J Abnorm Psychol* 78, (1971):292.
10. H. Merskey and F. Spear, *Pain: Pscyhological and Psychiatric Aspects.* (London: Bailliere, Tindol, and Cassell, 1967).
11. Marion Johnson, "Assessment of clinical pain," in Ada Jacox ed., *Pain: A Sourcebook for Nurses and Other Health Professionals* (Boston: Little, Brown & Co., 1977).
12. H. Merskey. "Psychological aspects of pain," in Ada Jacox, ed., *Pain: A Sourcebook for Nurses and Other Health Professionals* (Boston: Little, Brown & Co., 1977), 91.
13. J.D. Loeser, "Central pains," *Clin Med* 82, (4), (1975): 24–26.
14. Melzack and Wall, *The Challenge of Pain*, 96.
15. L. LeShan, "The World of the patient in severe pain of long duration," *J Chronic Dis* 17, (1964): 119–24.
16. M. Schmitt, "The nature of pain with some personal notes," *Nurs Clin North Am* 12, (1977): 621–29.
17. W.E. Fordyce, "An operant conditioning method

of managing chronic pain," *Postgrad Med 53* (6), (1973): 123–28.

18. M. Zborowski, "Cultural components in response to pain," *J Soc Issues,* 8:(4) (1952):16–30.

19. R. Wu, *Behavior and Illness* (Englewood Cliffs, NJ: Prentice-Hall, 1973).

20. J.M. Eland, "Children's experience of pain: A descriptive study." Unpublished data, 1976.

21. J.M. Eland, "The experience of pain in children," unpublished paper presented to the Mid-America Sigma Theta Tau Research Conference, Kansas City, Mo.: August 1976.

22. M.L. Stewart, "Measurement of clinical pain," in Ada Jacox, ed., *Pain: A Sourcebook for Nurses and Other Health Professionals.* (Boston: Little, Brown & Co., 1977).

23. J. Eland and J.E. Anderson, "The experience of pain in children," in Ada Jacox, ed., *Pain: A Sourcebook for Nurses and Other Health Professionals.* (Boston: Little, Brown & Co. 1977).

24. S. Loebach, "The use of color to facilitate communication of pain in children," unpublished Master's thesis, the University of Washington, 1979.

25. P. Schroeder, "Use of Eland's color method in pain assessment of burned children," unpublished Master's thesis, the University of Cincinnati, 1979.

26. D. Cummings, "Stopping chronic pain before it starts," *Nursing '81* 11 (4), (1981):60–62.

27. Z.J. Lipowski, "Physical illness, the individual and the coping processes," *Psychiatry in Med* 1, (1970):91–102.

28. L.A. Copp, "The spectrum of suffering," *Am J Nurs* 74:491–95.

29. Lipowski: "Physical Illness."

30. F. Cohen and R.S. Lazarus, "Active coping processes, coping dispositions, and recovery from surgery," *Psychosom Med* 35 (1973):375–89.

31. E.A. Mahoney, "Some implications for nursing diagnoses of pain," *Nurs Clin North Am* 12, (1977):613–19.

32. J.E. Meissner, "McGill-Melzack pain questionnaire," *Nursing '80* 10, (1980):50–51.

33. N.T. Meinhart and M. McCaffery, *Pain: A Nursing Approach to Assessment and Analysis* (Norwalk, Conn.: Appleton-Century-Crofts, 1983), 361.

34. J.E. Booker, "Pain: It's all in your patient's head (or is it?)," *Nursing '82,* 12 (3), (1982):46–57.

35. J.S. Mannheimer and G.N. Lampe, *Clinical Transcutaneous Electrical Nerve Stimulation* (Philadelphia: F.A. Davis Co., 1984).

36. J.G. Travel and D.G. Simone, *Myofascial Pain and Dysfunction: The Trigger Point Manual* (Baltimore: Williams & Wilkins, Co. 1984).

37. M. McCaffery, "Relieving pain with noninvasive techniques," *Nursing '80,* 10 (12), (1980): 54–57.

38. J.M. Richter and R. Sloan, "A relaxation technique," *Am J Nurs* 79 (1979).

39. J. Johnson, "Effects of accurate expectations about sensation on the sensory and distress components of pain," *J Pers Soc Psychol* 27, (1973): 261–75.

40. K.S. Billars, "You have pain? I think this will help," *Am J Nurs* 70 (1970):2143.

41. M. McCaffery, "When your patient's still in pain don't just do something: Sit there," *Nursing 81* 11 (6), (1981):68–61.

42. J. Tourville, personal communication, 1977.

43. A. Herz, K. Albus, et al., "On the central sites for the anti-nociceptive action of morphine and fentanyl," *Neuropharmacology,* 9 (1970):539.

44. J.D. French, M. Verzeano, and W.H. Magoun, "Neural basis of the anesthetic state," *Arch Neurol Psychiatry,* 69:519–93.

45. J. Tourville, personal communication, 1977.

46. Ibid.

47. Ibid.

48. G.G. Gebhart, "Narcotic and non-narcotic analgesics and relief of pain," in Ada Jacox, ed., *Pain: A Sourcebook for Nurses and Other Health Professionals* (Boston: Little, Brown & Co., 1977).

49. P. Hillman and P.D. Wall: "Inhibitory and excitatory factors influencing the receptive fields of lamina 5 spinal cord cells," *Exp Brain Res* 9 (1969):2814.

50. L.M. Mendell and P.D. Wall, "Presynaptic hyperpolarization: A role for fine afferent fibers," *J Physiol* 172 (1964):274.

51. J.H. Jaffe and W.R. Martin, "Narcotic analgesics and antagonists," in L.S. Goodman and A. Gilman, eds., *Pharmacological Basis of Therapeutics,* 6th ed. (New York: Macmillan Co., 1979).

52. M. McCaffery and L. Hart, "Undertreatment of acute pain with narcotics," *Am J Nurs* 76 (1976): 1586.

53. J. Porter and H. Jick, "Addiction rare in patients treated with narcotics," *N Engl J Med* 302 (1980): 123.

54. M. McCaffery, "Patients shouldn't have to suffer: How to relieve pain with injectable narcotics," *Nursing* 10, October 1980): 34–39.

55. R.R. Miller and H. Jick, "Clinical effects of meperidine in hospitalized medical patients," *J Clin Pharmacol* 18, (1978): 180.

56. H.K. Beecher, "Pain in men wounded in battle," *Ann Surg* 123 (1946): 96.

57. H.K. Beecher, *Measurement of Subjective Responses: Quantitative Effects of Drugs* (New York: Oxford University Press, 1959).

58. J.B. Knowles and C.J. Lucas, "Experimental studies of the placebo response," *J Men Sci* 106 (1960): 231.

59. A.K. Shapiro, "The Placebo response," in J.G. Howell, ed., *Modern Perspectives in World Psychiatry* (New York: Brunner/Mazel, 1971).

60. L. Halpern, *Neurophysiological Theories of Pain*, in Symposium: *The Management of Pain in Surgical Practice* (New York: Pfizer, Inc., 1979).

61. D. McDonnel, "Surgical and electrical stimulation methods for relief of pain," in Ada Jacox, ed., *Pain: Sourcebook for Nurses and Other Health Professionals* (Boston: Little, Brown & Co., 1977).

62. H.B. Crasilneck and J.A. Hall, "Clinical hypnosis in problems of pain," in Ada Jacox, ed., *Pain: A Sourcebook for Nurses and Other Health Professionals* (Boston: Little, Brown & Co., 1977).

63. Ibid., 270

64. W.E. Fordyce, "Operant conditioning: An approach in chronic pain," in Ada Jacox, ed., *Pain: A Sourcebook for Nurses and Other Health Professionals* (Boston: Little, Brown & Co., 1977).

65. T.H. Budzynski, "Biofeedback procedures in the clinic," in Ada Jacox, ed., *Pain: A Sourcebook for Nurses and Other Health Professionals* (Boston: Little, Brown & Co., 1977).

Annotated Bibliography

Booker, J.E. 1982. *Pain It's All in Your Patient's Head (or Is It?)*. Nurs 82 12(3):47–51. Pain can change the body's chemistry, and this article discusses techniques that will modify these biochemical responses.

Copp, L.A. 1985. Pain Coping and Typology. *Image* 17(3):69–71. Describes pain coping model that can be used as a guideline for nurses assessing pain. Also discusses client responses with use of model.

Horsley, J.A., Crane J., and Reynolds, M.A. 1982. *Pain: Deliberate Nursing Interventions*. New York: Grune & Stratton. Describes and defines knowledge base underlying nursing as an intervention for complaints of pain. Includes research studies.

Mannheimer, J.S. and Lampe, G.N. 1984. *Clinical Transcutaneous Electrical Nerve Stimulation*. Philadelphia: F.A. Davis. Discussion of current theories related to the use of electrical stimulation and the management of client with a stimulation unit.

Meinhart, M. and McCaffery, M. 1983. *Pain: A Nursing Approach to Assessment and Analysis*. East Norwalk, Conn.: Appleton-Century-Crofts. Complete discussion of pain assessment, evaluation, and decision making appropriate for application to the nursing process.

Melzack, R., and Wall, P.D. 1983. *The Challenge of Pain*. New York: Basic Books. Excellent basic text discussing the gate-control theory and other physiological and psychological aspects of pain.

McCaffery, M. 1980. How to Relieve your Patients' Pain Fast and Effectively . . . With Oral Analgesics. *Nurs 80* 10(11):58–63. This article compares and contrasts intramuscular (IM) and oral medications and proposes nursing actions to promote use of oral drugs instead of the more invasive IMs.

McCaffery, M. 1980. Patients Shouldn't Have to Suffer: How to Relieve Pain with Injectable Narcotic. *Nurs 80* 10(10):34–39. This excellent article describes the issues of most concern to nurses regarding narcotic administration and proposes solutions.

McGuire, L. 1981. A Short, Simple Tool for Assessing Your Patient's Pain. *Nurs 81* 11(3):48–49. This brief article proposes a pain assessment tool.

McGuire, L. and Shyane D. 1982. Managing Pain . . . In the Young Patient. *Nurs 82* 12(9):53–55. This article gives helpful tips for assessing pain in children from under two, up. It discusses some of the common problems in relieving pain in the very young.

Meissner, J.E. 1980. McGill-Melzack Pain Questionnaire. *Nurs 80* 10(1):50–52. This excellent article discusses the value of a careful pain assessment and includes the unique McGill-Melzack Pain Questionnaire.

Pageau, M.G., Mroz, N.T., and Combs, D.W. 1985. New Analgesic Therapy *Nurs 85* 15(4):46–49. It is possible for cancer clients to remain pain-free without hospitalization. This article describes the use of continuous pain medication infusion.

Panayotoff, K. 1982. Managing Pain . . . in the Elderly. *Nurs 82* 12(8):53–57. All clients in pain need to have nurses who are aware of their special needs. This article describes the needs of the elderly.

Wright, Z. 1981. From I.V. to P.O. Your Patient's Pain Medication. *Nurs 81* 11(7). A step-by-step procedure for the changeover from intravenous to oral medication is discussed in this article. A client situation is used as an example, and a pain medication flow sheet is presented.

Chapter 26

Anxiety, Fear, and Stress

Marie Rawlings

Chapter Outline

- Objectives
- Glossary
- Introduction
- Anxiety
    Theories of Anxiety
    Levels of Anxiety
    Physiological Responses
    Internal and External Behavioral Responses
    Adaptive and Maladaptive Behaviors Related to Anxiety
    Coping/Defense Mechanisms
    Nursing Considerations
- Fear
    Definition of Fear
    Types of Fear
    Responses to Fear
- Stress
    Theories of Stress
    Behavioral Responses to Stress
    Physiological Responses to Stress
    Adaptive Responses to Stress
    Maladaptive Responses to Stress
- The Nursing Process
    Assessment
    Planning
    Implementation
    Evaluation
- Summary
- Study Questions
- References
- Annotated Bibliography

Objectives

At the completion of this chapter, the reader will be able to:
▸ Define the concept of anxiety
▸ Define the concept of fear
▸ Define the concept of stress
▸ Describe physiological responses to anxiety, fear, and stress
▸ Describe the four levels of anxiety
▸ Identify four defense mechanisms
▸ Discuss the importance of the nurse–client relationship in regard to nursing intervention for anxiety

Glossary

Anxiety. Tension caused by an imagined threat to the self that affects physical and mental functioning.

Defense Mechanisms. Unconscious behaviors that a person exhibits to defend against pain and tension caused by anxiety.

Fear. Tension caused by a real threat to the self that affects physical and mental functioning.

Fight or Flight Response. The physiological response to a threat that consists of autonomic nervous system activation to provide strength and resourcefulness to fight or flee the threat.

General Adaptation Syndrome. Physiological pattern of response to stress consisting of an alarm reaction stage, stage of resistance, and the final exhaustion stage.

Intrapsychic. Pertaining to or originating from the mind.

Stress. The body's non-specific response to a variety of stimuli which interfere with the satisfaction of basic needs or which disturb the stable equilibrium.

Stressor. A stimulus that evokes the stress response; stressors may be physical, chemical, developmmental, or emotional.

Syndrome. A group of signs and symptoms occuring together that characterize a disorder.

INTRODUCTION

Anxiety, fear, and stress are terms most people are aware of, because they describe feelings that are commonly experienced by everyone. To many, they are dreaded conditions that hopefully will not have to be encountered. Avoidance of anxiety, fear, and stress, however, is not only impossible but also undesirable, as they can contribute to growth and productivity. On the other hand, uncontrolled stress and anxiety can have a detrimental effect on one's functioning ability and can even promote illness states.

All three concepts have been studied extensively in the realm of the physical and social sciences, and the findings indicate that there is a mind-body relationship associated with anxiety, fear, and stress. **Anxiety** is tension caused by an *imagined* threat to the self that affects physical and mental functioning. **Fear** is tension caused by a *real* threat to the self that affects physical and mental functioning. **Stress** is the body's physical, mental, and chemical reaction to any change in adaptation. Nurses must be aware of these mind-body relationships and interactions if they are to provide effective total nursing care.

ANXIETY

Anxiety is a condition the nurse frequently encounters. It is a natural response to situations in which one feels insecure. By definition, anxiety is tension felt in response to an *anticipated* threat to self-integrity. The awareness of the threat is perceived consciously or unconsciously, but the perception is vague and non-specific, as opposed to the real or specific threat associated with fear. The feeling of tension from anxiety can be described as an uncomfortable feeling of uneasiness, of impending danger, nervousness, or panic. The stimulus for anxiety may originate from psychic conflict when ideas, thoughts, or feelings threaten the individual's self-integrity. Consider, for example, a woman uneasy with close relationships because unconsciously she thinks she is unlovable and that men eventually will reject her. The stimulus also may originate outside the psyche, when something in the individual's biological or social environment threatens self-integrity. Examples would be an airline pilot faced with failing eyesight, or an individual with minimal education feeling anxious at social affairs where others are highly educated.

Throughout the life span, we experience anxiety in varying degrees. For most people, anxiety usually remains within the range of normal limits. For others, it is the basis of severe mental and emotional disturbances, some of which are situational and relatively short-term, while others last for years. Most clients in the health-care system experience some type of anxiety, since illness, hospitalization, medical tests, and procedures can all provoke feelings of insecurity. For example, surgical removal of a limb may threaten the security a client has with body image. Confinement to a wheelchair may threaten the role of a parent of small children. A lengthy recovery from an illness could threaten one's financial security. Clients may imagine countless ways that their future will be affected, as well as fantasies about how their medical plight came about. For example, a woman awaiting the results of fertility testing may be anxious that she will lose her husband if she cannot have children, or that infertility would be punishment for past promiscuous behavior.

The discomfort and energy that anxiety arouses motivates action in search of relief. Nurses may observe uncommon or fluctuating behaviors, such as anger or sudden crying outbursts, as a client attempts to cope with or avoid anxiety. The attempts can be adaptive, such as the tension relief provided by crying, or maladaptive, such as angrily throwing things or destroying property. Understanding anxiety enables the nurse to provide an environment conducive to the client's maintaining self-integrity, and to aid the healing and learning processes.

Theories of Anxiety

Probably the widest known theories of anxiety originate in psychoanalytic theory, with Freud's the most famous. Initially, Freud conceptualized anxiety as a state of unpleasure caused by repressed or pent-up sexual energy. Thus, the experience of anxiety originated within the individual. In later years, he viewed anxiety as tension resulting from internal or external threats to the ego. (Refer to chapters 18 and 19 for readings on Freud's psychic apparatus: the id, ego, and superego.) He viewed the occurrence of anxiety as a response to anticipated danger, based on an individual's past experience with traumatic events that remain with the individual on a conscious or preconscious level. Once the ego receives a threatening cue, it mobilizes protective measures to ward off danger. Freud believed anxiety resulted when the ego did not adequately defend against danger, and fears were externalized in symptoms such as phobias or obsessive-compulsive behavior. In psychotic states, the failure of the ego to defend against danger is even more complete, so that the ego is overwhelmed or destroyed, with a resultant loss of contact with reality.[1]

Harry Stack Sullivan, another psychoanalyst, also believed that an individual's past experiences influence present behavior. His concept of anxiety, however, pertained only to interpersonal relationships. He believed that the self developed, to a large extent, in relationship to approved, acceptable social norms and behavior patterns. An individual's self-esteem is incorporated in acceptance of society's norms. When the individual experiences disapproval by significant others, interpersonal security decreases. When one disapproves of one's own behavior or thoughts, the result is a decrease in self-esteem. A decrease in interpersonal security or self-esteem is called *anxiety tension*. Sullivan

viewed it as human nature that individuals constantly strive toward euphoria, or absence of tension. Subsequently, in the presence of anxiety tension, an individual will strive to modify his or her behavior in attempts to achieve an absence of tension.[2]

Portnoy speaks of anxiety as a normal reaction when we face our limitations, or the degree of our vulnerability. These traits are said to be inherent in the nature of human beings. They are brought to awareness in the face of realities such as death, old age, and illness. Portnoy points out that we also experience anxiety as we expand or move forward from the sheltered, the known, or the certain, to the new, unknown, untested, and uncertain. In this view, anxiety is an inevitable accompaniment of healthy growth and change. To Portnoy, a healthy involvement with normal anxiety would be to fight or flee to maintain the self. A neurotic involvement with anxiety would be to shrink or vanish as a self.[3]

Peplau views the cause of anxiety as any threat to an individual's security. Such threats fall mainly into two categories[4]:

- Threats to biological integrity—threats to maintenance of homeostasis through such processes as temperature control, vasomotor stability, and through actions taken to meet bodily needs
- Threats to the self-esteem—threats to maintenance of established views of self and the values and patterns of behavior used to resist changes in self-view

The theorists mentioned all agree that anxiety is the result of a threat to one's self-integrity. The theories differ in what they regard as precipitating a threat. Threats can arise from within the individual's psyche, from the social environment, and from loss of biological integrity.

Levels of Anxiety

Anxiety can be useful to an individual, depending on the amount or level, and whether behavioral responses are adaptive or maladaptive. Theorists see anxiety as a continuum similar to that in Figure 26–1. At each level, one's behavior is affected by the amount of tension because tension causes changes in perceptual awareness,

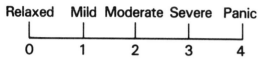

Figure 26–1. Levels of anxiety.

the ability to concentrate, and the ability to reason.

When *relaxed,* the individual is comfortable, unconcerned, and has a sense of well-being. This is the optimal state for healing to take place. During this state, however, one may lack motivation to change, learn, or expend energy.

With *mild anxiety,* there is slight tension and an accompanying increase in energy. The senses are more alert, and the perceptual field is widened. Thus, the individual is attentive to his or her own concerns as well as the environment. The person is able to concentrate and reason to full capacity. One is capable of effective problem solving with mild anxiety. During an average day, most people probably fluctuate between being relaxed and mildly anxious.

With *moderate anxiety,* the individual is more alert and tense. The perceptual field is narrowed. One is able to focus on events important to one in the environment but is less aware of peripheral details and forgets or ignores less important details. One can effectively reason or solve problems when moderately anxious, although usually not for prolonged periods of time. The average person is uncomfortable during this state, but some people can function effectively with moderate anxiety for prolonged periods of time without discomfort.

With *severe anxiety,* the perceptual field is gravely narrowed. The individual will focus on details, unable to see the larger picture of events in the environment. The person also is unable to make reasonable associations between the details of which he or she is aware. The person will be mostly unaware of anxious behavior but very aware of the discomfort from tension. The individual with severe anxiety cannot focus attention to solve problems and has difficulty reasoning. Severe anxiety is detrimental to the healing process and always should be considered a problem necessitating intervention.

In *panic* the perceptual field is completely disrupted. The individual focuses on detail, but the perceptions are enlarged or distorted. Consequently, perception of what is going on around the person is fragmented and distorted. Thinking is disorganized, and behavioral responses will be inappropriate. Individuals in panic feel overwhelmed and frightened. In essence, they are in a crisis state (see Chapter 28 for description of a crisis state). See Figure 26–2 and Table 26–1 for further understanding of anxiety levels.

Physiological Responses

When an individual is faced with a threat, the body systems adjust to provide the individual with more energy to confront or get away from the threat. This is known as the **fight or flight response.** This physiological response is a result of autonomic nervous system activation aided by pituitary stimulation, which together provide far greater strength and resourcefulness than is usual.

The autonomic response is activated once the brain perceives a threat. The brain, by way of the hypothalamus, triggers the sympathetic portion of the autonomic nervous system, which increases visceral and mental functions by stimulating increased secretion of adrenalin from the

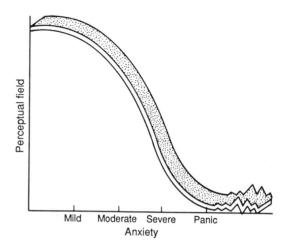

Figure 26–2. The effect of anxiety on the perceptual field. *(From C.R. Kneisl and S.A. Ames, Adult Health Nursing, Addison-Wesley Publishing Co., 1986, with permission.)*

TABLE 26–1. BEHAVIORAL PATTERNS RELATED TO LEVELS OF ANXIETY

Level	Behavioral Patterns
Mild anxiety	Alertness
	Quick eye movements
	Increased hearing ability
	Increased awareness
Moderate anxiety	Decreased awareness of environmental details
	Focus on selected aspects of self (or illness)
Severe anxiety	Disturbances in thought patterns
	Incongruency of thoughts, feelings, and actions
Panic	Distorted perceptions of environment
	Inability to see or understand situation
	Unpredictable responses
	Random motor activity

From B.C. Long and W.J. Phipps, Essentials of Medical-Surgical Nursing, C.V. Mosby Co., 1985, with permission.

adrenal medulla. Simultaneously, the sympathetic nervous system increases functioning in those organs that aid the fight or flight response. The functioning of organs that do not aid the fight or flight response is inhibited. This process of stimulation and inhibition results in the following physiological changes.

Activation of cardiopulmonary functioning results in increased heart rate, arterial pressure, and respirations to provide greater blood supply to the tissues. Increased innervation and cellular metabolism to muscles of the motor system result in greater strength and agility. Pupils are dilated to widen visual perception. The gastrointestinal and genitourinary systems are generally inhibited as they are not important in the fight or flight response. Increased blood flow to the brain increases mental alertness. Increased sympathetic nervous stimulation to the liver results in increased release of glucose for energy. Stimulation to the spleen increases the number of red blood cells in circulation. The increased autonomic nervous system functioning is aided by hypothalamic stimulation of the pituitary, which triggers production of hormones that act on the thyroid to produce growth hormones and on the adrenal cortex to produce hormones that aid in glucose production (Fig. 26–3).

Signs of the internal physiological response

may be observed externally. Because of the circulatory changes, the vital signs may increase. The increase in adrenalin and autonomic nervous system innervation may be observed in behaviors like trembling, restlessness, and dilated pupils. Dry mouth, perspiration, and menstrual changes are indicative of changes in glandular activity. Inhibition and stimulation of particular areas of the gastrointestinal and genitourinary systems may cause vomiting, loss of appetite, diarrhea, constipation, and urinary frequency.

Internal and External Behavioral Responses

Many internal and external responses typically are associated with anxiety. In order to gather data that indicate internal behavioral responses to anxiety, the nurse must rely solely on the client's subjective account of what is being experienced. The external behavioral responses to anxiety may be directly observed or measured. Table 26–2 lists the internal and external responses typically associated with anxiety. These responses reflect the physiological and psychological adaptation to anxiety.

Adaptive and Maladaptive Behaviors Related to Anxiety

Individuals experiencing anxiety consciously or unconsciously adapt their behavior to avoid, minimize, or eliminate the anxiety. The method depends on the intensity of the threat, current circumstances, and the individual's established repertoire for coping. Possible adaptive and maladaptive behaviors may be observed in the physiological, psychological, and social areas of the individual's self-system. Each of these areas of the self-system can be a cause of anxiety as well as the basis for adaptation.

The *physiological* adaptive response to the energy and tension of anxiety may be observed in disturbances in sleep. Some individuals may complain of insomnia, which is usually not a problem for short periods. Over prolonged periods, however, insomnia interferes with the healing process and can limit a person's reasoning and problem-solving abilities. Other individuals may sleep excessively in an attempt to avoid tension or in response to exhaustion from tension. This may serve to "recharge batteries" and allow the person to subsequently cope

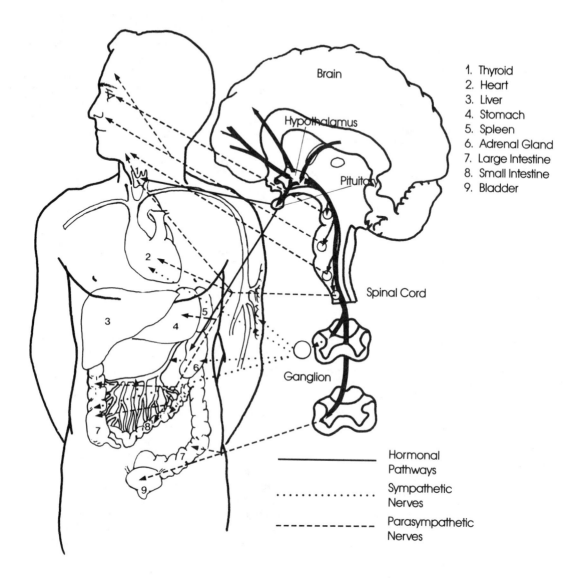

1. Thyroid
2. Heart
3. Liver
4. Stomach
5. Spleen
6. Adrenal Gland
7. Large Intestine
8. Small Intestine
9. Bladder

Brain

Hypothalamus

Pituitary

Spinal Cord

Ganglion

——————— Hormonal Pathways

· · · · · · · · · · · · · · Sympathetic Nerves

– – – – – – – – – Parasympathetic Nerves

Figure 26–3. Physiological responses to stress.

from a stronger position. Excessive sleeping for days, however, may indicate pathological withdrawal, such as that accompanying severe depression.

Many anxious clients experience headaches or vague aches and pains as the body goes through the circulatory and musculoskeletal changes of the adaptive fight or flight response. The client's awareness of anxiety and taking

appropriate measures for relief is an adaptive response. However, constant complaining may indicate a maladaptive response, as the client focuses on detail, and an inability or reluctance to focus on the broader source of tension.

Adaptive behaviors such as picking at clothing, twirling or pulling hair, and pacing the floor are indications of restlessness or anxious energy. These types of behaviors are fairly com-

TABLE 26–2. INTERNAL AND EXTERNAL BEHAVIORAL RESPONSES TO ANXIETY

Internal	External
Jittery or tense	Elevated blood pressure
More alert	Increased respiration
Headaches	Trembling
Chest pain	Vomiting
Tightness in muscles	Urinary frequency
Comprehension difficulty	Pupils dilated
Apprehension	Worry or preoccupation
Shame	Crying
Depression	Joking
Jealousy	Withdrawal
Uncertainty	Irritability
Feelings of worthlessness	Angry outbursts
Hallucinations	Slumped posture
Heart pounding	Increased pulse rate
Nausea, heartburn, gas	Sleep disturbance
Dry mouth	Restlessness
Loss of appetite	Diarrhea or constipation
Inability to concentrate	Perspiration
Confusion	Hypervigilance
Guilt	Sadness
Doubt	Talkativeness
Helplessness	Inquisitiveness
Suspiciousness	Dependency, clinging
Isolation or loneliness	behavior
Delusions	

mon in all individuals during stressful periods and the person is generally unaware of them. Constructive responses are directed toward effectively dealing with or avoiding the source. It also is constructive to work off excess energy through exercise or hard work. A maladaptive response may be observed in hostile aggression toward others or destruction of property.

Behaviors associated with anxiety can be constructive or destructive to the *psychological* integrity of the self-concept. Anxious persons, for example, may be observed to be deep in thought or daydreaming. This behavior is adaptive when it results in the individual gaining awareness of his or her feelings and an accurate perception of threatening events. However, excessive fantasizing ("what if—" or "if only—") and withdrawal from reality are maladaptive responses.

Verbal and emotional expression of feelings can be helpful in relieving psychic tension. Expression of feelings may be noted in behaviors such as crying, laughing, and swearing, or verbalization of guilt or anger. Resistance to expressing intense feelings generally increases or maintains psychic tension.

Attention to the physical and personal self can be constructive to the anxious person. Examples of adaptive response in this area would be taking necessary physiological precautions during an illness and attention to grooming and hygiene to preserve body image. Maladaptive responses would be self-destructive behaviors, such as suicide or mutilation attempts, apathy or avoidance behavior toward problem solving, and behaving in a manner that goes counter to one's own well-being, such as abuse of alcohol or drugs.

Adaptive and maladaptive behaviors can stem from anxiety affecting the *social* realm of the self-image. Anxiety often affects an individual's role. For example, a project engineer may be unable to complete a project because of his inability to solve problems. A student may be unable to study because of inability to concentrate. The failure to perform a role in a usual manner can contribute to anxiety. One may, at times, have to make adjustments in role functioning, in order to cope with anxiety. Maladaptive responses would be inability to make choices regarding role functioning, rigidly maintaining roles when adjustments should be made, or feeling alienated from established roles.

Many people turn to others to provide care and emotional support when they are anxious. The care and support of others can relieve tension by increasing an anxious person's self-esteem, lessening the burden of problem solving by offering different perspectives, or by handling stressful situations until the anxious person is better able to handle them. Maladaptive responses to these dependency needs could be behavior that is demanding of attention or rigidly denies the need for help.

Coping/Defense Mechanisms

Anxiety can result from **intrapsychic** conflict as well as from external threats. This conflict generally arises when an individual has desires, fears, or motives that threaten the concept of self. To defend against the pain and tension from the anxiety these conflicts cause, people learn to develop certain behaviors over time, to conceal these threats to self from their awareness. Hence, **defense mechanisms** are usually unconscious behaviors. Individuals may be aware that they use such mechanisms at times, but during the process of employing them, they are unaware. Table 26–3 lists the most commonly known defense mechanisms with examples of the desires, fears, or motives that may cause intrapsychic conflict.

Everyone uses defense mechanisms to some degree as a means of coping with anxiety. Individuals may unconsciously choose a particular mechanism for consistently defending against anxiety if it was successful in the past. However, occasions may arise when usual mechanisms of defense are ineffective. Panic or poor mental health can result when the usual mechanisms fail.

Nursing Considerations

In summation, anxiety is an intense emotion that can be constructive as well as destructive. Awareness of anxiety expands the role of the nurse beyond "hands on" care, and is included in total client care.

FEAR

Fear is another emotion that nurses observe during client care. It is similar to anxiety in many ways, yet different enough to warrant exploring. Understanding the difference between the two can help maximize the possibility of effective nursing interventions.

Definition of Fear

Fear is a strong emotional response to the threat of danger to one's well-being. The threat associated with fear is specific *and consciously perceived*. Fear is a response to a real or threatened danger. The intensity of the fear is usually proportionate to the perceived danger. This means that one who is fearful would be able to recognize what is causing the discomfort and why. This differs from anxiety, wherein the perception of threat is most often unconscious and vague. The experience of fear can be characterized as a feeling of dread, doom, or panic.

Types of Fear

Most fears are rational; that is, fear is a reasonable reaction to certain stimuli. For example, a woman who finds a lump in her breast may fear she will die from cancer. The reality may be that the lump is not cancerous and, if it is, the prognosis for her surviving may be excellent. However, since lumps in the breast can be cancerous, with the possibility of metastasis and death, her fears are not without basis. Our awareness of fearful or dangerous events is learned from past experiences with dangerous events, or from observing or learning of the danger associated with particular situations.

Sometimes fears are irrational, i.e. the fearful response seems unreasonable to the specific stimulus. This type of fear is exhibited in panic associated with phobic fear (of heights, germs, enclosures). These fears are the result of the projection of anxiety from inner conflict to external objects and are neurotic in nature. Illness, surgery, medical tests, and procedures all can signal a response of fear. There may be danger of pain, death, disfigurement, and loss of usual mode of functioning. Fear can be a useful emotional response, if the energy alerted is focused on preparing for the danger. If there is no preparation for danger, fears may be heightened and interfere with the healing process.

Responses to Fear

Fear triggers the same physiological response as that associated with anxiety. When the brain perceives a threat, it does not distinguish whether the threat is real (as in fear) or imagined (as in anxiety). In either case, the individual's need for "fight or flight" is the same.

The observable behaviors associated with anxiety are also associated with fear and are a result of the anticipation of danger. (Review internal and external behavioral responses to anxiety.) The behaviors that will be particularly associated with worry and feelings of fear are those of helplessness (agitation, preoccupation, dependency). The emotional responses associated with inner conflict (guilt, anger, shame) also may be observed in clients who ponder the origin of the danger. It is not unusual for clients with fear to initially "freeze" or respond with panic in a psychological attempt to deny or flee

TABLE 26-3. DEFENSE MECHANISMS

Compensation: Emphasizing or excelling at a certain personal feature to defend against anxiety stemming from perceived personal deficiency in another area. Example—a boy with below-average intellectual capacity may compensate by being the "class clown."

Denial: Refusing to accept, on a conscious level, the presence of a threatening event or personal attribute. Example—a person who is clearly alcoholic may insist that drinking is not a problem.

Displacement: Transferring emotional feelings toward something or someone to a substitute, because it would be too threatening or unacceptable to express them toward the originating source. Example—a child who is angry with a parent for refusing to grant permission to go out subsequently goes to his room and kicks his bed or smacks a stuffed animal.

Identification: When one incorporates attributes of someone one admires into one's own behavior to increase self-esteem. Also, when one is unusually sympathetic with someone else's plight because of one's own sense of guilt, conflict, or similar experience. Example of the latter—a student organizing a protest against the expulsion of another student found guilty of cheating because of his unconscious sense of guilt.

Projection: When one attributes one's own unacceptable motives, thoughts, or feelings to someone else. Example—a husband accuses his spouse of being unfaithful when actually he is defending against his own desire to be unfaithful.

Rationalization: When one gives a reason for behavior other than the real motivating desires or thoughts one feels guilty about. Example—a failing student withdraws from college early with the excuse that it was not a good college, rather than admitting personal failure.

Regression: Reverting to earlier successful methods of coping that have been outgrown in an effort to cope with a currently overwhelming situation. Example—an adult whose parents took responsibility for childhood difficulties when she cried and looked helpless, cries and looks helpless when the nurse coaches her to self-administer an insulin injection for the first time, as a way of coping with overwhelming conflict about having diabetes.

Repression: Not allowing undesirable thoughts or feelings to come to awareness. Example—a man who hates his father and has no awareness of it.

Sublimation: Gratification of an impulse through socially acceptable channels. Example—directing the energy from aggressive (anger) impulses into aggressive sports activities.

Suppression: The conscious or subconscious refusal to allow undesirable thoughts to come to awareness. Example—a woman who has strong feelings against divorce pushes from awareness any feelings of her own marital discontent.

Reaction formation: Handling the tension from undesirable thoughts by behaving in a manner that is the direct opposite. Example—a person who has a lot of hate and anger, constantly behaves as a kind, polite, friendly person.

Introjection: Incorporating into the ego system the standards and values of someone who is regarded with love, hate, fear, or guilt, in an effort to control the tension resulting from these feelings. Example—a woman begins to dress and act like her deceased mother in an effort to stay close to her.

Conversion: Relieving the tension of emotional conflict by symbolically expressing it through physical symptoms, thus drawing attention away from the conflict. Example—a person overwhelmed by guilt and shame, resulting from having committed a theft, develops paralysis in the hands for which there is no physiological basis.

---

the danger. Anxiety may be a response to fear when the individual anticipates a danger before actually experiencing danger.

Adaptive responses to fear foster preparation for the threat of danger and subsequently defend against overwhelming anxiety. Clients who ask questions about their illness or medical procedures and make plans for how they will deal with them are adapting to fear. Calling upon past experiences with similar dangers and appropriately applying learned methods of coping also show adaptation to fear. For example, a client recently diagnosed with a cardiac con-

dition may plan to have his wife attend his next visit to the doctor for emotional support and to gain knowledge to help with their future life adjustments. Another client, who has learned that taking deep breaths and relaxing muscles decreases pain, may apply that principle to a painful testing procedure. These adaptive responses assure that the client will be able to cope with the threat.

Maladaptive responses are those that do not prepare clients for danger and threaten to overwhelm them with anxiety. Those who deny or suppress worries about the danger are more apt to be anxious, overwhelmed, and helpless when confronted with the danger. Those who ruminate over frightening rumors and their own imagined exaggerations are likely to be overwhelmed with anxiety. These maladaptive responses do not prepare clients with mechanisms for coping and thus psychological and physiological integrity are further compromised. The nurse's understanding of and appropriate intervention regarding signs and symptoms of fear are important responsibilities for providing total nursing care.

STRESS

Stress is the reaction of the body to any threat or change in equilibrium and is therefore a direct result of adaptation to events in the social, physical, and emotional environment. A **stressor** is an event or activity that serves as the stimulus to evoking a stress response. Socially we are often confronted with stress when changes are made in our political, ethical, and technological systems. Our nation, for example, is moving through a complex series of cultural changes that are stress-producing: the breakdown of traditional sex roles, a climbing divorce rate, burgeoning technology, increasing mobility, and almost instant access to worldwide information on natural disasters, terrorist acts, and other stress-producing events. The impact of these changes can cause anxiety. In addition we are confronted with stress-related events such as maturation (i.e., change from one developmental stage to another), and family or interpersonal relationship difficulties. Stress also can be caused by the physical environment, such as skin and temperature changes caused by extreme weather conditions, air and noise pollution, and trauma to the body from injury or disease. These events can disrupt psychobiological functioning. Thus, a broad definition of stress is the body's physical, mental, and chemical reactions to any stimulus that causes change in adaptation.

Stress can be caused by events in our lives that are pleasant as well as those that are unpleasant. Getting married, for example, is a pleasant event, and getting divorced is an un-

pleasant event, but the process of accomplishing either is stressful. The events causing significant stress do not necessarily have to be "big events." A phone call from relatives, a minor car accident, a reprimand from the boss can all accumulate over varying periods of time and cause the body to experience a stress reaction.

Stress has a positive side also, in that it keeps us creative and productive. Low levels of stress act as motivators, as devices that challenge and promote interest. For example, the stress of failing a quiz can prompt a student to buckle down, study, and make an A on the final exam. Therefore, a goal is not to eliminate stress, but to manage or adapt to it successfully.

How one reacts to stress is an individual matter. It would depend on how one perceives the stressful event, the stressor, or the degree of change caused by it, and one's ability to adapt, such as one's health, genetic endowment, and available coping mechanisms. When the level of stress is more than the individual can handle, well-being is threatened. The nurse can play a significant role in helping clients avoid poor mental and emotional health by teaching effective stress management.

Theories of Stress

A theory of the biology of stress was introduced in the 1920s by Cannon. It was Cannon who discovered the "fight or flight" response as he observed responses to emergency situations, such as pain, fear, anger, starvation, and inadequate supply of oxygen. He saw the fight or flight response as the body's adaptive process to maintain homeostasis.[5]

In the 1930s, Hans Selye, a Canadian endocrinologist and the most widely recognized stress researcher, concluded that fight or flight was only the initial alarm reaction to stress, and that two other stages follow.[6] He identified these responses to stress as a **syndrome**. Selye called the first stage of the stress syndrome the *alarm reaction;* the second stage, *resistance;* and the third stage, *exhaustion.* His theory describing these stress responses is known as the **General Adaptation Syndrome** (GAS), which is described in Table 26–4. Selye also brought attention to the fact that, although the physiological response to stress is a specific syndrome, the stimulus for stress is nonspecific. This means

TABLE 26–4. THE GENERAL ADAPTATION SYNDROME

Stage 1: **Alarm reaction** is the fight or flight response. Selye emphasized the process of enlargement of adrenal cortex, enlargement of the lymphatic system, and increase in hormone levels, because these activities are responsible for disease symptomatology. The extent to which these activities are increased depends on the perception of the stressor.

Stage 2: **Resistance** is reached when the body fails to resist stress any longer. This stage is characterized by enlargement and dysfunction of the lymphatic structures and an increase in hormone levels, with eventual depletion of adaptive hormones.

Stages 1 and 2 are repeated throughout life. If an individual cannot sustain resistance to stress, exhaustion will occur with accompanying psychophysiological alterations.

Stage 3: **Exhaustion** occurs when the original stressor is so damaging that it is impossible for the defense mechanism to be effective or if the stressor is not removed and the energy needed to maintain resistance is depleted. Unless this stage can be controlled, mental dysfunction or death may result.

TABLE 26–5. THE SOCIAL READJUSTMENT RATING SCALE

Life Event	Mean Value
1. Death of spouse	100
2. Divorce	73
3. Marital separation	65
4. Jail term	63
5. Death of close family member	63
6. Personal injury or illness	53
7. Marriage	50
8. Fired at work	47
9. Marital reconciliation	45
10. Retirement	45
11. Change in health of family member	44
12. Pregnancy	40
13. Sex difficulties	39
14. Gain of new family member	39
15. Business readjustment	39
16. Change in financial state	38
17. Death of a close friend	37
18. Change to different line of work	36
19. Change in number of arguments with spouse	35
20. Mortgage	31
21. Foreclosure of mortgage or loan	30
22. Change in responsibilities at work	29
23. Son or daughter leaving home	29
24. Trouble with in-laws	29
25. Outstanding personal achievement	28
26. Wife begins or stops work	26
27. Begin or end school	26
28. Change in living conditions	25
29. Revision of personal habits	24
30. Trouble with boss	23
31. Change in work hours or conditions	20
32. Change in residence	20
33. Change in schools	19
34. Change in recreation	19
35. Change in church activities	18
36. Change in social activities	17
37. Mortgage or loan less than $10,000	16
38. Change in sleeping habits	15
39. Change in number of family get-togethers	15
40. Change in eating habits	13
41. Change in schedule (vacation)	12
42. Christmas	11
43. Minor violations of the law	10

Scores of 150–199 indicate a 37% chance of physical illness

Scores of 200–299 indicate a 51% chance of physical illness

Scores of 300 indicate a 90% chance of physical illness

From T. Holmes and R. Rahe, J Psychosom Res, 1967, with permission.

that whatever the stressor is, the physiological response is the same.

Harold G. Wolff, in the 1940s and 1950s, studied life situations and emotional stages associated with certain illnessess. He concluded that disease can be precipitated by stress in combination with other predisposing factors, such as genetic endowment, individual needs, and past experiences. This combination of stress and the aforementioned predisposing factors affect the body organs in stereotypical ways, and if the stress persists, the physiological changes become chronic.[7]

Holmes and Rahe conducted some interesting studies on thousands of patients. They noted that a number of significant life events tended to occur in a brief period prior to the onset of major illnesses. They gave a numerical value to each of these events to represent the amount, duration, and severity of change required to cope with the event. From their observations, they devised a scale, whereupon, adding the values for recent life events, one could determine what percent chance there was for the occurrence of a major illness in the next two years (Table 26–5).[8]

Behavioral Responses to Stress

The behavioral responses to stress are the same as those associated with anxiety. The most common of these are listed below:

- Increased vital signs
- Sleep disturbance
- Appetite disturbance
- Fatigue
- Tension
- Concentration difficulties
- Decreased ability to solve problems
- Irritability and emotional liability
- Body aches and pains
- Depressed mood

Physiological Responses to Stress

The general changes that occur in the body during adaption to stress were noted in the discussion of the "fight or flight" syndrome. However, if stress continues without remission, the body becomes exhausted, which can lead to structural changes in the organ systems. Consequently, many of the diseases the nurse comes in contact with are stress-related. The determinant for which organ system is particularly affected by prolonged stress is mainly based on genetic load. For example, if one's ancestors had cardiac problems, one is more likely to have distress in the cardiovascular system, if stress is prolonged. Table 26–6 lists some of the disorders that may be caused by stress.

Adaptive Responses to Stress

Many of the stressors in life can be positive, and, if managed appropriately, provide one with a sense of self-satisfaction and increased ability to cope. Examples of such stressors are career tasks, developing intimate relationships, political or academic pursuits, and any type of contest. Negative stressors, such as death of a loved one, may be unavoidable, but in the process of adapting positively to them, one's self-esteem and ability to cope are enhanced. Since stress is inevitable, an adaptive response would be to effectively manage what can be controlled, such as:

- Regular exercise: Strengthens the cardiovascular system, promotes healthy breathing for

TABLE 26–6. CLASSIFIED LIST OF STRESS-RELATED DISORDERS

System	Disorders
Cardiovascular	Arrhythmias, hypertension, coronary occlusions, migraine headaches
Gastrointestinal	Chronic constipation or diarrhea, colitis, gastritis, ulcers, unhealthy weight loss or gain
Genitourinary	Urinary frequency, nocturnal enuresis, disturbance in sexual functioning, menstrual difficulties
Musculoskeletal	Torticollis, back pain, arthritis, rheumatism, bruxism
Endocrine	Menstrual irregularities, thyroid conditions, diabetes, fertility problems, excessive sweating, hirsutism
Skin	Acne, hives, eczema, psoriasis
Respiratory	Asthma, chronic bronchitis, emphysema

better cell oxygenation and metabolism, helps to regulate hormonal activity, and increases muscular strength. Exercise provides energy and well-being to help cope with stress.

- Nutrition: Proper nutrition provides strength and energy to resist stress.
- Regular relaxation: Helps to decrease stress and cope by providing diversion from stress. Examples of techniques for relaxation include:

Yoga	Spectator sports
Biofeedback	Crafts
Meditation	Vacations
Hypnosis	Leisure interests
Progressive relaxation	Self-help groups
Hobbies	Psychotherapy

- Self-awareness and acceptance: Self-awareness regarding one's strengths and limitations is helpful in order to use available skills and avoid, if possible, those things one cannot cope with. Whenever possible, it is also helpful to control life stressors by setting priorities for accomplishment, scheduling or managing time well, and to some degree, regulating the amount of stress allowed into one's life. Self-awareness includes becoming familiar with body cues, such as tight muscles or headaches, that might indicate stress. These cues can alert one to the need for control measures.

Maladaptive Responses to Stress

Maladaptive responses to stress are responses that do not help a person cope with or minimize stress. We have mentioned the physiological maladaptive response in the discussion of the exhaustion phase of the General Adaptation Syndrome. Stress-related illnesses also have been mentioned as physiological maladaptive responses to stress.

Behavioral manifestations of maladaption to stress are, primarily, anxiety, depression, and mental confusion. There may be drug and alcohol abuse. Bizarre behavior, such as severe hostility, suspiciousness, and suicide attempts, also may be seen. These maladaptive behavioral responses do not necessarily mean that the individual has an emotional or mental disorder. Prolonged stress, however, can lead to emotional or mental disorders as well as physiological disorders.

THE NURSING PROCESS

The nursing process is the basis for effectively identifying and intervening in problems of anxiety, fear, and stress.

Assessment

Assessment is the first step in the nursing process. It involves collecting subjective and objective data for formulating a nursing diagnosis. The most important tool the nurse can use to assess the presence of anxiety, fear, or stress is skill in observation and interviewing. Indications of anxiety, fear, or stress may be noted in five general areas of the client's behavior and appearance:

- Motor activity: Physical signs of agitation, such as pacing back and forth, rapid limb movements, increased restlessness
- Mood: Angry, sad, anxious, pensive
- Vegetative signs: Changes in sleeping habits, appetite, or elimination
- Thinking processes: Forgetfulness, concentration difficulties
- Perceptual awareness: Loss of ability to see things clearly or realistically

(Review the list of internal and external responses in Table 26–2.)

Once the nurse has observed behavior indicating anxiety, fear, or stress, interviewing skills must be used to determine what factors are influencing the client's behavior. Thus, interviewing must be geared toward determining:

- What is the internal or external threat to the client's self-integrity
- Other factors present in the client's life that may be relevant to the present experience
- What past experiences or beliefs might help the client to cope with anxiety, fear, or stress, or what might hinder adaptation

After this data has been gathered, the nurse must identify and rank the problems that necessitate intervention. To do this, the level of anxiety, fear, or stress must be known, whether the behavior observed is adaptive or maladaptive, and what behaviors are most threatening or destructive to the client's self-integrity.

It is important for nurses to share with clients the results of the assessment. This provides them with some understanding of what they are experiencing and may help decrease any feelings of hopelessness, helplessness, or powerlessness. The client's understanding of maladaptive behavior also encourages change.

After gathering the data, nursing diagnoses are identified for problems necessitating intervention. The following are examples of possible nursing diagnoses:

- Anxiety: Mild, moderate, severe, panic
- Loss of appetite related to anxiety
- Coping, ineffectual, individual
- Sleep pattern disturbance related to stress

Once a nursing diagnosis has been formulated, goals for intervention must be planned.

Planning

Planning is the second stage of the nursing process. In planning for intervention in problems, the goals should be client-centered and focused on behaviors that maintain the client's self-integrity. In some situations of anxiety and fear, this may be accomplished with goals aimed toward eliminating, diminishing, or encouraging adaptation to the threat provoking the anxiety or fear. With stress, the focus of planning may be on avoiding, minimizing, or managing the stress. The goals may be to change maladaptive behavior to adaptive behavior. The following are examples of appropriate goals using the previously stated nursing diagnoses as reference:

Nursing Diagnosis	Goal (Outcome Criteria)
Loss of appetite in response to anxiety	Client will verbalize understanding of this response and its hazard to illness
Sleep pattern disturbance related to stress	Client will sleep 4 to 5 hours at night
Fear related to feelings of helplessness regarding illness	Client will discuss a plan for increasing sense of control in managing illness

After goals are established, the nurse is ready for the next stage of the nursing process, which is implementation.

Implementation

The most important tool for implementing the goals for intervention in problems of anxiety, fear, and stress is the nurse–client relationship. By being provided with a warm, trusting atmosphere, clients can be helped to talk about their concerns and can recognize how these concerns affect their behavior. The nurse's skill in observing, listening, interviewing, and teaching will help guide clients toward understanding the dynamics of anxiety, fear, and stress. The nurse's presence, strength, calmness, and control may help clients manage their own behavior. The nurse must use expertise and judgment in offering alternatives to maladaptive means of coping, taking into consideration individual client needs and circumstances. In instances of fear, a careful explanation of what the client can expect when confronted with a threat, as well as suggestions for how it may be dealt with, is often helpful. Implementation of plans for relieving stress most often will involve education regarding what caused the stress and how it can be managed. (Review adaptive responses to stress.) The client's self-integrity is supported by offering praise and encouragement for adaptive behavior.

Evaluation

To determine whether the interventions were effective or not, the nurse must evaluate the care plan. This last stage of the nursing process entails applying the outcome criteria to the continued observations of the client's behavior. Criteria for evaluating outcome should include the following:

- Does the individual express concerns related to anxiety? (fear? stress?)
- Is the client able to discuss the connection between concerns and behavior?
- Can the client verbalize adaptive methods of coping with anxiety? (fear? stress?)
- Did the client feel the nurse's interventions were helpful in changing maladaptive behavior?
- Was anxiety decreased? (fear decreased? stress decreased?) as evidenced by. . . .
- What goals were not met?

For those goals not met, the nurse must go through the nursing process again to reassess the problem and reformulate goals and interventions where necessary.

SUMMARY

Anxiety, fear, and stress result from human psychological and physiological interaction with the environment. The adaptation response to anxiety, fear, and stress is behavioral and physiological. The initial physiological response is the same with anxiety, fear, or stress and is known as the fight or flight response. This physiological response is a result of autonomic nervous system activation aided by pituitary stimulation, which together provide far greater strength and resourcefulness to the individual than is usual.

Certain behaviors are associated with certain levels of anxiety. The same behavioral responses are associated with fear and stress, with some variance in incidence and intensity. These behaviors reflect changes in perceptual awareness, the ability to concentrate, and the ability to reason. Maladaptive responses intensify and prolong anxiety, fear, and stress. This interferes with the healing process and can lead to poor mental or physical health. Adaptive responses relieve anxiety, fear, and stress. This aids in the healing process, and promotes individual growth by increasing coping skills. Nurses commonly encounter all three of these concepts in all types of clinical settings. The nursing process provides a basis for intervening in maladaption to anxiety, fear, or stress, and for supporting adaptive responses.

Study Questions

1. Identify personal sources of anxiety over a 24- or 48-hour period and rate your behavioral responses according to the levels of anxiety.

2. You are assigned to medicate a 13-year-old adolescent who begs you to stay away from him because he is afraid of needles. How would you use your knowledge of fear to intervene effectively?

3. Discuss specific ways that nurses can help clients understand how stress and illness are sometimes related.

4. Explain what is meant by the "fight or flight" response.

References

1. A. Freedman, H. Kaplan, B. Sadock, eds., *Comprehensive Textbook of Psychiatry*, 2nd ed. (Baltimore: Williams & Wilkins Co., 1976).
2. Ibid.
3. I. Portnoy, "The anxiety states," in S. Arieti, ed., *American Handbook of Psychiatry* (New York: Basic Books, 1959).
4. H.E. Peplau, "A working definition of anxiety," in S. Burd and M. Marshall, eds., *Some Clinical Approaches to Psychiatric Nursing* (New York: Macmillan, 1963).
5. W.B. Cannon, *The Wisdom of the Body*. (New York: W.W. Norton Co., 1932).
6. H. Selye, *Stress Without Distress* (Philadelphia: J.B. Lippincott Co., 1974).
7. H. Wolff, *Stress and Disease* (Springfield, Ill.: Charles C. Thomas, 1953).
8. T. Holmes and R. Rahe, "The social readjustment rating scale," *J Psychosom Res* 2 (4), (1967): 213–17.

Annotated Bibliography

Davis, A.S. 1984. Stress. *Am J Nurs* 84 (3):365–66. This brief and interesting article is a response to a letter from a nurse who has felt "stressed out" because of a new job in a new city.

Guzzetta, C.E. and Forsyth, G.L. 1979. Nursing diagnostic pilot study: Psychophysiologic stress. *Adv in Nurs Sci* 2(1):27–44. This study was designed to develop a typology of stress as observed from clients' suffering from acute illnesses.

Jasmin, S.A., Hill, L., and Smith, N. 1981. The art of managing stress. *Nursing 81* 11(6):53–57. This informative article provides tips for nurses in managing their own stress and helping clients to manage theirs.

Meissner, S. 1980. Measuring patient stress with the hospital stress rating scale. *Nursing 80* 10(8):70–71. This 49-item checklist was designed to measure stress, as it has been identified by hospitalized clients, and those experiences in the hospital that are viewed as stressors.

Peplau, H.E. 1963. A Working Definition of Anxiety. In Burd, S., Marshall, M., eds. *Some Clinical Approaches to Psychiatric Nursing*. New York: Macmillan, 323–27. This classic work on anxiety provides a working definition of anxiety formulated by a nurse author "from the experiences of experts." It is an operational definition presented in outline form.

Perley, N.Z. 1984. Problems in Self-Consistency: Anxiety. In C. Roy: *Introduction to Nursing*, 2nd ed. Englewood Cliffs: Prentice-Hall. Discusses the behavioral manifestations of anxiety and underlying states of mind usually associated with the threat that causes anxiety. Emphasis is on the nursing process, based on the adaptation model.

Rickles, N.S., and Finkle, B.C. 1975. Anxiety—yours and your patient's. *Am J Nurs* 73(3):23–27. The authors of this excellent article provide a list of suggestions for nurses to use when they find themselves in a stressful situation.

Selye, H. 1977. "Further thoughts on 'Stress Without Distress'" *Resident and Staff Physician* (June): 124–40. This article explains how, in the author's opinion, to achieve a balance for stress levels.

Sideleau, B.F. 1978. Stress and the Mind-Body Interrelationship. In Haber, J., Leach, A.M., Schudy, S.M., Sideleau, B.F., eds., *Comprehensive Psychiatric Nursing*. New York: McGraw-Hill, 407–17.

An excellent resource for the historical perspective on stress and understanding the stress syndrome.

Sideleau, B.F., eds., Physiological Maladaptation to Stress. In Haber, J., Leach, A.M., Schudy, S.M., Sideleau, B.F., eds., *Comprehensive Psychiatric Nursing*. New York: McGraw-Hill, 421–39. Discusses physiological maladaptations to stress in relation to psychosomatic illness. Considerable attention is given to nursing care planning and particularly to primary, secondary, and tertiary prevention in stress management.

Smith, M.J.T. and Selye, H. 1979. Reducing the negative effects of stress. *Am J Nurs* 79:1953–55. In this article a model for coping with stress is presented with suggested nursing interventions.

Wilson, H., and Kneisl, C. 1983. Disturbed Personal Coping Patterns. In *Psychiatric Nursing*, 2nd ed. Menlo Park, Calif.: Addison-Wesley, 291–301. Distinguishes anxiety from fear and provides data that indicate fear. Good diagrams of autonomic nervous system responses.

Chapter 27

Loss

Sally Laliberté

Chapter Outline

- Objectives
- Glossary
- Introduction
- Coping with Loss
  Grief
  Mourning
  The Mourning Process
- Factors Influencing the Grief Response
- The Nursing Process
  Assessment
  Planning
  Implementation
  Evaluation
- Summary
- Study Questions
- References
- Annotated Bibliography

Objectives

At the completion of this chapter, the reader will be able to:
- Define the terms loss, grief, mourning, anticipatory grief, maladaptive grief
- Describe various types of losses that affect persons at different points in the life cycle: age and development; life experience; illness; death

- Describe the physical and emotional responses that occur as part of an uncomplicated grief reaction
- Describe the stages of the mourning process along with characteristic responses of the person moving through each stage
- Identify factors that influence the type and severity of the grief reaction and mourning process
- Describe the nurse's role in dealing with persons experiencing loss
- Identify factors that influence the nurse's ability to work effectively with persons experiencing a loss
- Describe basic nursing interventions useful in assisting persons suffering from a loss

Glossary

Anticipatory Grief. The experience of a grief reaction and movement, either partially or completely, through the mourning process while under *threat* of a loss.

Bereavement. The period of grief following the death of a loved one.

Grief. A series of intense physical and emotional responses that occurs following a loss; an adaptive response.

Loss. Any situation either actual, potential or perceived in which a valued object is rendered inaccessible to an individual or is altered in such a way that it no longer has qualities that make it valuable.

Maladaptive Grief. A grief reaction complicated by an abnormal psychological response to a loss; the inability to allow oneself to experience grief or resolve a loss.

Mourning. The period of time in which the grief reaction is expressed and resolution and integration of the loss occurs, an adaptive process.

INTRODUCTION

In our modern world, we are constantly confronted with loss. Through advanced communication systems, we hear frequent reports of terrorism, war, and natural disaster. There is also a growing potential for loss through depletion of natural resources, advancing technologies, and the increasing stress of living in an advanced society. It can be overwhelming to contemplate real and potential losses. As members of a helping profession, nurses must be aware of the potential for loss in today's world, as well as the processes by which human beings adapt to them. These two factors, potential-for loss and human adaptive processes, become part of the environment surrounding each individual who must deal with a specific and personal loss.

At every point in the life span, we are faced with loss. Loss is an essential part of the human experience, for without it, we cannot continue to grow. With every loss there is always the potential for some gain. Just as a young man leaving home to begin a new job loses the security and support of his family, he also gains status in his new position and a sense of pride and accomplishment in his new role.

Often the concept of loss is linked only with illness and death. In reality, loss occurs daily. In fact, certain losses are necessary for human beings to maintain adaptation and to grow physically, psychologically, socially, and spiritually. For example, each day, the human body uses nutrients and disposes of wastes. Millions of cells are turned over daily, and through this process the steady state within the body as a system is maintained. Likewise, a toddler will gain an increasing sense of independence with the ability to manipulate certain parts of the environment. With the gain in mastery comes the loss of a sense of security that came from dependence on parents to maintain control over the environment. It is crucial to interpret the concept of loss in this broader context in order to understand that people deal with loss daily and, in so doing, establish certain patterns of response in an attempt to adapt to specific losses.

The study of loss as a concept for nursing is twofold: as a knowledge base from which to proceed, and in the context of our own personal experience with loss. How we have dealt with loss in our own lives will certainly have an impact on the nursing care we are able to give. In reading this chapter, be aware of your own feelings about loss. Reflect on your own experiences with loss and recall your reponses.

Loss is defined as:

> any situation either actual, potential or perceived in which a valued object is rendered inaccessible to an individual or is altered in such a way that it no longer has qualities that make it valuable.[1]

It is important to remember that a loss can be potential or perceived as well as an obvious or actual loss.[2] It is easy to understand the severity of the loss when a family member dies. It may be much less obvious when the loss involves an ideal, a life goal, or one's self-perception. For example, a young woman gives birth to her first child after a long, tiring labor. She had planned to use no medication but ended up having taken several injections during her labor. She and her infant are healthy and recovered, yet no one can understand why she feels a sense of loss within herself. She was not able to have the kind of experience she envisioned and so it is a loss of what might have been.

The various types of loss with which the nurse must be familiar are divided into four basic categories: loss related to age and development, loss related to life situation, loss related to illness, and loss related to death. Table 27–1 provides a list of losses by category. Although this list is certainly not exhaustive, it does recount many common losses that occur within

TABLE 27–1. CATEGORIES OF LOSS

I. Loss Related to Age and Development

Infants	Protective, warm environment in utero
	Breasts or bottle and comfort of sucking
Toddlers/preschoolers	Immediate and consistent meeting of needs as the toddler grows in independence and begins testing the environment
	Spontaneity of body function that comes with toilet training and acquisition of other social skills
	Familiar environment when leaving the home for daycare or nursery school
	Special place in family as the only child or the youngest child, with birth of sibling
School age	First set of teeth
	Friends and significant others (teachers, coaches, ministers) as they move through grades at school or as the family moves
	Loss of body function at various times with normal childhood illness and injuries
Adolescent	Spontaneity and freedom of childhood with increasing social pressures to act "grown up"
	Child's body with advent of puberty and secondary sexual characteristics
	First boyfriend or girlfriend with adolescent "crushes"
	Virginity with first sexual encounter
	Known, safe environment of family, friends, and community, with leaving home to work or continue education
Young adult	Loss of financial security through parents when leaving home
	Friends, through leaving school, changing jobs, or moving
	Childhood dreams, fantasies, expectations, and ideals
	Freedom, with increasing responsibilities of adulthood (e.g., marriage, family, job)
	Sexual partner for any reason
	A job
Middle adult	Spouse, through divorce or death
	Physical capacities with increasing age (especially stamina and strength related to athletic abilities)
	Children as they grow up and leave home
	Friends through moving, changing jobs, death
	"Youth," especially related to physical appearance, changes in libido, and physical capacities
	Fertility in women, with menopause
	Parents through death
Older adult	Sensory acuity
	Hair and teeth
	Sexual desire or function
	Intellect and memory
	Control over some bodily functions
	Job, through retirement
	Independence in living (moving in with children or to retirement home)
	Spouses and friends through death

II. Loss Related to Life Experience

Death of a spouse, child, relative, or friend
Separation or divorce
Breakup of a love affair or friendship
Loss of a job
Financial loss
Move away from friends, family, professional contacts
Change of teachers, school, neighborhoods
Loss of a personal goal or ideal
Robbery, assault, rape
Fire, flood, or other natural disaster
Status
Hope
Control
Self-confidence

(continued)

TABLE 27–1. (Continued)

III. Loss Related to Illness

Loss of:
    Good, general health due to chronic illness or repeated episodic illnesses
    Bodily function and control
    A body part or part of a body system
    The perception of oneself as whole and integrated
    The perception of oneself as independent and functional
    A positive self-image
    Independence and the ability to make choices about one's care and life
    Control over one's environment

IV. Loss Related to Death

Loss of:
    A cherished, significant person
    An interdependent relationship
    A significant support
    A defined role (in relation to the space left by the loss one)
    Sexual partner
    Chance to work out areas of conflict
    Hope (for future relationships)

each category. Review them and see if you can add any more, given your own personal experience with loss.

COPING WITH A LOSS

Grief

Loss of a significant and valued object is considered to be the precipitating factor for the state of acute grief. **Grief** is defined as a series of intense physical and emotional responses that occur following a loss. The lost object is defined as any person, place, or other entity (job, dream, hobby) that has significant value to the person suffering the loss. It is important that the nurse be aware of common responses in an individual dealing with a loss in order to assess accurately the behavior indicative of the normal grief state.

It has been postulated that even the use of the term "normal grief" is an erroneous one. Engle states that "the grief reaction corresponds to many other entities commonly regarded as diseases and fulfills all the criteria of a discrete syndrome."[3]

- There is a common etiologic factor (i.e., the loss)
- There is a predictable symptomatology and course

- There is impairment of capacity and function for a considerable time period
- The stricken person is acutely distressed and disabled

Engle offers the term "uncomplicated grief" to specify a grief reaction that normally occurs after a significant loss. This reaction runs a fairly consistent and predictable course and ends in the relinquishing of the lost object and the return to the client's previous, although not unaffected, life.[4]

Some of the common responses encountered in a person suffering from a recent loss are listed in Table 27–2. Not all people may experience all symptoms; however, those listed have been validated as the responses most often seen in individuals suffering from a recent loss.

Lindemann's classic paper on the manifestations of acute grief led the way for other clinicians working with grieving patients to validate and expand on his observations.[5] During Lindemann's interviews, patients who had recently lost a loved one described "waves" of discomfort that were precipitated by the mention of the lost one. These waves lasted about 20 minutes to an hour and including feelings of tightness in the throat along with a choking sensation, a need for sighing, shortness of breath, an empty feeling in the stomach, muscle weak-

TABLE 27–2. COMMON REACTIONS TO LOSS

Physical Reactions	Psychosocial Reactions
• Loss of appetite	• Helplessness
• Digestive intolerance	• Hopelessness
• Insomnia	• Severe "pangs" of loneliness
• Decreased libido	• Extreme sadness
• Loss of weight	• Denial
• Increased susceptibility to illness	• Guilt
• Lack of strength and physical exhaustion	• Hostility
• Restlessness	• Anger
• Inability to initiate or complete activities	• Tension
• Weeping	• Disturbing dreams or fantasies
• Other physical complaints (i.e., headache, backache, muscle tension)	• Feelings of emptiness
	• Preoccupation with lost object
	• Need for solitude mixed with need for social contact
	• Inability to concentrate

ness, and an "intense subjective distress described as tension or mental pain."[6]

Symptoms that are manifest in the acute grief reaction are both physically and emotionally draining. They are also variable in intensity and frequency and tend to be self-limiting. As the person experiences grief and begins to work through the loss, life takes on its previously normal patterns. The uncomplicated grief reaction related to death averages approximately six months—that is, the period in which the most intense physical and emotional reactions are felt and disorganization of the person's life occurs.[7] This time frame should be interpreted with great flexibility, because it varies depending on many different circumstances. The length of a grief reaction related to other types of loss is not well documented. It depends on the specific loss, its meaning to the individual, and many other influencing factors.

Mourning

Many terms have been used to describe the period of time in which grief is expressed. **Mourning** and **bereavement** commonly are associated with the period during which one expresses grief, when the loss is through death. However, it is important to remember that a person will express grief with any significant loss and will move through a process of mourning no matter how tragic or trivial the loss may seem. The difference is only in the length of time grieving

takes and the intensity of the feelings expressed.[8] A very simple example might be when a person misses the bus to get to work. Although this may seem trivial, the process is the same as for a major tragedy. The man who misses the bus for work one morning expresses *shock and disbelief* ("I can't believe I missed it, I ran all the way . . ."), a *developing awareness* ("If only the driver had slowed down I would have made it"), and *restitution and recovery* ("Oh well, I'll have to call a cab now"). Again the only differences are in the intensity of feelings expressed and in the length of time needed to resolve the loss. The process will always be the same.

Other important terms to keep in mind are *survival, healing,* and *recovery,* because they are three processes that mingle to produce growth through the experience of loss.[9]

The Mourning Process
The process of mourning has traditionally been associated with death; however, it will be used here in its broadest context, that is, *the period of time in which the grief reaction to some specific loss occurs, as well as the time it takes to integrate and resolve the loss.* We are faced daily with minor losses, and periodically with major ones. Each loss that occurs adds to our experience in dealing with loss and forms the basis of our ability to cope with future ones.

Separate and distinct stages characterizing

the process of mourning have been documented.[10–13] Although the occurrence of a major loss is usually the precipitating factor for triggering a grief reaction and the mourning process, clients may experience these under only threat of loss. This is known as **anticipatory grief.** This phenomenon was first observed in the spouses and other family members of military personnel who were stationed overseas during World War II. In anticipatory grief, a person experiences symptoms of grief and moves through the mourning process while anticipating a major loss. The advantages of anticipatory grieving is that it allows a client to begin working through an inevitable loss (i.e., a person who is terminally ill) or may prepare a person for the news of a possible tragic loss. The disadvantage is that sometimes a person may have worked so completely through the process and resolved the loss that, for example, they are unwilling to accept a loved one home again.[14]

This is a phenomenon seen today in the families of chronically or terminally ill clients. With advances in treatment modalities, many clients can live for long periods of time after diagnosis. Since they are usually under constant threat of death, families have considerable difficulty with prolonged grief and mourning periods. This can become a major nursing care problem when members of the family go through anticipatory grieving. The family may then isolate the client, sometimes so completely that the client's entire support system is gone.

The three stages of the mourning process, according to Engle, are an initial stage of *shock and disbelief,* a second stage of *developing awareness,* and a final stage of *restitution and recovery.*[15] Usually stage I is the shortest, lasting an average of six to eight weeks. Stage II is somewhat longer, six months to a year, and stage III, the longest, lasting possibly several years.[16–19] It is important to remember that not only is there a progression from one stage to another, there is also movement within each stage. Progression occurs, but only with many periods of regression. In other words, measurement of progress must be flexible and take into account the many variables that influence how each person may react to a loss.

Stage I: Shock and Disbelief. In this initial stage, the person discovers the loss. The person is unable to acknowledge that the loss is threatened or has occurred. People react to shocking news in a variety of ways, such as sitting or standing abruptly, fainting, crying out, moaning, pacing, wringing hands, inability to speak, or rhythmic body movements. The person usually will feel dazed, disoriented, and helpless.

The initial phase can be a time of intense physical and emotional pain, depending on how shocking the loss is. However, some clients find that they are numbed, as if they cannot feel anything. This can be quite upsetting and may cause a person to feel abnormal or "crazy." This period is a crisis point in which a person needs a lot of caring from family, friends, and professionals.[20]

During this stage and well into the second stage of developing awareness, a person may be excessively preoccupied with the lost object. If a loved one has died, the person suffering may keep "searching" for that lost individual.[21] "I keep expecting her to come through the front door." "I see his face everywhere I go, but it's never really him."

Parkes believes that this searching behavior is found in anyone who has lost a loved one. It has been observed that a person in an acute grief state is restless and seems to move about aimlessly. The person is unable to begin or finish any activity and is "continually searching for something to do." Parkes contends that there is a purpose to such behavior: the recovery of the lost one. Since recovery is usually irrational, especially in the case of death, many people will not admit to this need, for fear of sounding crazy.[22]

Part of this searching process may be manifest in the need, on the part of the client, to review over and over again the details of the time immediately preceding the loss. Trying to remember what happened, who was there, and what was said can be useful in helping the person begin to believe that the loss is real. In fact, intense preoccupation with a lost loved one is considered essential in eventually resolving the loss.[23,24]

Denial is an important and frequently found component of this stage of the mourning process. "Denial functions as a buffer after unexpected shocking news, allows the patient to collect himself, and, with time, mobilize other, less radical defenses."[25] Denial is used throughout each stage of the mourning process in various ways and to different degrees. In an uncomplicated grief reaction, denial is generally a temporary defense. When reality testing is done, the client knows that the loss has occurred. The client also realizes that it is not possible realistically to hold onto the belief that the loss is temporary.

Separation anxiety is also common in the stage of shock and disbelief. The death of a loved one naturally will evoke anxious feelings. The client may wonder how he or she will ever survive. A death is especially anxiety-producing because of the concomitant loss of a defined role, within which the client is used to functioning. Separation anxiety can occur with other losses, such as loss of a job or loss of friends, as one moves to a new place. In fact, it has been postulated that separation anxiety is at the very core of the grief experience.[26]

Stage II: Developing Awareness. The stage of developing awareness, in which the client must come to terms with the fact that the loss occurred, may be the most painful psychologically. The client not only will have to recognize the reality of the loss but attempt to understand the meaning of the loss in relation to the rest of life. As this happens, many of the feelings previously described will be experienced. Overwhelming feelings of the helplessness and frustration are common at first. The realization of having no power to change the loss contributes to these feelings.

Anger and hostility are common during this stage. The person often will try to blame others for what has happened. Many times, health professionals take the brunt of such hostility when loss is related to illness and death. Family members are often blamed, not only directly related to the loss, but indirectly in day-to-day living situations. The client may feel that no one can do anything right. "If only the doctor had operated two years ago." "He never gave me a chance, that's why I was fired." "Don't talk to me like that, I don't need your pity." Statements like these reflect a client's need to let someone else take responsibility for the loss, at least for a while.

Feelings of guilt also emerge during this stage and are closely related to anger. The client may feel guilty about something he or she said or in the manner in which he or she behaved, perceiving these as somehow contributing to the loss. Clients also may feel very guilty about any anger or hostility that was shown to health professionals, family, or friends who were trying to help.

Extreme sadness and feelings of isolation and loneliness are other components of this stage. Grief "pangs," which are periods of intense feelings of anxiety and psychological pain, are also common.[27] This is especially true with clients who have lost someone close to them through death, or with clients who are terminally ill and anticipating their own death. These pangs are extremely uncomfortable and are evoked when the lost one is mentioned or when the client is alone and thinking about the lost one. It is significant that a person feels such sorrow in order to be able to move toward integration of the loss. Initially, grief pangs occur quite frequently and are usually most acute in the months after the loss. Later they may occur around anniversaries of the loss or at other special times that remind the client of the loved one, such as holidays, birthdays, or vacations. This may happen for years following a major loss.

There is usually great variability in mood states during the time of developing awareness, since clients experience many intense feelings. Relatively normal behavior, in terms of daily living, alternates with periods of immobility and helplessness. Weeping and expressions of loneliness are common. There may be variable levels in activity, appetite, libido, and sleep. The person may also experience changed needs for solitude and social interaction. There will be many days when they feel as if they have made no progress and that they never will recover and be able to live their lives normally.

Stage III: Restitution and Recovery. In this final stage of the mourning process, the client continues to deal with the loss and its effect on his or her life. However, during this time, the client also does much of the work involved in the true healing process.

> Normal grieving involves a reintegration process which brings together the intellectual awareness of a loss, its implications and consequences, and the physical and emotional experience of deprivation, mourning and healing.[28]

The goal of this stage is the acceptance of the altered state and the relinquishing of the lost object. This is signaled by the formation of new relationships and patterns of social interaction.[29] Preoccupation with the loss continues but on a different level. There are no longer such extremes in emotion, but gradually a detachment and intellectualization of the loss. This is not to say that the lost object is forgotten or any less meaningful to the client, but rather that the client is coming to terms with the loss and managing to continue a normal life.

As this growing away from the loss occurs, less acute pain is felt. The client is able to tolerate ambivalent feelings about the loss. For example, a man who is fired from his job initially may be full of anger and resentment toward his boss. Only after he resettles into a new job and has had time to reflect and grieve does he allow himself to experience mixed feelings. Perhaps his former boss taught him many skills that helped him acquire his current job. He is now able to have positive as well as negative feelings about his loss.

How and when a client is ready to do this work depends on the type and severity of the loss. If the loss is related to the death of a loved one, for example, it may take considerably longer and be that much more difficult to tolerate such ambivalent feelings. We can probably each recall someone in our lives who has lost someone close, who can think only of the good qualities and good times related to the lost one. The importance of being able to experience ambivalence must be stressed, because a large portion of the work of integration and recovery is related to developing a realistic perception of the loss and its meaning for the future.

Another crucial part of the recovery has to do with the formation of new relationships and patterns of social interaction. This must be interpreted in a broad context. A person suffering a loss must be able to get on with life. This means interactions with family, friends, neighbors, co-workers, and others, that are changed as a result of the loss. This is not as easy as finding a new mate or simply getting a new job. It also means being able to see oneself as a normal, whole, worthwhile human being. A loss can and will affect any of these self-perceptions, and, in turn, affect social interaction.

> A 19-year-old woman training to be an olympic skater lost her leg in an accident. She recovered well physically but had a great deal of trouble establishing friendships with anyone her own age for about 2 years after her accident. She worked in a preschool day-care center and volunteered occasionally in a nursing home. She found that she could not relate to her former friends, and she never dated. She said the reasons were because they didn't want to be around a "cripple" and because she could no longer skate. Only through the establishment of new relationships was she able to see herself more realistically. She subsequently went to work as a skating coach for handicapped children.

The client has to be willing to take some risks and look at the loss realistically. It can be quite painful to acknowledge what a particular loss means in terms of one's future. When this is done, however, comfort and relief usually follow, and movement toward recovery occurs. Sometimes it takes trying to establish new social patterns to force a person to look at the loss more realistically. Letting go may then be easier in light of the reward of new relationships.

Since a loss causes such tremendous changes in a client's daily life, at least for a period of time, the opportunities for renewal of relationships and establishment of new ones may be quite limited. The social networks we build center mainly around our likes and dislikes, physical abilities, jobs, and family or other personal ties. When a loss occurs, these networks can be severely disrupted. Many adjustments and perhaps major changes will have to be made. In light of the disruptions caused by a major loss, changes may be very difficult tasks to accomplish.

A 34-year-old man lost his wife and was left with their three young children. He continued working but had to cut back his hours somewhat due to the demands of his children. This caused quite a bit of friction at work. He was unable to socialize with friends from work because of his new responsibilities at home. He rarely saw any of the friends he and his wife used to associate with. He and his children lived some distance from both sets of grandparents, so he became isolated from his family, friends, and co-workers.

Because of this man's life situation, including responsibilities to his children and need to continue working, his "normal" life was severely disrupted. Not only did he have to deal with losing his wife and missing an intimate and interdependent relationship with another adult, but also with very little opportunity for any new, adult social interaction. Even if a client can reach a point where he or she is willing to try to renew normal relationships or to develop others, he or she may truly be hindered by either limited opportunities or limited knowledge of opportunities. This can be a source of considerable frustration and may require professional intervention.

During this process of attempting to adjust to the loss and form new relationships, the client also may be dealing with periods of denial, anger, guilt, and sadness. Although these are certainly less acute than in the stage of developing awareness, they may still be present. This is especially true around times that remind the client of the loss, such as birthdays, anniversaries, and holidays. It is important to remember that mourning is not simply a gradual, one-way process, from shock to recovery, but rather is full of "ups and downs, progression and regression, dramatic leaps and depressing backslides."[30] For the client, adjustment in this stage can be difficult, because on the surface life appears to be back to normal, when in reality the client is still dealing with many feelings and changes in his or her life brought about by the loss. This

is why restitution and recovery may be such a slow process, and indeed, why it is the longest stage of mourning.

FACTORS INFLUENCING THE GRIEF RESPONSE

Numerous factors influence the type, severity, and length of a specific grief reaction. Since these factors play a key role in how a particular client will experience and cope with grief, it is important that the nurse be aware of them.

One basic influencing factor will be the client's self-concept. Self-concept is how a person sees her- or himself in the world, what the client values about self. It is a constantly evolving phenomenon, and just as the self-concept will affect how a person copes with a loss, so too will it be further shaped by the loss. The major components of a client's self-concept are *physical self* and *personal self*.[31]

The physical self encompasses the client's body image, which includes both physical appearance and functioning. Other important components are sexual identity and general health state.[32] Body image is developed over the course of a lifetime and will vary depending on age, developmental task mastery, and life experience. When the loss of a body part or function occurs, a threat to the physical self follows. A loss of this type will have profound implications, depending on how positive or negative the client's body image is. For example, the self-concept of a 43-year-old woman who loses her breast following diagnosis and treatment for cancer may be severely threatened because of the impact of the loss on her physical self: her appearance and function, sexual identity, and perception of herself as ill.

The personal self encompasses the client's moral values, self-expectations, regulatory behaviors, and self-esteem.[33] This part of the self-concept is involved in every experience of loss, especially in a client's coping mechanism. For example, expression of emotion during the grief reaction may be distasteful to certain men. For many years society has dictated that men should be "strong" and unemotional, and so men traditionally cry much less than women. A man may feel inhibited about weeping after a loss because his value system tells him men should not cry, therefore his expectation of himself is not to show emotions publicly. Self-regulation requires that he "be in control," so his self-esteem will be maintained only if he can refrain from weeping.

Another important component of the self-concept is the mastery of age-appropriate developmental tasks. Depending on where a client is along the age-development continuum, the impact of a major loss will be experienced differently. Children may be able to adapt to changes in their lives more easily than adults, provided the adults around them handle the situation and the child's feelings in an appropriate manner. This means recognizing the child's or adolescent's level of understanding and helping the child to express, not repress feelings about the situation. However, certain kinds of loss at key developmental points in life may have a profound effect on a person's progression through task mastery.

It has been observed that both children and adults can regress or fixate at a level of development as a result of certain types of loss.[34] This is especially true with children and adolescents, since they are still in the process of mastering basic tasks necessary for positive ego functioning.

When a major loss occurs, such as the death of a parent or sibling, or parental divorce, the potential for maladaptation in a child or adolescent can be great. This will depend on the developmental level, family functioning, and how the situation is handled by key adults in the child's or adolescent's life. Unfortunately, problems may go unnoticed for many years, because feelings may be repressed, or because adults around the child do not recognize the child's needs. Only when a situation such as some other major loss (or potential loss) triggers recall of feelings can a problem be discovered.

A 25-year-old woman became pregnant with her first child. She and her husband were excited and had planned the pregnancy. Yet during her fourth month she developed hyperemesis, a syndrome of severe vomiting in pregnancy. She was then hospitalized for dehydration and eventually went home apparently well. She was subsequently readmitted twice for the same

problem. During a psychiatric evaluation it was discovered that her mother had died during the birth of a sibling when the client was five years old. She had never resolved her grief over her mother's death and it took becoming pregnant herself to trigger those feelings. With some counseling, she was able to work through her delayed grief reaction and go on to have a healthy pregnancy and birth.

It is important to understand how a child's concept of death develops, since it is tied to developmental task mastery and is different at various levels. There is a wide variety of opinion related to exactly when a child becomes cognizant of death and is able to grieve. It is generally recognized that children are aware of death after the age of at least two years but are not cognizant of the finality of it. From then until age five or six, the child's understanding is at the level of a temporary separation.[35] Children understand that there is something special and significant about death, probably in large part because of the behavior of adults around them. However, at this age a child cannot acknowledge the inevitability or finality of death. Preschool children may be especially apprehensive about death because they are increasingly aware that it is both an important and disruptive event. The child searches to find causes of death and may misinterpret certain phenomena as being involved with death.[36] The formation of unrealistic associations are common. For example, the notion that going to sleep may mean that the child will die. An all too common response of parents when children ask what happened to someone who died is, "She's sleeping with God in heaven." Often, when a child's pet dies the child is told that the pet was "put to sleep," and then sees that the pet never returns. It is crucial that the issue of death be handled with reassurance and realistic explanations in order to prevent the formation of completely erroneous ideas about death. This would certainly be true of other major losses, such as separation of a child and parent or sibling through divorce or illness. Children also tend to blame themselves, and this can have tremendous effects on their feelings of self-worth, unless they are reassured that they are not responsible for the loss.

For children between the ages of 5 and 10,

a gradual understanding that death is both inevitable and final develops. During this time the child tends to personify death. The child fantasizes that death is a person who has the power to take the child away. This personification has been called the "death-man."[37] Children will devise all sorts of ways of avoiding the death-man. Behaviors such as hiding under the bed covers, looking behind doors and in closets may be indicative of this avoidance behavior.

After about age ten, the child is able to recognize death as the final cessation of body function and the ultimate outcome of human life.[38,39] As children move toward adolescence and its many new developmental tasks, they develop their concept of death more fully. Death becomes an issue as adolescents begin to intellectually analyze the world and understand where they fit in it. Kastenbaum believes that the intellectual tasks of adolescents are important to their developing concept of death:

> At the very time that everything is changing inside and around him, the adolescent must begin to develop a comprehensive and stable conception of the adult-world-with-him-in-it.[40]

This includes thoughts about the individual's end. As the adolescent begins to take on increasingly adult responsibilities and thoughts, he or she begins to see loss as a potential in many life situations. Table 27–3 provides a summary of the child's and adolescent's perception of death.

Any type of major loss that occurs at key points in the life span has the potential for interfering with the mastery of specific developmental tasks. Children and adolescents can be quite vulnerable to complications after a loss, owing to the number of age-specific tasks to be accomplished. However, in adult life, the self-concept continues to evolve with increased responsibilities and life experience. In addition, during the adult years the potential for loss through illness and death is much more profound, especially in middle and late adulthood. Thus, it is crucial to assess age-appropriate developmental task mastery as an integral part of the evolving self-concept when looking at factors influencing loss.

Another factor that influences a person's reaction to a specific loss is the person's perception of the magnitude of the loss. This perception will be influenced by self-concept and developmental level, religious and cultural orientation, and relationship to the lost object. Self-concept and developmental level have been discussed as the basis on which a person perceives self and the world and will not be further delineated here. See Chapter 19 for further discussion of self-concept.

Religious and cultural orientation as well as previous experience with loss can have a significant effect on the perception of all types of loss, especially major ones, such as death or separation from a loved one and illness. Each culture and the religious sects within it have certain beliefs about birth, death, and illness. Many dictate mourning rituals and, to a certain extent, normal conduct for men, women, and children at various points in the life cycle. Beliefs in God, afterlife, and redemption of the soul have been observed as important components in helping clients move through the mourning process when the loss is or will be death.[41] Depending on the type of loss and when it occurs, cultural and religious orientation has varying degrees of influence.

Finally, the client's relationship with the lost object will have profound influence on perception of the loss. It is also important to understand that the loss may be replaced, to some extent, in the client's life. Certainly people and our interactions with those we love can never really be replaced. However, the needs met by key people in our lives can be met in other ways and by other people. Of course, this issue is at the very core of the grief experience: enough healing must take place so that new relationships can be initiated.

The amount of interdependence involved with the lost object will influence the perception of the severity of loss. The change in a client's daily life may be great depending on the amount of daily interaction and interdependence.

> Mr. and Mrs. J. had waited until their late 30s to begin their family, and after a few years of infertility problems, had a daughter, C. Mrs J. stayed out of work for 11 months to be home with C. She was ambivalent about leaving her with a sitter but

TABLE 27–3. CHILDREN'S AND ADOLESCENTS' PERCEPTIONS OF DEATH

Age	Perception/Developmental Disruptions
Birth to 2 years	Not aware of death. Can react to parent and family's emotional response to death. Can appreciate disruption in normal routines. May have significant psychosocial problems if mother or surrogate is lost in first two years of life.
2 to 6 years	Sees death as a temporary separation. Can understand and react somewhat to the gravity of death, but this is greatly influenced by the reaction of parents or other caretakers. Many have significant psychosocial problems if either parent is lost at this stage, especially from ages 4 to 6 and with parent of same or opposite sex depending on where child is in relation to sex patterning and identification.
6 to 10 years	Can appreciate that death is inevitable and final. Fantasizes and tends to personify (i.e., the "death-man"). May have nightmares normally, even without experiencing death firsthand. Death-man avoidance behavior common, such as leaving on lights at night, closing closet doors, hiding under covers. At this age a child may feel intense guilt surrounding a loss and responsibility for death of a close relative (parent or sibling).
10 years to adolescence	Able to recognize that death means the cessation of bodily functions and is the ultimate outcome to human life. Adolescents tend to deny that death could ever happen to them, whereas preadolescents may still worry about death to some extent. Loss of a parent at this stage may have a profound effect on adolescents' movement into young adulthood and their ability to form intimate relationships with members of the opposite sex.

finally decided to return to work on a full-time basis. She was called home one day by her frantic baby-sitter. The woman had been carrying C. down the stairs and accidently dropped her. Upon arrival at home, Mrs. J. found her daughter barely conscious. The child was immediately helicoptered with her parents to a regional trauma center and underwent surgery for several hours. She never regained consciousness and died two days later.

The loss of a child will have a tremendous impact on the parents' lives. So much of everyday living is centered around young children, since they are dependent on parents for meeting basic survival needs. In the above example, there are additional factors to consider, such as the couple's infertility problems, their age (a factor in considering future children), and the mother's ambivalence about leaving her child in the care of another person. A high degree of interdependence with the lost object is usually associated with a more severe although not necessarily a more complicated grief reaction.

Other important factors that influence the grief reaction are the meaning of the loss in relation to past experience with loss and the client's normal methods of coping with any crisis. Clients that nurses work with experience numerous kinds of loss in their lives. In addition,

they may have had vastly different life experiences and have formed methods of coping that have been significantly influenced by those experiences. A client's usual methods of coping with any stressfull life situation will serve him or her during the mourning process. This is why, for some people, denial works best initially and for others hostility is encountered first. Some people need to be close to others immediately following a loss. Some need space and time.

Resolution of a loss is a painful process and must be done by the client in the client's own way. As professionals, nurses can care, assess, advise, and assist, but the client will have to follow his or her own course, depending on many influencing variables, as he or she moves through the process of mourning.

THE NURSING PROCESS

Nurses in all specialties will deal with clients recovering from many different types of loss. In almost any situation that requires nursing intervention, loss of control and independence will be manifest. In addition, many other situation-specific types of loss will be encountered. Hospital-based nurses generally will deal with clients experiencing loss through acute, episodic illnesses or though acute phases of chronic or terminal illness. On the other hand, community health nurses more often deal with loss related to chronic illness and loss of function, as well as those types of loss related to life situations resulting from poverty. The nursing process is an excellent framework for the delivery of nursing care.

Assessment

The initial client assessment should be quite thorough in order to make an adequate care plan. Figure 27–1 offers the major areas in need of assessment for a client suffering a loss. When describing a client's loss, try to see it from the client's viewpoint, because that is crucial to the planning phase.

In addition to assessment of the adaptive grief reaction, the nurse must look for signs of **maladaptive grief.** Differentiation may be very difficult at times. Because a major loss causes such disruption of the client's daily routine, minor physical illnesses may be precipitated. Because of problems such as insomnia, poor appetite, and lack of exercise during the period after a loss, the client will not maintain regular activities. The client may then be more susceptible to colds, intestinal problems, headaches, and muscular aches and pains. The client's weight may increase or decrease depending how food is used in times of stress. This can lead to an even further susceptibility to physical problems and decreased self-esteem caused by a change in body image.

Certain diseases have been specifically associated with the stress after the death of a loved one. These include ulcerative colitis, rheumatoid arthritis, and asthma.[42] Exacerbation of other illnesses diagnosed previously, such as hypertension, diabetes, heart disease, stomach ulcers, migraine headaches, skin problems, and various neuromuscular disorders may occur in clients under stress.[43,44] These will cause additional problems to be dealt with in planning care.

Important components in the differentiation of adaptative from maladaptive behaviors involves the duration and intensity of the reaction as well as the perception of resolution on the part of the client. Some basic behavior patterns that are indicative of a prolonged or maladaptive grief reaction include[45–48]:

- Gross disruption of the client's daily life, lasting longer than about six months
- Serious suicidal thoughts or any suicide attempt
- Acquisition of symptoms belonging to the last illness of a deceased loved one
- Extreme weight changes; a loss or gain of 30 to 50 lb.
- Extreme social isolation, inability to renew and maintain relationships or to form new ones
- Extreme hostility toward a person or group
- No apparent reaction in relation to the loss
- Severe insomnia with early morning waking
- Extremely low self-esteem
- Inability to see lost object as really gone
- Use of present tense in speaking of loss.

If any of these behaviors are noted, and they more often are groups of behaviors, the client may need additional intervention by someone experienced in handling a maladaptive grief reaction.

An important reminder here is that, when confronted with a client suffering a major loss, the nurse needs to consider her or his own feelings about the specific loss. Those feelings can either positively or negatively affect how the nurse is able to care for the client.

> A 22-year-old graduate nurse was reassigned from the surgical floor where she usually worked to the pediatric unit because of a staff shortage. The first day was enjoyable for her, since she liked being around children and usually worked exclusively with adults. On her second day on the new unit, she was assigned a 10-year-old boy who was dying of leukemia. She was able to finish her morning care of the child, which took almost three hours, since he was unable to do very much for himself. At lunchtime she told the head nurse that she was feeling too ill to finish her shift and requested to be sent home. She was unable, however, to tell the head nurse that she had had a younger brother who had died of leukemia when he was 8 years old.

Many times in your nursing career, you will be confronted by clients with such tragic personal losses that they seem almost overwhelming. All the factors that we assess in our clients,

Assessment Tool for Loss

A. Type of Loss (describe) _____

_____

When did it occur? _____

B. Client Characteristics

Name: _____

Age: _____ Sex: _____ Occupation: _____

Place of employment: _____

Developmental Stage: _____

Cultural Orientation: _____

Religion: _____

Affiliation (church/synagogue) _____

C. Support System

1. Family members: _____

_____

_____

2. Friends: _____

_____

_____

3. Other Relatives: _____

_____

4. Religious: _____

5. Problems: _____

D. Activities of Daily Living (note specific problems)

Diet: _____

Exercise: _____

Sleep: _____

Elimination: _____

Social Interaction: _____

Personal Hygiene: _____

Sex: _____

Work: _____

E. Community Resources _____

_____

_____

F. Assessment _____

_____

Problem Areas to Address _____

Figure 27–1. A written assessment tool can aid the nurse in assessing loss.

such as age, sex, developmental stage, religion, etc., also have an impact on us as nurses and the care we are able to give. There may be many times when feelings of anger, frustration, hopelessness, and guilt must be first worked through in order to help our clients. Many times these feelings are subtle, and since it is not really our loss, they are difficult to recognize. Sometimes we may notice a simple resistance to going into that one client's room, or putting off that one home visit until next week. It is helpful to think about loss in its broadest context, so that in our dealings with all clients, we are cognizant of loss as an issue each one deals with to some extent.

At the conclusion of the assessment phase of the nursing process, nursing diagnoses are formulated. Examples of nursing diagnoses for loss include:

- Grieving related to amputation of a leg
- Grieving: Anticipatory secondary to impending death
- Grieving reaction related to a loss of a significant other

Planning

To effectively develop a plan of care for a client experiencing loss, the nurse must be familiar with the types of interventions appropriate for such clients. Three main categories of intervention are: physical and psychological assessment, education and guidance, and mobilization of resources.

Goals should be developed within these three categories. Mutual goal setting with the client may be difficult in the initial phase after a loss. However, after the initial shock period, goal setting may be helpful, for example, helping a client learn to resocialize, find a new job, or join a therapy group.

Use knowledge of the normal grief reaction and phases of mourning in the nursing care plan. Take into account regression as well as progress toward adaptation. The care plan is dynamic and needs to be flexible to account for this.

Implementation

Intervention within the three categories identified above will be discussed. In addition, since communication is at the very core of any type of intervention, techniques specific to intervening with clients suffering a loss also will be delineated.

Intervention is generally not needed in the course of an uncomplicated grief reaction. Usually a caring, understanding approach is sufficient. The nurse's demeanor is important in allowing the client to feel comfortable to discuss feelings related to the loss. Above all, the natural healing process must be allowed to progress.

Listening and attending skills are useful in dealing with grieving clients, especially in the initial period after a loss. When a great personal loss does occur, or is threatened, there is really not much anyone can say, although most caring people will feel the need to do so. At this point, the client needs empathy and understanding offered within his or her own frame or reference.[49] At times, silence and just being with a client is all that is necessary and communicates effectively the notion of not knowing what to say, but still caring.

Denial is a reaction that emerges initially after a loss and warrants special attention in discussing communication. It will continue throughout the mourning process in varying degrees. Since it is an important defense against intense feelings of separation anxiety, the client may need to experience denial, depending on the loss and its meaning. Vigorous confrontation of the person experiencing denial may be harmful, because the person may not be ready to confront the reality of the loss. The nurse should not, however, support unrealistic ideas or fantasies. Most grieving clients understand that their loss is real. Denial is used simply as a way of insulating themselves from the initial shock.

Some clients deny a loss because they were never able to realistically experience it. For example, a woman delivered a stillborn infant under general anesthesia and was never allowed to see her child. Perhaps the family held the funeral while she was in the hospital, or perhaps there was no formal acknowledgment of the infant's death through a funeral. Too often, in an effort to make the client "feel better" or "feel less pain," family, friends, and health professionals deny someone the chance to acknowledge their loss and begin the healing process.

In fact, it is inappropriate at any time to try to suppress normal expressions of grief, which involve many feelings and defense mechanisms. Often clients are given the message that their feelings are abnormal or, at the very least, that other people cannot tolerate such expressions. An example is overmedication of clients because the health professionals caring for them are unable or unwilling to deal with their feelings. This deprives the person of full awareness and of experiencing the real significance of his or her loss.[50] This a good opportunity for the nurse to act as a role model for the client, family, and other health professionals, in order to facilitate attitudes of acceptance toward expression of the pain associated with loss.

Along with role modeling, another communication technique that may be helpful is appropriate sharing of personal experience. There are times throughout the mourning process when this technique is very useful. Having personally experienced a similar loss may enable the nurse to understand more fully the intense pain associated with a client's specific situation. The nurse may be aware of certain resources, such as a particular type of support group that could be of benefit to the client. Certainly, through both personal and professional experience, the nurse will be able to share experience and resources for dealing with specific problems associated with certain types of loss.

Another communication technique that is often used is facilitation of decision making. This is more often done during the stage of restitution and recovery, since this is the time when the patient has to deal most concretely with the effects of the loss. The client may need to make many decisions. There will be many changes in the client's life that will require some additional problem solving. Exploration of the problem begins the process, followed by focusing on the various alternatives available. The nurse then assists the client in evaluating each separate alternative and facilitates the client's choice of the best one.

Reflection and clarification are also important communication techniques. See Chapter 14 for examples of using reflection and clarification techniques. One of the goals of the mourning process is to assist the client and family to express their feelings of anger, guilt, doubt, and sadness. Reflection and clarification can be useful in encouraging such expression. It may be extremely uncomfortable and threatening for many people to be able to express such intense feelings. It has been observed that although great relief usually follows weeping and expression of feelings, the client often feels compelled to apologize for letting go in front of another person.[51] The nurse must communicate a sincere attitude of personal acceptance and respect for the client and family in order to facilitate emotional expression.

Communication patterns between nurse and client are best facilitated by the establishment of rapport, by a caring, empathic attitude, and by allowing the client to progress through this mourning process at the client's own pace based on his or her special needs. It is important to point out that nurses are not always able to follow a client through the entire mourning process, because of limited contact and the length of the mourning process. We usually only see clients at certain points in the process. Knowledge of normal progression through the process will help the nurse to use the most appropriate, situation-specific patterns of interaction within each category of intervention.

Category I: Physical and Psychological Support. In nursing care, we usually strive for complete physical independence (or as much as possible) on the part of the clients with whom we work. Generally, we can more readily accept the need for psychological dependence. However, the person who is grieving after a loss may need substantial physical and psychological support for a period of time following the loss. As in any major crisis, the impact may immobilize some individuals. It is not uncommon for a person to forget to eat, to be unable to maintain even the simple activities of daily living, or to take care of other family members who are dependent on them. The nurse must make an adequate assessment of the client's physical needs and then plan for meeting those needs either through direct action or delegating certain tasks to family, friends, or other health-care workers. For example, many people lose their appetite during the early traumatic period after a loss. Taking the client for a walk prior to meals and keeping the menu simple but nutritious may encourage a lagging appetite. Eating with the client or sitting with the person during meals may also be helpful.

Personal hygiene is another area that may be neglected. This can be harmful to a client if severe. Skin and scalp problems and even breakdown of the skin barrier allowing for entry of pathogens can occur. This also perpetuates a cycle of a negative body image and low self-esteem. Assisting a client in maintaining adequate personal hygiene tells the client that he or she is a person worth caring about. It also gently lets the client know that life continues after a loss, and that it is important that he or she move on. This is a subtle but powerful suggestion.

Adequate rest is another area in which a client may be lacking. Certain individuals deal with trauma by sleeping much of the day. Others find it difficult to fall asleep. Rest is crucial, since the body and mind are healing. So much emotional energy is being spent that even though a person may be "doing nothing," the person will feel exhausted for some time. Suggesting the time-honored remedies for insomnia may be helpful. Warm baths, warm milk, relaxing music, or reading can aid insomnia.

There are many conflicting opinions regarding the prescription of tranquilizers and sedatives to induce relaxation and sleep. Certainly there are advantages for certain clients, depending on the type and severity of the loss.

However, this must be weighed against the idea that sleeplessness is very common to the grief reaction and in essence may represent the extra emotional work being done in an effort to adapt. Medications are more often used with inpatients and are frequently prescribed on an outpatient basis. The nurse's observations may be extremely important to a physician managing the client's medical care and in deciding for or against the use of drugs as an adjunct to other therapies.

Another physical problem that may occur is changes in pattern of elimination. Diarrhea and constipation are frequent developments. They are probably due to a combination of change in diet, exercise, and sleep patterns. Certain people notice gastrointestinal problems whenever they are under stress, such as stomach pain, gas, cramping, and change in stools. Helping the client return to as normal a pattern of daily living as quickly as possible usually will relieve these problems.

Clients who are ill or who have suffered exacerbation of a previously diagnosed illness concurrent with a major loss may need substantial physical support for some period of time. A diabetic, for example, may need to be given insulin injections, even though normally, the client manages self-care. An elderly man living alone may need a male home health aide to assist him with personal care following his loss of sight. These clients are especially susceptible to the development of complications to their illnesses and need to be closely monitored for adverse signs and symptoms.

> A 37-year-old woman was just finishing divorce proceedings after a struggle of several months regarding child custody and support. She had been diagnosed with multiple sclerosis several years earlier during her first pregnancy but had been quite well with only a couple of mild flare-ups of her symptoms. She now began to notice increasing weakness in her right leg and some occasions of urine incontinence. She eventually had to be hospitalized for stabilization and was successfully treated with steroids. She was referred for counseling to assist her in transition to single parenthood, her return to full-time employment, and working through her feelings surrounding the divorce.

In this case, the woman's multiple sclerosis symptoms were aggravated as a direct result of the loss that occurred with its concurrent stress.

When a client's loss involves any physical limitation, such as loss of a body part or body function, the nurse needs to assist in adaptation to a new body state as well as maintaining and increasing body function. In this type of loss situation, the client not only must accept and integrate the loss, but also must learn many new skills that will be strange and awkward at first. There may need to be a period of considerable physical dependence during this learning phase.

At times, it is difficult to separate physical and psychological support. Much is conveyed in the nurse's physical actions that can be viewed as supportive. A client will feel understood and helped as the nurse offers physical support when necessary, encourages and accepts expressions of feeling, and is able to anticipate the client's and family's need for information and guidance.

Category II: Education and Guidance. Education, along with anticipatory guidance, is necessary to help the client understand the normal grief reaction and period of mourning. Many people who suffer a major loss and consequently go through an uncomplicated grief reaction feel that they are abnormal. They may never have experienced such extremes in emotion or such disruption of their personal lives. Some patients express feeling "crazy," or worse, feel crazy and are not able to tell anyone. Educating the client and family about common reactions to loss may offer them reassurance. Including family and friends is also important, because they then may be even more sensitive to the client's needs. Anticipatory guidance about what to expect in the months to follow a loss also will be helpful.

Some specific information that will be useful to share with any client or family suffering from a loss follows[52]:

- The healing process takes time. Allow yourself time to experience the pain you feel. It is healthy to do this.
- Use your family and friends. Let them know how you are feeling and how they can best help you.

- Try and stick to your normal schedule. Make certain you eat right. Allow yourself some extra time off from work or school, if possible.
- Do not make any major changes in your life right now. Keep decision making to a minimum. Your judgment won't be what it is normally.
- Many people experience thoughts that they would be better off dead, rather than feeling such emotional pain. If you seriously consider hurting yourself, talk to someone immediately.
- Don't be afraid to let out your emotions. Crying is useful to some people. Screaming in the shower or in your car can be good ways to let out feeligs of anger and frustration. Beating up pillows is another.
- Physical exercise can also be helpful. You have a right to feel terrible; a terrible thing has happened to you.
- Avoid addictive behaviors, such as smoking, drugs, or overeating. These are escape mechanisms.
- It's a healthy idea to seek help from a counselor if you feel the need for more support than you're getting from family and friends.
- Some people find keeping a journal of thoughts, feelings, and dreams helpful in working through this disruptive time.
- Prepare yourself for changes in your life that may be frustrating, sad, or scary. As you heal, the changes may become exciting or fun. Allow yourself to feel good. Sometimes you may feel guilty about feeling good again. When this happens, you are truly recovering.

These suggestions should not necessarily be given to clients as a list. The client may be ready to hear them only at different points in his or her own process of recovery. Keep them in mind and be ready to share them appropriately.

Category III: Mobilization of Resources. Mobilization of resources is an important component of caring for clients suffering a major loss. It includes using family, friends, relatives, church and civic organizations, other healthcare professionals, and appropriate community resources. Planning for use of additional resources must be an integral part of total care to provide the client and family ongoing support once the crisis is past. Very often, the only time a client receives help is during this initial trauma, when he or she simply cannot function alone. As we have seen in the discussion of mourning stages, once a person has recovered from this early period of shock, the true healing process begins. Significant and ongoing physical and emotional support is critical in the client's making an adaptive response.

> Mrs. J., a 63-year-old, insulin-dependent diabetic was sent home from the hospital after a below-the-knee amputation of her left leg. She was to be fitted for an artificial limb two months after surgery but never kept her appointment. Six months later she presented through the emergency room with multiple skin ulcerations of her right lower leg. She was brought in by a neighbor who said he found her hopping around the ground of her apartment. Her physical exam revealed a thin, poorly kept woman who was unable to follow the physician's questioning. Mrs. J. was readmitted to the hospital for stabilization, and it was subsequently discovered that her son, who was her only relative, had died in a car accident three months earlier. Mrs. J. had no support system.

In this case, many preventive measures should have been instituted prior to Mrs. J.'s discharge after surgery. Referring her to a visiting nurse association or the public health nurse in her area could have prevented the problems that followed. Most communities have some sort of "meals-on-wheels" program and public nursing service facilities for elderly, homebound people. A little educational planning along with referral to the appropriate agency can make all the difference in assuring clients some continuity of care and prevention of further disability.

Evaluation

The ultimate evaluation of the impact of nursing care given to clients suffering from a major loss is that the client moves through the process of mourning. Although the general symptomatology relative to grief and mourning has been documented in the literature, it is impossible to generalize any specific time frame in which all people suffering all types of loss will adapt. The broad range of influencing factors that contribute to anyone's private experience with grief and mourning make specificity impossible.

However, in order to evaluate a client's progress, we must have some criteria by which to measure the reaction. The estimate of six months to one year following a sudden, major loss has been postulated as a time frame in which an otherwise healthy person is well on the way toward integration of the loss.[53] It must be emphasized that this estimate requires great flexibility relative to the individual, the type of loss, the perception of loss in relation to the client's specific life situation, and any concurrent physical or psychological illness. If, after that time, any symptoms previously described as maladaptive grief response are exhibited along with or in addition to signs of depression or extreme anxiety, professional psychiatric help is warranted.

Some general criteria to evaluate movement through grief and mourning from the onset related to a major loss are:

- Grief symptomatology—i.e., extreme sadness, depression, anxiety—in which the client is in a crisis state. This should be close to the time the loss occurred.
- Requests for help from family, friends, health professionals. Most people will ask someone for help.
- As time progresses after the loss, the client should be returning to a more normal pattern of living. Most people can verbalize that they feel less pain.
- There are definite periods of regression when the client feels awful again, but these are usually brief and happen less frequently with the passing of time.
- Establishment of new patterns of social interaction is a crucial signal that the client is adapting to the loss.

Evaluation of a person moving toward adaptation of a loss is critical throughout the entire recovery period. By continual evaluation and reassessment, we can anticipate and prevent problems from occurring and better deal with maladaptive behaviors as they do occur.

SUMMARY

The concept of loss has been presented in a broad context, affecting clients at all points along the life span. A sound knowledge base related to the concept and its manifestations in the people we care for will help us to assess, plan, intervene, and evaluate our nursing care.

Methods of coping with a loss involve the acute grief state and the process of mourning. This process is divided into three overlapping stages: shock and disbelief, developing awareness, and restitution and recovery. The many factors that influence the type and severity of a particular grief reaction were delineated and are important in helping us to maintain a flexible approach. The nursing process framework was used to outline the basic approaches to nursing intervention with clients suffering a major loss. The three categories of nursing interventions are physical and psychological support, education and guidance, and mobilization of client resources.

Coping with loss has become so much a part of our existence that, as health-care professionals, we must be aware of the many types of loss that our clients face. The relationship between loss as a stressor and resulting physical illness is a critical area to pursue, both in clinical practice and in the promotion of research. Through these efforts we may be able to make the grief experience easier to bear and can maintain and enhance a high level of wellness in the populations we serve.

Study Questions

1. Identify at least three types of loss an 18-year-old boy might experience following amputation of his lower leg because of a bone cancer.

2. Name two major losses that occur during the life experience of a 45-year-old woman.

3. What is meant by an "uncomplicated" grief reaction?

4. Denial is used throughout the entire process of mourning. In which stage is it most common?

5. Describe a grief pang.

6. Acceptance of the altered state and relinquishing the lost object is the goal of which stage of the mourning process?

7. How do age and developmental level affect the type and severity of the grief reaction?

8. What is probably the most significant influencing factor that affects the severity of the grief reaction?

9. Describe the three categories of interventions used with clients suffering from a loss.

10. Identify five behaviors that are indicative of a maladaptive grief reaction.

References

1. Baccalaureate Curriculum Committee, Catholic University of America. "Adaptation as a Model for Nursing Curriculum and Practice," unpublished, (Washington, D.C.: Catholic Univeristy of American, 1978), 16.
2. M. Colgrove, H. Bloomfield, and P. McWilliams, *How to Survive the Loss of a Love* (New York: Bantam Books, 1976), 16.
3. G.L. Engle, "Is grief a disease?" *Psychosom Med,* 23, (1961):18–22.
4. Ibid., 18.
5. E. Lindemann, "Symptomatology and management of acute grief," *Am J Psychiatry,* 101, (1944):141–48.
6. Ibid., 141.
7. V. Volkan, "Re-grief therapy," in B. Schoenburg, I. Gerber, A. Wiener, A.H. Kutscher, and A.C. Carr, eds., *Bereavement: Its Pscyhosocial Aspects,* (New York: Columbia University Press, 1975).
8. Colgrove, Bloomfield, and McWilliams, *Loss of a Love,* 16.
9. S. Freud, "Mourning and melancholia," in W. Gaylin, ed., *The Meaning of Despair* (New York: Science House, 1968).
10. Lindemann, "Symptomatology," 147.
11. Engle, "Is grief a disease?"
12. Elizabeth Kübler-Ross, *On Death and Dying* (New York: Macmillan Co., 1969).
13. Lindemann, "Symptomatology," 147–48.
14. Ibid., 148.
15. Engle, "Is grief a disease?"
16. Volkan, "Regrief."
17. Lindemann, "Symptomatology," 147–48.
18. J.M. Schnieder, "Clinically significant differences between grief, pathologic grief, and depression," *Patient Counseling Death Educ* 2:161–66.
19. Collin M. Parkes, *Bereavement: Studies of Grief in Adult Life* (New York: International Universities Press, 1972).
20. Ibid., Chapter 4.
21. Lindemann, "Symptomatology," 42.
22. Parkes, *Bereavement.*
23. Lindemann, "Symptomatology," 147–48.
24. Schneider, "Significant differences," 161–66.
25. Kübler-Ross, *On Death and Dying,* 39.
26. David K. Switzer, *The Dynamics of Grief* (New York: Abingdon Press, 1970), 105.
27. Parkes, *Bereavement.*
28. Schneider, "Significant differences," 166.
29. Lindemann, "Symptomatology," 148.
30. Colgrove, Bloomfield, and McWilliams, *Loss of a Love,* 16.
31. Baccalaureate Curriculum Committee, "Adaptation," 16–17.
32. Ibid., 16.
33. Ibid.
34. Perihan A. Rosenthal, "Short-term family therapy and pathological grief resolution with children and adolescents," *Fam Process* 19, (1980): 151–59.
35. Robert Kastenbaum, "The child's understanding of death: How does it develop?" in E.A. Crolhonan, ed., *Explaining Death to Children* (New York: Springer Publishing Co., 1967), 89–108.
36. Ibid., 101.
37. Maria Nagy, "The child's view of death," *J Genet and Psychol* 73 (1948):3–27.
38. Kastenbaum, "Child's understanding of death," 103.
39. Sharon Roberts, *Behavioral Concepts and Nursing Throughout the Life Span* (Englewood Cliffs, N.J.: Prentice-Hall, 1978), 145–71.
40. Kastenbaum, "Child's understanding of death," 105–106.
41. Kübler-Ross, *Death and Dying.*
42. Lindemann, "Symptomatology," 145.
43. R. Rabe, "Social Stress and Illness Onset," *J Psychom Res* 8, (1964):35–43.
44. Hans Selye, *The Stress of Life* (New York: McGraw-Hill Book Co., 1956).

45. Ibid., 144–46.
46. Volkan, "Regrief."
47. Parkes, *Bereavement.*
48. Schneider, "Significant differences," 161–66.
49. Lynette Long and Penny Prophit, *Understanding/Responding: A Communication Manual for Nurses* (Monterey, Calif.: Wadsworth Health Sciences Division, 1981), 19.
50. Schneider, "Significant differences," 162.
51. Maurice J. Barry, "The prolonged grief reaction," *Mayo Clin Proc* 48, (1973):329–35.
52. Colgrove, Bloomfield, and McWilliams, *Loss of a Love.*
53. Schneider, "Significant differences."

Annotated Bibliography

Bowen, F.L. 1980. *Nursing and the Concept of Loss.* New York: Wiley. This volume is a collection of learning modules of various types of loss that the nurse encounters. It provides an excellent opportunity for independent study or as a basis for education related to loss.

Colgrove, M., Bloomfield, H.H., McWilliams, P. 1976. *How to Survive the Loss of A Love.* New York: Bantam. This superb book offers ways of dealing with loss.

Donnelley, K. 1982. *Recovering from the Loss of a Child.* New York: Macmillan. An essential reference for nurses, this book provides descriptive data about the experience of the death of a child as well as invaluable references for referral to supportive organizations.

Engel, G.L. 1964. *Grief and grieving. Am J Nurs* 64(9):93–96. This classic article discusses the adapative grief process and suggests ways to help individuals suffering loss.

Finn, W.F., et al., eds. 1985. *Women and Loss.* New York: Praeger Scientific. This collection of essays deals with the specific types of losses with which women deal throughout the life-span.

Friedmam, R. and B. Gradstein. 1982. *Surviving Pregnancy Loss.* Boston: Little, Brown. This book provides crucial information to both clients and health-care professionals about the emotional response to pregnancy loss. A crucial reference for those providing health care to women.

Kübler-Ross, E. 1969. *On Death and Dying.* New York: Macmillan. This excellent classic book identifies and describes the five stages of dying and gives many examples.

Kübler-Ross, E. 1975. *Death: The Final Stage of Growth.* Englewood Cliffs, N.J.: Prentice-Hall. This book is a collection of articles about death and dying.

Lindemann, E. 1944. Symptomatology and Management of Acute Grief. *Am J Psychiatry* 101:141–48. This classic article discusses grief and the grieving process.

Parkes, C.M. and Weiss, R.S.: 1982. *Recovery From Bereavement.* New York: Basic Books. This book is an actual study of how a sample of widows and widowers under age 45 coped with their bereavements. It is wonderfully descriptive of grief and the process of mourning in the first year after the loss of a spouse.

Ramsay, R.W. and Noorberger, R. 1986. *Living with Loss: A Dramatic Breakthrough in Grief Therapy.* New York: William Morrow. This is a most thorough review of grief therapy and its relation to stress. It provides a clear outline of the detrimental effects of severe stress on the human body.

Schneider, J. 1984. *Stress, Loss and Grief: Understanding their origins and growth potential.* Baltimore: University Park Press. This excellent, comprehensive book dealing with the broad context of loss in our lives is essential reading for nurses and other health care professionals. A superb reference.

Smith, W.J. 1985. *Dying in the Human Life Cycle.* New York: Holt, Rinehart, Winston. A comprehensive text covering death and other losses throughout various points in the human life cycle.

Weizman, S.G, and Kamm, P. 1985. *About Mourning.* New York: Human Services Press. This excellent book is not about death, but about life: The emotional life of one who has suffered the loss of a loved one. A profound and deep look at mourning, its process and promise. Essential reading.

Werner - Beland, J.A. 1980. *Grief Responses to Long-Term Illness and Disability.* Reston, Va.: Reston Publishing. This book addresses the effects of physical and emotional losses and how resolutions can be found by nurses and other health-care professionals.

Chapter 28

Crisis Intervention and Suicide

Linda Manglass

Chapter Outline

- Objectives
- Glossary
- Introduction
- Theoretical Development
- Types of Crises
  Developmental Crisis
  Situational Crisis
- Predicting Crisis
- Identifying Individuals in Crisis
- Suicide as a Response to Crisis
  Survivors of Suicide
- Crisis Prevention
- The Nursing Process
  Assessment
  Planning
  Implementation
  Evaluation
- Summary
- Study Questions
- References
- Annotated Bibliography

Objectives

At the completion of this chapter, the reader will be able to:

▶ Define crisis
▶ State developmental theories of crisis
▶ Identify elements of a crisis
▶ Differentiate between maturational and situa-

tional crisis
▶ Identify factors that indicate a crisis state
▶ Use a crisis intervention model as a framework for providing nursing care to clients experiencing a crisis
▶ Identify suicidal behaviors as a maladaptive response to crisis
▶ Recognize prodromal clues to suicide
▶ Assess client lethality when presented with suicidal behavior
▶ Describe steps taken when intervening with suicidal clients
▶ Predict behaviors in family members and significant others following a suicide attempt
▶ Describe resources available on a primary, secondary, and tertiary level for the client in crisis

Glossary

Adventitious Crises. Accidental, uncommon, and unexpected crises that result in multiple losses and environmental changes.

Anticipatory Guidance. A process that aims to help persons cope with a crisis by discussing the details of the impending difficulty and intervening before the event occurs.

Anxiety. A diffuse apprehension that is vague in nature and is associated with feelings of uncertainty and helplessness; an emotion without a specific object, subjectively experienced by the individual and communicated interpersonally. Anxiety occurs as a result of threat to a person's being, self-esteem, or identity.

Crisis. A situation in which customary problem-solving methods are no longer adequate; a state of psychological disequilibrium. A crisis may be a turning point in a person's life.

Crisis Intervention. An intervention process aimed at reestablishing the individual's functioning to a level equal to or better than the precrisis level.

Developmental Crises. Crises that occur in response to stresses common to all people in particular phases of human development and transition.

Grieving. A process of separating from a highly valued person, place, object, or ideal.

Lethality Assessment. An estimation of the probability that a person experiencing suicidal impulses actually will succeed in an attempt based on the method described, the specificity of the plan, and the availability of means.

Primary Prevention. Biological, social, or psychological intervention that promotes emotional well-being or reduces the incidence and prevalence of mental illness in a community by altering the causes before they have an opportunity to do harm.

Secondary Prevention. Early recognition and detection with rapid intervention.

Situational Crises. Crises that occur when a person is confronted with stressful events of unusual or extreme intensity or duration and habitual methods of coping are no longer effective.

Survivors of Suicide. Individuals, usually family or close friends, who are at risk after the death by suicide of someone close.

Tertiary Prevention. The elimination or reduction of residual disability following illness.

INTRODUCTION

Individuals vary in their ability to adapt adequately to anticipated and unanticipated events in their lives. Most of the time, people live in some degree of balance or homeostasis. Individuals usually are able to cope with the every-day stressful events that occur and maintain an adaptive balanced state. Sometimes, however, there is an imbalance between the problem facing an individual and the individual's perception of it and the repertoire of adaptive behaviors available. In such situations a **crisis** may be precipitated.

A crisis is defined by Gerald Caplan as "a psychological disequilibrium in a person who confronts a hazardous circumstance that for him constitutes an important problem which he can, for the time being, neither escape nor solve with his usual problem solving resources."[1] A crisis occurs "when a person faces an obstacle to important life goals that is, for a time, insurmountable through utilization of customary methods of problem solving. A period of disorganization ensues, a period of upset during which many abortive attempts at solution are made."[2] A person in crisis is at a turning point. The usual methods of coping are not available or are not working. The person experiences helplessness and increased anxiety. In the search for a solution and relief, the individual may move toward healthy adaptation or increasingly maladaptive behavior.

Crisis intervention is a direct, goal-oriented approach to help the individual resolve the crisis as quickly as possible and return to a level of functioning at least as functional as prior to the crisis.

THEORETICAL DEVELOPMENT

The study of crisis, crisis theory, and the crisis intervention approach to the treatment of emotional disturbances is relatively new when compared to psychoanalysis, psychotherapy, and other traditional approaches to providing care.

The theory of crisis intervention rests heavily on the early formulations of Erich Lindemann and the subsequent works of Gerald Caplan.[3,4] In 1944, Erich Lindemann studied 101 individuals in crisis. These were survivors and the families of those killed in the Coconut Grove nightclub fire in Boston. Hundreds of people lost their lives in this fire, and Lindemann's observations of and work with survivors and families provided the basis for crisis intervention theory and practice. Lindemann believed that the concept of intervention during bereavement could be applied to intervention during other kinds of crisis situations.

Also of significance in the development of the crisis approach was the report of the Joint Commission on Mental Illness and Health published in 1961.[5] A result of this publication, which was based on massive analysis of the nation's mental health services and resources, was the Community Mental Health Centers Act of 1963. Between 1963 and 1972, the population of state institutions across the nation declined by almost half. Local community mental health centers were to be created to meet the mental health needs of communities. This act was supposed to create several thousand such centers. However, fewer than 500 were formed by 1973. Thus, a direct, brief, cost-effective treatment approach based on the concepts and principles of crisis intervention began to be used in an effort to meet the demands of this increased population in need of mental health services.

The problem of providing adequate mental health and social services to those in need is still a problem today. Long-term care facilities continue to have budgets reduced with subsequent reductions in services available. Programs to meet community members' mental health needs are often inadequately planned and administered.

One means to bridge the gap between availability of resources and demand is crisis intervention. Crisis intervention serves as a link but is not the only solution.

Gerald Caplan's preventive approach to psychiatry was instrumental in the articulation of key definitions, terms, and concepts of crisis intervention. According to Caplan, a crisis is composed of the following characteristics[6]:

- It is a threat or danger to life goals
- It creates mounting tension or anxiety and the effects of fear, guilt, or shame are felt subjectively
- It evokes or awakens unresolved problems from the past
- It is a turning point in which the person may achieve emotional growth or become further disorganized

A crisis does not occur automatically as a result of a particular set of circumstances, nor does it develop quickly. There are identifiable phases of development that lead to an active state of crisis. Caplan describes four phases in the development of extreme **anxiety** and, finally, crisis. Recognition of these phases and timely intervention may help prevent a full-blown crisis.[7]

Phase I   The individual is faced with a crisis-provoking situation. Attempts are made to cope with the anxiety and tension by using behaviors that have worked successfully in the past.

Phase II   The crisis-provoking situation continues to cause anxiety and tension as usual coping mechanisms and problem solving techniques fail. The person feels increasingly upset and perplexed. At this stage, since there is greater stress, the possibility of a crisis state occurring increases, but is still not inevitable, depending on what happens next.

Phase III   Emergency problem-solving mechanisms are brought into play; the individual searches for assistance and calls on all reserves of strength. As a result, the problem may be solved and equilibrium restored.

Phase IV   If the problem is not solved, an active crisis state will result. A person in crisis feels helpless and does not know where to turn or what to do. Internal strength and social supports are unavailable or lacking. Unbearable anxiety and tension are experienced.

Howard Parad and Harvey Resnik identify a crisis sequence that involves three time periods: precrisis, crisis, and postcrisis. An individual in precrisis functions in the usual manner to ensure the achievement of needs. The person in crisis experiences a period of disorganization and disequilibrium. Attempts are made to reduce the discomfort and anxiety experienced. The resolution of the crisis or postcrisis period can result in either an increase or decrease in the person's level of functioning or a return to a precrisis level of functioning.[8] The three periods of crisis sequence are pictured in Figure 28–1.

Obviously a person cannot stay in crisis indefinitely. The feelings experienced are far too uncomfortable and distressing. It is generally accepted that there is a limitation to the amount of time an individual can remain in a crisis state. The emotional discomfort stemming from the extreme anxiety moves the person to reduce the anxiety to a more manageable level as quickly as possible. Experience with persons in crisis has led to the observation that the acute emotional upset lasts from a few days to a few weeks.[9] Several outcomes are possible for the individual experiencing a crisis state.[10]

- The person can return to a precrisis state. This happens as a result of effective problem solving, made possible by one's internal strength and supports.
- The person may not only return to the precrisis state but can grow from the crisis experience through discovery or new resources and ways of solving problems.
- The person reduces intolerable tension by lapsing into maladaptive patterns of behavior. For example, the individual may become very withdrawn, suspicious, or depressed. Others in crises may reduce their tension, at least temporarily, by excessive drinking or

other drug abuse, or by impulsive, disruptive behavior. Still others resort to more extreme measures by engaging in suicidal or homicidal behaviors.

TYPES OF CRISES

In an attempt to differentiate types of crises, two broad categories are considered. Developmental crisis, also referred to as maturational or internal crisis, is one, and situational or external crisis is the other.

Developmental Crisis

Developmental crises are expected life events that occur in most individuals' life span. They have been described as normal processes of growth and development. As one grows and develops one constantly is faced with new situations, challenges, and influences to which one must adapt biologically, psychologically, and socially. Potential crisis areas occur during these periods of change and stress.

Erik Erikson's psychosocial maturational tasks provide a theoretical framework for the understanding of maturational crisis (Table 28–1) and developmental task achievement.[11] Others, such as Piaget's development of intellectual abilities, H.S. Sullivan's stages of personality development, and Maslow's basic human needs theory, also provide frameworks for assessing maturational growth and task achievement.

Facing the challenges of developmental task achievement can be and, in fact, is usually somewhat stressful and anxiety-provoking. Coping behaviors that until now have been adequate and appropriate are no longer effective. Adjusting to previously unexperienced biological changes in adolescence or old age, for example, may precipitate concern over body image and physical functioning. Adjusting to new societal expectations regarding role changes—from single to married, childless to parent—requires energy, understanding, and nurture from others.

With adequate support, individuals usually are able to successfully meet the tasks required in the normal process of growth and development. It is in this sense that maturational crises are considered normal. Because maturational

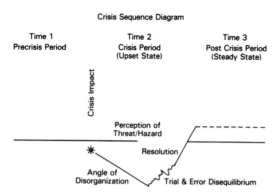

Figure 28–1. Crisis sequence diagram. *(From H. Parad and H. Resnick, "A crisis intervention framework," in H. Resnick and H. Ruben, eds., Emergency Psychiatric Care, (Bowie, Md.: Charles Press, 1975) 4.)*

TABLE 28–1. ERICKSON'S EIGHT STAGES OF MAN

Developmental Stage	Area of Resolution	Basic Attitudes and Behaviors
Infancy (0 to 18 mo)	Trust versus mistrust	Developing a sense of trust in oneself and others; hopefulness Withdrawal from others
Early childhood (18 mo to 3 yr)	Autonomy versus shame and doubt	Ability to express oneself and cooperate with others; self-control without loss of self-esteem Defiance; compulsive self-restraint or compliance
Late childhood (3 to 5 yr)	Initiative versus guilt	Purposeful behavior with a sense of reality; beginning ability to evaluate one's own behavior Self-denial and self-destruction
School age (6 to 12 yr)	Industry versus inferiority	Believing in one's abilities and competencies; perseverance Self-doubt and a feeling that one can never do well at things; withdrawal from school and peers
Adolescence (12 to 20 yr)	Identity versus role diffusion	A clear sense of self; plans to actualize one's abilities Confusion and indecisiveness about oneself; a crisis of identity; may lead to antisocial behavior
Young adulthood (18 to 25 yr)	Intimacy versus isolation	Capacity for reciprocal love relationship; commitment to work and relationships Impersonal relationships; prejudices
Adulthood	Generativity versus stagnation	Capacity to care for others; creativity and productivity Impoverishment of self; self-indulgence
Old age (65 yr to death)	Integrity versus despair	Acceptance of one's life as worthy and unique Sense of loss; contempt for others

crises are expected, there is opportunity to prepare for them. No amount of preparation can eliminate the crisis, but preparation can increase control over the event, thus reducing the amount and severity of disequilibrium experienced. This kind of preparatory education is an important aspect of crisis intervention.

Situational Crisis

Situational crises occur when a specific external event upsets an individual's psychological equilibrium. Some situational crises may stem from anticipated life events, such as beginning school, changing schools, success or failure in school. Family-related events may be the addition of a family member through birth or adoption, separation, divorce, remarriage, or a change in the family's financial status. Examples of anticipated events related to self are outstanding personal achievement, beginning to date, the breakup of a relationship, an unwanted pregnancy, physical deformity, or involvement with drugs or alcohol.

Unanticipated life events (sometimes referred to as **adventitious crises**) are distinguished from anticipated life events by the variable of prediction. Caplan defines unanticipated life events or situational crises as chance events that are viewed by the person as unpredictable.[12] It is often a traumatic event that is beyond one's control. Some common situational crises are loss of a loved one through death or divorce, loss of financial security, imprisonment, rape, assault, hospitalization, and natural disasters. The occurrence of one of these events does not automatically mean that a crisis will occur. As is true of developmental crisis, much depends on the individual's personal and social resources. Another factor influencing whether a crisis results is the person's stage of development. An individual confronting a major developmental task is already vulnerable. It is more likely that the added stress of a traumatic event will precipitate a crisis.

PREDICTING CRISIS

Herbert Schulberg and Alan Sheldon identified a number of factors helpful in predicting the probability of a crisis occurring. According to them, several factors should be considered in assessing which persons are crisis prone and at risk[13]:

- The probability that a disturbing and hazardous event will occur. For example, death of a close family member is highly probable, whereas natural disasters are very improbable
- The probability that an individual will be exposed to the event. For example, every adolescent faces the challenge of adult responsibilities, whereas only some face the crisis of an unwanted pregnancy
- The vulnerability of the individual to the event. The mature adult, for example, can more easily adapt to the stress of moving than a child in the first years of school

In looking at the probability of any one individual experiencing a crisis, one needs to consider the degree of stress stemming from a hazardous event, the risk of being exposed to the event, and the person's vulnerability or ability to adapt to stress.

IDENTIFYING INDIVIDUALS IN CRISIS

Nurses, by virtue of where they work, and as health-care providers, are often in positions of meeting individuals experiencing crises. Hospitalization has the potential to provoke crisis because of the many changes with which the individual is confronted. It is always an anxiety-provoking and stressful experience. The reason for the hospitalization itself has crisis potential—loss of physiological integrity, loss of independence, or a change in role and functioning are examples.

Individuals experiencing maturational crisis can be identified in settings such as maternal-child health, pediatrics, young adult health, and gerontology. It is in these age groups where individuals make transitions in life-style behaviors. Nurses in emergency units frequently see people experiencing unanticipated events, such as disasters, suicide attempts, unexpected life-threatening accidents, and illnesses.

Nurses who work in the community are in a position to recognize maturational and situational crises occurring in the home—the child

who refuses to go to school, the parents of a new baby, the family that has experienced a recent death.

The ability to accurately assess and intervene with individuals' crises is a learned skill, and it is invaluable for nurses in almost every health-care setting. Nurses in positions of assessing and providing care to clients experiencing crisis can use the crisis intervention model, which is a problem-solving approach and closely follows the steps in the nursing process.

SUICIDE AS A RESPONSE TO CRISIS

There are instances when an individual responds to crisis by attempting to commit or committing suicide.

Nurses, as health-care providers, find themselves in situations where an individual is responding to crisis by engaging in suicidal thinking or behavior. A knowledge of facts about suicide, demographic characteristics of suicidal individuals, how to assess suicide lethality, and intervention approaches is, therefore, necessary.

There are numerous myths regarding suicide that influence how we think about and act with suicidal individuals. The following statements are examples of some of the myths about suicide. True or False?

1. An individual serious about killing himself leaves a note. False. A note may or may not indicate seriousness of intent.[14]
2. At one time or another almost everyone contemplates suicide. True. Suicide is common enough that everyone is familiar with it as a behavior and thinks about it at some point, although not necessarily with intent.
3. Only "crazy" people or those with weak moral characters attempt or commit suicide. False. Suicide, as a response to crisis, is used by all kinds of people.
4. People who talk about suicide never do anything about it. False. People who give verbal indications of suicidal feelings and intentions should *always* be taken seriously. Studies have shown that as many as 75 percent of persons who commit suicide have contacted their physicians for some reason within three to six months prior.[15]

5. Suicidal persons are fully intent on dying and nothing you can do or say will stop them. False. Suicide is a behavior, and there is communication in any behavior. Persons who engage in suicidal behaviors are attempting to communicate their helplessness and despair. Suicidal people are ambivalent; they are struggling with a desire to live and a desire to die. As long as an individual has ambivalent feelings, it is possible to work with him or her in considering alternatives. Individuals who are no longer ambivalent seldom come into contact with others willing and able to offer help.

6. Asking a person if he or she is suicidal only puts ideas into his or her head. False. Even if you have no indication that a person is considering suicide as an alternative to crisis, you should ask about it as part of your assessment. "Sometimes people under a lot of stress have thoughts of hurting themselves. Have you had any thoughts like that?" "Are you so upset you're thinking of killing yourself?" Comments made by individuals that should be explored include such statements as, "If it weren't for the children, I wouldn't be going through this," "Sometimes I wish I'd just fall asleep and never wake up," "I can't live with myself," or "There's nothing left for me now."

Behavioral clues that should be addressed are actions such as giving away possessions, taking out a life insurance policy, and a "tidying up" of one's personal affairs. Asking a person outright about how the person is feeling, if he or she is experiencing any self-destructive thoughts, is appropriate and necessary. Having someone pick up the cues being sent and providing an opportunity to talk can be helpful and reassuring.

Suicide has been recognized as a serious problem in the United States for many years. In 1962, a grant from the United States Public Health Service was awarded to the University of Southern California to open a suicide prevention center in Los Angeles. Much of what is known about suicide has been discovered through the research done at this center.

A major task in preventing suicide is accurate assessment of the seriousness of suicidal intentions. This **lethality assessment** is the process of determining the likelihood of suicide for an individual. The nurse's first goal in working with an individual responding to crisis with suicidal thinking is to determine how likely the person is to engage in suicidal behavior in the immediate future, so that appropriate action can be taken. Lethality assessment techniques are based on knowledge obtained from the study of completed suicides. Research about suicide is a difficult area, and the knowledge available, although extremely useful, is by no means absolute.

Survivors of Suicide

The **survivors of suicide**—those left after someone commits suicide—are a crisis-prone population. In addition to the usual feelings associated with loss, there is the tragic aspect of it, the anger at the individual who is no longer a part of one's life, and the surviving person's guilt about the experience. The guilt is over not having been able to prevent it from happening or even seeing it beforehand. Sometimes there is a sense of relief, especially if the individual had been having difficulties for a long time.

Some suicide prevention centers have established programs for survivors of suicide. One plan developed is termed *"postvention"* and occurs in three phases. The first phase is *resuscitation*. This occurs within 24 hours of the suicide. Usually the survivors are in shock at this time and another follow-up visit is in order within three days. At this point, the intervenor can expect to deal with feelings of guilt and blame.

The second phase lasts two to three months and is *resynthesis*. Explaining grief reactions— Are the survivors grieving appropriately? How are they adjusting?—is the focus at this time.

The last phase is *renewal*. This is the period, from six months on, when the survivors will be forming new relationships and finding substitutes for the loss. This phase ends with the anniversary of the death. This can be a particularly vulnerable time for survivors, and a last contact should be made at this time.[16]

CRISIS PREVENTION

Nurses are offered many opportunities to intervene with individuals facing crises or crisis-provoking situations, including suicidal crises. The first step in helping individuals and their families deal with such situations is through **anticipatory guidance** and education. This is an aspect of primary prevention. **Primary prevention** is designed to reduce the occurrence of mental disabilities in a community through education, consultation, and crisis intervention.[17] Examples of ways nurses can be involved in primary prevention are educative groups such as prenatal classes, parenting groups, and groups formed to deal with major life events like adolescence and aging. Community health nurses and those in schools are in unique positions to engage in primary prevention. These types of situations afford nurses opportunities to recognize and intervene with individuals at risk.

Secondary prevention includes early recognition and detection with prompt, timely intervention, such as offering support and guidance to the newly bereaved spouse (the postvention approach previously described), or intervening with the client who has recently been diagnosed with a life-threatening illness. Emergency units, outpatient departments, and occupational health settings are just a few places where early recognition and intervention is appropriate and necessary to prevent the client from harm.

The **tertiary prevention** includes intervening to prevent any further maladaptation and helping the individual to achieve or regain a maximum level of adaptive functioning. This usually occurs in inpatient settings, but also occurs in the community and some outpatient settings.

THE NURSING PROCESS

The *crisis* approach to problem solving, articulated by Morley, Messick, and Aguilera, involves an assessment of the individual and problem, planning of therapeutic intervention and resolution of the crisis, and anticipatory planning.[18] This model is pictured in the paradigms depicted in Figure 28–2 and in Figure 28–3. Thorough assessment of suicidal thoughts and/or behaviors is essential for client well-being.

Assessment

Assessment begins before or on initial contact with the person. It is often possible to anticipate that an individual may be experiencing *crisis* behaviors by being familiar with events surrounding contact with the health-care system. For instance, an emergency unit receives a call from the highway patrol that persons will soon be arriving who have been in a serious accident. Family or friends accompanying these persons may also be in need of crisis intervention. The news of serious illness, injury, or death always brings with it the possibility of difficulties in adaptation. A phone call to the community health nurse may reveal a distraught mother of a new infant who is having problems with breastfeeding. An adolescent confides to the nurse practitioner that he or she is failing in school and can't seem to make any friends. These are all situations nurses face that call for careful assessment and intervention.

Basic to carrying out the steps in the nursing process is establishing an alliance with the individual. This is facilitated by conveying to the client that you want to help him or her. It is useful to remember that the goal of crisis intervention is to reestablish psychological equilibrium as quickly as possible. The first step in crisis assessment is to identify events that led to the person's distress. Naomi Golan has made a workable differentiation between the hazardous event and the precipitating factor, both important concepts in crisis intervention.[19]

The *hazardous event* is the initial shock or internal rise in tension that sets in order a series of reactions leading to the crisis. The hazardous event may be anticipated or unanticipated and may be related to maturational or situational events. To determine the hazardous event, the question, "What happened?" should be asked. The process of talking about the event and recalling time sequences, circumstances surrounding it, and others involved is often helpful for the individual. The opportunity to put the events in order and make some sense out of what is often chaos has a calming effect and gives the person a sense of control. Simple, direct questions and clarifying comments are useful in assisting the individual.

The *precipitating event* is the "straw that broke the camel's back." It is usually the focal

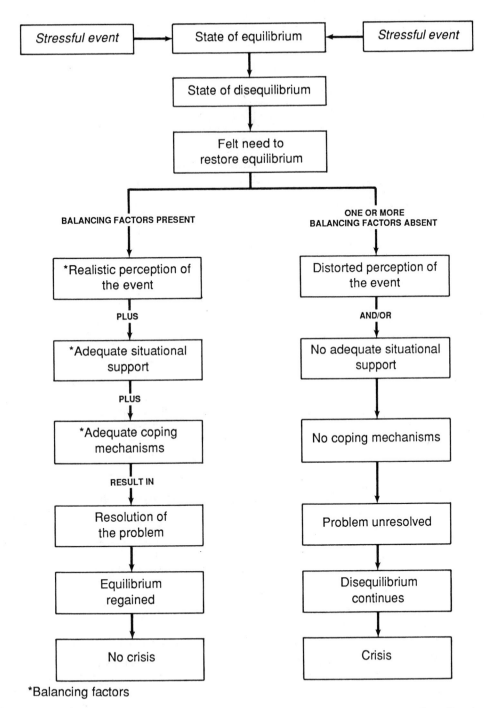

*Balancing factors

Figure 28–2. Master paradigm of crisis. *(From D. Aguilera and J. Messick, Crisis Intervention, 4th ed. [St. Louis: C.V. Mosby Co., 1982.])*

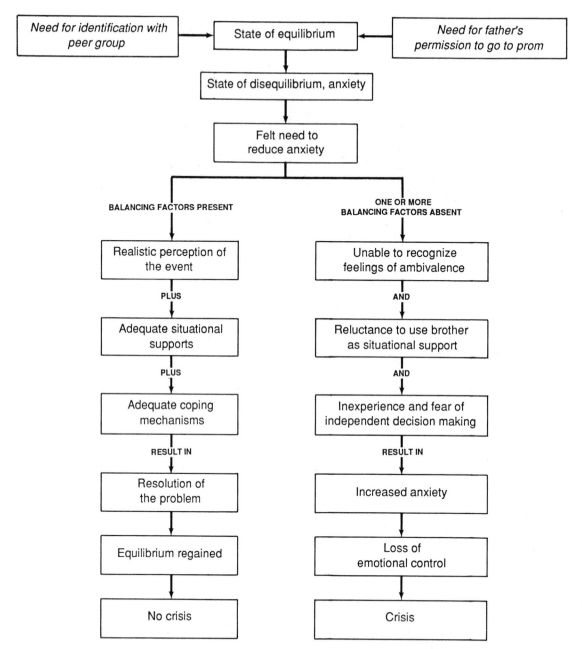

Figure 28–3. Example of a paradigm of a crisis (Case study: Mary). *(From D. Aguilera and J. Messick, Crisis Intervention, 4th ed. [St. Louis: C.V. Mosby Co., 1982.])*

point that prompted the person to seek help at that particular time. It is not always clear to the person what the precipitating event is, and the question, "What happened today that made you seek help?" is often a useful one. The crisis event usually has occurred quite recently; however, people will sometimes be dealing with issues related to the crisis weeks or even months after it has occurred. In many situations where nurses are involved, the situation is one that just occurred at that very moment. In attempting to identify the precipitating event, look for themes of loss. Often a recent loss (i.e., threat of a boyfriend breaking off a relationship) will precipitate or reawaken feelings of another loss (death of mother a few months earlier). On occasion, individuals will not make the connection between a crisis event in their lives and problems they are experiencing.

It is imperative in the assessment process to determine the individual's perception of the event. How does the individual (or family) view the event? What significance does it have for the individual? What is the impact of the event on the rest of his or her life and future? How this event fits into the client's view of the world may be very different from how the same event would fit into the nurse's world. Nurses will not be able to intervene in a manner that is useful or helpful to the client unless they are able to establish meaningful communication with their clients. It is necessary to develop an awareness and understanding of what needs (particularly developmental needs) are important in the client's life and how these needs and values influence his or her perception of the event and the response to it.

A thorough assessment of the client in the crisis also includes identifying other balancing factors that influence an individual's response to the crisis-provoking event. Identification of these balancing factors also aids the nurse in planning intervention strategies.

Aguilera and Messick state that between the perceived effects of a stressful situation and the resolution of the crisis are three recognized balancing factors that may determine the state of equilibrium. Stress or weakness in any one of these areas can be directly related to the onset of crisis or its resolution. These are perception of the event, available situational supports, and coping mechanisms.[20] By assessing these stimuli, the nurse identifies areas in which to intervene.

In addition to the individual's perception, it is necessary to determine whether the individual views the event realistically or in a distorted manner. If the event is perceived realistically, there will more likely be recognition of the relationship between the event and the distressed feelings. In this case, intervention can be directed toward relief of anxiety and

tension, and successful resolution will be more probable.

Identification of *situational supports* is important in assessing the individual or family and planning for intervention. Who are the significant people in the person's life? Has the event been discussed with them? If not, why not? If so, how have they responded so far? Is there anyone with whom the person feels safe and comfortable at this time? It is not unusual for individuals in crisis to be underutilizing the support systems they do have. This, in fact, may be a determining factor in whether an individual handles a situation adaptively or goes into crisis and is valuable information for planning interventions.

The third set of balancing factors is related to *coping mechanisms*. What kinds of coping mechanisms does the individual usually use to handle stressful situations? How has the person handled stressful situations in the past? Coping mechanisms are conscious and unconscious ways of relieving and dealing with anxiety and tension. An individual, because of the newness of the situation or the severity and shock of the event, may not be able to use those coping mechanisms that have worked in the past. Exploring with the client what has worked previously, how the client can try using those behaviors again, or what other kinds of coping behaviors could be tried (i.e., clients confined to bed in a hospital often are not able to use mechanisms that have worked for them in the past), is a nursing intervention strategy. (For more information on coping behaviors and intervention strategies see Chapter 26).

Suicide Risk. Assessing the degree of suicide risk is an important aspect of nursing practice. The following information about suicide potential assessment is a compilation of the results of much research done in the area, most notably, Schneidman, Litman, and Faberow[21] from the Suicide Prevention Center in Los Angeles, California, and also Beck, Resnick, and Lettieri,[22] and Linden and Breed.[23]

It is known that men commit suicide three times more frequently than women and are higher risks. The exception to this is among urban black males between the ages of 20 and 25. The suicide rate among this group is twice as high as for white males of the same age group.

Women, however, attempt suicide more frequently than men.

Certain population groups are higher risks than others. The elderly (over age 65) constitute an estimated 25 percent of all suicides. Considering that the elderly only account for 12 percent of the total population, this is a disproportionate number. The elderly can kill themselves in ways not likely to be detected as suicide, e.g., neglecting to take life-sustaining medication, falls, or accidents. The crises of old age that lead to suicidal behavior in some elderly individuals have most to do with irreversible losses. The least likely to be able to deal successfully with these crises are white males in the age group 70–84. As men reach age 85, their suicide rates quadruple the national rate.

Suicide is the third leading cause of death. The crises of adolescence and young adulthood are among the most difficult.

Suicide among the young, especially teenagers, has come to the attention of the public and the media in recent years and is of grave concern to professionals and families. More than three times as many 15- to 24-year olds committed suicide in 1980 than did in the mid 1950s.[24] Available statistics show increasing trends toward use of more lethal means but do not identify definite risk factors associated with suicidal behavior. In other words, it is not known for sure why young people are taking their own lives in ever-increasing numbers.

One of the factors that is important in assessing the risk of suicide in the young adult is the presence of depression. As with adults, depression is a significant precursor of suicide among both adolescents and young adults.

A study of 108 adolescent suicide attempts over a two-year period found the attempts to be a combination of long-standing problems coupled with the impact of a recent precipitating event. More than half of these precipitating events involved problems with parents.[25]

As with adults, alcohol and drug abuse are significantly linked with suicidal behaviors. A history of suicidal attempts by family members and relatives is prevalent among young adults who attempt or commit suicide. This tendency is attributed to the strong identification that a young person may have had with a family member who committed suicide.[26] This "identifica-

tion" hypothesis may, in part, explain the multiple suicides that occur in schools, for example.

For many years, experts questioned whether young children could really suffer emotional pain to the point of intentionally seeking relief through death. Research has shown that they do. The data available have shown suicidal thinking most often associated with depression and related to the crises of loss (loss of parents), fear of loss, and abandonment. It is important to know that the wish to die for some children may be a misconception, since most children do not comprehend the finality of death before age 8.

Influencing Factors. A crisis that involves a *loss* is a very significant indicator for risk. Loss through death of a loved one or friends and loss of physical and mental capabilities are prime examples.

Contact with others is critical in crisis situations involving suicidal behavior. If a person has family, friends, a job, or a therapist, the danger is reduced. Studies have shown that people are less likely to commit suicide while in contact with others. Suicide occurs less frequently among the married and people who have never been married. The risk is higher for divorced or widowed people who live isolated lives, either emotionally or physically.

The state of an individual's health is an indicator in predicting suicide. People who are physically ill, particularly those with recently diagnosed illnesses that affect self-image or lifestyle, are a high risk.

Alcohol and drug usage increase the risk of suicide. It is estimated that at least one in five suicides is alcohol-related. Suicide among drug abusers is three times as high as for the rest of the population.

Personality structures and degree of emotional health are important influencing factors. Studies of completed suicides at the Suicide Prevention Center show that 40 percent of completed suicides have a retrospective diagnosis of depression. Compared to the nondepressed people, the incidence of suicide is 50 to 100 times greater.[27] An individual who is depressed or experiencing emotional problems such as psychosis (hearing voices telling him to kill himself), an alcoholic, or drug addict may be a high risk.

Probably the most significant factor in assessment of suicide lethality is the individual's plan. Suicide is rarely an impulsive act. Studies of completed suicides show deliberate planning. If it is determined through questioning that the person is not considering suicide as a response to crisis, or if the person has thought of it but has no plan or intent, there is probably no need for further assessment in this area. If the person says he has a plan, you must find out what it is by asking, "What are you thinking of doing?"

The methods by which individuals choose to commit suicide fall into high-lethal and low-lethal categories. High-lethal methods include guns (a plan to shoot oneself in the heart or head is more lethal than planning to shoot oneself in the abdomen), jumping out of a window ("What floor do you live on?"), drowning (determine nearness to water), carbon monoxide poisoning, barbiturates, aspirin or Tylenol (acetaminophen) in high doses, or automobile accidents. Low-lethal methods include wrist cutting, house gas, nonprescription drugs, and tranquilizers.[28] The person's knowledge about the lethality of the chosen method is important. For instance, does the person know how many pills it will take to kill?

The availability of means or access to a lethal method may be the single most alarming criterion. Does the person have a gun and know how to use it? The more available the method, the higher the risk and the more lethal.

How specific are the plans? Has the person thought out how to do it, where, and when? A plan that includes precautions against discovery, for instance, is more lethal than one that takes no precautions.

Does the individual have a previous history of attempts? Has the person ever acted on suicidal feelings? How? A move from a history of low-lethal to high-lethal indicates seriousness of intent.

The following case studies are examples of the significance of demographic factors, method, plan, assessing suicide potential, and intervening appropriately.

Carol (age 28) was brought to the emergency unit of the community hospital by her husband. When he had arrived home that evening at his usual time, he found Carol asleep and only partially responsive. There was a half-empty bottle of Valium (diazepam) in the bathroom. After medical intervention, more information was obtained from Carol. It was learned that she had recently discovered that her husband was having an affair with another woman. She felt alone and helpless to deal with this. She was embarrassed to share with friends and had no family available to her. She said she did not want to die but wanted to be able to talk with her husband about her despair and knew of no other way to communicate. She was responsive to an appointment made for the next day at the crisis service.

Carol was a low risk. She expected her husband home at the usual time. Timing made discovery likely. There was little planning involved, the intent being to bring about a change in her environment.

Warren (age 54) had recently been diagnosed as having metastatic cancer. His wife died six months ago, unexpectedly, and he had had a difficult time adjusting to that change. He had not been able to use support systems available to him because of his depression, and the news of his illness was "the last straw." He lived alone, and called a crisis hotline because he was thinking of going to a cabin he owned and shooting himself. He had been drinking.

Warren was a moderate-high risk. He had experienced a recent loss. He had a plan with available means. He was a high risk in terms of age, sex, race, and marital status. The influence of alcohol was involved.

Beck and associates developed a scale for assessing the seriousness of suicide intent.[29] This scale ranks various categories from zero to 20. Examples of some of the categories are shown on the continuum in Figure 28–4.

Before going on to the planning and implementation phases of the nursing process, nursing diagnoses should be formulated. Examples of nursing diagnoses for crisis and for the two previous suicide case examples might be as follows:

- Anxiety moderate: related to mothering role
- Disturbance in self-concept, low self-esteem: related to unanticipated job loss

High Risk _____ Low Risk
Gravely serious . . . . **Extreme ambivalence**
Timing and Isolation
No one near or   **Someone nearby**
expected . . . . **and in contact**
Precautions Against Discovery
Extensive precautions . . . . **No precautions**
Acting to Gain Help
No attempt . . . . **Attempt to get help**
Plans for Attempt
Elaborate plans . . . . **No plans; impulsive**
Communication of Intent
Note, letter, message . . . . **No note, no message**
Purpose of Intent
Remove self from   **Bring about change**
environment . . . . **in environment**

Figure 28–4. Circumstances related to suicide attempt.

- Ineffective coping, individual: related to developmental crisis of marriage
- Ineffective coping, individual: with suicide attempt (Carol)
- Potential for self injury: suicidal thoughts, with plan, available means and alcohol abuse (Warren)

Planning

Throughout the process of assessment, plans should be formulated as to how to intervene with individuals experiencing a *crisis* state. It should be kept in mind that the goal of crisis intervention is the establishment of equilibrium and a return to the precrisis state. Plans should, therefore, be specific and time relevant. Examples of planning goals for an individual in crisis might be as follows:

- The client will experience a decrease in anxiety by the end of the interaction as evidenced by:
  verbalization of an increase in comfort level and a decrease in restlessness
  ability to state what he is going to do and with what kind of support, over the next 24 hours

- The client will identify one person who can be contacted as a support system
- The client will identify two new coping behaviors he can try this week to aid in reducing anxiety, e.g., exercise, relaxation program

Once the plan has been developed it should be written on the client's chart or cardex, and the implementation and evaluation phases of the nursing process can begin.

Suicide Prevention. In the case of suicide prevention, however, implementation may be going on during the planning stage in order to prevent harm to the client.

Implementation

Intervention in *crisis* actually begins with the establishment of an alliance with the client. Conveying a caring, concerned attitude is, in itself, helpful and reassuring. Providing an opportunity for the client to verbalize, clarify, and organize is useful in gaining a sense of control over the situation. General principles of crisis intervention include:

- Decrease the intensity of the crisis experience. This is accomplished primarily through anxiety-reducing techniques (see Chapter 26).
- Keep intervention brief and goal-oriented. The goal is to reestablish equilibrium and return the client to at least a precrisis level of functioning as quickly as possible. This is not the time for in-depth intrapsychic exploration or resolution of chronic emotional problems. It is not unusual to have to differentiate the crisis the client is experiencing from other more chronic kinds of emotional difficulties the client brings up.
- Identify and use client strengths. How has the client been coping with the situation so far? The client may, in fact, be dealing with the situation very well. The emotional pain and distress being experienced can easily get in the way of recognizing that one is doing all right. Reassuring the client that the **grieving** process he or she is going through, although very painful, is in fact normal and necessary, is an invaluable tool in helping the client cope with the situation. Focusing on strengths

helps raise self-esteem, making the person feel more confident and capable of coping.

Another aspect of using strengths has to do with support systems. As soon as significant others can be brought in and those ties cemented, the nurse may assume a less active role and move out of the situation. Ways to achieve this may include calling a family member or friend to be with the client or making sure the client can name someone to contact, and have him or her do so. Before you leave the crisis situation, you must replace yourself, depending upon the severity of the situation, with another person or with the availability of another person to help the client, should help be needed.

- Environmental manipulation is an intervention aimed at altering the environment that is influencing the client in crisis. It usually involves changing the individual's personal or interpersonal situation, which in turn will decrease stress and provide support. For example, moving people into the home environment temporarily may provide support (as in the case of an individual alone during crisis), or moving some children out of the home to relieve the pressure on a mother may be appropriate.

Throughout the process of assessment and intervention, the nurse conveys an attitude of concern and caring. Crisis intervention requires that expertise, responsibility, and knowledge be communicated to the client. Specific communication skills necessary in working with a client in crisis include:

- Listening. Listen to find out what the crisis is and the meaning it has for that person. Putting your perception of the situation into words and summarizing for the client is a way of assuring you have an accurate understanding.
- Focusing. Keep the client focused on issues relating to the problem causing the disequilibrium.
- Questioning. Ask questions to clarify, to find out details, and to refocus.
- Observing and acknowledging feelings. This aids the individual in sorting out feelings, expressing them, and having them validated as normal and acceptable.

- Solving problems and exploring alternatives. Discuss new ways to deal with the problem. Offer suggestions and provide opportunities to try new behaviors, if possible.

In many situations, the nurse's involvement with a client experiencing crisis may stop when the nurse assesses that a client is in crisis and needs further help. In such situations, a referral made for the client is appropriate. Referrals for clients in crisis should be expeditious, with as much help from the nurse as is necessary to ensure followthrough.

Suicide Intervention. Intervening with clients who are thinking of *suicide* as a response to crisis situations requires knowledge of assessment techniques including identification of demographic characteristics and use of lethality scales. It also requires that the intervenor has access to expert consultation.

As beginning practitioners of nursing, you should be able to accurately determine whether an individual is experiencing suicidal thoughts and assess the seriousness of intent and suicidal lethality. Unless you have an opportunity to become confident of your skills in this area through experience and supervision, these judgments should always be made in consultation with an experienced clinician. Occcasionally, a situation may occur when it is necessary to intervene in some way even before consultation can be sought. Some general guidelines that are helpful in immediate intervention follow. All the techniques for intervention in crisis are applicable in intervening in suicidal crisis.

An attitude of acceptance, hope and encouragement may help offset the hopelessness and despair the person is experiencing. It is important to recognize that the hostility and anger that may be expressed is a reflection of the despair and may have pushed everyone else away.

Involving others (other professionals, family members, friends, co-workers) in the identified client's crisis situation is imperative. Suicide is a solitary act, and the more quickly others become involved, the faster the risk is decreased. In some situations, this may involve getting a friend or family member to remove the lethal weapon.

Encourage the person to avoid making such a final decision during this time of crisis. Maintain contact with the individual until a plan is worked out.

There may be occasions when a nurse must use *telephone intervention* with an individual who is expressing thoughts about suicide. Intervening when face-to-face contact is not possible is very difficult, because the benefits of nonverbal attending behaviors (see Chapter 14) are unavailable. Norman Faberow outlines a plan for telephone intervention that is a useful guide[30]:

- Establish a rapport with the individual as quickly as possible. Maintain contact and obtain as much information as possible in a nonthreatening, accepting manner.
- Identify the central problem and maintain the focus on this concern.
- Evaluate the potential for action.
- Assess the individual's strengths and resources as evidenced by: an improvement of mood during the call, even the ability to listen to you and focus on the conversation.
- Formulate and initiate plans; call an ambulance, get the person to go to an emergency unit or crisis center, arrange for an appointment the next day. Contact should be maintained until a plan is worked out and some change has occurred in mood or tone.

Evaluation

The evaluation phase of *crisis* intervention is fairly simple. The client should be experiencing a more tolerable level of anxiety as evidenced by verbalizations of such and the ability to use more effective coping mechanisms. There should be other people actively involved in offering support and problem solving. The person should be functioning at least at a precrisis level. Crises have inherent growth-producing potential. People who master crisis situations have the opportunity to develop a broader repertoire of coping skills that will help them deal more effectively with life situations in the future.

Suicide Prevention. Evaluation of suicide prevention is obvious, in that the client should demonstrate and verbalize a reduced desire to harm her- or himself. Evaluation should be based on the goals and objectives delineated in the planning stage of the nursing process. If the client is meeting these, then the plan is working. If

not, the client needs to be reassessed and the plan altered, implemented, and reevaluated in a cyclic process until positive outcomes of interventions can be measured.

SUMMARY

This chapter has discussed the development of crisis intervention historically and theoretically. Crisis as a concept, the elements of a crisis, and characteristics of individuals in crisis were presented to provide the basis for using the nursing process in assessing clients in crisis, planning and implementing nursing care for clients experiencing crisis, and criteria for evaluating the effectiveness of nursing strategies implemented.

As we have seen, crisis can be viewed as an opportunity for growth and the development of new, more effective problem-solving skills, or it may be a time when individuals resort to maladaptive, growth-inhibiting behaviors.

Study Questions

1. Describe characteristics of a crisis state including feeling, state, and sequence of events.

2. How does crisis intervention differ from other types of intervention?

3. Under what circumstances and in what types of settings might a nurse see individuals or families in crisis and utilize a crisis intervention model?

4. Differentiate between developmental and situational crisis and give examples of each.

5. Describe factors necessary to adequately assess and plan in a crisis.

6. Discuss goals and intervention strategies in helping an individual in crisis.

7. State demographic characteristics useful in assessing suicide potential.

8. Discuss the concept of lethality.

9. Describe intervention strategies in helping the individual experiencing suicidal thoughts and feelings.

10. Discuss and give examples of primary, secondary, and tertiary prevention.

References

1. Gerald Caplan, *An Approach to Community Mental Health* (New York: Grune & Stratton, 1961).
2. Caplan, *Community Mental Health.*
3. Erich Lindemann, "Symptomatology and management of acute grief," *Am J Psych* 101, (September 1944), 101–48.
4. Gerald Caplan, *Principles of Preventive Psychiatry* (New York: Basic Books, 1964).
5. *Action for Mental Health, Report of the Joint Commission on Mental Illness and Health* (New York: Basic Books, 1961).
6. Caplan, *Principles of Preventive Psychiatry.*
7. Ibid.
8. Howard Parad and Harvey Resnick, "A crisis intervention framework," in Harvey Resnick and H.L. Ruben, eds., *Emergency Psychiatric Care* (Bowie, Md: Charles Press, 1975).
9. Lindemann, "Symptomatology."
10. Lee Ann Hoff, *People in Crisis: Understanding and Helping* (Menlo Park, Calif.: Addison Wesley Publishing Co., 1978), 21.
11. Erik Erikson, *Childhood and Society,* 2nd ed. (New York: W.W. Norton & Co., 1963), 247–74.
12. Caplan, *Principles of Preventive Psychiatry.*
13. Herbert Schulberg and Alan Sheldon, "Probability of crisis and strategies for preventive intervention," *Arch Gen Psychiatry* 18, (May 1968):558.
14. Robert Litman, Edwin Schneidman, Norman Faberow, and N.D. Tabachnick, "Investigation of equivocal suicides," *JAMA* 184,(1963):924–29.
15. Robert Litman, "Actively suicidal patients: Management in general medical practice," *Calif Med* 104,(1966):168–74.
16. Harvey Resnick and Berkley Hawthorne, eds., *Suicide Prevention in the 70's,* Department of Health Education and Welfare, Publication No. (HSM) 72–9054 (Washington, D.C.: U.S. Government Printing Office, 1973).
17. Gerald Caplan and Henry Grunebaum, "Perspectives on primary prevention: A review," *Arch Gen Psychiatry* 17,(1967):331–46.
18. Wilbur Morley, Janice Messick, and Donna Aquilera, "Crisis, paradigms of intervention," *J Psychiatr Nurs* 5, (November-December 1967), 538–40.
19. Naomi Golan, "When is a client in crisis?" *Soc Casework* 50, (July 1969):389–94.
20. Donna Aguilera and Janice Messick, *Crisis Intervention,* 2nd ed. (St. Louis, Mo.: C.V. Mosby Co., 1974).
21. Edwin Schneidman, Norman Faberow, and Robert Litman, eds., *The Psychology of Suicide* (New York: Science House, 1970), 165–228, 259–92.
22. Aaron Beck, Harvey Resnick, and Don Lettieri, eds., *The Prediction of Suicide* (Bowie, Md.: Charles Press, 1974), 59–141.
23. Leonard Linden and Warren Breed, "The demographic epidemiology of suicide," in Edwin Schneidman, ed., *Suicidology: Contemporary Developments* (New York: Grune & Stratton, 1976).
24. Susan J. Blumenthal and Robert Hirschfeld, with assistance from other staff members of ADAMHA, NIAAA, NIDA and NIMH, "Suicide among adolescents and young adults," Oct. 19, 1984.
25. Ibid.
26. Tischler, L., P.C. McHenry, and K.D. Morgan. "Adolescent suicide attempts: Some significant factors," *Suicide Life Threat Behav* 11, (Summer 1981):86–92.
27. Psychiatric Research Interview with Robert E. Litman, MD. *Depression Notes No. 23* (Cinncinati, Ohio: Merrell-National Laboratories, January 1978).
28. Hoff, *People in Crisis,* 119.
29. Aaron Beck, Dean Schulyer and Ira Herman, "The Development of a Suicidal Intent Scale," in Aaron Beck, Harvey Resnick, and Don Lettieri, eds., *The Prediction of Suicide* (Bowie, Md.: Charles Press, 1974), 45–56.
30. Norman Faberow, Samuel Heilig, and Robert Litman, "Evaluation and management of suicidal persons," in E. Schneidman, N. Faberow, and R. Litman, eds., *The Psychology of Suicide* (New York: Science House, 1970), Chapter 16.

Annotated Bibliography

Faberow, N., and Schneidman, E., (eds.), 1961. *The Cry for help.* New York: McGraw-Hill. Something of a classic in the field of suicide, this work covers all aspects of suicide and is highly recommended reading.

Hall, J., and Weaver, B., (eds) 1974. *Nursing of Families in Crisis*. Philadelphia: Lippincott. A valuable resource for nurses covering many different types of family-related crises.

Hendin, H. 1986. A review of new directions in research. *Hosp Community Psychiatry* 37(2):148–54. An update and review of research done on suicide. The findings are summarized, making it a very informative resource.

Maslow, A., 1962. *Toward a Psychology of Being*. Princeton: Van Nostrand. This psychologist presents a theory of human functioning based on needs. It is an easily used theoretical framework and is highly applicable to nursing.

Russianoff, P., ed. 1981. *Women in Crisis*. New York: Human Sciences Press. Addresses aspects of and issues relevant to women in crisis, including intervention problems and approaches.

Slaikeu, K.M. 1984. *Crisis Intervention: A Handbook for Practice*. Boston: Allyn & Bacon. A comprehensive book on crisis intervention and its use as a treatment approach in different settings and by different care providers. Excellent bibliography.

Smith, K. 1986. Research-informed comments on the treatment of suicidal inpatients. *Psychiatr Hosp* 17(1):21–25. This article includes the results of studies at the Menninger Foundation over a period of eight years with 400 clients. It particularly considers clients during inpatient hospitalizations but includes information applicable to all suicidal persons.

Part VI

Social Systems, the Environment, and Nursing

In nursing, family and community concepts have traditionally been viewed apart from concepts related to the individual in the acute care setting. Likewise, the importance of understanding global environmental issues and group dynamics has often been directed toward specialty areas such as community and psychiatric nursing. Clearly these concepts are unique and expand beyond the scope of the individual. Equally clear is that the health status of the individual, whether on the illness or wellness end of the continuum, is profoundly affected by family and community relationships, and their importance cannot be minimized in the delivery of quality nursing and health care in any setting.

This section provides an awareness of how group and family concepts and community and environmental issues can be used in the nursing process. Community concepts are presented both generally and in the context of community health nursing, giving the reader an understanding of community roles and responsibilities as well as broadly applicable concepts. The family chapter presents selected historical aspects of the American family as well as therapeutic concepts and techniques that provide a base from which to understand and work with present day families. Environmental issues such as air pollution and the control of toxic substances are presented in the context of significance to health and disease prevention. Factors of environmental control and safety within the hospital are explored.

Chapter 29

Group Concepts

Nancy S. McKelvey
Sally Laliberté
Phyllis B. Heffron

Chapter Outline

- Objectives
- Glossary
- Introduction
- Theoretical Foundations of Group Concepts
- Characteristics of the Group
    Holistic Characteristics of Groups
    Boundaries
    Equilibrium
    Open Versus Closed Systems
- Group Structure, Function, and Process
    Group Structure
    Functions of Groups
    Group Process
- Types of Groups
- The Nursing Process
    Assessment
    Planning
    Implementation
    Evaluation
- Summary
- Study Questions
- References
- Annotated Bibliography

Objectives

At the completion of this chapter, the reader will be able to:

▶ Define the following terms: group, group process, group cohesion, and group dynamics

▶ Discuss the contributions of at least two group dynamics theorists
▶ Explain the purpose for nurses working with groups
▶ Describe the group as a system
▶ Differentiate between formal and informal group structure
▶ Describe the communication processes that occur in groups
▶ Compare and contrast the three main types of group leadership
▶ List the task and maintenance functions in a group
▶ Describe typical member behavior in each of the three phases of group process
▶ Identify four types of groups nurses work with
▶ Discuss the application of the nursing process to working with the group as the client

Glossary

Boundaries. Delineations that separate members and nonmembers of a group (external boundaries) or that differentiate between the members of a group (internal boundaries).

Cohesiveness. The attractiveness of a group for its members; the force that develops to give a sense of belongingness and a desire to participate in the group.

Group. A system composed of two or more individuals engaged in repeated interaction within an interdependent relationship and sharing a need or goal.

Group Dynamics. Scientific study of groups; the forces in group situations that are determining its nature and the behavior of the group and its members.

Group Process. Conflicts of forces that result from attempts to disrupt or change the structure of a group; the stages that a group moves through.

Maintenance Functions. Actions that encourage harmony and meaningful social interaction between members in the group.

Norms. Rules about or standards of appropriate behavior in a group.

Primary Group. Informal social group that generally functions with spontaneous communication, e.g., family group.

Secondary Group. Formal group generally existing for a specific purpose, e.g., postmastectomy support group or a professional association.

Task Functions. Actions that encourage the group to do the work necessary for goal achievement.

INTRODUCTION

Groups have always been important in society. Beginning with the earliest experience of the family group, all persons become naturally and increasingly associated with friendship groups, school and church groups, work groups, and other clusters of people.

The family group is known as a **primary group.** Primary groups are generally established through involuntary means, such as common heritage or geographic location.[1] Members communicate over long periods of time in face-face interactions and have a high degree of influence over the behavior of individuals within the group. Neighborhood cliques and adolescent peer groups, as well as families, provide examples of these informal groups.

Individuals also function within **secondary groups.** These groups usually are established for a specific purpose, and they involve a more formal pattern of interaction. They generally exert less influence on their members than primary groups do. Examples of secondary groups include committees, therapy groups, and professional associations.

A simple definition of a **group** is two or more people engaged in repeated interaction who are in an interdependent relationship and share a need or goal. Various disciplines and people who have studied group concepts have given definitions relative to kinds of groups or to group functions. Lewin, a psychologist and eminent researcher in group therapy, defines a group as "a dynamic whole based on interdependence."[2] Bion, another major group researcher, defines a group as "an aggregate of individuals who have a specific function or set of functions."[3] Murray and Zentner, nurse authors, define a group as an "assembly of people who meet over a period of time."[4]

An important concept regarding the definition of group is the differentiation between a group of people and an aggregate of people. A group refers to associations between people in an interdependent relationship.[5] This chapter addresses the ways that people organize this interdependence and how they accomplish their goals as a result of their interactions.

The use of groups in the general population has mushroomed in recent times. There are, for example, groups designed to help people lose weight and control eating behaviors, groups that teach stress management and assertiveness, groups to help recently divorced or widowed persons cope with loss, and groups to assist smokers quit their habit. The intensiveness of the group experience movement in the United States has made it a social phenomenon.[6]

The concept of working with groups in the health-care setting also has expanded, particularly in the past decade. Nurses have worked therapeutically with groups in the inpatient psychiatric setting for many years. In addition to working with hospitalized clients, nurses in the mental health field who have additional training and supervision also work as group psychotherapists. Community health nurses work with family groups, either as health counselors or family therapists.

There are vast opportunities for group work with clients in all types of clinical settings, and both hospital and community health nurses are increasingly taking advantage of this. Examples of group work by nurses include prenatal teaching groups, groups for postoperative clients such as amputees and persons who have undergone colostomies or mastectomies, groups to prepare post-heart-attack clients for discharge from the hospital, and motivational groups for clients in extended care facilities.

In addition to direct clinical involvement with groups, nurses frequently participate in other personal and professional groups, such as leading team conferences and serving on planning committees. Because so much of the nurse's personal and professional time is spent with groups, it is highly desirable for them to develop skills and knowledge about **group dynamics.** Knowing how to participate effectively with groups enables nurses to facilitate behavior change and to accomplish goals in the group setting.

This chapter provides an overview of the theoretical basis of group study, identifies types and characteristics of groups, and discusses the use of groups in carrying out the nursing process.

THEORETICAL FOUNDATIONS OF GROUP CONCEPTS

One of the first recorded research efforts on groups took place in the health field in 1905. Dr. Joseph Pratt, a Boston physician, worked with a group of tuberculosis patients and recorded his observations of their behavior and reactions over time.[7] Early sociological investigations of groups centered around behavior in crowds (mobs, fads, cliques, and public gatherings) and approaches toward understanding the dynamics of groups have evolved since that time.[8]

Jacob L. Moreno introduced the term *group psychotherapy* in 1932 and developed a special kind of therapy called psychodrama, which was group theory and dramatic techniques to achieve psychotherapeutic goals.[9] During World War II and since that time there has been tremendous growth in the use of groups for psychotherapy.

Kurt Lewin, a German psychologist and gestaltist, conducted early research on group dynamics and group behavior in the 1940s. His research demonstrated that learning occurred

productively in groups and that groups assisted active participants to develop new attitudes, learn new skills, and make behavioral patterns more effective.[10] Lewin developed what is known as field theory and did considerable research on group leadership style.

Small group theory, as a conceptual entity, has been widely studied in education, business, and industry for a number of years. The term *small group* is generally referred to in the literature as stemming from the basic training group (T-group), which was a group experience invented by the National Training Laboratories in 1947 for the purpose of helping persons become more sensitive to social reality.[11] Bion, a British psychiatrist, contributed to small group theory by studying group leadership and extending group concepts to institutions and organizations.

The study of groups draws on a wide range of theoretical frameworks. The practice of group therapy, for example, can be based on any of the theoretical approaches to psychotherapy—Freudian, transactional analysis, or gestalt.[12] The scope of this book limits a comprehensive listing or in-depth discussion of all the contributions to research on groups and group dynamics. Group dynamics is the scientific study of groups.[13] The term describes the forces in the group situation that are determining the behavior of the group and its members.[14] Group dynamics is the net result of what has been learned about groups through research, and through an understanding of this knowledge, nurses will increase their effectiveness as they participate in group activities.

CHARACTERISTICS OF THE GROUP

The group is a system composed of elements or individuals who are its members. These individuals come together because of a common interest or need, to accomplish a task, or because of situations they find themselves in (e.g., workplace, neighborhood, family groups).

Holistic Characteristics of Groups
As individual members interact and develop a sense of interdependence, a group begins to form. The members acting together become

greater than and different from any individual member. The group is thus said to exhibit the property of *summativity,* in which the whole becomes more than the sum of its parts.[15] Members of a task group attempting to influence legislation on the use of seat belts may be willing to behave more aggressively than any individual. This group would be acting in a different way from the way any of the individuals would act.

Boundaries

As group members continue to meet, communicate, and work together, the group gradually assumes its own character. Goals become apparent, special communication patterns develop, and behavior standards are established. The group members grow more interdependent and the group values and limits become apparent. While this is happening, the group is increasingly developing its own identity. **Boundaries** separate members of the group from nonmembers. "We" and "they" can be delineated.

Equilibrium

Not only do unique communication patterns and behavioral **norms** help to maintain the group's identity, but they provide the basis for sustaining the group's equilibrium, steady state, or sense of balance. Members will adapt to changes that occur within the group. If the psychotherapy group member who usually assumes a scapegoat role is absent, the other group members will adapt their behavior to adjust to this situation. For instance, the remaining group members may keep their communication superficial at that meeting because they fear unpredictable circumstances. The group maintains its equilibrium when an internal change occurs.

Open Versus Closed Systems

Groups also attempt to maintain their equilibrium in response to external influences. A group is said to be an open system, because it engages in an exchange relationship with the environment.[16] It responds to input from the environment, uses that input for change, and then produces output that affects other groups in the environment.

Input, throughput, and output are referred to as the three major processes of groups.[17] *Input* involves bringing energy or information into the group from outside its boundaries. *Throughput* refers to the process that occurs within the group in response to the input. *Output* is the result of accomplishing the group goal and provides the purpose for the group. The group's output provides input for groups in the environment as well as for the original group. When the output comes back and provides input to a group, we call that input *feedback.* Characteristics of the group as an open system must be remembered as one examines group structure, function, and process factors in greater detail.

GROUP STRUCTURE, FUNCTION, AND PROCESS

The three major components of groups, as a concept for nursing, are *structure, function,* and *process.* It is important to have a clear understanding of each of these major aspects of group before using the nursing process in group work. From a systems perspective, structure, function, and process are inseparably linked and serve to maintain equilibrium within the group as a system. However, for clarity, the three will be discussed individually.

Group Structure

Structure provides a system within which a group can meet its goals in some fairly predictable fashion. It offers the group an operational form from which relationships and boundaries within the group will develop. The relationships and boundaries occur between group members individually and between the group and the outside environment in which it functions.[18] Structure maintains constancy within a group over time so that, even as members move in and out, the basic group structure remains the same.

Members can and do have an impact on group structure. Again, structure is dynamic and constantly evolving; therefore, a change in membership or leadership will have some effect on structural aspects of the group. There are certain constants relating to structure, however, that need to be understood.

Group Boundaries. Berne has identified important sets of group boundaries.[19] The *major external boundary* separates the group leader and members from the outside environment. The *major internal boundary* separates the group leader from the group members. The *minor internal boundary* establishes vertical communication patterns between members, in which a type of hierarchical class system for interrelating develops. Assessment of group boundaries reveals important information about group roles, power, prestige and ability of members, group identity, stability, and group communication patterns.

Structual Forms. Group structure can be divided into two basic forms: formal and informal. A *formal* group structure consists of the explicit or readily apparent arrangements of the group. These include who the members are, the meeting time and place, length of group meetings, agendas, specific rules and duties, and responsibilities and rights of both the membership and the leadership. The formal structure is open, visible, and quite easily assessed.[20]

Informal group structure refers to the implicit or less readily apparent networks within the group, especially those related to power, prestige, and ability.[21] This informal group structure differs from the formal in that it pertains to how individuals within the group see themselves in relation to other members. Depending on members' perceptions of their own needs and goals within the group, as well as their past experiences, informal structures can be similar to formal structures but more often are quite different. They also may be important to group functioning and development.[22] For example, in many groups, certain individuals are seen as quite powerful, perhaps because of personal qualities such as assertiveness or aggressiveness. The formal structure may delineate the leadership as rotating each week, but the informal structure reveals one member consistently taking on the leader's role. Assessment of structure necessitates looking beyond the readily apparent formal structure, or much valuable information will be lost in the process.

Group Roles. The role network of a group is another important aspect of group structure. It has been described aptly as an interlocking network formed by many different roles.[23] Each group member will take on various roles over the lifetime of a group, depending on his or her own needs and past experience. The interaction of these roles within the role network of a group serves as a basis for the group to function and develop.

Many roles are inherent in any group. These will become manifest at various times, depending on the type of group and the specific work being done. Three basic categories of roles have been identified.[24–26] *Individual roles* meet the individual member's personal needs and are not aimed at group task and maintenance functions. *Task roles* deal with the actual work of the group, i.e., accomplishing group tasks and working toward meeting group goals. *Maintenance roles* deal with the social and emotional aspects of group work, such as support and nurturing of members, easing communication, and socialization of group members. Specific task and maintenance functions within the group will be delineated under group function.

Communication Patterns. Communication structure forms the basic patterns by which group members will interact. In addition, communication within a group is significantly different from communication between two individuals because of the number of possible interactions between group members. The basic axioms of communication, however, apply within the group format.

There are two levels of communication: verbal and nonverbal. Communication involves four components: sender, receiver, message, and context. (Refer to Chapter 14 on communication for greater detail.) It is impossible not to communicate. Communication patterns are learned. These factors are critical. Because communication patterns are learned, they also can be unlearned and replaced with more effective ones. In fact, learning how to communicate effectively can be one of the greatest advantages of group work.

There are four basic structural patterns of group communication networks (Fig. 29–1). In analyzing group communication patterns, a key concept is *centrality*.[27] This is the position of dominance in a communication network from

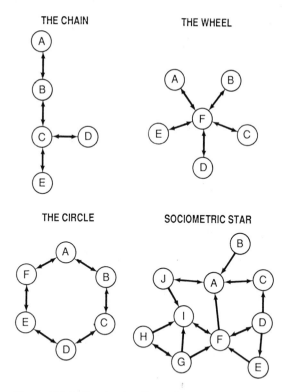

Figure 29–1. Structural patterns of group communication networks.

which and through which most communication flows. For example, the most central position in the chain is C, whereas in the circle all positions are equally central, since all are equidistant.

Research on group communication structures has shown that the more highly centralized group communication structures (chain, wheel) are most efficiently used in simple task-oriented groups. When the task is very complex, a more decentralized structure (circle) is more efficient.[28] For example, in a group of people conducting a telephone poll, the wheel would be quite effective. Each member is given a list of numbers to call and a tally sheet for recording the results. By having one person in a central position to give information, make sure members get their calls done, and then collect tally sheets, the task can be accomplished in an organized, efficient manner. On the other hand, in a support group for overweight adolescents,

the circle would be a more effective communication structure to meet the group's goals.

Another important type of communication structure within groups is the sociometric star.[29] This will be noted more in the informal structure, since it is based on attraction of group members to others in the group.[30] Generally, one member is known as the *sociomeric star*, or the person chosen most often with whom to communicate. In Figure 29–1, that person is A. There is also a member known as the *sociometric isolate*, who communicates with A, but with whom no other member communicates. Within this type of structure, we also can see different pathways and subgroupings. Certain individuals may communicate with each other but not with other members, such as G, who communicates with H, I, and F but no one else.

The communication structure of a group may involve overlapping of one or two structures. This is especially true in therapeutic groups, which are more process oriented. Evaluation of the communication structure yields valuable information, and the formation of *dyads* (two individuals who interact exclusively) and *subgroups* (three or more individuals who interact excluding other members) can be assessed by looking at both formal and informal communication structures. These components are extremely helpful in evaluating the group's progress.

Leadership Structure. Group leadership is a critical factor in the overall structure of a group. It helps guide, direct, and develop the group's progress. Depending on the leadership model and style, it is crucial to an adaptive group process.

There are three basic models for group leadership. In the *single* leader model, a group functions with the same leader throughout all group sessions. In the *coleader* model, two persons share the leadership, and in the *rotating* leader model, a different leader is designated from the membership at each group session. There are advantages and disadvantages to the three models, and each will influence a group in different ways depending on the specific type of group. Table 29–1 compares the advantages and disadvantages of the three different models of group leadership.

TABLE 29–1. ADVANTAGES AND DISADVANTAGES OF THREE GROUP LEADERSHIP MODELS

Leadership Model	Advantage	Disadvantage
Single leader	Leader gives total attention to the group; does not need to concentrate on a co-leader relationship Timing of intervention and follow through is facilitated Economical	Entire burden of responsibility for leading and evaluating group falls on one person
Co-leader	Leaders can model effective communication patterns Interpretation and evaluation of the group is improved with two leaders combining impressions Complementarity of styles may increase effectiveness of group. Permits working through anger at one therapist Facilitates training for an inexperienced therapist Simulates the family group situation and allows members to work through problems One leader may work intensively with a member of a group's problem, while the other monitors the general group process	May be difficult for co-leaders to develop an egalitarian or good working relationship If strain between co-leaders, group may exhibit tenseness and inhibition Widely divergent styles can cause problems Subgrouping may occur if a small group aligns itself to one therapist or if a "splitting" arrangement occurs Expensive
Rotating leader or leaderless	May foster independence and responsibility of group members In self-help groups, members feel a particular affinity to a leader who has the same type of problems	Generally, little opportunity for working through conflict or authority issues Difficult to facilitate behavior change

Style is another important component of leadership structure. Three basic styles have been described.[31] The *democratic* leader operates within a member-centered framework. This type of leader acts primarily as a facilitator of the group's participation in forming goals, decision making, problem solving, and evaluating member participation. The democratic leader sees the strengths and resources in group members and tries to develop a climate in which these qualities can flourish and thereby accomplish the work of the group.

The *autocractic* leader is very much leader-centered. This type of leader assumes the position of "leader knows best." The leader determines group goals, tasks, norms, and frequently the roles members should take within the group. This type of leader is not necessarily aggressive or hostile. The autocratic leader may also foster excessive dependency, hostility, passive–aggressive behavior, and apathy in group members.

The third style of leadership is the *laissez-faire* approach. This is the least active type of leadership. The leader takes a very passive role in the group, allowing members to do what they will, when they want to, for whatever reasons they choose. The laissez-faire leader believes the group will produce without intervention. The effects of this style on group interaction tend to be confusion and frustration or dissatisfaction with the group. The group may never form goals or be able to function.

Some characteristics of an effective leader are[32–34]:

- Conveys security and acceptance of own limits; in turn, accepts others and helps them feel safe
- Demonstrates friendliness, empathy, and concern for others
- Watches carefully for unspoken as well as listening for verbal messages
- Insists on freedom rather than perfection within the group
- Is capable of using humor kindly and appropriately
- Permits dissent from group members
- Does not resort to and does not permit blaming or persecution of members
- Does not anticipate immediate release from

conflict but strives to cope with and gain meaning from the conflict as part of the resolution

- Does not permit himself or herself to be used as a means to an end and does not use others in this manner (manipulation)
- Does not assume superiority over others

Functions of Groups

Purpose and Goals. A group originates and continues for some specific purpose. That purpose generally defines, and to some extent is defined by, the type of group. For example, one type of task group may have a purpose of developing a client classification system for direct reimbursement for nursing care. A therapeutic group's purpose will be very different, for example, to prevent excessive emotional trauma to a group of elderly clients who are relocating to a new resident facility. The purpose of any group should be understood clearly at the beginning of group work.

Again, we see the interdependence of structure and function. Purpose gives form to function; without it, there is no reason for the group to function and grow. Purpose is also linked to structure; it is a key element that allows the group to form, develop, and eventually terminate.

Purpose will remain fairly constant throughout the life of the group. Goals and tasks, which flow directly from purpose, are dynamic and will continually change as they are met and subsequently new goals and tasks evolve.

Whereas purpose is explicit at the beginning of a group's life, goals and tasks are not. Part of the initial phase of group interaction and development is a definition of group goals. This should be a joint enterprise between membership and leadership.

One factor that will certainly influence group goal setting is the personal goal orientation of both members and leaders. These need to be clearly identified and articulated in the beginning phases of group work. Unfortunately, this is not always done, because either members are not consciously aware of their personal goals or are not comfortable enough in the

group to share them. In task-oriented groups, a lot of personal needs sharing is not usually tolerated, so this may be a problem in these groups. **Group process** can be severely inhibited if personal goals are not identified early, because members' needs will not be met, and members may not be able to fulfill the task and maintenance roles required for adaptive group functioning. For example, Nurse X agrees to become a member of the above-mentioned task group to set up a nursing classification system. The nurse's personal goals include acquiring expertise in nursing classification systems and fulfilling requirements of committee work for a promotion from staff nursing to nursing administration. Nurse X knows that two influential administrators are also on this committee and wants to impress them. The nurse chooses to share only the first goal, the acquisition of expertise. During the initial meeting, Nurse X is assigned the duty of collecting client records from nursing units and reviewing them for certain data. To do this, Nurse X will have very little contact with the influential administrators she is trying to impress. Her group role assignment does not meet her needs, and so in her group work, she may actually hinder the group process toward meeting its goals because she is too busy trying to meet her own.

Group goals are related to and develop from the purpose. They are objectives defined by the group to be met within the group. Group tasks, on the other hand, are the actual work that must be done in order to meet the group goals. The purpose, goals, and tasks of the nursing classification system committee are differentiated in Table 29–2.

The distinction between purpose, goal, and task is important to an understanding of group process and evaluation of the ability to function as a group.

Another related functional issue is motivation, which has been described as a system of internal tension that is aroused within a group member and is not relieved until the group goal has been met.[35] The need for congruence between a member's personal goals and the overall group goals has been addressed. The key point here is that without such congruence, a member will lack the motivation needed to perform tasks necessary for goal achievement. Commitment of

Table 29–2. PURPOSE, GOALS, AND TASKS OF THE NURSING CLASSIFICATION SYSTEM COMMITTEE

Purpose	The development of a client classification system in order to receive direct reimbursement for nursing care.
Goals	1. To develop a client classification system ready for pilot testing within one year.
	2. To develop an operational definition of professional nursing care.
	3. To identify various levels of professional nursing care.
	4. To define outcome criteria for evaluating different levels of nursing care.
	5. To identify two nursing units that are best suited for a pilot study of the newly developed system.
Tasks	1. Hold biweekly group meetings to share information and report on progress.
	2. Send out a memo to all nursing units to inform them of group purpose.
	3. Meet with nursing units coordinators to share ideas.
	4. Review the literature related to nursing classification systems.
	5. Spend time on each nursing unit and chart observation of direct nursing care.
	6. Review medical records of clients in the last year to identify levels of care used.

members to accomplish group goals will be influenced by several factors:

- The desirability of the goal
- The likelihood of group accomplishment
- The challenge of the goal—what is the risk of failure?
- The abilities of the group to delineate when and if the goal has been achieved
- The satisfaction or reward the group will receive with goal achievement
- The working relationship among members necessary to achieve goals

Task and Maintenance Functions. Once goals are developed by the group and the tasks are identified, certain functions are necessary for the actual work of the group to proceed. These have been described as task maintenance functions. **Task functions** encourage the group to do the work necessary for goal achievement. **Maintenance functions** encourage harmony and meaningful social interaction between members (Table 29–3).[36]

Group Process

Group process refers to the stages through which a group passes during its existence. These stages are characterized by specific group behaviors and feelings.[37] They also are influenced by the structural and functional properties of the individuals who comprise the group. The three basic stages that all types of groups go through are beginning, working, and termination.[38]

The *beginning* stage is an initial orientation period for the group. Generally, the formal structure is delineated early, usually by the leader. Expected behavior related to group norms and roles, as well as general operational components of the group, are dealt with during this time. Goals and tasks are developed, and members become acquainted, at least superficially.

Initial sessions may be uncomfortable for group members because of fears of exposing their inner feelings and thoughts. These may be even more pronounced in therapy groups, in which the basic purpose is self-disclosure. In task-oriented groups, members may be better able to hide behind the tasks to be accomplished.

During this stage, several important group themes arise. Themes are the issues underlying specific content being discussed. Some of those important to this stage of group development are:

- Exclusion versus inclusion
- Trust versus mistrust
- Control
- Safety
- Resistance

A new member will be concerned about being accepted as a member. Can the new member trust the others not to reveal what he or she discloses in the group? Will other members or the leader recognize his or her vulnerability? Will the group like him or her and care about his or her participation? Will he or she lose emotional control? What will happen in that case? Will he or she turn out to be abnormal? Should he or she risk any of these?

The idea of group work is frightening to many people; therefore anxiety is common to this stage. Generally, the group will look to the

TABLE 29–3. TASK AND MAINTENANCE FUNCTIONS OF A GROUP

Task Functions	Maintenance Functions
Information- and *opinion-giver*: Offers facts, opinions, ideas, suggestions, and relevant information to help group discussion.	*Encourager of participation*: Warmly encourages everyone to participate, giving recognition for contributions, demonstrating acceptance and openness to ideas, is friendly and responsive to group members.
Starter: Proposes goals and tasks to initiate action within the group.	*Tension reliever*: Eases tensions and increases the enjoyment of group members by joking, suggesting breaks, and proposing fun approaches to group work.
Summarizer: Pulls together related ideas or suggestions and restates and summarizes major points discussed.	
Energizer: Stimulates a higher quality of work from the group.	*Evaluator of emotional climate*: Asks members how they feel about the way in which the group is working and about each other, and shares own feelings about both.
Evaluator: Compares group decisions and accomplishments with group standards and goals.	*Process observer*: Watches the process by which the group is working and uses the observations to examine group effectiveness.
	Trust builder: Accepts and supports openness of other group members, reinforcing risk taking and encouraging individuality.

leader as an authority and sit back waiting to be told what to do. Members also tend to be unable to focus on themselves. Situations outside the group are discussed at length, but there is resistance to concentrating on their own feelings and perceptions within the group.[39]

There is no sharp dividing line between the stages of group development. It is, therefore, somewhat arbitrary to divide them into distinct entities. Nevertheless, there are behaviors that signal a transition from the beginning to the *working* stage.

Trust is a crucial issue for a group, for without a sense of trust among the membership, the true work of a group can never take place. There are many indications of trust. When members begin to take risks by sharing their feelings and reacting to others in a "here-and-now" focus, they are trusting the group.[40] When conflict is recognized and resolved or members can agree to disagree, trust is operational within the group and it is truly in a working stage.

In addition to the themes underlying group work in the beginning stage, ambivalence and caring emerge in the working stage of a group. Members are now sharing more of themselves, yet they may have ambivalence about just how far they can go. At this time members also begin to really care about the feelings and perceptions of the rest of the group. The problem of one member becomes the problem of the entire group. Members are able to give of themselves without necessarily needing to receive anything. A sense of belongingness is present. The work of the group progresses, and members seem to care about it. Attendance at group meetings is good and in-group participation is high. At this point the group is said to have **cohesiveness**.

Cohesion may take quite a while to develop depending on the type and purpose of the group. It is essential, if a group is to continue to grow and to be able to meet its goals effectively. Cohesion also allows the membership to work with less dependence on the leader. Members can deal with difficult issues with much less leader participation. Qualities that promote positive group interactions are recognized in members within the group, and task and maintenance roles are operational over and above individual roles.

As the group moves along, the third stage of group development is recognized. The *termination* stage is not simply the last meeting or two. It is really a distinct process in its own right. In reality, termination begins with the first few group meetings, when goals are developed. There is always an end in mind, a place where the group members want to be eventually. Dealing with issues surrounding termination usually begins at some point during the working stage of the group. As members develop a sense of cohesion, dependence becomes a major theme. With dependence also comes the idea of loss. What happens to me in the future, without this group? Many times, this issue comes to the surface when the first member or leader leaves the group. Separation anxiety is present due to the loss of a significant, interdependent relationship with its concomitant role. At this point, the group tends to revert back to needing more direction from the leader, because termination can be a painful process. In a highly cohesive, well-adjusted group, termination also can be a very important growth experience.

Other behaviors noted in this stage are a need to review what has been accomplished in the group, expression of caring and appreciation of group members and the leader by group members, as well as resistance to termination. This stage may be marked by regression of members and the entire group in an attempt not to have to deal with good-byes.

In very task-oriented groups, there may be a celebration party or formal dinner to acknowledge the completed work of the group. Certain psychotherapy groups may be ongoing, and the group never completely dissolves. Members may come and go. In other therapeutic groups, final termination may be simple, with each member expressing to the group what the group has meant to him, prior to disbanding.

TYPES OF GROUPS

Nurses work with clients and colleagues in many types of groups. They can be categorized into four types, according to purpose.

A *task group* has the purpose of accomplishing a designated task. For example, the rehabilitation team meets to develop discharge planning protocols for clients with spinal cord injuries. The group has a particular task to complete.

A second type of group has been termed a *therapeutic group* by Marram.[41] The purpose of this type of group is to support and maintain adaptive behaviors for people involved in change or crisis situations. A therapeutic group for newly diagnosed diabetics, for example, may have the purpose of preventing maladaptive coping behaviors while adjusting to the idea of having a chronic disease that requires medication, dietary changes, and so forth. Therapeutic groups also may be used for clients experiencing developmental or situational crises. Groups for new parents or recently widowed men provide examples of groups where support, sharing of feelings, and developing new coping behaviors would be stressed.

The third type of group is the *therapy group*, intended for clients needing treatment for an emotional disturbance.[42] The purpose of the therapy group is to provide the group members with insights into themselves and help them change their behavior. Therapy groups are used in psychiatric hospitals, mental health clinics, and in the community. Groups of narcotic addicts or depressed individuals may meet for psychotherapy in the group situation, for example.

A fourth type of group is called the *training group*, or T-group, popularized in the early 1960s. It was designed to teach people about developing interpersonal skills and group processes. Members participate in the group and gain cognitive and experiential knowledge about group processes. Encounter groups, such as those associated with the women's movement, also foster self-awareness and development of interpersonal competence.

This classification of groups provides a convenient way to identify the purpose of any group the nurse might work with. The classification is not rigid, however, and many groups overlap in purpose, and fall into more than one category. Table 29–4 provides a summary of the types of groups with their purposes, membership, and leadership characteristics.

THE NURSING PROCESS

Once nurses have obtained knowledge and experience with groups, they may wish to use group intervention to assist their clients. Nurses use the nursing process to guide their practice with groups just as they use it with individuals. The nursing process provides a framework for the nurse, once a problem amenable to nursing intervention has been perceived. The four phases of the nursing process provide a systematic way to proceed.

TABLE 29–4. TYPES OF GROUPS

	Task Group	Therapeutic Group	Therapy Group	Training Group
Purpose	Accomplish designated task	Support and maintain adaptive coping behaviors	Provide intrapersonal insight, reeducate, remotivate, or support behavior change	Learning cognitively and experientially about group process
Membership characteristics	People assigned or volunteer for job	Emotionally healthy Experiencing stress related to physical illness or maturational or situational crisis	Individuals experiencing emotional disturbance; desire to learn new ways of coping	Basically healthy individuals desiring to improve knowledge and skills in interpersonal relations
Leader role	Facilitates progress toward desired goal Maximizes problem solving capabilities of the group	Facilitates group process; provides supportive climate Information giver Role model; select and prepare clients	Stimulate member interaction; reinforce appropriate behavior; select and prepare new clients	Facilitates group process. Resource person, catalyst. Maintain educational focus
Requirements for leadership	Knowledge of task Acceptable to members	Knowledge and skills for group therapy Ability to identify appropriate levels of intervention and interaction	Knowledge and skills for doing psychotherapy in group; knowledge of group and individual dynamics	Knowledge of group, interpersonal, and individual dynamics Ability to maintain appropriate level of interaction and focus

Adapted from B.W. Spradley, Community Health Nursing, 2nd ed. (Boston: Little, Brown, 1985), 289–98; J.E. Hall and B.R. Weaver, Distributive Nursing, 2nd ed. (Philadelphia: Lippincott, 1985), 120–24; and G.D. Marram, Group Approach (St. Louis: C.V. Mosby, 1978), 9–72.

Assessment

Once nurses perceive problems, they enter into the assessment phase of the nursing process. In this phase, nurses systematically review the situation in order to formulate the nursing diagnoses.

Maxine Loomis provides the following set of questions that can be used during assessment to determine whether the use of group intervention would be appropriate[43]:

- What are the client needs I am attempting to meet?
- Can these needs be met in a group?
- What are my expectations for the group?
- What are the expectations of the system relative to the proposed group?

If the answers to these questions are consistent with group intervention, the nurse formulates appropriate nursing diagnoses.

As an example, consider how one nurse used the nursing process to work with a group of new parents:

Ms. Marcus teaches childbirth education classes. When she talks to her former students after their babies are born, she consistently perceives a need for support and further education for new parents. Some of these new parents seem frightened about the responsibility of caring for a new infant; others just seem to need reassurance. Because our society is transient, extended family support systems are frequently missed. Also, since family size continues to decrease, the chances are increased that one or both of the parents have had no experience with or exposure to new babies. The parents may have no friends with babies.

The nurse, Ms. Marcus, has recognized potential client problems that she feels may be helped by nursing intervention. She begins assessing the problem in order to determine how to proceed. Ms. Marcus uses the questions proposed by Loomis to begin her assessment.[44]

What are the client needs I am attempting to meet? Ms. Marcus reviews what she knows about the needs of new parents. She considers their developmental stage. From her studies about human development, she realizes that new parenthood may initiate a maturational crisis if the couple is not supported in acquiring the adaptive behaviors necessary for this developmental stage.[45]

She decides that the new parents need information about infant development and the wide range of normal infant behavior. They may need practice with infant care skills. In addition, the parents may need an opportunity to express their feelings about being parents. The mother and father may need help in communicating and working on their own relationship.

On the basis of the feedback she receives from new parents and her knowledge of the new parents' developmental tasks, Ms. Marcus feels the major client need is for support and education: support with developing adaptive coping behaviors to their new situation, and education about the new baby.

Can these needs be met in a group? Ms. Marcus feels that group intervention would be the best approach to meeting the new parent needs. She recognizes that as group members share information about their own parenting experiences, they will realize the commonality of their situation and difficulties, as well as the different approaches that can be used in problem solving.

The needs of the parents may be more economically met in the group situation. In addition, the couples have already demonstrated willingness to work in groups by participating in childbirth preparation groups.

What are the objectives for the group? Ms. Marcus decides that she wants to focus on learning and practicing communication skills and expression of feelings. Learning about the infant will be secondary. She feels that other resources are available for learning about infant care. Also, the nurse can give information when the situation is appropriate.

Based on this assessment, Ms. Marcus arrives at the following nursing diagnoses for the group:

- Potential alterations in good parenting behaviors related to lack of experience regarding infant development and care
- Knowledge deficit regarding growth and development and infant care
- Role modification related to the gain of a new family member
- Anxiety related to change in interaction patterns and change in role function
- Potential for compromised family coping secondary to arrival of new infant

Planning

The planning stage for group intervention first involves clearly articulating the purposes and objective for the group. The purposes will determine what type of group is being planned.

In the clinical example described above, Ms. Marcus lead a therapeutic group for new parents. Its purpose was to maintain adaptive or healthy coping behaviors during a new developmental stage. The group also had an educational component. The objective for the group provided the framework for planning, implementing, and evaluating the group. The objectives for the parenting group follow:

- Parents will communicate their feelings about the baby and being a parent as evidenced by verbalization in the group
- Parents will improve communication skills between one another as evidenced by verbalization and body language and measured by a preassessment and a postassessment
- Parents will feel confident about their ability to care for their child as evidenced by parenting behaviors such as comfort with feeding and dressing infant and appropriate attention and stimulation
- Parents will be able to identify age-appropriate behaviors for their child in the first year of life as measured by observation and by post test

Once the purpose and objectives are determined, nurses address group process considerations. They decide who will be admitted to the group. One should avoid a very large or a very small number of members. Six to ten members is thought to allow for a variety of interactions, experiences, and opinions but is not so large that it prevents all members from fully participating in the group.

Planning also involves deciding on an open or closed group structure. Will members be permitted to join as others terminate, or will there be a predetermined number of meetings that all members are expected to attend?

Planning the physical arrangements for the group must include a convenient and consistent meeting place with adequate space, ventilation, and lighting. Any special requirements, such as access and additional space for a group involving clients in wheelchairs, should be planned for.

Other planning activities have to do with leadership. What will the role of the leader be, and what are the leader's goals? What reimbursement if any, will the leader receive?

In addition, planning involves preparing the clients for what will happen in the group. Some leaders prefer to have a pregroup interview with each member to discuss group goals. The interview can explain generally what goes on in a group, what is expected of members, and what members can expect to gain from the group experience. A group contract may be used to formalize this part of the planning process.

Finally, deciding how to measure whether the group objectives are being met must be considered. Documentation may be necessary before the group begins. For instance, it may be very important to document the members' blood pressure prior to the group experience if one is expecting to lower the blood pressure through a group stress reduction scheme. An outline of Ms. Marcus's plan for the parenting group follows:

1. Structure
   a. Group member characteristics
      Male/female couple with an infant who is two weeks to three months of age at the beginning of the group
      Couples will attend group voluntarily
      Selection of appropriate couples
   b. Closed group to meet for eight weeks
   c. Physical variables

Meet for two hours one evening per week
Group size: five to six couples
Meet in a well-lighted, comfortable room, large enough to accommodate six couples with their babies, the leader and infant-care equipment
   d. Leader reimbursement: $80.00/couple/8-week series
   e. Leader role
      Support
      Facilitator of group process
      Educator/information-giver
2. Function: the nurse will prepare each couple for what they might expect from this group
3. Process: the nurse and the couple will agree on a contract with mutual goals and designated responsibilities
4. Plan to measure whether the objectives are being met

Implementation

After the planning phase is complete, the nurse will begin implementation of the group intervention. The implementation phase involves use of leadership skills and knowledge of group processes. Relying on her knowledge of the three stages of group development, the nurse acts as the leader in the implementation phase.

In the *beginning* stage the nurse attempts to provide both caring and stimulation to group members, providing enough structure to allow both the members and the nurse to become acquainted with each other in order to build a sense of trust and to protect members from the embarrassment of divulging too much information. In addition, the nurse teaches members how to use the group to redirect their questions and focus their attention on the group.

As the group moves into its *working stage,* the leader encourages the members to express their feelings, be aware of their behavior patterns, respond to one another, share experiences, work through conflicts, and turn to the group for help.

Another leader role in the implementation phase is to prepare the group for termination. This process must begin before the last session, and group members should be encouraged to recognize what has been achieved.

Ms. Marcus identified the following steps and actions for carrying out her plan:

1. Demonstrate awareness of the three phases of the group process and the leader and member roles in each phase
2. Attempt to have the group exhibit balance of task and maintenance functions
3. Promote group cohesiveness
4. Act as supporter and information-giver

Evaluation

The final phase of the nursing process is evaluation. Plans for measuring the objectives for the group is started in the planning phase, when the nurse states goals and outcome criteria. At this time, the nurse appraises the changes experienced by group members as a result of the group experience and applies outcome criteria.

The following plan for evaluating the nursing intervention in the parenting group was devised:

1. Administer pretest and posttest to measure knowledge about infant development
2. Obtain verbal or written feedback on an ongoing basis about progress toward meeting objectives
3. Observe factors, such as attendance, prompt arrival, and participation, for information on member attachment to the group
4. Keep anecdotal records on observed couple communication and infant handling so that behavior change can be measured
5. Have a colleague review tapes of selected meetings to provide feedback on the effectiveness of leadership skills
6. Obtain written information about each group member's perceptions of ability to communicate with his or her partner and about feelings of being understood by the partner; measure this information before and after the group experience

SUMMARY

Everyone participates in groups throughout their life spans. Nurses can be more effective as group members and as group leaders if they use more than "intuitive" knowledge as a basis for participation and actions.

Group dynamics is the scientific study of groups. Using knowledge from this study and from other theoretical frameworks provides a basis for practicing with groups.

One of the major theoretical frameworks used in group work is systems theory. The group is an open system that engages in constant interchange with its environment. It is composed of members who, when they behave independently, provide the group with its own identity and boundaries. Input, throughout, output, and feedback are the group's processes.

Each group exhibits structure, function, and process characteristics. Structure provides the group with an operational form or system that allows the group to meet its goals in a particular fashion. Structural components include group roles, communication patterns, and leadership roles.

The function component of a group includes the group's purpose, tasks and goals. The group members' motivation and performance of appropriate task and maintenance functions help the group to achieve its purpose.

The process component describes the stage of the group. Beginning, working, and terminating stages have definite characteristics that group members and leaders should be aware of.

Four types of groups are described. The task, therapeutic, therapy, and training groups are classified according to their main purpose. Leadership and membership characteristics may differ or they may overlap from group to group.

In all types of groups nurses use the nursing process. This approach provides a systematic and comprehensive process for nursing intervention. The assessing, planning, implementing and evaluating steps supply the framework for the process of working with groups as clients.

Study Questions

1. Identify five groups that you belong to. Classify each group as a primary or secondary group. Specify the purpose of each secondary group.

2. Explain the difference between group process and group dynamics.

3. Describe how your clinical nursing group works as a system.

4. Observe the communication that occurs in your next group meeting (study group, social group, dormitory unit meeting). Describe the nonverbal communication patterns you observe.

5. Think about a task group that you have participated in recently. Did task or maintenance functions predominate? What happened to goal achievement as the result?

6. Differentiate between the role of the leader in the task, therapeutic, therapy, and training groups.

7. Identify three health problems that you feel need nursing intervention. Assess each problem to determine whether group intervention would be appropriate. Plan an implementation strategy for one problem with a potential group solution.

8. Describe the evaluation methods you could use if you were leading a support group for homesick freshman students.

References

1. Joanne E. Hall and Barbara R. Weaver, *Distributive Nursing: A Systems Approach to Community Health*, 2nd ed. (Philadelphia: J.B. Lippincott Co., 1985).
2. Kurt Lewin, *Resolving Social Conflicts* (New York: Harper & Row, 1948).
3. Margaret Rioch, "The work of Wilfred Bion and groups," in Arthur D. Coleman and W. Harold Bexton, eds., *Group Relations Reader* (San Rafael, Calif.: Associates Printing and Publishing Co., 1975), 3–8.
4. Ruth Murray and Judith Zentner, *Nursing Concepts for Health Promotion*, 3rd ed., (Englewood Cliffs, N.J.: Prentice-Hall, 1985).
5. Edward E. Sampson and Marya Marthas, *Group Process for the Health Professions*, 2nd ed. (New York: John Wiley and Sons, 1981), 120.
6. Ann W. Burgess, *Psychiatric Nursing in the Hospital and the Community*, 4th ed. (Englewood Cliffs, N.J.: Prentice-Hall, 1985).
7. Murray and Zentner, *Nursing Concepts for Health Promotion*.
8. Malcolm Knowles and Hulda Knowles, *Introduction to Group Dynamics* (Chicago: Follet Publishing Co., 1972), 18.
9. Holly S. Wilson and Carol R. Kneisl, *Psychiatric Nursing* (Menlo Park, Calif.: Addison-Wesley Publishing Co., 1979), 435.
10. D. Johnson and F. Johnson, *Joining Together: Group Theory and Group Skills* (Englewood Cliffs, N.J.: Prentice-Hall, 1975).
11. Lawrence Solomon and B. Berson, eds., *New Perspectives on Encounter Groups* (San Francisco: Jossey-Bass, 1972).
12. Darwin Cartwright and Alvin Zander, *Group Dynamics Research and Theory* (New York: Harper & Row, 1968), 19.
13. Marvin E. Shaw, *Group Dynamics*, 3rd ed. (New York: McGraw-Hill Book Co., 1976), 14–15.
14. David H. Jenkins, "What is group dynamics," in Leland Bradford, ed., *Group Development* (LaJolla, Calif.: University Associates, 1974), 5.
15. Sampson and Marthas, *Group Process*, 121.
16. Ibid., 120.
17. Hall and Weaver, *Distributive Nursing*, 123–24.
18. Eric Berne, *The Structure and Dynamics of Organizations and Groups* (New York: Grove Press, 1963), 53–64.
19. Ibid., 54–56.
20. Hall and Weaver, *Distributive Nursing*, 124–26.
21. Ibid., 124.
22. Ibid., 125.
23. Sampson and Marthas, *Group Process*, 52.
24. Kenneth Benne and Paul Sheats, "Functional roles of group members," *J Soc Issues* 4 (1948).
25. Robert F. Bales, "Task roles and social roles in problem-solving groups," in E.E. Macoby, T.M. Newcomb, and E.L. Hartley, eds., *Readings in Social Psychology*, 3rd ed., (New York: Holt, Rinehart & Winston, 1958).
26. Hall and Weaver, *Distributive Nursing*, 128.
27. Shaw, *Group Dynamics*, 140.
28. Ibid., 139–42.
29. J.L. Morens, *Sociometry, Experimental Method and the Science of Society* (New York: Beacon House, 1951).
30. Sampson and Marthas, *Group Process*, 62.
31. Ronald Lippitt and Robert White, "An experimental study of leadership and group life," in E.E. Macoby, T.M. Newcourb, and E.L. Harley, eds., *Readings in Social Psychology*, 3rd ed. (New York: Holt, Rinehart & Winston, 1958).
32. Murray and Zentner, *Nursing Concepts for Health Promotion*.
33. Edward Lindman, *The Meaning of Adult Education* (Montreal: Harvest House, 1961).

34. Robert Wicks, *Counseling Strategies and Intervention Techniques for the Human Services*, 2nd ed. (Philadelphia: J.B. Lippincott Co., 1984).
35. Johnson and Johnson: *Joining Together*, 88.
36. Ibid., 26–27.
37. Gerald Corey and Marianne Corey, *Groups: Process and Practice*, 2nd ed. (Monterey, Calif.: Brooks/Cole Publishing Co., 1982).
38. Hall and Weaver, *Distributive Nursing*, 137–41.
39. Corey and Corey, *Groups: Process and Practice*, 92–94.
40. Ibid., 102.
41. Gwen D. Marram, *The Group Approach in Nursing Practice* (St. Louis: C.V. Mosby Co., 1978), 18, 19.
42. Barbara W. Spradley, *Community Health Nursing: Concepts and Practice*, 2nd ed. (Boston: Little Brown & Co., 1985), 298.
43. Maxine Loomis, *Group Process for Nurses* (St. Louis: C.V. Mosby Co., 1979), 18, 19.
44. Ibid., 22.
45. Donna C. Aguilera and Janice M. Messick, *Crisis Intervention: Theory and Methodology*, 5th ed., (St. Louis: C.V. Mosby Co., 1986).

Annotated Bibliography

Adrian, S. 1980. *A Systematic Approach to Selecting Group Participants. J Psychiatr Nurs* 18(2):37–41. Nurses may use this article to assist in selecting or referring clients for participation in health care groups. An assessment tool is presented and can be used to determine appropriate candidates for group participation by using inclusion and exclusion criteria.

Corey, G., Corey, M. 1977. *Groups: Process and Practice*. Monterey, Calif: Brooks/Cole Publishing Co. The first section of this book reviews information necessary for working with groups in a leadership role. The second section provides examples of various therapeutic groups one would use for clients throughout life. Each of these latter chapters describes the leader's considerations for the particular type of group.

Johnson, D., Johnson, F. 1975. *Joining Together*. Englewood Cliffs, N.J.: Prentice Hall, Inc. This is a general book about working with groups in a membership or leadership role. It contains many assessment tools used to gain knowledge about how one functions within the group setting.

Johnson, R., et al. 1982. *The Professional Support Group: A Model for Psychiatric Clinical Nurse Specialists. J Psychiatr Nurs* 20(2):9–13. This article describes how psychiatric clinical nurse specialists use the group intervention model to provide practical help to one another, stimulate ideas, and share personal and professional information. The description suggests how nurses can use groups to support their professional and personal growth. This journal issue is devoted entirely to group therapy.

Larson, M., Williams R. 1978. *How to Become a Better Group Leader. Nurs* 78(8):8. Nonfunctional problem behaviors are identified and illustrated in this article. Suggestions of how the leader may deal with the "smoke screener," "interrogator," "rescuer," etc., are provided. The authors also describe the situations in which the behaviors are likely to occur.

Loomis, M. 1979. *Group Process for Nurses*. St. Louis, Mo.: C.V. Mosby Co. This is a very helpful book for nurses who plan to work with groups. It provides frameworks for the nurse to follow from the time she perceives a problem and determines that it may be appropriate to intervene through leading a group.

van Servellen, G.M. 1984. *Group and Family Therapy*. St. Louis, Mo.: C.V. Mosby Co. This book describes the scope of group work in which nurses may function effectively as group leaders and outlines various theoretical frameworks that guide the nurse's interventions and interpretations. Also, there are sections on the application of theory to practice, common objectives, and on group membership.

Sampson E, Marthas M. 1981. *Group Process for the Health Professions*. New York: John Wiley and Sons. The book deals with why health professionals need to understand the group's role in health promotion and illness. It describes the group process and the health professional's role as member and leader in groups. Change theory and its relationship to the group process are discussed.

Sines, D. and Moore, K. 1986. The Magic Shop, *Nursing Times* 82(11):50–56. The article describes how group techniques are used with a group of mentally handicapped individuals. Emphasis is on themes, support, group process, and termination.

Tucker, C.M., et al. 1986. Assessment Based Group Counseling to Address Concerns of Chronic Hemodialysis. Patients *Patient Education and Counseling* 8(1):51–61. The article provides a good example of how nurses can use group intervention to address problems of the chronically ill. Methods of involving clients in establishing objectives and participating in groups are discussed.

Yalom, I.D. 1975. *The Theory and Practice of Group Psychotherapy*. New York, Basic Books, Inc. This is a comprehensive but easily read book on group psychotherapy. The nurse who is just beginning to study group work will find the sections on the curative factors in group, group process, group cohesiveness, and problem patients particularly enlightening.

Chapter 30

Family Systems Concepts

Phyllis B. Heffron
Eliza M. Wolff

Chapter Outline

- Objectives
- Glossary
- Introduction
- Historical Perspectives
    Early Family History
    The Industrial Revolution
    The Space Age Family
- Theoretical Approaches to Family Study
- The Systems/Adaptation Approach
    Types of Family Organization
    Family Processes
- Family Functions
- Family Life Cycle
- The Nursing Process
    Assessment
    Planning
    Implementation
    Evaluation
- Summary
- Study Questions
- References
- Annotated Bibliography

Objectives

At the completion of this chapter, the reader will be able to:

- Describe briefly the history of the family
- Identify four distinctive approaches to family study
- Discuss the relationship of systems theory to family study
- Describe at least six organizational structures of families
- Describe three types of boundary regulations in families
- Identify at least six major roles families must perform for effective family functioning
- Identify two types of role conflict in families
- Identify six bases of power in families
- Describe at least six major functions performed by the family
- Identify the major components of the family assessment
- Discuss at least four general methods of nursing intervention with families

Glossary

Ecomap. A family assessment tool that consists of a graphical representation of a family's relationship with its environment.

Extended Family. A nuclear family group with the inclusion of additional related members such as grandparents, aunts, and uncles.

Family of Orientation. The family group into which a person is born.

Genogram. A family assessment tool that consists of a family tree diagram depicting family dispersals, losses, roles, and organizational patterns over three or more generations.

Monogamy. The practice of being married to only one spouse at a time.

Nuclear Dyad. A husband and wife with no children.

Nuclear Family. A family grouping that consists of a husband and wife and their children.

Polyandry. A family unit in which there is one wife with two or more husbands at the same time.

Polygamy. The practice of having two or more spouses at a time.

Polygyny. A family unit in which there is one husband with two or more wives at the same time.

Single-parent Family. A family grouping consisting of only one parent; the single parent may be the mother or the father, who may be widowed, separated, divorced, or never married.

INTRODUCTION

The family system is the most basic and primary unit of every human society. It is universally recognized as primary because of its reproductive and parenting functions. In addition, it is the most stable of primary groups and endures the longest. All of us, as newly born infants, are first received by the family group, and we develop and experience many crucial "firsts" within its boundaries.[1]

Families have been studied by several disciplines, most notably sociology, biology, anthropology, and psychology. At the most fundamental level, a family can be defined in terms of its biologically central members, the mother, father, and dependent children. Called the **nuclear family,** this baseline biosocial definition is what many people think of when thinking about families. However, many different kinds of family groups exist within our society and in other cultures.

Beyond the very traditional definition of the nuclear family, families can be defined in terms of domestic living arrangements, roles, functions, and personal relationships. These criteria, among others, may vary even further from culture to culture and within geographic or religious boundaries within the same culture.

Despite all the definitions, viewpoints, and structural and functional variations of families that will be discussed in this chapter, there are certain basic concepts and assumptions applicable to almost all family groups. These assumptions and concepts have been derived primarily from the social sciences and help to illustrate why family study is so important to the nursing profession.[2–5]

- The family is a complex social system and is the basic unit of all societies
- The family is a primary group in the sense that it gives the individual the earliest and most complete experience of social unity and initiates self-concept formation
- The family is an adaptive open system that is constantly influenced by exchanges with its environment
- All family systems have goals in the areas of reproduction and the meeting of physical needs, love and affection, economic survival, and socialization
- The family is the locus of health beliefs, practices, values, and attitudes and is often the greatest single influence on the health of the individual

Throughout its history, the nursing profession has maintained an interest in families, particularly in the areas of public health nursing, community nursing, and maternal and child health nursing. As the holistic approach to health and health care has increasingly advanced, nurses in all specialties have found a need for family study.

Nurses are taking responsibility for coordinating and giving expert professional services in areas about which families have special needs and concerns. Home birthing experiences, family planning services, and the provision of adequate parenting skills are some of the topical issues that maternal-child health nurses and nurse-midwives are helping families with. In traditional hospital settings, for example, the impact of the birth of a new baby on family members has long been ignored. Staff nurses are encouraged to foster the importance of family interaction at this time by facilitating the opportunity for sibling visitation.[6]

Psychiatric nursing is increasingly involved with families and their mental health concerns.

These concerns may range from relatively mild situational anxieties or depressions related to a role change by one family member to more serious issues of coping with chronic alcoholism or child abuse. The community mental health movement, which began in the 1960s, has led to nurse involvement with families of newly discharged former psychiatric inpatients, and the services may include family therapy as well as individual and marital counseling. Community mental health nursing has been described as favoring a holistic approach, of which family analysis is a vital part.[7]

HISTORICAL PERSPECTIVES

Families have existed in one form or another since the beginning of time. Duvall categorizes family history in terms of four major transition periods. The first period, which took place about 10,000 years ago, describes families as hunters and food-gatherers until the time when they became dwellers in farming villages. The growth of cities some 5000 years later marks a second transition period, followed by an industrial and technological growth period. The fourth and present transition period is marked by profound advances in science and technology, and changing ideas, attitudes, and beliefs.[8]

The family system can be traced back at least 3000 years, though there are no written comprehensive accounts or recorded models of family behavior prior to the twentieth century. Much of the early information on family issues is derived from historical documents, folklore, and myths.

Only recently have efforts escalated and research been undertaken to look more specifically at resources that can help build a composite picture of the history of the family.[9]

Early Family History
Anthropologists and archeologists give very early evidence of the family as the center of individual and community life, regardless of its form.[10]

These early sources show the focus of family systems and their functions shifting. The ancient family, for example, was strongly patriarchal, with the father the supreme head of the household and family heritage traced through his lineage only. The practice of polygamy was common. This patriarchal orientation has shifted back and forth through the ages to a nearly egalitarian, monogamous, and conjugal family situation.[11,12]

In early family sociology, there were several different models or frameworks proposed as ways to view the family. They were based on various political, religious, and philosophical ideologies and fostered studies that sought to uncover whether human societies were originally matriarchal or patriarchal, whether they were monogamous or promiscuous, etc. These early studies failed to produce any concrete patterns or widely accepted viewpoints, and posed conflicting ideas and issues, actually helping to create more interest in the family.[13]

The rapid social changes that took place in Europe, and later in America, brought attention to the family through the many problems created by poverty and its resulting suffering. Mass immigration to the United States led to overcrowding in urban areas, and the family faced increasing problems with juvenile delinquency, crime, and disease. Industrialization and specialization began to affect the family profoundly, as technological advances mushroomed and the family, as a unit of production, began to disappear. The following discussion of the impact of industrialization on the family is based largely on material presented by Hawley, Gordon, Goode, and Murray and Zentner.[14–17]

The Industrial Revolution
The industrial revolution, which began to flourish in America in the latter part of the nineteenth century, was characterized by centralization (from home to factory) of the production of goods and services, growing reliance on machines and other technological advances, and a shift away from an agrarian way of living to an urbanized society. Factories, the primary institutions of this movement, were uniquely specialized and market oriented. They created many new consumer goods and services, particularly in the areas of food-processing, garment manufacturing, recreational facilities, home construction, education, and health care.

The functional role of the family changed dramatically from a production unit (producers) to a unit of consumption (consumers). As producers, families had spent all of their time together working jointly toward the prosperity of the household. With the introduction of the factory, the father began to work outside the home and contribute finances to the family system. Women were freed from some of their domestic chores, e.g., they no longer had to spin cloth and sew everything from scratch, do all the laundry by hand, or harvest and prepare food on a daily basis. Children were no longer viewed as a valuable resource to the family prosperity, as future members of the household labor force, but as a charge against a wage or salary income.

The role of the elderly changed with the coming of industrialization, and the family was faced with a number of new problems in this area. Before industrialization, the **extended family** was more common. Elderly members remained a part of the family household and contributed as they were able. Young adult children remained at home, and generations shared a common base. As work options increased, young people had greater independence and could go outside the family to work and live. The organization of factories, along with the growth of corporate industry and government regulations led to forced retirement and an altered role of senior family members. Burnside, a contemporary nurse-author, presents a listing of some 43 psychosocial needs of the elderly today in which things such as role reversal, isolation, fear of being unwanted and no longer useful, no interested family, loss of status, difficulty in adjustment to institutional living, boredom, and self-devaluation are major headings.[18]

During this same time, other social problems affecting families became apparent. The middle class was increasing and family forms changing. Divorce and separation increased and the birth rate declined. Babies, on the average, were born earlier and were more closely spaced, leaving more leisure time for the parents. Families became mobile because of greater choices in jobs and industry-controlled moves, and it was uncommon for families to stay in one community permanently. Thus, kinship ties were potentially weakened. Within communities and neighborhoods, the higher turnover rate of residents lessened the probability of emotional friendships developing through long-term associations. The family had to devote a great deal of energy to constant adaptation to new surroundings.

Families were affected by numerous new stresses and strains that were imposed on participants in the industrial work force. Mass production, for example, required workers to become specialized in a single task and perform it over and over in the course of a workday. Closely aligned were the concepts of assembly line production and automation, all of which tended to result in workers becoming bored and frustrated as they were denied the pleasures of creativity and a sense of fulfillment in completing a whole task. In addition, automation led to the reduction of some jobs, as machines became more sophisticated and able to perform tasks previously done by hand. Increasingly, the primary responsibility for relieving these stresses and strains and satisfying the emotional needs of the worker rested with the family.[19]

Because the employed adult became one of the primary supportive structures of the family, there emerged a great deal of pressure to compete for favorable jobs, perform in a satisfactory manner, and seek avenues for upward mobility. When job security became threatened in any way, workers were highly susceptible to depression and emotional and physical illnesses, all of which affected the family system.[20]

Industrialization and modern technology have contributed to changes in traditional family value systems. Achievement of the individual is highly valued in our society and often takes precedence over birthright. As young people moved to jobs outside the family, jobs were no longer passed down from father to son or to other family members, and the individual was forced to make his own way. Johnson states that technology has influenced the nature of contemporary social organization by substituting more individualistic striving to gain a paycheck in place of duty to the family group.[21] Materialism has been identified as a central value in American life and, theoretically, an individual with enough money can live a life completely apart from his family.[22] There is great pressure to purchase and consume and to judge others by their ability to do the same; family relationships are easily manipulated under these circumstances.[23]

A great deal more has been written about the industrial revolution and its relationship to the evolution of the family. There has been considerable debate on the causes, and whether the technological advantages outweigh the disadvantages. Most scholars agree that it is a very complex relationship. Although it is clear that the industrial revolution fostered many changes in family behaviors and organization, it is still unclear as to the *degree* of change that it has contributed.[24]

The Space Age Family

The effects of social changes on the modern twentieth century family have been so vast, particularly since 1950, that characteristics and life styles between one family generation and the next are often totally dissimilar. The rapidity of these changes has been unparalleled in human history and has required the family to be extremely adaptive and flexible.[25]

Economic and educational changes, technological advances, and political shifts all have contributed to changes in family structures, roles, attitudes, and life styles.

Economic change, and in particular the economic relationship between families and society, continues to be a central factor in shaping family life today. The basic changes in economic patterns that industrialization brought to the family have become more and more complicated. Production and distribution of goods have increased, and there is more to buy. In nuclear families, not only does the father go outside the home to work every day, but he may commute an hour or more each way and be accompanied by his working wife. Economic welfare for the family becomes the focal point of the family's existence. Families feel pressured to consume material goods, as perpetuated in advertising and other media communications, and competition with other families often produces stressful consequences. Frequent relocation to new communities has become a way of life, and the cause of this mobility is most often job-related. Family stability and security, especially for school-age children, can be severally jeopardized.

The changing roles of women in American society, particularly in regard to employment, have had far reaching effects on the family. More women are working than ever before, and many have children and maintain a family life, as well. In 1980 there were 45.6 million working women, an increase of 173 percent since 1947.[26] In this same year (1980) 66 percent of married mothers were working, and 78 percent of single mothers were employed.[27] These statistics account for growing concerns about modern day child rearing, child abuse, and an increase in depression among children. Stress is greatly increased in both a **single-parent family** and in a family in which both parents work, and children often end up spending less and less personal contact time with parents.

Much has been written about the effects of such stressors as economic uncertainty, dual career family situations, single parenthood, and high technology on the stability and quality of family life. Some authors are very pessimistic about what is happening to the American family and feel its strength and unity is declining.[28] Others take a more conservative view and look at the enduring history of the family as a guide for predicting the future.[29]

One thing certain throughout the ages and very much in evidence today is the need for adaptation in families. Today, families' adaptive abilities are being tested, perhaps more than ever before, as they cope with the impact of changes in functions and roles within the context of our urban society.

THEORETICAL APPROACHES TO FAMILY STUDY

The study of families and the theoretical approaches used to describe how they function are many and varied. These approaches can be classified in a variety of ways. One method is to look at family study in terms of the disciplines within which they were developed. In this context, anthropological, sociological, psychological, and psychoanalytic family frameworks can be delineated. Other frameworks for family analysis that have been identified include the structural-functional approach, the interactional approach, the systems approach, and the institutional approach. Family study has been viewed from a purely developmental approach, as well as philosophical and legal points of view.[30,31]

This chapter focuses on the family as viewed from a systems and structural-functional approach. An overview of other selected theories and conceptual frameworks of the family appear in Table 30–1.

THE SYSTEMS/ADAPTATION APPROACH

Viewing the family as an adaptive system gives us an orderly and structured way of describing families and their characteristics. It allows us to "break down the whole" and look at each part individually as well as learn how the parts relate. In this approach, the "parts" of the family system are viewed in terms of individual members of the family and in terms of traditional system parts, such as boundaries, roles, and subsystems. By looking at families in this way, nurses can focus on one member in relation to the whole group or on the entire family.

The systems approach defines a family as an open, living, social system.[32] It has distinct structures, functions, and patterns of communication, power, and decision making. Family systems are adaptive by nature and continually communicate with environmental subsystems in the community and world. Within the context of being a social system, families have certain tasks, such as biological reproduction, socialization of members, and maintenance of order.[33] Within an adaptive framework, family systems continue to grow and change.

Although the family is viewed in this chapter as an adaptive system, selected ideas and research findings from other family studies using other approaches are included.

Types of Family Organization

As we have noted earlier, there is a wide range of definitions of a family. Friedman says that "a family is a group of people emotionally joined together who live in close geographical proximity."[34] Nye and Berardo write that a family is "two or more people related by blood or marriage who customarily maintain a common residence."[35]

Scientists who have studied the family have noted a variety of forms families may take. These include the nuclear family, the extended family, the nuclear dyad, the single-parent, and the single adult. Other varieties of family forms include homosexual pairings, common-law marriages, communes, group marriages, and cohabitation without marriage. Nurses may encounter any of the above family forms in their nursing practice, and understanding of the organizational arrangement is important. Stresses and health needs may be very different in a single parent family than in a homosexual pairing.

The *nuclear family* consists of a husband and wife and their children. This is the family form with which most people have had the most experience. "Although the classic form continues to, and most probably always will exist, there are now many variations of the nuclear model as well as emerging new patterns of family structure. Each requires recognition and acceptance by the professionals who wish to help actualize family health potential."[36]

The *extended family* includes the nuclear family and other related members of the family, such as grandparents. Other people who may be included are siblings of the husband and wife and the siblings' children. Extended families living together were once common in America, but mobility, industrialization, and a changing economy have led to a decline in this pattern. The extended family in several households, however, is an important part of family life in Native American culture. Non-kin may be incorporated into Indian family life through formal and informal processes. Non-kin for whom a child is named participate in a formal ritual. That individual is expected to participate in child rearing and role modeling.[37]

When clients have special health needs, members of the extended family may be able to offer care and support if they live with the family or nearby.

The **nuclear dyad** refers to the husband and wife with no children. This may become an increasingly common family form, as more couples choose to remain childless. The nuclear dyad also refers to the couple whose children have moved away.

The *single-parent family* is becoming increasingly common. Single parents include di-

TABLE 30–1. OVERVIEW OF THEORETICAL FRAMEWORKS FOR FAMILY STUDY

Framework	Key Features
Interactional	• The family is defined as a set of interacting personalities, each having self-defined roles • The general approach is psychosocial, in which personality and socialization are key • The family is studied by assessing roles and relationships within the family system • Intervention is based on analysis of communication patterns and other internal family dynamics as they affect relationships
Structural/functional	• The family is defined as a social system whose members have specific roles geared toward maintaining internal and societal stability • Family fucntions are defined primarily in terms of societal needs • The nuclear family and traditional sex roles are seen as universal and timeless • Families are assessed in terms of fulfillment of roles and functions
Institutional	• The family is defined as a social unity that functions in accord with established social institutions • Primary concerns of family study are cultural values and how family functions have adapted in response to societal changes
Systems	• The family is viewed holistically as an open system made up of various subsystems, all working toward common goals • Family members are interdependent and relate through communication and feedback • Adaptation is ongoing in families, and there is a tendency toward growth and differentiation • Family study and assessment depend on analysis of all the parts of the system, patterns of communication, and adaptive abilities
Psychoanalytic	• The family is defined as a natural group whose members have complementary needs • The family is seen as the root of human behavior, and there is a strong correlation between individual personality development and the growing up experiences in the family • There is emphasis on the importance of intrapsychic conflict between individual needs to remain close to the family group versus establishing self-identify • Feelings, attitudes, and values are transmitted from one family generation to the next through an unconscious process of assimilation
Developmental	• The family is viewed as it evolves over time • Families have a predictable life cycle that can be divided into chronological stages of development • Specific tasks and role assignments are associated with each developmental stage • Assessment and family study is based on analysis of task fulfillment with major considerations given to physical maturation, social and cultural factors, and individual personality and values

Adapted from A.S. Skolnick and J.H. Skolnick, Family in Transition (Boston: Little, Brown, 1971); M.M. Friedman, Family Nursing, Theory and Assessment (New York: Appleton-Century-Crofts, 1981), 44–47; C.W. Tinkham and E.F. Voorhies, Community Health Nursing (New York: Appleton-Century-Crofts, 1972), 146, 147.

vorced, widowed, unmarried, and adoptive parents, as well as step- and foster parents. The most common type of single parent family is that headed by a woman.[38] In the United States, this family form constitutes 12 percent of households.[39] The single-parent family may be subjected to unusually high stress levels. This parent often works and combines the role of mother and father in caring for children at home. The parent may have to curtail social life because of other responsibilities. According to the 1980 census, about one half of families below the poverty line were composed of women and chil-

dren with no husband present in the home. The poverty rate in this type of family was 32.7 percent. For single men with children, the poverty rate was 11.1 percent, while the rate for couples was 6.2 percent.[40]

Single adults are another family form. Approximately 6 percent of adults live alone.[41] Although they live by themselves, they are part of a family referred to as the **family of orientation**, the family into which the person is born.[42] Single adults may be young and recently separated from their parents, or they may be elderly and without any immediate family left. They may be lonely and may not have ready support systems available. Nurses need to be alert to these possiblities. People who live alone may have no one to care for them if they are sick or disabled, or they may have no one to talk with in times of crisis.[43]

Additional family forms include common-law couples, communes, and group marriages. *Common-law couples* are those who are eligible to marry but don't. They maintain a common residence. Such couples are recognized in a number of jurisdictions by the law as a family.[44] *Communes* refer to households where adults live together but are not necessarily monogamous. The latter example is a group marriage.

Characteristics of family structure are affected by cultural norms and values. Nye and Berardo describe the kinship system in the United States according to the following characteristics[45]:

- There is an incest taboo
- Monogamy is the prevailing pattern
- As far as location of household, choosing a mate, or inheritance patterns are concerned, there is no preference shown to maternal or paternal kin
- No particular preference is shown to lines of descent of either the husband or the wife
- Major emphasis is on the immediate conjugal unit (the mother, father, and children)
- The nuclear family is a fairly autonomous unit
- The family is a consumptive rather than a productive unit
- There is relatively little emphasis on tradition because of the emphasis on the nuclear family and the multilineal kinship system
- Free dating and mate selection is the norm
- There is widespread dispersion of adult children

These characteristics of our society may vary considerably among families in other countries and cultures. The one exception is the incest taboo. This characteristic is common to family life in nearly all societies. Whereas **monogamy** is a common feature in our culture, **polygamy** (plural spouses) may be a common feature of other cultures. **Polygyny** refers to one husband with two or more wives at the same time. **Polyandry** refers to one wife with two or more husbands at the same time. This latter form has been recorded in only four societies.[46] Murdock studied 565 societies of the world; he found that about 75 percent favored polygyny and 25 percent favored monogamy. Less than 1 percent favored polyandry. No society practiced group marriage.[47]

It is important for nurses to understand as much as they can about the structure of the families under their care and of the families of their specific clients. With more and more people living in family structures other than the nuclear or extended type, the kind of and need for nursing services is changing. Support groups and needs differ from one type of family to another, and some of these family types are more dependent on the health-care system than others.[48]

Stresses, health needs, and health practices may vary considerably according to these structures, and an organizational knowledge will help guide the nurse in carrying out the nursing process.

Family Processes

All family systems, regardless of their structure or stage of development, possess certain characteristics that help define them and maintain their viability. These characteristics or processes make it possible for families to function as whole units and include the basic systems concepts of boundaries, roles, power, decision making, energy, communication, and feedback. Various subsystems exist within the family system. Some of these subsystems include dyads, such as husband–wife, parent–child, or sibling–sibling. In any subsystem, the individual learns interpersonal skills, performs roles, and has varying levels of power. Adaptation is constantly taking place within families, and through an interplay between family coping mechanisms and family processes, equilibrium can be maintained and growth can take place.

Boundaries. All subsystems have semipermeable boundaries, and clarity of these boundaries in families is very important. Boundaries are the rules that define how participation takes place in subsystems.[49] Boundaries also serve to foster differentiation of family members.

All families are involved in distance regulation in order to attain goals of affect (love and intimacy), power (freedom to decide what they want and the ability to get it), and meaning (a philosophical framework by which to order events). Families attain these goals as they regulate boundaries applying to space, time, and energy.[50]

Regarding the issue of space, family members are continually engaged in the task of developing and maintaining spatial relationships with one another. As they interact, decisions must be made about how close to be.[51] The desire for and tolerance of close physical proximity varies from person to person and culture to culture.[52] Much has been written about how individuals communicate through body language. Boundary and distance regulation are important facets of this communication. Physical space boundaries may be quite specific in families—a person's bedroom or favorite spot at the dining table. Every individual also maintains what is called "personal space," which can be violated when there is poor communication or a lack of sensitivity among family members. Assessment of a family's use of space may be very helpful in the overall analysis of family interaction and function. Such things as the actual physical design of a house may have a strong effect on how much closeness or distancing is attained by the members.[53]

In addition to spatial boundaries, families erect temporal boundaries in order to help them attain their goals.[54] Aspects of boundaries concerning time include frequency, rate, sequencing, duration, calendar time, and clock time. How individual members use their time and how the family uses time together give clues to these kinds of family boundaries. Schedules for going to bed, getting to work or school, and going shopping are also examples of time boundaries. Family members all need a certain amount of solitude or "private time." This kind of privacy involves temporal as well as spatial boundaries. Other types of temporal boundaries involve feelings and thoughts about past experiences and future plans. Information such as this can be helpful in assessing family functioning and in helping families organize their time efficiently.

Boundary Maintenance. An important role for nurses working with clients and families is to support clear and appropriate boundaries within subsystems of the marital dyad, the parental dyad, and the sibling dyad. Where there are problems with boundaries, enmeshment (diffuse boundaries) or disengagement (rigid boundaries) may occur.[55] An overprotective mother who keeps her son home from school when he is able to go is an example of enmeshment. In some chaotic families, there are no links between members and boundaries are rigid. They come and go with no regard for others in the family system. Both types of families may need counseling to alter their boundaries. The psychiatric nurse who has specialized in family therapy has special skills in helping families attain more satisfactory boundaries.

Energy. *Energy* is defined as the capacity to do work. All family activities require the expenditure of energy to attain goals. Energy within a family system refers to psychic and physical energy. Psychic energy refers to attitudes and feelings of motivation that precede the action. The capacity to show an interest, to want to get involved in something, or to go through the mental steps of organizing and managing an action are some general examples of psychic energy. The mother who takes the initiative, for example, to call for an appointment with the pediatrician, find out how to get to the office, call the bus for a schedule, and arrange for a change in her own work schedule is expending considerable psychic energy. How the family obtains energy and with what frequency are important for nurses to understand when they are working with families.[56] Chronic illnesses, depression, and situational crises within families can affect family energy levels.

The regulation of energy flow to attain energy balance or imbalance is the major energy issue in families.[57] Community nurses and others who work with families in depth often can provide this kind of intervention.

Roles. Role refers to an expected set of behaviors. It is a dynamic family aspect, the acting out of behaviors expected of the occupant of a particular status or position. "Role is referred to as more or less homogeneous sets of behavior which are normatively defined and expected of an occupant of a given social position."[58] Nye emphasizes that these expectations are based not just on present-day role behaviors, arising out of social interaction, but on the behavior of those previously occupying the roles.[59] Roles include not only behavior but attitudes and values.

How are duties or roles in families assigned? Who takes out the trash, cooks the meals, works outside the home, and cares for the children?

Role enactment is necessary for the fulfillment of family functioning.[60] Roles we commonly think of in families include those of husband-father, wife-mother, and child-sibling. These roles are associated with expected behaviors. Some of Mrs. Jones' roles as wife and mother include housekeeping, child care, child socialization, and sexual partner. Because Mrs. Jones works, she shares the provider role with her husband.

TYPES OF ROLES. Roles must be negotiated. They may be decided on the basis of tradition, competence, or what the husband and wife each like best or least. Families commonly perform the following roles:

Provider	The occupant of this role provides income to secure material resources
Housekeeper	Cleaning house, obtaining food, and preparing food are some of the expected behaviors of this role
Sexual partner	In addition to the act of sexual intercourse, part of the expected behavior of this role for both men and women today is to provide pleasure to the partner
Therapeutic	Role behavior in this category includes the provision of emotional support, sustenance, and reassurance
Child care	Providing the basic needs of a child through feeding, changing, and clothing are components of this role[61]
Recreation and kinship	Providing recreational activities and keeping in touch with relatives[62]

Women traditionally have been involved in housekeeping, child-care, and child socialization roles, while men have filled the provider role. More and more women, however, are entering the work force. In the 20 years from 1960 to 1980, one-earner households decreased by 27.2 percent. These households declined from 49.6 to 22.4 percent. At the same time, the percentage of married working women increased from 32 to 51 percent. While 26.3 million mothers stayed at home, 31.8 million went to work.[63]

In a study of attitudes and practices of roles among 1518 cases (759 husbands and their wives), Albrecht, Bahr, and Chadwick found greatest acceptance of the female provider role among younger study participants (under 30 years of age). Most respondents favored the traditional role of greater wife involvement in the child-care and housekeeper roles. A majority of participants felt that kinship roles should be shared.

When role enactment (the actual carrying out of a role) was investigated, a higher percentage of older respondents (over 65) shared the provider role. Women of all ages were more likely to have a larger role in housekeeping, kinship, and child care. Most role sharing was seen in the kinship role. Some was seen in the child-care role.

Women made decisions about housekeeping and child-care. Some shared decision making was seen in the child-care and provider roles. Husbands under 30 were more likely to be involved in decision making about children. Most shared decision making was seen in the kinship role.[64]

Smith states, "Research indicates that although dual career couples may have egalitarian attitudes, women are still responsible for the majority of domestic tasks. Further, both partners generally relegate the wife's career to secondary status—second to her husband's career and second to her roles as homemaker, wife, and mother."[65]

FORMAL AND INFORMAL ROLES. Roles may be formal or informal. "Whereas formal roles are explicit, roles which each family role structure contains (father-husband, etc.), informal roles are implicit, often not apparent on the surface, and are played to meet the emotional needs of individuals and/or to maintain the family's equilibrium."[66]

Examples of informal roles include the following[67]:

- Encourager
- Initiator-contributor
- Blocker
- Dominator
- Martyr
- Pal
- Harmonizer
- Compromiser
- Follower
- Recognition-seeker
- The Great Stone Face

ROLE VARIATION. Families may base their roles on the pattern the culture provides. They also arrive at decisions about roles through interaction, negotiation, and trial and error.

Roles may vary considerably, within and across cultures. This is true for the husband-father, wife-mother, and child-sibling roles. Expectations concerning role performance may be strong or weak. To determine importance of role expectations, sanctions applied for not meeting expectations are a good indicator.[68]

Lisa was supposed to be in from her date at midnight on the weekend. While attending a party, she didn't notice the time and arrived home at two hours past her curfew. Her parents had waited up for her. Lisa was grounded the following weekend.

Role complementarity is the match between role performance and the expectations of the partner in the role relationship. When complementarity doesn't exist, conflict occurs.[69] This conflict may arise from within or outside the person. *Intrarole* conflict occurs when there

are conflicting expectations about one role the individual holds. *Inter-role* conflict occurs when two or more roles of the individual conflict with each other.[70]

The concept of roles is important in understanding and promoting adequate family functioning. There is wide variation in the way families enact roles. Roles can be changed if they are not satisfying and if the family is willing to negotiate. A frequent nursing role is to help families maintain healthy roles and to learn new ones when they are needed. Families can be helped to learn new roles by teaching, role modeling, and role playing.

Power. When boundaries and roles are decided, the method of decision making is an indicator of power in the family. Various authors have described power as the ability to influence the behavior of another, to influence a decision, to achieve intended outcomes or goals, or to influence the emotions of others.[71–74] Power is a concept with multiple dimensions. In all systems, it is dynamic, not static.

Friedman says that there are six bases of power.[75] *Legitimate power*, also called primary authority, is the shared belief that one person in the system has the right to make decisions for others in the system. Such power is traditionally based. The power of elected members of Congress to enact laws for the health of the nation is legitimate power. Another example is found in the Smith family. Mr. Smith, the breadwinner, makes all the decisions. Mrs. Smith regards this decision making power as her husband's right. This is a traditionally based power, which has the status of legitimacy in such a family. In families where women work, it is less commonly seen.

Referrent power is the influence of one person over another. This occurs through positive identification with the person possessing power. In this situation the person with less power adopts behaviors and attitudes similar to those held by the person in power. Referrant power may be seen when clients positively identify with good role models in the health-care system. This can be a sound influence in fostering the adoption of positive health behaviors such as stopping smoking.

Expert power, based on the perception that a person or group has particular knowledge or skills, is important in the health-care system. One of the reasons Mrs. Stokes consented to having her baby delivered by a nurse-midwife is because of her belief in the knowledge and skill of the nurse-midwife.

The expectation that a person has the resources to reward others is *reward power.* In the practice of nursing, the nursing supervisor will have reward power because of her ability to grant time off and to recommend promotions and merit pay increases. Clients may be vested with a certain amount of reward power in their appreciation of the nurse's efforts, although this should not influence quality of care.

Coercive power is the expectation that punishment will occur if something is not done. Husbands and wives who physically abuse one another are using coercive power. Nurses may have to use it when telling a mother that her child is not allowed in school without immunizations.

Informational power is the power of a message to convince the recipient of the message that change is necessary. Television commercials have strong informational power. Health brochures may have informational power.[76]

Decision Making. An important way to gain understanding of the dynamics of family power is to analyze decision making within the family. Decision making is necessary for the family to fulfill its functions. Areas of decision making include[77,78]:

- Who decides who will be involved in the decision?
- Who is actually involved? How did this come about?
- What is the relative power of each member?
- What processes are used in decision making? (Processes may include assertiveness, control, persuasion, negotiation, and influence.)
- Who makes the final decision?
- What is the significance of the decision?
- How is it implemented?
- What are its effects on relationships?

Decision making reflects how the family meets the needs of its individual members. In the Stokes family, members felt very differently about a decision made on the basis of discussion and consensus as opposed to a decision made on the basis of threatened punishment.

TYPES OF DECISION MAKING. Families may arrive at decisions through consensus, accommodation, or just by allowing things to happen. *Consensus* is a type of decision making achieved through discussion and consideration of all viewpoints. Everyone agrees on the course of action. There is equal commitment to and satisfaction with the decision made. This kind of decision making is seen more in families where power is shared. It requires the ability to communicate and solve problems.[79]

Accommodation, another type of decision making is "always an agreement to disagree, to adopt a common decision in the face of irreconcilable differences."[80] Accommodation may occur through coercion, bargaining, or compromise.

In *coercion,* one or more family members agree because of an implied threat if they don't go along with the decision. When Suzanne angrily refused to join her family for Thanksgiving dinner unless her boyfriend was invited, she was using coercion to influence decision making.

In *bargaining,* the decision reached may involve each side's giving up something, but there are elements in the final decision that are satisfying to all concerned. Each party expects sacrifice to be reciprocated. It is a tit-for-tat arrangement. Joanna and her mother agreed that if Joanna helped her mother with housework in the morning, her mother would take Joanna shopping in the afternoon.

Compromise involves a decision making process where involved parties agree on a course of action that was not the original one. The new course of action has satisfying elements for all. In the Parson family, everyone agreed on a movie to be seen that was not anyone's first choice; compromise had been reached.

De facto decision making occurs when things are just allowed to happen. Archer refers to decision making by default, in which all options except one are exhausted. Only one recourse is left open to the family. This leads to crisis management. Those involved can only react and not participate in shaping events.[81]

What factors influence decision making?

Cultural norms and social class can both play a part. Power may increase, for example, as the husband or wife's income increases. The family life cycle also influences decision making. Women with young children have less power. Their power increases when the children leave home. When men retire, women's power also increases.[82]

Other factors that affect decision making include:

- The communication network in the family. If members talk to each other only through a mediator in the family, the person in the mediating role has more power.[83]
- Implementation control. Power resides in the person who must implement the decision.
- Interpersonal resources. These resources can be influential in the decision making process:

> *Self-confidence*
> *The meaning and importance of the issue to the individuals involved*: People who are more emotionally involved in the decision will put more energy into bringing about a resolution they want.
> *Restrictive norms*: Cultural norms may inhibit certain kinds of behavior in individuals.
> *Attitudes toward conflict*: Where conflict is viewed as wrong, families may not work at decision making.
> *Importance of relationships*: An individual may avoid conflict or alter behavior in situations where the relationships are important to him or her.
> *Formation of coalitions*: When the majority side on an issue, it may influence the outcome of the decision.

Decision making may be autocratic (decision making for the group by only one person), syncratic (shared), autonomic or atomistic (making decisions for oneself alone or independently of one another), or chaotic.[84]

Power in the family may be demonstrated by decision making. Culture, the family's ability to communicate with each other, the importance of the decision to various family members, and the influence and numbers of those involved in the decision making process influence family decision making.

Adaptation and Communication. All of the processes that take place in a family system are related. Adaptation, as a process, is dependent on the existence of boundaries and how they are maintained, on the availability and use of energy, and on the use of power and decision making within various role structures. Adaptation in the family is the ability of members to change their responses to one another and to the outside environment as the situation dictates.[85] Adaptation is essential in the survival of any system, and in family systems it often makes the difference between functional and dysfunctional families.

Communication processes in the family are closely aligned with adaptation and are frequently the single most important factor influencing equilibrium. Communication in families can be viewed as a subprocess of adaptation.[86] Family communication is the giving and receiving of messages among family members and between members and the environment.

In addition, communication in a family tends to take place within the context of its structures. Family members have a tendency to communicate in terms of their roles and how much power or status they have.[87] Families also have distinct styles of communication that can be related to cultural norms, social class standing, and age.[88]

Nurse therapists and community health nurses who work in depth with families can draw more specific conclusions about communication in families from authors with family expertise such as Virginia Satir. Satir uses communication theory as a basis for her practice in family therapy and outlines many assessment and intervention techniques for working with communication problems in families.[89] Later in this chapter some further examples of assessment of communication in families are given.

Growth and Differentiation. The term differentiation is a systems concept that describes the system's tendency toward growth and advancement.[90] Families, particularly those that are well adapted and functioning within a healthy environment, are continually in a state of change and growth. This growth and change may be manifested physically, emotionally, and socially. Families vary in their ability to grow and change, and the rate of change is particularly affected by various life crises. Each time a family goes through a developmental crisis, such as a birth in the family, new roles are formed, new methods of coping are learned, and behavior and communication patterns change. In therapeutic situations in which the nurse is in the role of family counselor or therapist, growth can take place similarly through changes in communication style, life style, interpersonal relations, and interpersonal transactions.[91]

FAMILY FUNCTIONS

Most families have specific and fundamental functions in common. These functions can be broadly categorized into biological, economic, educational, affectual, status-conferring, recreational, religious, and protective.[92] Friedman views family functions as outcomes or consequences of the family structure and identifies the following additional and more specific functions: socialization of children and social placement function, family coping function, and physical and health-care function.[93] Basically, functions describe what the family does to meet its goals and maintain a balance, both within itself and in relation to outside systems.

The biological function of the family is primarily reproductive and provides for the creation of family members, the society, and continued human survival. This most basic function traditionally has been seen by many families and groups of people as a moral obligation to society, a requirement or necessity in which all families participate. Increasingly, however, the birth of children is not viewed within such rigid boundaries, and families feel more freedom to choose whether or not they will participate in this function.

Meeting the sexual needs of adult partners in the family is also part of this biological function. In the past, the sexual relationship was taken somewhat for granted and often not identified explicitly as a responsibility. Heightened public and professional awareness about sexuality and sexual functioning has been very positive in regard to understanding this function and promoting its healthy adaptation in families.

The economic function of the family is to provide financial resources to meet the needs of the family. As discussed earlier in this chapter, American families are extremely dependent on financial income. With few exceptions, most goods, services, and other resources needed by the family are obtained through financial arrangements. This function entails allocation of resources as well as attainment of them. Family values, educational level, personal needs, and a host of other circumstances contribute to how families decide to spend their money and balance income with expenditures. There are considerable health-care implications related to the economic situations of families, such as the high incidence of disease and prevalence of ill health among poor families.[94] Unemployment and work-related disabilities also have health-care implications and pose great threats to this vital function.

The educational function of the family pertains primarily to the socialization of children and helping them to fit into the structure of society. The socialization process helps children form acceptable behavior patterns and skills, develop a personal value system, learn about cultural traditions, and learn to live satisfactorily with their fellows. More specifically, this function provides children with a sense of right and wrong, of what is normal and appropriate, and what is accepted in the way of role and status.[95] This crucially important process is one of the most significant family functions and provides influences that mold basic attitudes and personality characteristics for life.

The family function of protecting and nurturing is interrelated with all other functions of a family. In the United States, this function is recognized legally as well as traditionally; all states have laws requiring parents to support their children, and many laws broadly support parental authority.[96] Families function to provide a safe environment for their members, especially young children. Physical and mental health is protected by providing basic nutritional needs, a safe and warm shelter, love, affection, emotional interaction, and health care. Another term used to describe much of the essence of the protective function is *parenting*. Parenting behaviors are child rearing functions passed down from generation to generation and include roles of teaching and modeling as well as protection.[97] Also, adult members of the family frequently need protection, particularly from some of the stresses and strains of modern life. The family unit can function as a haven or safe retreat where people can feel trust and regain their equilibrium.

Meeting recreational needs is another function that families perform. Recreation refers to activities that take place during leisure time and that are not connected to obligations of work or school. These activities vary greatly from family to family and within families and may include religious, educational, civic, cultural, sports, or entertainment activities.[98] Helping younger family members to use their free time constructively and develop special interests or hobbies is an essential aspect of this function. The fostering of pleasurable and diverting activities also helps the family to relax and reduce day-to-day stresses. Whether quietly reading alone, enjoying a family picnic, or playing a vigorous game of handball, it is important that the family sanction and support these kinds of activities.

The religious functions of a family vary according to individual beliefs and cultural traditions within the family's history. Many families are members of a particular religion and identify strongly with its teachings and practices. Other families may not espouse a specific religion but follow a special philosophy of life or set of beliefs. An exact definition of the religious function in families is difficult to generalize. It is a function that centers around maintaining a faith or philosophy of life that allows for growth beyond one's personal and immediate needs; it gives a more futuristic and comprehensive framework from which families and individuals view themselves.[99] A religious environment can support and encourage growth and service to mankind.[100] The religious or philosophical element in a family can be a strengthening bond that helps people cope with and understand more about peak life events such as birth, death, serious illness, marriage, and divorce.

Families function to provide each other with love, affection, and emotional support. All human beings have strong needs to be cared for and nourished by others. Just as young children need affection and nurturance for their development, adults need it for continued feelings of security, self-esteem, and emotional growth. From earliest infancy to the most advanced age, the feeling of being deeply loved and valued is an important precondition to meeting life's challenges and expectations, to doing one's best without unhealthy stress.[101] Families carry out the affective function through verbal communication, touch, empathy, and numerous other gestures that convey messages of love.

All of the above family functions are related and interdependent. They are all part of a system that works together to achieve goals and relate to other environmental systems and subsystems. In addition, these functions are highly individualized and vary from family to family and culture to culture (Fig. 30–1). They are subject to unique situations, such as economic circumstances, natural disasters, health, and illness. The amount of energy available and the type of decision making in the family system also affect functions and what priority is given to each of them. One of the most helpful ways to understand family functioning is to consider the natural life cycle of families, their predictable stages, and related tasks.

FAMILY LIFE CYCLE

Families are dynamic social systems that go through predictable stages of development and rhythmic cycles of behavior and activities. As

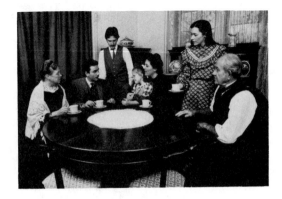

Figure 30–1. Family structure varies within and across cultures.

two people come together to share their lives, a family is born. Typically, the family increases over time with children, and each child, along with the parents, continues growth and development patterns. Chronologically, there are births and deaths in the family, and the cycle is repeated. "The family life cycle is a composite of the individual developmental changes of its members and the cyclical changes of the marital relationship itself."[102]

Duvall has identified an eight-stage family life-cycle framework that has corresponding developmental tasks (Table 25–2).[103]

Although this framework is limited to families with a nuclear structure, it can be very useful in understanding family dynamics and assessing family functioning. It begins by identifying a young couple as they establish their relationship and adjust to forming a household. The second stage begins with the first pregnancy, and the next four stages correspond to events in the developmental years of the children until they marry or leave home. The last two stages focus on the couple after all the children have gone.

In families with more than one child, the stages will overlap, and tasks from several stages may be going on simultaneously. Other factors and situations result in variations of the order of stages or completion of tasks. Among these are foster families, families who adopt older children, or those who wait until later in life to have their first baby. A couple may have a 10- or 20-year age difference, for example, and the husband may be planning retirement at the time of the first pregnancy. Divorce, single parenthood, remarriage, and changes in child custody also affect the order and emphasis of the family life cycle (Fig. 30–2). Some individuals or groups never do fit into Duvall's framework. Among these are most homosexual pairings, nontraditional group marriages, communal households without children, and childless couples.[104]

THE NURSING PROCESS

The nursing process is equally applicable in the care of individuals, families, or communities. An understanding of family processes and family dynamics helps nurses to care for family units,

TABLE 30–2. DEVELOPMENTAL STAGES IN THE FAMILY LIFE CYCLE

Stage	Developmental Tasks
1. Married couple	Establishing a mutually satisfying marriage Adjusting to pregnancy and the promise of parenthood Fitting into the kin network (in-laws)
2. Childbearing	Having, adjusting to, and encouraging the development of infants Establishing a satisfying home for parents and infant
3. Preschool age	Adapting to the critical needs and interests of preschool children in stimulating, growth-promoting ways Coping with energy depletion and lack of privacy as parents
4. School age	Fitting into the community of school-age families in constructive ways Encouraging children's educational achievement
5. Teenage	Balancing freedom with responsibility, as teen-agers mature and emancipate themselves Establishing postparental interests and careers as growing parents
6. Launching career	Releasing young adults into work, college, marriage, military service, etc., with appropriate rituals and assistance Maintaining a supportive home base
7. Middle-aged parents	Rebuliding the marriage relationship Maintaining kin ties with older and younger generations
8. Aging family members	Coping with bereavement and living alone Closing the family home or adapting it to aging Adjusting to retirement

Reprinted by permission from E.M. Duvall, Marriage and Family Development, 5th ed. (Philadelphia: J.B. Lippincott Co., 1977), 179.

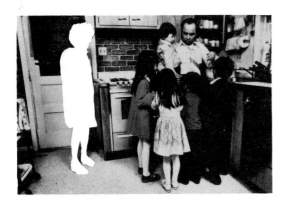

Figure 30–2. The role of a single parent may pose special stresses.

to assess the role of the family in caring for ill individuals, and to be aware of the impact of an individual's illness on the family.

Each subsystem in the family influences the other subsystems. Because of these influences, the family is an important determinant in health-care practices. Families decide when members are ill, whether care will be sought, and what care will be sought. The family also decides whether to implement prescribed health care. Friedman states that 75 to 85 percent of health care is given by the family.[105]

The following discussion of the four components of the nursing process as it applies to family theory focuses primarily on the whole family as the unit of care.

Assessment

Family assessment is the collection of data that give a comprehensive and graphic description of a family's structure and cultural makeup, conditions of living, financial resources, communication and emotional support systems, and physical and mental health status of each member. The family is assessed in terms of its internal functioning and its relationship to the external environment. This serves as an important guide in formulating nursing actions, based on family strengths as well as needs or imbalances in the family system.[106] The family assessment is an ongoing process requiring a great deal of trust and open communication between the nurse and the family. Community health and visiting nurses are usually fortunate enough to assess the family in the home setting over a period of time. Each time there is contact with the family, the health status continues to be assessed; the information base grows and changes over time, and the nurse–family relationship deepens.

Information Sources. Information sources for the family assessment include the family interview, physical examination of members or the identified client, information in the family or client record, videotapes of family interaction, and staff and other community agencies that have worked with the family.[107] An important principle in the ongoing process of conducting a family assessment is to obtain and review available information before the family interview, if possible. This will help to organize the interview, save the family time, and avoid repetitious reporting of information.

Information for the family assessment can be gathered in any setting, but every effort should be made to interview the family at least once in the home. In this way, the nurse can observe living conditions, the neighborhood, and community characteristics on a first-hand basis and acquire a better understanding of family values and priorities.

Making a Home Visit. Making a home visit is quite a different experience from interviewing a client in the hospital or clinic setting. For nurses who are accustomed to caring for clients in these latter settings or for student nurses making their first home visit, there may be feelings of role reversal or confusion. A person's home is a private domain, a space where the individual is usually in control, and where the person exercises power over who visits and what they do there. On the contrary, the hospital or other health-care facility is the domain of the health-care worker, and the client is subject to power and control by nurse and doctors. Being aware of some of these feelings and using guidelines presented in the following discussion will help to make home visiting experiences more successful.

Preparatory guidelines that can help organize the home visit and increase chances for things to go smoothly include the following:

- Call the family ahead of time to verify the convenience of the time and make sure they will be at home
- Verify the family's address and directions for getting there
- Review the purpose of the visit and make notes regarding your goals
- Assemble any equipment including health and family assessment forms and educational materials

Upon arrival at the family's house, observe the neighborhood. Look for such things as safety, conditions of the buildings, and accessibility to shopping and transportation. Are there rodents? Is play space available? Are there trees, grass, and flowers? If so, are they well tended? Look at the family's house. Is it a single family dwelling, a group home, or an apartment building? Are window panes knocked out? Are screens broken? Such factors are important, because they enhance entry of disease-carrying vectors as well as cold and rain.

It is important to ensure that initial contact with the family is as nonthreatening as possible and starts off positively. An amiable introduction to the person who answers the door sets the tone for establishing trust and cooperation (Fig. 30–3). The nurse's attitude should reflect the fact she is a guest in the client's home and considers it a special privilege to visit.

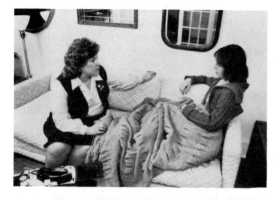

Figure 30–3. An appropriate introduction helps set a good tone for the home visit.

In beginning the interview, it is important to let the family know the purpose of the visit in terms they can understand. The nurse "contracts" with the family regarding what she would like to do in the assessment process, why the actions are necessary, and what expectations and outcomes there are for all involved.

Information obtained from the family interview is a combination of subjective and objective data. Subjective data are all the things the family verbalizes. Objective data are observable things, such as skin color, household odors, and patterns of communication. Family assessment tools are constructed in varying formats, but they all contain basic categories of subjective data (biographical information, family history, family health practices, income data, and so forth) and sections for the nurse to record her observations and other objective data. The remainder of this section discusses the important categories of family assessment as carried out in the ideal setting—a home visit where the nurse can interview family members and observe them interacting.

The Household Roster. The household roster is a listing of all the members of the family and any other persons residing permanently in the home. Biographical information, such as sex, date and place of birth, education, and occupation are included for each person. It is customary to identify the heads of the household first, followed by children, in order of birth. Other relatives and individuals who live with the family are listed last. It is important to clarify the first and last names of each member of the household. Children of divorced or remarried parents often have different last names. Also, mothers of illegitimate children may give the child the last name of the father.[108]

The Family's Health Picture. To begin determining areas of nursing need, it is necessary to find out about illness in the family and about health practices that are health-promoting. This will help draw conclusions about what the nurse and the family see as problems, needs, and strengths. The questions below serve as guides for assessment[109,110]

- Who is currently ill in the family?
- What is wrong with them?

- How long have they been ill?
- What medicines and treatments are being used in their care?
- What is the family pattern of care giving?
- What feelings has the family expressed about their situation?
- What is the frequency of illness among various family members?
- What symptoms of poor health are present in the family—chronic fatigue, pain, abuse, or neglect?
- Are children immunized?
- What is the family's source of medical care? Dental care?
- When did family members last have a physical exam?
- When did family members last have a dental exam?
- Who smokes?
- Is there alcohol or drug abuse of which you are aware?
- What plan of care does the family have in case of emergency?

Family Health Practices: Nutrition. A good method of assessing nutritional status is to ask the family to do a 24-hour food recall. Each person who is able to lists everything eaten in the past 24 hours and at what time. On the basis of this information, conclusions can be drawn about adequacy of the diet in relation to the body's daily requirements. Other questions helpful in assessing nutrition include[111]:

- What knowledge does the family show about food?
- Is refrigeration available?
- What cooking facilities are available?
- Who buys and prepares the food? Is the person who buys the food literate? (This affects ability to read food labels.)
- Does the family have particular food likes and dislikes?
- Are there food allergies?
- Is anyone on a medically prescribed diet?

Safety in the Home. During the home visit, the nurse can be alert to any home hazards. Providing tactful guidance to the family is a very important facet of preventive care. Accidents are a major killer of young children (Fig. 30–4).

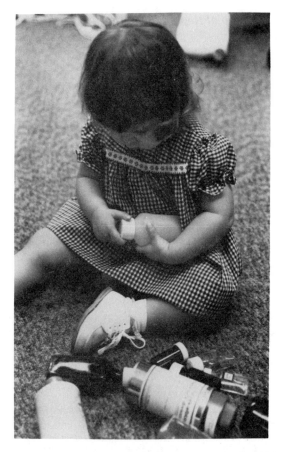

Figure 30–4. Drugs within reach of children are an invitation to disaster. Families need to provide a safe environment for their members. *(Courtesy of the Food and Drug Administration.)*

The checklist below will guide you in determining safety in the home[112,113]:

- Are drugs and poisons kept out of reach of small children?
- Do drugs have safety tops?
- Do you see peeling paint? Peeling paint may have lead in it, and ingestion by young children may lead to lead poisoning.
- Are there guardrails at steps to protect toddlers from falls?
- Are there nonskid mats and bathtub and toilet handrails for elderly members?
- Is lighting adequate?
- Are matches kept out of reach of children?

Provision of Rest and Sleep. Adequate rest and sleep contribute to feelings of mental and physical well-being (Fig. 30–5). In assessing this aspect of family life, it is useful to note[114]:

- How much sleep does the family get at night?
- What are the sleeping arrangements?
- What provision is made for rest and naps during the day?
- Does anyone have insomnia? How is this treated?

Emotional Environment. The family provides a vehicle through which individual members develop self-images and feelings about themselves and others. The quality of personal relationships is important in overall life satisfaction.[115] Lockhard asks, "Are family members able to support one another in their daily lives?"[116] When observing the emotional climate in the family, test for the following[117]:

- Is the communication clear?
- Are feelings and words congruent?
- What are the interaction patterns like? Is anyone consistently ignored? Who speaks to whom?
- Is differentness accepted? How is it handled?
- Do family members support and encourage one another?
- How is labor divided?
- How is conflict resolved?
- How are the decisions made?
- What stresses are the family experiencing?

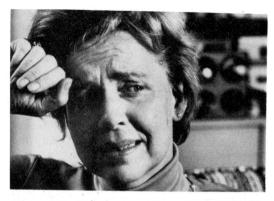

Figure 30–5. Fatigue can be a stressor affecting the performance of family tasks.

- What coping behaviors do they employ to deal with stresses?
- What functional patterns of interaction does the family use?
- What dysfunctional patterns of interaction do you observe in the family?

Dysfunctional patterns of communication may occur in a family when stress is present, a family member's self-esteem is threatened, and family members don't feel free to communicate. When this happens, Satir says one of the following four communication patterns emerges:

- Placating
- Blaming
- Computing
- Distracting

The *placator* invariably tries to please the other person. He uses ingratiating behavior and apologies. He fears to disagree. The *blamer* constantly finds fault and plays the boss. If the blamer can feel superior to others, he feels better about himself. The *computer* gives a cool, calm, ultrarational appearance. This belies his feelings of vulnerability. The *distractor* uses words and does things that are not relevant to what is going on. He feels there is no place for him.[118]

Where lack of honesty is present in communication, problems exist. Dishonest communication may hide an ulterior motive and is destructive. The following list gives some examples of dysfunctional communication between couples:

Concerning the partner	John consistently puts Susan in positions where she looks wrong or undesirable. This communication is dysfunctional. Its result is a "damned if you do; damned if you don't" position for Susan.
Tell me your problem	In this case, Ann encourages Ted to reveal vulnerable emotion-laden areas and then uses this information with family, friends, and neighbors. She uses Ted's perceived inadequacy to shore up her own feelings of inadequacy.

Doing something for the other	Instead of being able to communicate her own desires or needs to William, Mary comunicates that these should be obtained because he needs them.
Placing the burden of decision making on the partner	Although Bob is interested in the outcome of a decision, he often avoids responsibility for participating and then places the consequences of a bad decision on his wife.
Courtroom behavior	Steve often verbally attacks Jean. This puts Jean in the role of defendant. She tries to justify her behavior. If a third party is present he might be called on to act as a judge. Each spouse is more interested in proving her- or himself right than solving the conflict.[119]
Camouflage	In Alice and Mark's marriage, messages are not communicated directly but are so veiled they can barely be recognized. In this way, the person giving the message does not have to deal with rejection of the message or with conflict.

Game playing runs in familes and can be passed on through generations.[120] Such games represent manipulation and exploitation.

Couples that avoid discussing their conflicts display dysfunctional behavior. Tensions build in such situations. Tension also builds when couples focus on the conflict and not on the issue. Person-centered attacks are common in this situation. The persons involved need to learn that it is more constructive to focus on the issue and respect the right to disagree. It is important, too, for them to learn to discuss alternatives and the pros and cons of these alternatives.[121]

Social Influences. Social influences are an integral part of a family assessment. They include culture, ethnicity, and religious practices (Fig. 30–6). "Spiritual beliefs still affect the lives of most individuals. They influence such things as contraceptive practices, dietary habits, developmental transitions through rites of passage, selection of marriage partners, and reactions to health and illness."[122] Information that is helpful to gather about social influences includes the following:

- Is there a particular ethnic group with which this family identifies? What influence does this have on the family's health practices?
- Does the family practice a particular religion?
- Where does the family attend church? How frequently? What influence does religion have on the family's health attitudes, beliefs, and practices?

Recreation. "Recreation refers to activities apart from the activities of work, family, and society to which the individual and family turn at will for their relaxation, diversion, self-development, or social participation."[123] It is helpful to assess how each member of the family uses leisure time and how each one feels about it. In addition, you can note what the family group does for fun and whether they share activities, or each does his own thing.

Income. Lack of income can be a stressor that enhances the family's susceptibility to illness. It may mean the family is unable to provide adequate food, clothing, medical care and shelter for its members. Questions about money are sometimes difficult to ask. Ann, a student nurse, asked about income in the following way:

> "Mrs. Jones, some families have financial needs that it's helpful to share with the health department, because we may know of some community resources that can help you. Often families haven't had an opportunity to learn about these resources. I wonder if you feel your income is adequate in meeting your family's needs. Perhaps we could talk about it."

Family income may come from jobs, pensions, insurance payments, investments, or public assistance. In some situations, it is important to know the family's specific income for eligibility determinations; a number of government

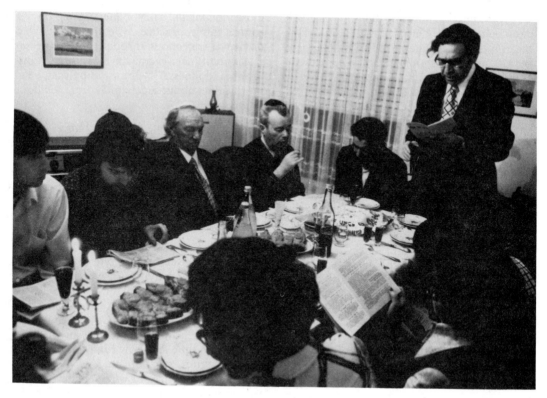

Figure 30–6. Spiritual practices may provide a rich heritage and form cohesiveness in families.

resources and programs require such information. Other factors to consider in determining a family's financial health are whether the family owns or rents its living quarters and what its patterns of debts and expenditures are.[124]

Home Environment. The home in which the family lives provides clues about factors that may or may not be conducive to health. Relevant questions and observations include the following[125]:

- How many rooms does the home have?
- What provision is made for privacy? Privacy provides space for autonomy, a place for self-exploration, and a place for protected communication.
- How is the home heated?
- Does ventilation seem adequate?
- Is there indoor plumbing?

- Are towels and soap available?
- What laundry facilities are available?

Community Resources. "Part of a family's successful coping is its ability to secure compliance from the environment, meaning that within the community the family is able to seek out, receive, and/or accept the appropriate resources to meet their needs for food, services, and information.[126]

- What community resources does the family use? How often?
- What are the family's feelings about the resources it uses? What are their areas of satisfaction and dissatisfaction?
- What extended kin does the family see?

Family Strengths. As data are gathered for the family assessment, it is very important to get an understanding not only of problems but also of strengths. Family strengths are those things that help the family function as a unit and feel better about itself.[127] Characteristics of strong families include the following[128]:

- There is a facilitative process of interaction among family members
- Families enhance individual member development
- Relationships are structured effectively
- Families actively attempt to cope with problems
- There is a healthy home environment and lifestyle
- They establish regular links with the broader community

Otto is a well known family researcher who studied family strengths extensively. He listed the following characteristics as family strengths[129]:

- Having enough time together
- Freedom to be alone
- Common interests
- Liking/loving/caring for each other
- Mutual commitment
- Shared faith
- Sharing of feelings
- Lots of mutual support
- Common goals, values
- Agreement on handling family finances
- Willingness to forgive
- Fostering spiritual growth in each other
- A good circle of friends
- Having a lot of fun together
- Having a sense of mission
- Good communication
- Freedom of expression
- Good sense of humor
- Respect
- Affirmation
- Shared dreams
- Sharing the work
- Self-awareness
- Good food
- Encouragement of talents
- Developing responsibility
- Capacity to reach out to the family
- Family traditions, celebrations
- Willingness to accept other life-styles
- Freedom to grow as persons

- Sensitivity to each other's needs
- Fostering creativity in each other
- Self-worth and self-reliance building
- Structures for problem solving
- Interest in world community
- Concern

Nurses can be instrumental in helping families to recognize and use their strengths. The very act of pointing out strengths to the family can often be therapeutic and enhance coping skills and self-esteem.

Tools in Family Assessment. Numerous tools exist to help in conducting a family assessment. One tool is called an **ecomap** and is useful in depicting a family's relationship with its environment. It shows the systems with which a family relates and the strengths or weaknesses of those relationships. Developed for caseworkers by Dr. Ann Hartman, the ecomap "examines boundary maintenance aspects of family functioning. It dramatically illustrates the amount of energy used by a family to maintain its system as well as the presence or absence of situational supports and other family resources."[130]

To develop an ecomap (Fig. 30–7), draw a large circle, and place the nuclear family members inside it. Squares represent males and circles represent females. Put name and age of each person in the center of the circle or square. To represent systems with which the family relates, draw circles around the family circle, just as though you were drawing planets around the sun. Examples of systems external to the family include school, work, church, the police department, and the recreation department. Depending on where the relationship exists, connect these systems to the family system or to individuals in the family. A solid line represents a strong relationship, and a line with slashes through it represents a conflict-laden relationship. Use arrows drawn along these lines to indicate direction of the flow of energy. An arrow going in only one direction indicates a unilateral energy flow. The nurse and the client can complete an ecomap together. This joint effort can foster collaboration and help the family achieve greater self-understanding. The use of the ecomap over time can show client life changes in a graphic manner.[131]

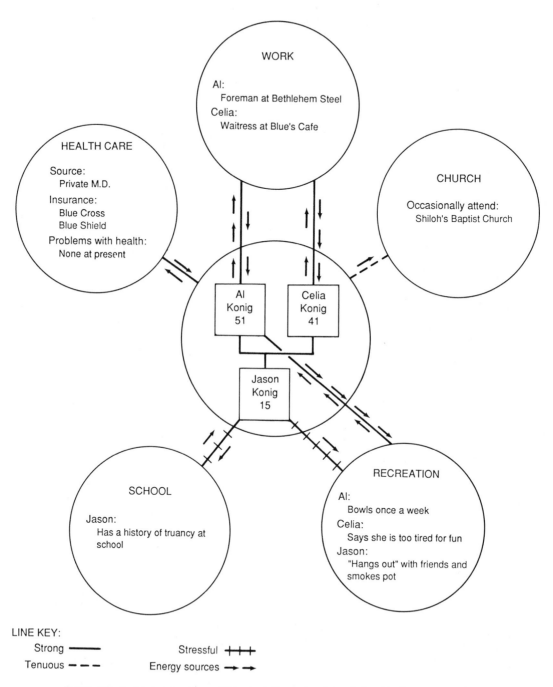

WORK

Al:
   Foreman at Bethlehem Steel
Celia:
   Waitress at Blue's Cafe

HEALTH CARE

Source:
   Private M.D.
Insurance:
   Blue Cross
   Blue Shield
Problems with health:
   None at present

CHURCH

Occasionally attend:
   Shiloh's Baptist Church

Al
Konig
51

Celia
Konig
41

Jason
Konig
15

SCHOOL

Jason:
   Has a history of truancy at
   school

RECREATION

Al:
   Bowls once a week
Celia:
   Says she is too tired for fun
Jason:
   "Hangs out" with friends and
   smokes pot

LINE KEY:
   Strong ——————
   Tenuous — — —
   Stressful ┼┼┼
   Energy sources ——▶ ⟶

Figure 30–7. An ecomap is useful in depicting a family's relationship to its environment.

Another useful tool in family assessment is the **genogram** which depicts three or more generations of a family. The genogram shows family dispersals, losses, roles, and organizational patterns. Hartman says, "Not only is each individual immersed in the complex here-and-now life space, but each individual is also part of a family saga, in an infinitely complicated human system which has developed over many generations and has transmitted powerful commands, role assignments, events, patterns of living and relating down through the years."[132]

The basic structure of the genogram is depicted in Figure 30–8 with suggested symbolic representations. Other symbols may be used as long as a clear key defines the meaning of each symbol.

Nursing Diagnosis. Data gathered about the individual and family is the precursor to developing an informed opinion about the family's health status. In the process of nursing assessment, health needs and strengths the family can use to meet those needs will have been identified. Using facts from the data base and principles of client self-determination and client participation in care, the nurse and family can arrive at a list of needs and problems in the family. Because of differing backgrounds and experiences, client and nurse perceptions may not be the same. In any case, a mutually developed set of family needs is always preferable because clients will be more apt to cooperate and assist in resolving problems that they have had a part in identifying.

It is possible that you will find no health problems. It is also possible that you will find *potential* stressors and problems that indicate the need for anticipatory guidance. Your nursing diagnosis may indicate the family's health status in terms of anticipated stressors, dysfunctional communication, or role conflict, for example. Problems may overlap. Gordon suggests describing problems and listing the etiologic factors and their symptoms. This provides a more detailed framework for reaching goals and intervening.[133]

Efforts are under way, in several nursing practice areas to develop specific guidelines for identifying nursing diagnoses. The following are examples of nursing diagnoses as related to the family[134]:

- Children not receiving health care: acute, secondary to divorce and a legal custody struggle
- Difficulty in reallocating family roles: acute, secondary to serious illness and hospitalization of an adult family member
- Inability to accomplish stage-specific developmental tasks: chronic, secondary to dysfunction family communication patterns
- Economic hardship: potential, secondary to prolonged union strike
- Acceptance of a new family member: potential, secondary to plans for adoption
- Abuse: intermittent, secondary to spouse's emotional illness
- Acute medical emergencies: intermittent, secondary to family's lack of knowledge
- System input deprivation: chronic, secondary to living in a nursing home
- Anger: chronic, secondary to being identified as a cultural minority
- Disruption of family transactions: acute, secondary to family reaction to discovery that a member is homosexual

As you and the family sort out the problems, rank them in order of importance to the family. This will help you to know where to begin. In multiproblem families, a long list of problems can seem overwhelming. When the client's life is at stake or community safety is jeopardized, you may not be able to begin where the client wishes.

Miss Goodwin visited the Scoloni family to find out why Mrs. Scoloni hadn't brought 1-year-old Tina to the clinic for her checkup. The Scolonis had no telephone. When Miss Goodwin arrived she found Mrs. Scoloni in tears. Mrs. Scoloni feared she was pregnant, their 3-year-old needed to be hospitalized for a hernia repair, and Mrs. Scoloni's mother had just died. Mrs. Scoloni said she needed to talk to someone about how much she missed her mother and how she feared she couldn't manage without her. Miss Goodwin wisely decided not to discuss Tina's clinic visit with Mrs. Scoloni. She listened while Mrs. Scoloni verbalized her fears. After a while Mrs. Scoloni

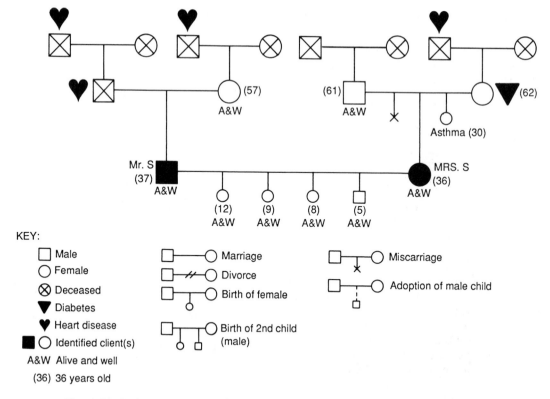

KEY:

☐ Male	
○ Female	
⊗ Deceased	
▼ Diabetes	
♥ Heart disease	
■ ○ Identified client(s)	
A&W Alive and well	
(36) 36 years old	

Marriage
Divorce
Birth of female
Birth of 2nd child (male)

Miscarriage
Adoption of male child

Figure 30–8. A genogram may show patterns of family functioning across generations.

began to relax. Miss Goodwin pointed out some of the strengths she had noticed in Mrs. Scoloni's care and warm concern for her children. She made an appointment to return in a few days to discuss Mrs. Scoloni's other concerns.

Part of problem identification is to sort out those problems you can do something about, those more effectively handled by other members of the health team, and those that can't be handled because of agency or client constraints.

When Miss Goodwin was reviewing Mrs. Scoloni's case, she decided to counsel her about her feelings of loss in relation to the death of her mother. Miss Goodwin referred her for pregnancy testing. It turned out that Mrs. Scoloni was pregnant. Although there were abortion services in the community, abortion was not an option for Mrs. Scoloni. She was a deeply religious woman, and her religion prohibited abortion.

Planning

When problems or needs in the family have been identified, the next step is to develop a plan. "The nursing care plan serves as a blueprint for action."[135] Developing a plan with the family involves mutual goal setting and strategy formation. "A strategy is a plan, method, or series of actions designed to lead to a desired outcome. In nursing, strategies represent the general plan or methods by which nursing action may be brought to bear so as to improve the health of families."[136] Goals must be clear, acceptable to the family, specific, and measurable.

Miss Goodwin was working with Mrs. Asher on improving her communication patterns. Mrs. Asher recognized that she had a tendency to make unilateral decisions in her family. She didn't give others a chance to speak. The family was going to start making vacation plans, so Mrs. Asher developed the following goals with Miss Goodwin's help: "When our family meets this Friday night to discuss vacation plans, I will not give my opinion until I have heard what others in the family think. I will let others know I have heard what they say by restating their opinions. If anyone has not spoken up, I will ask them what they think."

It is useful to set goals according to psychomotor, affective, and cognitive areas. In this way goals can be set according to what the client wants to do, feel, or know. Goals should reflect whether they are client- or nurse-focused.[137] The former refers to goals the client is to achieve; the latter refers to goals for the nurse to achieve.

Miss Goodwin and Mrs. Asher developed the following client-centered goals for Mrs. Asher:

"On Miss Goodwin's next visit, I will demonstrate knowledge of good communication by listing principles of good communication (cognitive goal). I will demonstrate ability to correctly apply knowledge of congruent communication through role playing (cognitive and psychomotor goals). I will work on increasing my self-esteem by discussing at least three strengths I think I have with Miss Goodwin (affective and cognitive goals)."

Miss Goodwin's goals were the following:

- In relation to Mrs. Asher's cognitive goals of learning the principles of good communication, I will review these principles with her on my next visit.
- In relation to Mrs. Asher's cognitive and psychomotor goals of being more congruent in her communication, I will review the use of "I feel" messages with her on my next visit.
- Regarding Mrs. Asher's affective goal of feeling better about herself, I will review a tape on self-affirmation with her on my visit after next.

When goals are decided, the next part of the nursing process is to list alternatives and resources for reaching them. These may include the family, the nurse, and other community resources. Pros and cons of alternatives are listed. The nurse must continually ask herself whether the alternatives will enhance the coping ability of the family and whether the family understands the various courses of action. As part of the goal-setting process, the nurse and the family may develop a contract that includes the goals, the length of the contract, family and nurse responsibilities, and fees if they are charged. Not every client has the motivation, insight, or ability to participate fully in a contract setting, but many can. A contract helps clarify the purpose of the visits and encourages self-care.

Implementation

Implementation is the third component of the nursing process and an important area for the family's involvement in its own care. Client desires, agency constraints, and cultural variables do interact to influence implementation. Components of the nursing roles in implementation are[138]:

Surveillance
Your surveillance of the family's health status involves screening, monitoring through observation and interview, and physical examination.

Teaching
Teaching a family about illness prevention, health maintenance, and skill development to implement a therapeutic regime are important parts of the nursing role. In teaching families, a cardinal rule is to assess learning needs first.

Counseling
You may interact with the client system to help facilitate effective communication or change a behavior the client wishes to change.

Referring
There are a number of health resources in the community to which you can refer the family. These resources may provide financial, educational, vocational, medical, and social services.

Case finding
Determining exposure to communicable disease in family members is often the first step in preventing harmful effects of the disease.

Collaboration
Working with other members of the health

team is essential in providing multidisciplinary care that the family needs to achieve its optimum level of functioning.

Direct care

Laying on of hands is an important part of the nurse's role.

The Life Cycle. Part of the nursing intervention is based on the position of the family in the life cycle.

> For about two years the average family will be childless; for the next twenty years or so, childbearing and child rearing will be central concerns, followed by about six years when children are leaving home for college, marriage, or careers. For approximately 13 years the older couple will be living alone once more, and for the following 16 plus years, the family will be reduced to a widow or widower.[139]

Friedman says that health concerns vary according to stages of the family life cycle.[140] In the beginning, family sexual adjustment, role adjustment, family planning, and prenatal education are primary concerns. For a homosexual couple, sexual and role adjustment are areas of concern.

In the early childbearing stage of the family life cycle, maternity and postpartum care, family planning, well-baby care, childproofing the home, obtaining knowledge about child development, and developing communication skills may be needs. Parents with preschool children have other health concerns. These include protecting children from accidents, arranging for time alone and time together, encouraging socialization of the child, integrating new family members, and caring for children who may have communicable diseases.

When the child enters school, parents need to encourage realistic school achievement for the child as well as work on maintaining a satisfactory marital relationship. As children enter their teen years, automobile, drug, and sex education are important. Parents must also tend to factors such as diet, rest, and exercise in their own lives.

When children leave home, parental health concerns may center around menopause and emerging chronic health conditions. Parents may need help adjusting to changes brought about by their roles as grandparents and also by their aging parents. They may need assistance in reestablishing communication in their own marriage.

The family in retirement may need the nurse's help in dealing with economic, housing, social, and work losses. Health problems may pose special needs. A family member's approaching death may require skilled intervention.[141]

Evaluation

The last step in the nursing process is to evaluate the outcome of care. This means determining if objectives and goals of care have been achieved. Some goals can be measured objectively. A reduction of 20 points, systolically, in a client's blood pressure is an example. Other objectives are measured on a more subjective basis, such as when a client tells you he feels more confident about his ability to relate well to others. Questions to aid you in evaluation include the following:

- What does the family see as outcomes of care? With what areas are they satisfied and dissatisfied? Why?
- Are there any unintended results of care? What are they? (When Mrs. Sebastian went for a blood pressure checkup, the noise, crowding, and long wait in the clinic contributed to a blood pressure increase. This was an unintended outcome of care.) Unintended outcomes can be positive as well as negative.
- Could other members of the health team have intervened more effectively? What would have been the outcome in terms of cost? What benefits would have occurred in the family?

Supervisors, peers, and the nurse's own critical self-awareness are all useful components in evaluating care. This evaluation is fed back into the system and is a basis for altering care, if necessary.[142]

The nursing process is used in caring for families whether you are a community health nurse, a hospital nurse, a psychiatric nurse specializing in family therapy, or a nurse practitioner. Whenever anyone in the family is hospitalized, the client and his family can experience it as a crisis. It is inevitable that the family will experience some disorganization. Whatever support and assistance the nurse can provide to help reestablish equilibrium and maintain family integrity will be helpful.[143] The community health nurse functions as a highly skilled generalist. Where behavioral or emotional problems are severe, she or he may refer the family to a colleague specializing in psychiatric nursing. Where physical problems are intractable, the nurse may use the skills of the family nurse practitioner. All have an important role to play in helping the family to maximize its health. Most important of all is the family itself.

SUMMARY

The family system, as a concept, is very important for professional nurses to study, understand, and appreciate. All individuals have been influenced and shaped to a large degree by their family history and family relationships. Most individuals are vitally linked to some kind of family system. Patterns of health and illness frequently correlate with the strengths, emotional climate, and functional status of the family.

The structure and functions of families have evolved over the ages. Early history gives us a very sketchy view of the particulars of family life, but the concept of families being strong unifying forces within the society is evident. Historic events that have had an impact on the family include urbanization, industrialization, and science and technology. Understanding the history of and changes in family functions, values, and attitudes gives the nurse a baseline perspective from which to better understand present day families.

Families can be studied from a variety of theoretical frameworks. Each of the six frameworks presented in this chapter provides useful ideas and approaches to family study. General systems theory and adaptation theory describe the family as an open, living, social system. The family system has distinct boundaries, functions, and patterns of communication and feedback. As an adaptive system, the family continues to change and grow within a predictable life cycle.

There are specific and fundamental functions that all families participate in. These functions can be broadly categorized into biological, economic, educational, affectual, protective, religious, and recreational. All of these functions are related and interdependent. They are carried out by various members, and by working together, family goals are achieved.

The nuclear family goes through a natural life cycle in which changes in functions and roles can be predicted. Duvall has identified an eight-stage family life cycle that begins with the young married couple and ends with retirement and death. Each of these stages has corresponding developmental tasks that are useful for family assessment and planning.

Understanding family relationships and influences on individuals is inherent in the nurse's ability to carry out the nursing process. This knowledge helps nurses to care for family units, to assess the role of the family in caring for ill members, and to be aware of the impact of illness and hospitalization on the client's family. Family assessment is a logically planned process of gathering data about the family's physical, emotional, and social situation. It is best carried out in the home setting. The nurse focuses on family strengths as well as dysfunctions. Nursing diagnoses are statements of problems in the family or areas of need or concern. They are mutually arrived at and serve as a basis for planning and intervention.

Developing a plan for caring for the family involves mutual goal setting and strategy formation. Goals are specified both in terms of nursing and client goals. Intervention with families is carried out through health surveillance, teaching, counseling, referring, and casefinding. Evaluation is accomplished by measuring criteria to determine if objectives and goals have been achieved. Whatever the outcome of the evaluation is, it is fed back into the system as a basis for continuing or altering nursing care, as necessary.

The care of families and their indiviaul members is practiced by nurses in every setting. The degree to which family assessment and intervention is carried out varies. Whatever the circumstance, involvement with family groups is a challenging and rewarding part of the nursing experience.

Study Questions

1. Give several examples of how the nurse might use knowledge of family history in clinical situations.

2. Explain why families are often referred to as open living systems.

3. Give three examples of family subsystems.

4. Analyze the power and decision-making structure in a family you know. How does it compare with your own family experience?

5. Give an example of a communication problem in a family. What are some ways in which the nurse might help the family overcome the problem.

6. Draw a genogram of your family or a family you know.

7. Why is it important and therapeutic for the nurse to assess family strengths as well as problem areas?

References

1. John Biesanz and Mavis Biesanz, *Modern Society* (Englewood Cliffs, N.J.: Prentice-Hall, 1968), 209–210.
2. Dennis H. Wrong and Harry L. Gracey, *Readings in Introductory Sociology* (New York: Macmillan Co., 1972), 72.
3. Evelyn Rose Benson and Joan Quinn McDevitt, *Community Health and Nursing Practice* (Englewood Cliffs, N.J.: Prentice-Hall, 1980), 239.
4. Cynthia J. Leitch and Richard V. Tinker, *Primary Care* (Philadelphia: F.A. Davis Co., 1978), 4, 23.
5. Jean R. Miller and Ellen H. Janosik, *Family-Focused Care* (New York: McGraw-Hill Book Co., 1980), 6.
6. Celeste R. Phillips, *Family-Centered Maternity-Newborn Care* (St. Louis: C.V. Mosby Co., 1980), 207.
7. Jeanette Lancaster, *Community Mental Health Nursing* (St. Louis: C.V. Mosby Co., 1980), 265.
8. Evelyn Millis Duvall, *Marriage and Family Development*, 5th ed. (Philadelphia: J.B. Lippincott Co., 1977).
9. Michael P. Farrell and Madeline H. Schmitt, "The American family: An historical perspective," in D.P. Hymovich and M.U. Barnard, eds., *Family Health Care*, 2nd ed., Vol. 1 (New York: McGraw-Hill Book Co., 1979), 57.
10. Miller and Janosik, *Family Focused Care*, 16.
11. Gerald R. Leslie, *The Family in Social Context*, 4th ed. (New York: Oxford University Press, 1979), 147, 148.
12. Ruth Murray and Judith Zentner, *Nursing Concepts for Health Promotion* (Englewood Cliffs, N.J.: Prentice-Hall, 1975), 348.
13. *Ibid.*
14. Amos H. Hawley; *Urban Society* (New York: Ronald Press Co., 1971), 120–23.
15. Michael Gordon, *The Nuclear Family in Crisis* (New York: Harper & Row, 1972), 6, 10.
16. William J. Goode, "Industrialization and family structure," in Norman W. Bell and Ezra F. Vogel, eds., *Family* (New York: Free Press, 1968), 113–20.
17. Murray and Zentner, *Nursing Concepts for Health Promotion*, 348, 362.
18. Irene Mortenson Burnside, *Psychosocial Nursing Care of the Aged* (New York: McGraw-Hill Book Co., 1980), 2–3.
19. Robert E. Rakel, *Principles of Family Medicine* (Philadelphia: W.B. Saunders Co., 1977), 249.
20. Edgar W. Butler, *Urban Sociology* (New York: Harper & Row, 1976), 389.
21. Elmer H. Johnson, *Social Problems of Urban Man* (Homewood, Ill.: Dorsey Press, 1973), 188.
22. *Ibid*, 97.
23. Miller and Janosik, *Family-Focused Care*, 28.
24. Goode, "Industrialization and family structure," 113.
25. Evelyn M. Duvall and Brent C. Miller, *Marriage and Family Development*, 6th ed. (New York: Harper & Row, 1985), 47.
26. Duvall, *Marriage and Family Development*, 136.
27. *Ibid*, 220.
28. "The calamitous decline of the American family," *The Washington Post*, January 2, 1977, C1.
29. Mary Jo Bane, *Here to Stay: American Families in the Twentieth Century* (New York: Basic Books, 1976).
30. I. Nye and F. Berardo, *Emerging Conceptual Frameworks in Family Analysis*, (New York: Macmillan Co., 1966).
31. Marilyn M. Friedman, *Family Nursing, Theory and Assessment*. (New York: Appleton-Century-Crofts, 1981), 45.

32. Friedman, *Family Nursing, Theory and Assessment*, 75.
33. Carrie Jo Braden and Nancy L. Herban, *Community Health: A Systems Approach* (New York: Appleton-Century-Crofts, 1976), 36.
34. Friedman, *Family Nursing, Theory and Assessment*, 8.
35. F. Ivan Nye and Felix W. Berardo, *The Family* (New York: Macmillan Co., 1973), 16.
36. Barbara Spradley, *Community Health Nursing—Concepts and Practices* (Boston: Little, Brown & Co., 1981), 239.
37. John G. Red Horse, "Family structure and value orientation in American Indians," *Soc Casework* 61, (September 1980), 462–63.
38. Friedman, *Family Nursing, Theory and Assessment*, 9.
39. Spradley, *Community Health Nursing*, 239.
40. Jay Cocks, "How long till equality?" *Time* (July 12, 1982):24.
41. Spradley, *Community Health Nursing*, 239.
42. Friedman, *Family Nursing, Theory and Assessment*, 8.
43. Nick Stinnett and James Walter, *Relationships in Marriage and Family* (New York: Macmillan Co., 1977), 36.
44. Nye and Berardo, *The Family*, 16.
45. *Ibid.*, 43–46.
46. *Ibid.*, 36.
47. *Ibid.*
48. Red Horse, "Family structure and value," 462.
49. Susan L. Jones, *Family Therapy—A Comparison of Approaches* (Bowie, Md.: Robert J. Brady, 1980), 76.
50. David Kantor and William Lehr, *Inside the Family* (New York: Harper & Row, 1976), 37.
51. *Ibid.*, 42.
52. Robert Sommer, *Personal Space* (Englewood Cliffs, N.J.: Prentice-Hall, 1969), 39–57.
53. Kantor and Lehr, *Inside the Family*, 42.
54. *Ibid.*, 42–44, 82–89.
55. Jones, *Family Therapy*, 63–64.
56. Kantor and Lehr, *Inside the Family*, 44–46.
57. *Ibid.*, 91.
58. Friedman, *Family Nursing, Theory and Assessment*, 149.
59. F. Ivan Nye, *Role Structure and Analysis of the Family* (Beverly Hills, Calif.: Sage Publications, 1976), vii.
60. Friedman, *Family Nursing, Theory and Assessment*, 149.
61. Nye and Berardo, *The Family*, 265.
62. F. Ivan Nye and Viktor Gecas, "The role concept: Review and delineation," in F. Ivan Nye, *Role Structure and Analysis of the Family* (Beverly Hills, Calif.: Sage Publications, 1976), 13.
63. Cocks, "How long till equality?", 21.
64. Stan L. Albrecht, Howard M. Bahr, and Bruce Chadwick, "Changing family and sex roles: An assessment of age differences." *J Marriage Fam* 41, (February 1979):41–50.
65. Audrey D. Smith, "Egalitarian marriage implications for practice and policy," *Soc Casework*, 61, (May 1980):288–95.
66. Friedman, *Family Nursing, Theory and Assessment*, 156.
67. *Ibid.*
68. *Ibid.*, 151.
69. Nye, *Role Structure*, 24.
70. Friedman, *Family Nursing, Theory and Assessment*, 151.
71. *Ibid.*, 130.
72. Nye and Berardo, *The Family*, 307.
73. Gerald W. McDonald, "Family power: The assessment of a decade of theory and research, 1970–1979," *J Marriage Fam*, 42, (November 1980):843.
74. Letha Scanzoni and John Scanzoni, "Progress in marriage: power, negotiation, and conflict," in Helene Lopata, ed., *Family Factbook* (Chicago: Marquis Academic Media, 1978), 132.
75. Friedman, *Family Nursing, Theory and Assessment*, 131–32.
76. *Ibid.*
77. McDonald, "Family power," 844.
78. Friedman, *Family Nursing, Theory and Assessment*, 132.
79. *Ibid.*, 133.
80. *Ibid.*, 134.
81. Sara E. Archer, "Politics and economics: How things really work," in Sarah E. Archer and Ruth P. Fleshman, eds., *Community Health Nursing—Patterns and Practices*, 2nd ed., (North Scituate, Mass.: Duxbury Press, 1979), 286.
82. Nye and Berardo, *The Family*, 305.
83. Friedman, *Family Nursing, Theory and Assessment*, 134–35.
84. *Ibid.*, 135–38.
85. P.H. Glasser and L.N. Glasser, *Families in Crisis* (New York: Harper & Row, 1970), 8.
86. Joanne E. Hall and Barbara R. Weaver, *Distributive Nursing Practice* (Philadelphia: J.B. Lippincott Co., 1977), 110.
87. *Ibid.*, 111.
88. Miller and Janosik, *Family-Focused Care*, 141.
89. Virginia Satir, *Conjoint Family Therapy* (Palo Alto, Calif: Science and Behavior Books, 1967). 1967).
90. Friedman, *Family Nursing, Theory and Assessment*, 74, 78.
91. Rosemary J. McKeighen, "Principles of family counseling," in Debra Hymovich and Martha

Underwood, *Family Health Care,* 2nd ed., vol. 1. (New York: McGraw-Hill Book Co., 1979), 312.

92. Rakel, *Principles of Family Medicine,* 264.
93. Friedman, *Family Nursing, Theory and Assessment,* 84.
94. Harold Herman and Mary Elisabeth McKay, *Community Health Services* (Washington D.C.: International City Managers' Association, 1968), 180.
95. Friedman, *Family Nursing, Theory and Assessment,* 85.
96. *Parenting: A Parent's Workbook:* (The American Red Cross, 1978), 13.
97. Bane, *Here to Stay,* 100.
98. Friedman, *Family Nursing, Theory and Assessment,* 97.
99. Evelyn Duvall, *Faith in Families* (Chicago: Rand McNally & Co, 1970), 32.
100. *Ibid.*
101. Daniel A. Prescott "Role of love in human development," *Marriage and Family in the Modern World* (New York: Thomas Y. Crowell Co., 1960), 191.
102. Rakel, *Principles of Family Medicine,* 279.
103. Duvall, *Marriage and Family Development,* 137–48.
104. *Ibid.*
105. Friedman, *Family Nursing, Theory and Assessment,* 229.
106. Claire Tuchalski, "Identification of needs of goals," in Ilse R. Leeser, Claire Tuchalski, and Rosine Carotenuto, eds., *Community Health Nursing* (Flushing, N.Y.: Medical Examination Publishing Co., 1975), 76–83.
107. *Ibid.*
108. Helen Cohn and Joyce Tingle, *Manual for Nurses in Family and Community Health,* 2nd ed. (Boston: Little, Brown, & Co., 1974), 10.
109. Paulette Robischon and Judith A. Smith, "Family assessment," in Adina M. Reinhardt and Mildred D. Quinn, eds., *Family Centered Community Health Nursing,* vol. 1 (St. Louis: C.V. Mosby Co., 1977), 45.
110. Friedman, *Family Nursing, Theory and Assessment,* 303–04.
111. *Ibid.,* 303.
112. Tuchalski, "Identification of needs and goals," 76.
113. Friedman, *Family Nursing, Theory and Assessment,* 303–04.
114. *Ibid.,* 303.
115. *Ibid.,* 99.
116. Carol Lockhart, "Family-focused community health nursing in the home," in S.E. Archer and R.P. Fleshman, *Patterns and Practices,* 2nd ed.

(North Scituate, Mass.: Duxbury Press, 1979), 165.
117. Friedman, *Family Nursing, Theory and Assessment,* 302–03.
118. Virginia Satir, *Peoplemaking* (Palo Alto, Calif.: Science and Behavior Books, 1972), 59–79.
119. Stinnett and Walter, *Relationships in Marriage and Family,* 129–33.
120. *Ibid.,* 136.
121. *Ibid.,* 155–62.
122. Susan A. Clemem, Diane G. Eigsti, and Sandra McGuire, *Comprehensive Family and Community Health Nursing* (New York: McGraw-Hill Book Co., 1981), 159.
123. Friedman, *Family Nursing, Theory and Assessment,* 97.
124. *Ibid.,* 95–96.
125. Robischon and Smith, "Family assessment," 95.
126. Friedman, *Family Nursing, Theory and Assessment,* 102.
127. Spradley, *Community Health Nursing,* 181.
128. *Ibid.,* 182.
129. Herbert A. Otto, "Developing human and family potential," in Nick Stinnett, Barbara Chesser, John DeFrain, eds., *Building Family Strength* (Lincoln: University of Nebraska Press, 1979), 39–50.
130. Clemen, Eigsti, and McGuire, *Family and Community Health,* 163.
131. Ann Hartman, "Diagrammatic assessment of family relationships," *Soc Casework,* 59, (October, 1980):465–72.
132. *Ibid.,* 472.
133. Friedman, *Family Nursing, Theory and Assessment,* 33.
134. Lillie M. Shortridge and Juanita Lee, *Introduction to Nursing Practice* (New York: McGraw-Hill Book Co., 1980), 496.
135. *Ibid.,* 35.
136. Ruth B. Freeman and Janet Heinrich, *Community Health Nursing Practice,* 2nd ed. (Philadelphia: W.B. Saunders Co., 1981), 100.
137. Clemen, Eigsti, and McGuire, *Family and Community Health,* 202.
138. Friedman, *Family Nursing, Theory and Assessment,* 37.
139. Freeman and Heinrich, *Community Health Nursing Practice,* 101–19.
140. *Ibid.,* p. 93.
141. Friedman, *Family Nursing, Theory and Assessment,* 50–62.
142. *Ibid.,* 38.
143. Janet M. Barber, Lillian G. Stokes, and Diane Billings, *Adult Child Care* (St. Louis: C.V. Mosby Co., 1977), 162.

Annotated Bibliography

Duvall, E.M. 1985. *Marriage and Family Development,* 6th ed. New York: Harper & Row. This is a classic textbook on the family and is widely known for the author's original work on the concept of the family life cycle and family developmental tasks.

Friedman, M.M. 1986. *Family Nursing, Theory, and Assessment.* East Norwalk, Conn.: Appleton-Century-Crofts. This is an excellent nursing text on family concepts and family theory. Family health assessment is covered in detail with separate sections devoted to communication patterns in the family, power, structures, roles, family values, and numerous functions within the family. The appendix provides guidelines for family assessment including case studies and sample care plans.

Kantor, D., Lehr, W. 1976. *Inside the Family.* New York: Harper & Row. This book presents family dynamics with an excellent section on all types of boundaries within families. It is clearly written and gives a thorough analysis of the necessary processes that go on within a family system.

McGoldrick, M., Gerson, R. 1985. *Genograms in Family Assessment.* New York: Norton. This book presents thorough and detailed instructions in how to interview families for genogram construction and how to draw the genogram. Examples are given using famous families.

Miller, J.R., Janosik, E.H. 1978. *Family-Focused Care.* Philadelphia: F.A. Davis. This general text on families and family health care uses a general systems theory framework. It provides a good overview of family theory and family development and discusses the common events with which families often need professional intervention and help. Sections on assessment, planning, and intervention processes by health-care workers are delineated.

Miller, S.R., Winstead-Fry, P. 1982. *Family Systems Theory in Nursing Practice.* Reston, Va.: Reston. This book presents an introduction to Bowen's family systems theory, which was developed from psychiatric clinical practice as a treatment plan for dysfunctional families. It is somewhat high level for beginning students but clearly illustrates how systems theory can be utilized in practice.

Chapter 31

Community Concepts

Eliza M. Wolff

Chapter Outline

- Objectives
- Glossary
- Introduction
- Concepts in Studying the Community
    The Community as a System
    Types of Communities
    The Concept of Community Health
    Epidemiology
- Community Health Nursing
- Settings for Community Health
  Nursing Practice
    Official Agencies
    Voluntary Agencies
    Other Settings for Practice
- The Nursing Process
    Community Assessment
    Planning
    Implementation
    Evaluation
- Summary
- Study Questions
- References
- Annotated Bibliography

Objectives

At the completion of this chapter the reader will be able to:

▶ Define the concept of community
▶ Describe the epidemiological framework of the host-agent-environment
▶ List rates commonly used in community health to describe the health status of a community
▶ Describe the purpose of community health nursing
▶ Describe the role of community health nurses
▶ Apply the nursing process to a community health problem

Glossary

Agent. That factor without which a disease cannot occur.

Community Assessment. The determination of health needs of a community based on its health status, its ability to deal with its health problems, and ways in which it is likely to handle these problems.

Community Health Nursing. Nursing of population groups that emphasizes prevention and health promotion, comprehensiveness and continuity of care, and application of current nursing and public health principles.

Epidemic. The outbreak of a disease above that statistically expected in terms of numbers of people affected.

Epidemiology. The study of the determinants and distribution of health, injury, and disease.

Evaluation. Determination of the achievement of a goal or objective, or determination of the worth of something.

Host. A species capable of being infected by a disease.

Incidence. New cases of disease occurring in a particular time period.

Planning. The development of an interrelated series of steps to achieve a certain goal or objective.

Prevalence. Cases of a disease existing at a particular point in time.

Primary Prevention. The prevention of an illness before it occurs.

Secondary Prevention. The early detection and treatment of an illness or condition to prevent further damage.

Tertiary Prevention. Maximum rehabilitation and prevention of further damage from an illness or condition.

INTRODUCTION

Understanding the basic concepts and characteristics of communities is important to nurses in any setting. A person's community often has a great deal to do with that person's overall health status and ability to seek care and stay healthy. Nurses will be better able to understand, assess, plan, and evaluate nursing interventions if they can appreciate what the client's community is like. Nurses trained in community health nursing often plan broadly based nursing interventions involving the health of an entire community. For this kind of nursing, understanding community concepts is crucial, since large numbers of people are affected.

CONCEPTS IN STUDYING THE COMMUNITY

The Community as a System

A *community* is a group of people living together in a particular place. These people may share interests, values, and purposes in addition to common boundaries. Relationships as well as boundaries may bind them together. Most definitions of community emphasize people, place, and resources and the relationships that hold these elements together. Groups, organi-zations, towns, and countries can all be considered communities.[1]

Communities are unique systems, each having suprasystems, subsystems, and varied inputs, throughputs, outputs, and feedback.[2] Suprasystems of a city are the state, the nation, and the world. Some subsystems of the city are its health, welfare, police, fire, and recreation departments. Suprasystems and subsystems of any community interact to give each community its unique identity.

Types of Communities

Archer and Fleshman categorize communities as emotional, structural, and functional. They stress that these categories are not mutually exclusive. *Emotional communities* are characterized by a special feeling. Such communities may be "belonging" communities, the place where a person feels at home. Another type of emotional community may be special interest groups. People committed to one another are a powerful tool in obtaining needed care for individuals and groups in that community. Family members, volunteers, churches, and philanthropic organizations may provided needed resources for clients.[3]

Structural communities, those with temporal and spatial boundaries, are divided into six categories: aggregates, face-to-face communities, communities of problem ecology, geopolitical communities, organizations, and communities of solution.

Aggregates are any group of people. They may simply be a group of people waiting for a bus. This concept is important when considering disease transmission. *Face-to-face communities* are close-knit, relatively small groups, such as neighborhoods and parishes. *A community of problem ecology* is a geographic area with a common problem. *Geopolitical communities* have definite legal as well as geographic boundaries. Census tracts, wards, and counties are geopolitical communities. *Organizations* are communities having purpose and structure that bind members together. A health department is an example of an organization. *Communities of solution* are those within which a problem may be defined, confronted, and resolved.

It is important to be aware of community boundaries because culture, policies, services, and reimbursement may vary according to these boundaries. Vital statistics are collected from geopolitical communities such as counties and states. Surveys of health and illness are conducted within clearly defined areas. Differences reflected in morbidity (sickness) and mortality (death) may reflect vulnerable groups needing nursing intervention.[4]

In addition to emotional and structural communities, Archer and Fleshman's third type of community is the *functional community*. The emphasis in these communities is on achievement for the common good rather than on geographic boundaries. Similarities can be seen in the concept of functional communities and the concepts of communities of special interest and problem ecology. Archer and Fleshman break functional communities into communities of identifiable need and critical mass communities. A *community of identifiable need* includes all people with a common problem but does not include boundaries. An example of such a community would be families of abused children. A *critical mass community* implies achievement. It is that combination of resources (manpower, money, equipment, and supplies) needed for the solution of a problem. The concept is an important one when considering the multiple resources that may be used in health care.[5]

The concepts of community emphasize emotion, structure, and function. Knowledge of community characteristics and their relationship and impact on clients will help the community health nurse to deliver effective client care for individuals, families, groups, and larger populations within the community.

The Concept of Community Health

The terms community health and public health are used interchangeably. In 1920, Winslow defined public health. His definition is still applicable today. Winslow said,

Public health is the Science and Art of (1) preventing disease, (2) prolonging life, and (3) promoting health and efficiency through organized community effort for

(a) the sanitation of the environment
(b) the control of communicable infections

(c) the education of the individual in personal hygiene
(d) the organization of medical and nursing services for the early diagnosis and preventive treatment of disease, and
(e) the development of the social machinery to insure everyone a standard of living adequate for the maintenance of health,

so organizing these benefits as to enable every citizen to realize his birthright of health and longevity.[6]

Epidemiology

Epidemiology is one of the basic disciplines of community health. Epidemiology comes from several Greek words: *epi* meaning down or on, *demos* referring to people, and *logos* meaning study of knowledge. Thus, epidemiology refers to the study of what comes down on the people.[7] Epidemiology is the study of the distribution and determinants of health, injury, and illness in populations. The term **epidemic** is derived from epidemiology and refers to the outbreak of a disease or harmful process that affects a higher-than-expected number of people. Epidemiological studies provide evidence about the severity and impact of disease and the effectiveness of preventive and treatment measures. This information is vital for planning and evaluation purposes.[8]

In the nineteenth and early-twentieth centuries, epidemiology focused on cholera, plague, other acute infectious diseases, and nutritional deficiencies. Today it focuses additionally on determinants of health and ills that affect mankind. Death, disease, disability, defects, social discord, and wellness come under its purview.[9] Investigations of personal and environmental factors related to an increased risk of heart attacks, cancer, and strokes; factors relating to more effective coping in activities of daily living among arthritis victims; studies of factors associated with compliance to medication regimens; studies of accident patterns; and investigations of determinants of suicide, homicide, and violence are some examples of epidemiological investigations. The most recent and dramatic example of present-day epidemiological study is inquiry into the epidemiology of acquired immune deficiency syndrome (AIDS).

Host, Agent, and Environment. The triad of host, agent, and environment is the framework used in epidemiological investigations. Epidemiologists study the interaction of host, agent, and environmental factors and their relationship to health outcome. Intervention may occur in any of the three areas.

HOST. The **host** is that species capable of being affected by disease. Host factors to be discussed in this section include demographic (population) characteristics, health status, genetic susceptibility, body defenses, and health behavior. *Demographic characteristics* include age, sex, ethnicity, occupation, and marital status. Each of these factors may be related to disease. For example, the risk of stroke increases as age increases. Cancer is more common in women. Black males have the highest incidence of hypertension, and black lung disease is associated with the occupation of mining.

Another important host characteristic is *health status.* "Street people," those who have no homes and sleep on the streets, are vulnerable to poor health status. They have an increased disease risk caused by lack of shelter, exposure to harsh climatic elements, and poor nutrition.

Other important host factors to consider are *genetic susceptibility* and *body defenses* such as skin, mucous membranes, and the immune system. In addition, the *health behavior* of the population is an important host factor to consider. This includes the population's dietary patterns, hygiene characteristics, recreation, and means of handling stress.

AGENT. In the host-agent-environment triad, **agent** refers to the presence or absence of an etiologic factor or factors. Agents may be biological, physical, or chemical. Living organisms, such as bacteria, viruses, helminths, and arthropods are examples of *biological agents. Physical*

agents include temperature, noise, and radiation. *Chemical agents* includes gases, dusts, liquids, and vapors. An example of an *absent agent* leading to disease would be the lack of vitamin C, causing scurvy. Sometimes agents influencing health and illness are unknown.

Agents require a habitat (or reservoir), a portal of exit, means of transmission to the host, and portal of entry.[10] The reservoir may be human or animal—a rat, squirrel, or bird. The diagram in Figure 31–1 illustrates the chain of causation.

In many illnesses today, the pathway is not so straightforward. Diseases are caused by many factors that interact.

ENVIRONMENT. "Major components of the environment may be identified as *physical, biological, social, cultural,* and *economic.* The status of these variables within the environment may enhance or inhibit the interaction between the host and the agent."[11] *Physical* features of the environment include such factors as climate, geography, weather, and terrain. For example, the incidence of muscular dystrophy increases in cold climates.

Biological features include animal and arthropod reservoirs and food supply.[12] *Social* features may include density and crowding, for example. *Cultural* features may include knowledge, customs, language, values, and institutions transmitted from one generation to the next. *Economic* features include income level of the population, level of employment, and sources of production, distribution, and consumption.

The concept of a vulnerable host, a harmful agent or agents, and factors in the environment interacting to influence a community's health and illness patterns are important in understanding a community's health status

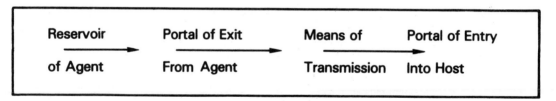

Figure 31–1. The chain of causation in disease transmission.

and providing a framework for intervention.

Methods of Epidemiology. The essence of epidemiological investigation is comparison. How does a group with a disease differ from one without the disease? Epidemiologists investigate the who, what, how, when, where, and why of death and disease.

Epidemiological methods encompass descriptive, analytic, and experimental studies. In *descriptive* studies, the epidemiologist describes patterns of health or illness in terms of occurrence, place of occurrence, and personal characteristics of the population affected. By studying these patterns, the scientist may develop hunches about wellness or disease causation.

In *analytic epidemiology,* the epidemiologist employs prospective (forward-looking), retrospective (backward-looking), or experimental studies to test hypotheses about the determinants of health or illness. Inferences are made on the basis of comparisons.

Prospective (forward-looking) studies are known as cohort studies. In these studies, the investigator studies selected characteristics of a population over time in terms of exposure to or existence of certain factors. The Framingham study is an example of a prospective study.[13] In this study, a population was studied over a number of years to dtermine who developed heart disease in relation to cigarette smoking, weight, levels of systolic and diastolic blood pressure, serum lipids, and other selected biochemical factors.[14] Prospective studies are a valuable means of gaining information but are time-consuming and expensive to conduct.

Retrospective (backward-looking) studies are referred to as case control studies. They refer to the comparison of recorded cases with a particular health pattern or illness with those without it. Individuals without the condition are called controls. Studying past records to determine smoking history among patients with lung cancer and those without it is an example of a retrospective or case control study. Retrospective studies are not as expensive as prospective studies, but problems with the data may be caused by missing data and incomplete recall on the part of study subjects.

Experimental studies are conducted to determine the effectiveness of a therapeutic or preventive mode of treatment. Study subjects are assigned randomly to treatment (experimental) and control groups.[15] The experimental and control groups are similar on major variables affecting the outcome of the study, but the experimental group is given the treatment and the control group is not.

Terms Used in Epidemiology. Incidence and *prevalence* are terms commonly used in epidemiological investigations. **Incidence** refers to new cases of a disease occurring within a particular period of time. Where incidence is short lived, as in outbreaks of food poisoning, incidence rates are referred to as attack rates.[16] **Prevalence** refers to number of cases at any one point in time. Prevalence depends on the number of people having the disease and the duration of the disease and is important to know in determining resources needed for health care.[17]

Facts about the health of a community may be displayed numerically with statistics. The term *biostatistics* refers to the use of statistics applied to biological data. Vital statistics are those events affecting the lives of population groups: births, illnesses, deaths, marriages, and divorce. They are collected on the local level and compiled on both a state and national level.

Statistics are expressed as percentages, ratios, or rates. All of these are useful in comparing one group with another. Percentages are used to clarify relationships between numbers based on 100.[18] If 10 out of 40 children contract measles, that is 25 percent. Ratios show the proportion of one group to another and are useful in comparing data. Rates are indicators of community health. They are proportions expressed in terms of the population at risk. Specific rates that are commonly used in community health are found in Table 31–1.

The *crude birth rate* is an important indicator in determining population increase or decrease. The estimated midyear population is used to account for population immigration and emigration through the year. The midyear usually is July 1. Crude birth rates are important as one indicator in determining need for programs, such as family planning, childbirth education, obstetrical hospital beds and manpower, schools, and recreational facilities.

Crude death rates require caution in their interpretation because they do not give information about cause of death, whether the death

TABLE 31–1. SPECIFIC RATES COMMONLY USED IN COMMUNITY HEALTH

1. Crude birth rate $= \dfrac{\text{number of live births in a given year} \times 1000}{\text{estimated midyear population}}$

2. Annual crude death rate $= \dfrac{\text{number of deaths in a given year} \times 1000}{\text{estimated midyear population}}$

3. Infant mortality rate $= \dfrac{\text{number of deaths of infants under one year of age in a given year} \times 1000}{\text{number of live births during the same year}}$

4. Neonatal mortality rate $= \dfrac{\text{number of deaths under 28 days of age in a given year} \times 1000 \text{ or } 10,000}{\text{number of live births during the same year}}$

5. Fetal mortality rate

$= \dfrac{\text{number of fetal deaths of specified period of gestation in a given year} \times 1000}{\text{number of live births plus number of fetal deaths of specified period of gestation during that same year}}$

6. Perinatal mortality rate $= \dfrac{\text{fetal deaths plus neonatal deaths in a given year} \times 1000}{\text{fetal deaths plus live births in the same year}}$

7. Maternal mortality rate

$= \dfrac{\text{number of deaths attributed to maternal conditions in a given year} \times 10,000 \text{ or } 100,000}{\text{number of live births in that same year}}$

8. Annual age-specific mortality $= \dfrac{\text{number of deaths in a specific age group} \times 1000}{\text{midyear population of the age group}}$

9. Case-specific fatality rate $= \dfrac{\text{number of deaths in a given time period} \times 100}{\text{total number of people with the disease in the same time period}}$

10. Annual cause-specific death rate $= \dfrac{\text{number of deaths from a specific cause in a given year} \times 100,000}{\text{estimated midyear population}}$

^{a}Expressed in terms of the population at risk.

was preventable, and who actually died. More specific information is needed for program planning purposes and for comparing death rates of one group to another.

The *infant mortality rate* is regarded as a highly sensitive indicator of a community's health status. A high rate may reflect poor nutrition, inadequate sanitation, lack of knowledge, inadequate health-care practices, inadequate shelter, and high infection rates. Rates vary from one location to another and from one ethnic group to another. A high infant mortality rate is a red flag signaling a need for community health intervention.[19]

The *neonatal mortality rate* reflects infants dying in the first month of life. Many infants who die in the first month of life have congenital malformation and are poorly equipped for survival. They are a highly vulnerable population.

The *fetal death rate* is derived from fetal deaths that are categorized according to period of gestation. An early fetal death refers to death

prior to the 20th week of gestation. An intermediate death refers to death from the 20th to less than 28th week of gestation. A late fetal death refers to the gestational period of 28 weeks or more. A death is described as a fetal death if there are no signs of life after expulsion by the mother. Fetal deaths are often underreported because definitions vary from state to state, and abortions are often not reported.[20]

Fetal deaths and neonatal deaths are used to derive the *perinatal mortality rate*. The risk of death is greatest in the perinatal period and then later again in old age.[21]

The *maternal mortality rate* measures deaths associated with pregnancy, delivery, and the puerperium and extends to 90 days postpartum. You will note that in this rate, the numerator is not derived from the denominator. This rate is expressed in terms of 10,000 or 100,000 live births. Because the maternal mortality rate is so low, in order for the number to be meaningful, it must be multiplied by these larger figures.[22] Maternal mortality is an important indicator of community health status.

The *annual age-specific mortality rate* refers to the proportion of people in a particular age group who die in a given time period.

The *case-specific fatality rate* refers to the proportion of people with a particular disease who die from the disease. Note that this proportion is multiplied by 100.

The *annual cause-specific death rate* refers to the proportion of the total population dying from a particular cause. Note that this proportion is multiplied by 100,000.

In addition to percentages, ratios, and rates, other statistical indices that are useful in analyzing data pertaining to groups include means, ranges, medians, and modes.

COMMUNITY HEALTH NURSING

Health care outside the hospital setting is becoming increasingly necessary because of the rising cost of hospital health care; the increase in the aging population; and the need to learn to live with chronic illness, manage stress, prevent illness, and enhance the quality of life. The 1979 Surgeon General's Report stated, ". . . of the 10 leading causes of death in the United States, at least seven could be substantially reduced if persons at risk improved just five habits: diet, smoking, lack of exercise, alcohol abuse, and use of antihypertensive medications."[23] Community health nurses can make an important contribution to their clients' health as they teach them about the importance of a healthy life style and help them prevent illness and cope more effectively.

The purposes of **community health nursing** are to prevent illness, promote health, and provide care to individuals, families, and groups of various ages and health needs in the community. Community health nursing had its beginnings in 1859 in England when William Rathbone established visiting nurse services for the sick poor. Florence Nightingale assisted in training these nurses. In 1879, the New York Mission employed the first visiting nurses in America.[24] One hundred years later, it was estimated that there were 80,523 registered nurses working in community health in America. This was 6.5 per-

cent of the nation's 1,235,152 employed nurses. These community health nurses worked primarily at the local level, particularly for health departments and visiting nurse associations. It was estimated that another 43,539 (3.5 percent) worked for student services, and 28,112 (2.3 percent) worked in occupational health.[25] Community health nurses, whether in a health department, school, industry, clinic, or other type of setting, have an important opportunity to emphasize the importance of preventive, continuous, and comprehensive care as they carry out the nursing process. Community health nurses work with other disciplines and play a key part in promoting the physical, social, and mental health of individuals, families, groups, and communities.

Preventing illness involves implementing and fostering three kinds of prevention. **Primary prevention** is the prevention of an illness before it occurs. **Secondary prevention** includes early detection and treatment of an illness or condition to prevent further damage. **Tertiary prevention** includes maximum rehabilitation and prevention of further damage from an existing illness or condition.

Immunizing an infant against diphtheria, pertussis, tetanus, polio, and mumps is an example of primary prevention. Screening programs for hypertension, diabetes, or glaucoma, are also examples of primary prevention.

Coordinating school screening programs to detect possible vision and hearing abnormalities is an example of secondary prevention (Fig. 31–2). Prompt referral and subsequent treatment of children who fail screening programs are important in the prevention of learning difficulties.

Helping a client revise his work schedule, minimize stress, and follow his diet after a heart attack exemplify tertiary prevention. This type of nursing care fosters rehabilitation and lessens chances of further damage to the client's heart.

In community health nursing, prevention of illness and the care of population groups are emphasized. Interdisciplinary care is rendered to promote the health of the whole group. Needs in the population may fall anywhere on the health–illness continuum and may be acute or chronic. Although community health care is usually given to clients outside the hospital, nurses may work in ambulatory care settings

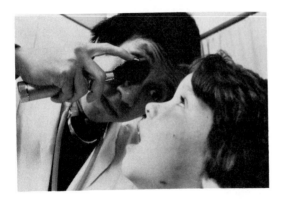

Figure 31–2. Screening programs are important in the detection of health problems.

and in discharge planning within hospitals. The following example illustrates community health workers in action (Fig. 31–3).

> After the Vietnam War, a large number of Indo-Chinese refugees came to the United States. Many suffered severe economic and emotional hardships in leaving their homeland. They came with no possessions; some had lost their entire family. Many were infected with tuberculosis, malaria, and parasites. They arrived in immediate need of food, shelter, clothing, and health care. Community health nurses participated in screening and health programs for these newly arrived refugees as part of a complete health-care team. Nursing and medical efforts involved primary prevention (immunizations), secondary prevention (early detection of tuberculosis), and tertiary prevention (treatment of social, emotional and physical illnesses).
>
> Through training in public health and the physical and social sciences, community health nurses and other community health workers were sensitive to the fact that these uprooted people now faced Western values and customs totally new to them. The community health nurses prepared brochures for health-care workers on Indo-Chinese customs and, for the refugees, materials on health department services. One way in which nurses assisted refugees in their cultural adaptation was by helping them find stores selling Asian foods. The nurses assisted the reguees in their social adaptation by listening carefully and helping them meet

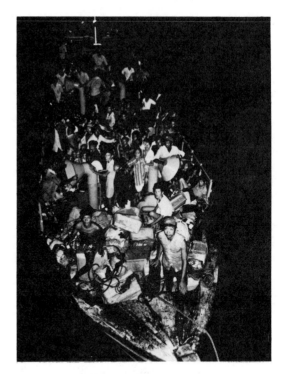

Figure 31–3. Refugees are a group with special health needs.

> other Asian families within the community. Helping refugees to adapt physically and socially was accomplished by providing care in health department clinics and by referring them for language training, schooling, and other needed services. Community health nurses provided care to meet ongoing needs that spanned the health-illness continuum.

Community and Role. This example illustrates a tenet of community health nursing—that role is shaped by health needs of the community.[26] If tuberculosis is rampant, much time may be spent in casefinding and follow-up. Where neonatal and infant mortality rates are high, the nurse may spend more time in maternal and child health programs stressing prenatal teaching and counseling, postpartum follow-up, anticipatory guidance, and family planning. The community health nurse's role encompasses *all* facets of a community's health, from rodent control to enforcement of housing codes.

The American Nurses' Association describes community health nursing in the following way:

> Community health nursing is a synthesis of nursing practice and public health practice applied to promoting and preserving the health of populations. The nature of this practice is general and comprehensive. It is not limited to a particular age or diagnostic group. It is continuing, not episodic. The dominant responsibility is to the population as a whole. Therefore, nursing directed to individuals, families, or groups contributes to the health of the total population. Health promotion, health maintenance, health education, coordination, and continuity of care are utilized in a holistic approach to the family, group, and community. The nurses' actions acknowledge the need for comprehensive planning, recognize the influences of social and ecological issues, give attention to populations at risk, and utilize the dynamic forces which influence change.[27]

SETTINGS FOR COMMUNITY HEALTH NURSING PRACTICE

Community health nurses practice nursing in a variety of settings. These include official and voluntary agencies, private corporations, ambulatory care settings, schools, and industry.

Official Agencies

The Local Health Department. Official agencies are run by local, state, or Federal government and are funded by taxes. Functions are mandated by legislation.

The official agency responsible for delivering services at the local level is the local health department. It may provide services to a city, county, or a municipality. Historically, local agencies have provided programs based on the health needs of communities.[28]

Services of local health departments may include immunizations, maternal and child health care, environmental protection, vector control, family planning, school health, tuberculosis control, home care, chronic disease control, and ambulatory care.[29] The following example illustrates a typical role for a nurse employed by a local health department.

> Mrs. McKelvey worked as a community health nurse for a county health department. She conducted periodic well-child clinics where children were screened for health problems and mothers were given anticipatory guidance about feeding, discipline, growth, and development of their children, time management, and stress.
>
> Mrs. McKelvey also had a caseload of families needing health supervision. Some of these families had members with chronic illness. Others were limited in their intelligence and needed community support. Mrs. McKelvey coordinated their care with members of other social agencies providing services to these families. She made referrals as necessary.
>
> Part of Mrs. McKelvey's role was working as the nurse one day a week in the local school. She coordinated vision, hearing, and prekindergarten screening programs. She counseled teachers on signs of illness in the classroom and conducted health teaching.
>
> Mrs. McKelvey was fortunate that her health department was well staffed. Other community health workers in the health department where she worked included physicians, sanitarians, laboratory workers, nutritionists, physical therapists, occupational therapists, speech therapists, and administrators. A multidisciplinary effort could be brought to bear on community health needs and problems. The funding for programs in which the nurses and other members of the health department worked came from local, state, and federal sources.

The State Health Department. State health departments are less involved in giving direct care to the population, but occasionally they do provide services when these services are not available at the local level. Mobile clinics may travel to local areas with needed services. Health education, environment control, licensing, administering laws, regulating providers and insurers, financing services given by others, and supporting education and research are some of the services provided by state health departments.[30] State health departments are agencies run by health officers, ideally with training in public health. The following is an example of a nursing role at the state level.

> Miss Godfrey was a nurse who directed the Division of Child Health and Development of the state health department. She participated in policy development for child health at the state level, reviewed legislation having an impact on child health in her state, and supervised program directors in her division. She also directed budget development and deployment of resources, and supervised nursing consultants and other community health workers in her division. The nurse consultants gave inservice education programs for nurses throughout the state, often in conjunction with the assistant commissioner of health, the immunization representative, the child development specialists, and the nutritionist. The nurse consultants conducted health programs with professionals from the mental health department and the social services department. Under Miss Godfrey's direction, the nurse consultants also reviewed and commented on legislation and assisted in the development of the child health standards for the state.

The Federal Level. At the Federal level, numerous departments are concerned with various aspects of the nation's health. Most health programs are under the jurisdiction of the Department of Health and Human Services (HHS), formerly the Department of Health, Education, and Welfare (HEW). This department administers the Public Health Service, which at this writing is comprised of the National Institutes of Health (NIH), the Center for Disease Control (CDC), the Health Resources and Services Administration (HRSA), the Food and Drug Administration (FDA), and the Alcohol, Drug Abuse, and Mental Health Administration (ADAMHA). Each of these agencies is concerned with setting policy, providing information and direction for the development of health legislation, giving technical and financial assistance to states, and monitoring health trends.

Other departments at the Federal level are concerned more directly with United States health. The Veterans Administration (VA), for example, operates the single largest health care system in the United States. The VA provides direct medical and nursing care and other health services to veterans through a network of hospitals, outpatient clinics, and other health-related facilities. The Department of Defense provides a wide range of health services through each of its branch services to military men and women and dependents.

Nursing is an integral part of the health system at the Federal level. Policy development, legislative direction, and monitoring trends in nursing takes place in the Division of Nursing, part of the HRSA in HHS. Specific funding for nursing education and practice is provided by the Division of Nursing. The Office of the Chief Nurse of the Public Health Service also participates in the development of policy and legislation and monitors trends. The National Center for Nursing Research, housed within NIH, was opened in 1986. The Center will provide national leadership in nursing research and administer funding for nursing research projects and research training programs.

Voluntary Agencies

In addition to working for local, state, or Federal government, community health nurses may work in voluntary agencies. Voluntary agencies are funded through donations from individuals, professional organizations, and philanthropic foundations. It is estimated that there are over 100,000 voluntary agencies in the United States. The most common activities of a voluntary agency are[31]:

- To raise funds for research and educate the public about specific diseases
- To launch vanguard programs to demonstrate the value of having the government institute certain services
- To provide professional advisory services on a specific disease program
- To support official agencies

Voluntary agencies can be described according to those concerned with specific diseases, such as The American Diabetes Association; those concerned primarily with a part of the body, such as The American Heart Association; those concerned with the health of special groups, such as The American Child Health Association; and those involved with particular aspects of health, such as Planned Parenthood.[32]

One well-known community health voluntary agency is the Visiting Nurse Association, which is concerned with the care of the sick at home. Community health, physical and occupational nurses, speech therapists, and social workers work as visiting nurses. Funding comes from private contributions, third-party payers, and fees for service. In some localities, visiting nurse associations combine with local health departments so that care is given both to the well and the ill. Such agencies are referred to as combination agencies.

Other Settings for Practice

Other settings for community health nursing practice include ambulatory care settings, such as college clinics, industrial settings, neighborhood health centers, proprietary (for profit) home health agencies, health maintenance organizations (HMOs), hospices where care to the dying and their families is provided, and prisons.

Occupational Health. Occupational health nursing involves care to individuals in the work setting. Its purpose is to prevent disease and injury and to promote health, productivity, and social adjustment.[33]

Occupational health nurses have a long history of participating in the protection of the American worker. In 1888, Betty Moulder was employed as a nurse by a group of coal mining companies to care for the sick and injured.[34]

There is a definite need for occupational health nursing in America today. The National Safety Council stated that in 1981, 12,300 people were killed in work accidents and 2,100,000 suffered on-the-job disabling injuries. The total cost was $32.7 billion.[35]

The occupational health nurse may work in mining centers, manufacturing plants, in construction industries, or with migrants. The work includes assessing the health status of workers, monitoring the environment, assessing and reporting hazards, caring for the sick and injured, educating the work force about preventive measures, and assisting workers in rehabilitation efforts. Giving preemployment physicals, keeping records pertaining to accidents, and observing the workers and their environment provide important data in planning to meet employee health needs (Fig. 31–4).

In large industries, members of the health team include the nurse, the physician, the industrial hygienist, and the safety officer. The industrial hygienist has special skills in environmental analysis and monitoring. The safety officer has responsibility for accident hazards. Small industries may have a one-nurse unit. Companies with fewer than 500 people may not have a nurse.

The nurse working in an occupational health center deals with health problems of workers that are common to the American population, such as heart disease, cancer, stroke, accidents and health needs peculiar to particular subgroups. Pregnant women are one example. Maisenbacher described an occupational health program for pregnant women in which she gave classes in growth and development of the fetus and community resources. Periodic weight and blood pressure checks were done.[36]

Other health needs requiring the skills of the occupational health nurse may result from the stress of shift work and exposure to particular hazards of the workplace, whether this is coal dust in the mines, carcinogenic asbestos and beryllium, extremes of temperature, or noise. Conflict, harsh competition, and monotonous work may produce stress.[37] Other stresses may arise if workers are heads of single-parent families. The occupational health nurse has an

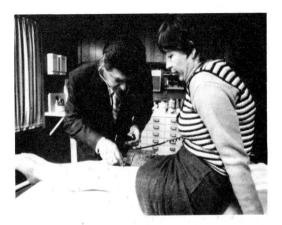

Figure 31–4. Pre-employment physicals are an important part of health maintenance.

important role to play in helping workers and their families manage stress. The nurse's role will be determined by health needs of the labor force, administrative support, professional standards, the law, and policies and resources of the company.[38]

School Health. In 1902, Lillian Wald and Linda Rogers of the Henry Street Settlement showed that decreased absenteeism in the schools occurred with nursing intervention and follow-up among children with communicable diseases. As a result, 12 nurses were hired for the schools.[39] Today there are almost 20,000 nurses to care for a large group of students with actual or potential health needs.[40] In 1977, over 60 million people were enrolled in educational programs through postsecondary school.[41]

School nurses may be employed by health departments, departments of education, or visiting nurse associations. An increasing number of nurse practitioners are working in the school setting. The school nurse assesses and monitors environmental hazards, appraises health status of children and refers them for needed treatment, assists teachers in recognizing and meeting health needs of students, and coordinates health programs for students (Fig. 31–5). They also serve as a liaison between the school and community health agencies, provide necessary emergency care to children who are injured or

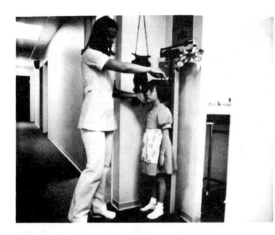

Figure 31–5. The school nurse has a special role to play.

ill at school, and work as a member of a team in meeting health needs of handicapped children.[42]

THE NURSING PROCESS

In community health nursing, the nursing process is practiced both on an individual level and a level involving families, groups, and communities. The following standards for integrating the nursing process into community health nursing were developed by Helvie and illustrate a systems approach.[43]

- The nursing process is a systematic and continuous collection of data about the health status of the system; this data should be accessible, communicated, and recorded
- The health-status data provide the data for nursing diagnosis
- Nursing diagnosis forms the basis for goals and nursing care
- Plans for nursing care include priorities and nursing measures to achieve the goals derived from nursing diagnosis
- Nursing actions provide for a system's participation in health promotion, maintenance, and restoration
- Nursing actions assist systems to maximize their health potential
- The system's progress toward mutually determined goals is determined by the system and the nurse
- Nursing actions involve ongoing reassessment, reordering of priorities, new goal setting, and revision of the nursing plan

In presenting the nursing process as applied in the community, the components of assessment and planning will be discussed primarily in terms of the community as a whole. Intervention will be looked at from the viewpoint of nurses working with individual clients. In this way, the diversity of settings in which nurses can use the nursing process in the community can be illustrated.

Community Assessment
The purpose of **community assessment** is to determine needs. These needs are based on an imbalance in the system.[44] Assessment involves

collection of appropriate data, interpretation of these data, and diagnosis as a basis for nursing intervention. Community health assessment is the process of "defining a community as a system, identifying the attributes of its components and describing the pattern and organization of the community in reference to its levels of wellness."[45] Implicit in this definition of assessment is an emphasis on strengths as well as needs. There is also an emphasis on data pertaining to the population of the community as a whole. Community assessment is important in understanding influences from various systems that have an impact on individuals, families, and groups in the community. In applying concepts from the epidemiological framework of host-agent-environment, this means analyzing influences from the agent and the environment on the host system. Understanding the interaction of various influences in the community gives a stronger foundation for nursing interventions. Interventions may be direct care (immunizing infants) or indirect care (testifying at a court hearing in behalf of a neglected or abused child).

In any community assessment, observations of the community are important and so are data describing the population, its health and illness patterns, health-care usage patterns, health resources, and the interaction of these factors.

Observing the Community. Questions useful to ask in conducting a community assessment include the following: What does the community *look* like? Are the people pale, wan, and listless or robust? Are there a number of vacant homes? What is their condition? Are there rodents? How do people spend their time?

What does the community *sound* like? What are the major sources of noise? When is it noisiest and quietest?

What does the community *smell* like? Are the smells from lush vegetation, from industrial pollution, from sewage, or cooking pots in a small village?

Is this an urban or rural community? What is the climate like? What is the topography like?

What clues arise from the observations in terms of assets and health liabilities that exist in the community?

Using Statistics in the Assessment. In addition to observations, *statistics* are important in community assessment. They may be available from the census, the health department, or local planning groups. Other sources include the Chamber of Commerce, the police department, and the welfare department. Statistics give a numerical picture of people in a community. They show potential groups that may be at high risk.

Particular statistics the nurse will want to know are the age, sex, race, and ethnic groupings within a community. Other important population data include information about education, income, marital status, occupation, and employment rates of the population. These are important in an assessment because of their relation to health and illness. They point to groups needing certain kinds of health-care services. For example, populations with large numbers of women in their childbearing years will need maternal and child health services. The elderly will need greater access to hospitals. They are likely to use three times as many hospital days as the younger population.[46]

Employment data are important, because there is increasing evidence of the relationship between exposure to harmful substances in the work environment and health.[47,48] Not only workers but families and communities are affected by hazards of the workplace. Contaminated clothing and pollution from factories may have a harmful impact on members of the community.

Health and Illness Data. Health and illness community data are important in community assessment. Although these data are useful, the nurse should know their limitations. Measuring the health status of a community is difficult because definitions of health vary. Although there are commonly accepted definitions for mortality (death) and morbidity (sickness), errors in diagnosis creep in, and this is compounded when dealing with less precise terms such as physical or social health.

Mortality and morbidity rates and health resource usage data all have been used as indicators of community health. Mortality data show the risk of dying and may be depicted by life tables or death rates. What are the causes of death in the community? How many deaths could have been prevented? How do birth and death rates compare? When considering immigration and emigration patterns as well as birth and death rates, is the community growing or shrinking?

In order to get additional data about the community's health, other questions to ask include: What is the impact of disease on this community and the community's way of dealing with the impact? How many days has the population lost from work? How has school absenteeism been affected? What can people no longer do that they were formerly able to do? How are they meeting their needs? What health resources are available to people in terms of hospitals, doctors, nurses, dentists, physical therapists, occupational therapists, social workers, clinics, nursing homes, and health departments? Are they accessible? Accredited? What is the level of care provided? Is licensing of personnel provided? Are faith healers or witch doctors used? What political, economic, and legal subsystems affect the services provided? What other subsystems contribute to health and are available, such as recreation facilities and religious institutions? What patterns of diet, exercise, rest, and alcohol and tobacco use exist in the population? Personal habits and genetics have been noted as major determinants of health outcome.[49]

SOURCES OF DATA. Although data are available for the United States and for specific states and counties, data may not be available for smaller areas. There may be an opportunity for the nurse to become part of a team effort to acquire data through a survey. In such a case, the survey organizers may obtain statistical consultation to determine study subjects to be included in the sample. The team may seek advice, too, about the most appropriate tools to use for data collection.

Some data are available from local health departments, the Chamber of Commerce, law enforcement agencies, and other community agencies. Neighborhood residents may have valuable information. One source of data that may be useful to you is information from the census. The census gives a great deal of information about the population, for example, age, sex,

race, and median monthly rental. Census data are collected every ten years in the United States.

Vital statistics (births, deaths, marriages, and divorces) are collected on standardized forms developed by the National Center for Health Statistics (NCHS) of the United States Public Health Service (USPHS). They are gathered on the local level. County, state, and national data are compiled frequently to examine trends in the United States. Classifications for cause of death are based on terminology in the *International Statistical Classification of Diseases, Injuries, and Causes of Death* (ICD), which is revised every 10 years. When classifications change, it may appear that there has been a change in mortality when this is not the case.

The NCHS publishes a great deal of health information about the population that is available from the Government Printing Office (GPO). The GPO health information is based on surveys and provides a rich source of data about health patterns and practices in the United States.

Another source of data that may be useful to you is *Morbidity and Mortality Weekly Reports* (MMW). This publication provides trends on outbreaks of diseases reported to the Center for Disease Control. The World Health Organization publishes worldwide information about infectious diseases in *Weekly Epidemiological Reports* and *WHO Statistics Annual*. Volume 2 of the Annual is entitled *Infectious Diseases: Cases, Deaths, and Vaccinations.*[50]

Occasionally, a state or local area maintains a registry with information about individuals with a particular condition. This is helpful in determining incidence and prevalence of a disease although problems of definition and follow-up are common. Cancer registries exist in Connecticut, upstate New York, Utah, parts of California, and Seattle (King County).[51] Other records that may contain useful information about various segments of the population are insurance records, school health records, and results of screening exams.

Before making the nursing diagnosis, the nurse should compare the community statistics to statistics of comparable communities if such data are available. This will help determine the magnitude of a particular problem. Examining trends over time is extremely important in seeing whether a problem is on the rise or on the decline.

Problems may be categorized according to size; seriousness in relation to death, illness, and disability; economic loss to individuals and the community; potential number of people affected; effectiveness of existing and potential programs; and urgency according to public health officials and the public at large.[52] Categorization is useful because it provides a framework for looking at the magnitude of the problem. In addition to Hanlon and Pickett's framework, categorizing needs according to whether they are physical, social, cognitive, or environmental provides a framework for the nursing diagnosis. Several examples of nursing diagnoses that might be found in the community setting are as follows:

- Limited access to health care by homebound residents related to discontinuing visiting nurse services
- High incidence of venereal disease in teenagers secondary to a lack of health education and follow-up programs
- Inadequate social services secondary to a lack of information and committment by city officials

Any assessment involving the health of a community must look at the interplay of environmental, political, social, psychological, and biological factors within the system. Each must be weighted for its relative contribution to a problem, and judgments must be made as to which factors are amenable to change. Community assessment is a prelude to understanding forces having an impact for sound health **planning** and intervention for community health.

Planning

When a community assessment is completed, the next step is to develop a plan. In community health nursing, planning may be directed to the nursing needs of an individual or a larger group. The influences of the community on the individual or group must be kept in mind in order that the health plan be realistic. Planning involves ranking needs, developing goals and ob-

jectives, and recording the plan. Planning is important in determining needs, allocating resources, avoiding fragmentation, eliminating waste, improving organization and integrating health into other community needs.[53] "Planning is like a system in which each step is a subsystem in itself. The interdependence and inter-relatedness of subsystems should prepare us to expect that any step of the process will be subject to change as a result of feedback from the activities in any other step."[54]

The first step in planning is to rank needs of the individual, group, or community. Prioritizing needs on the basis of the nursing assessment, the client's priorities, and where nursing intervention can be most effective is essential.[55] Ranking may be on the basis of numbers of people affected; seriousness of the problem in terms of death, disease, and disability; economic, social, and psychological impact of the problem; and resources available to deal with the problem. Other factors to be considered include cultural acceptability of funding, manpower, and propriety and legality of treatment.[56] Political considerations also come into play.

Goals and Objectives. After ranking the client's or community's needs, the next step is to develop goals and objectives. Goals and objectives give direction to nursing interventions. Goals are ultimate ends to be achieved. Objectives (or subgoals) are specific accomplishments or targets to achieve in realizing the goals.

An example of a specific goal for a defined population group is:

> In 1985 the health goal in Sawyer Elementary School is to increase immunization levels of new students by 30 percent.

Written goals are often accomplished by a needs statement or statement of justification. This is always done if the nurse is developing a formal proposal requesting additional resources in terms of nurses, money, equipment, or continuing education. An example of a needs statement follows:

> The literature indicates that elementary school children are particularly vulnerable

to communicable diseases. In 1984, communicable disease absenteeism of 100 children at Sawyer Elementary School totaled 90 percent of all absenteeism. School days lost amounted to 400. A plan is needed to reduce susceptibility to communicable disease, reduce absenteeism, and thus maximize classroom learning.

Supporting documentation from the literature and from actual experiences are both important in citing needs. When writing a formal proposal, indicate how the data were obtained. It is helpful to cite examples from the community. This lends depth and validity to the needs statement.

After writing the goals, the next step is to write objectives. Detailed material on writing objectives is given in Chapter 15, on teaching and learning. An example of an objective for the community health nurse is:

> The school nurse will screen 100 percent of the health records of school enterers in Sawyer Elementary School to determine which children are behind in their immunizations.

Objectives must be related to goals, because achievement of goals is measured by achievement of objectives.

Once goals and objectives are selected it is time to examine and decide on alternatives for reaching them. These alternatives, or strategies, should be outlined with their associated costs and benefits. The nurse may not know the actual costs and benefits of various approaches so there may be a need to consult expert nurses, health planners, or other experts. In deciding alternatives, do not forget to seek input from client groups, too. An alternative that is not acceptable to clients is not viable. When a decision is reached about the best alternative, another statement of justification is needed for writing a formal proposal.

When the alternative is selected, steps and resources necessary to ensure its completion should be drawn up. What is needed in terms of manpower, supplies, and equipment?

List dates for completion of the various tasks necessary to achieving the objective, and schedule a periodic review of accomplishments to date. It is wise to have an experienced person review the plan. Such a person will have valuable suggestions.

Implementation

The next step is implementing the plan. Implementing the plan is putting it into action. It involves carrying out strategies to meet goals and objectives and may require action on both the nurse's and the client's part.

Direct intervention requires a basis of trust between nurse and client. It is important to keep the client's goals in mind and try to see things through his or her eyes. Careful attention to communication skills and relationship building is essential.

Three types of nursing intervention that are particularly applicable in the community have been described. These are called: supplemental, facilitative, and developmental.[57] *Supplemental* intervention means doing things for clients that they cannot do for themselves. It should be remembered that intervention may be not only at the individual level but also at the larger level of family, group, or community.

> Mr. Stevens made weekly visits to Mr. Smith, a 65-year-old diabetic. Mr. Smith had poor vision and was not able to draw up his insulin. Mr. Stevens drew up the insulin for Mr. Smith, who stored the filled syringes in his refrigerator. Mr. Stevens provided supplemental intervention for Mr. Smith by filling his syringes, an activity he was not able to do for himself.

Facilitative intervention means removing barriers to care whether they are physical, emotional, cultural, cognitive, or economic.

> Mrs. Cary made a home visit to Mr. and Mrs. Jones. Mr. and Mrs. Jones had recently given birth to a premature infant, Wanda. When Mrs. Cary finished her family assessment, she was concerned about Mr. and Mrs. Jones' lack of nutritional knowledge. Mrs. Cary knew the family was eligible for a supplemental feeding program in the community. She explained the program to Mr. and Mrs. Jones and told them how the foods would be beneficial to the health of their family. Mrs. Cary completed a referral to the supplemental feeding program for the

Jones' family. Mr. and Mrs. Jones were able to obtain milk, juice, cereal and eggs for their family at reduced cost. By removing cognitive and economic barriers, Mrs. Cary intervened so that the family could meet its nutritional needs more effectively.

Developmental intervention is directed to helping the client act more positively in his or her own behalf.

Mrs. Schroeder was concerned about the obesity among a group of high school girls in one of her schools. The girls were continually downgrading themselves. Their self-esteem was low. They wanted to lose weight and increase their confidence. Through a program of weight control and counseling, Mrs. Schroeder helped the girls lose weight, focus on their strengths, and increase their self-esteem. Mrs. Schroeder provided developmental intervention in helping the girls act more positively in their own behalf.

In supplemental, facilitative, and developmental interventions, the nurse's role may require *referring* clients to other resources for needed care. These resources may include health, counseling, welfare, and educational resources. When making a referral, it is important for the nurse to introduce the client, either on the phone or through a referral form, summarize the client's needs, and state the expectation of the referral.

The nurse's role also may require *coordination* with other health-care workers in providing care to clients. This prevents fragmentation and duplication of services. Care may need to be *delegated* to other members of the health-care team such as a home health aide. Other jobs of the nurse may be *screening, casefinding, follow-up,* and *research*. In screening programs, the nurse tests clients for the presence or absence of disease. In casefinding, the nurse looks for contacts of persons with a particular disease, such as TB or hepatitis, in order to screen them for disease and refer them for needed treatment. Follow-up of such clients involves seeing that they obtained treatment. Research might involve investigating those factors that influenced the client's seeking care and complying with treatment.

Evaluation

The next step in the nursing process is **evaluation,** "the process of determining value or the amount of success in achieving a predetermined objective."[58] It is important in determining which interventions are most effective with particular groups. Determining how well objectives have been met with client groups necessitates the development of criteria and tools to measure attainment of objectives. It means determining the success level of nursing care and client achievements.

When evaluating nursing care, questions useful to ask include: Was the care effective? Was it efficient? What was the quality of nursing performance?

Effectiveness means looking at what was accomplished in terms of the objectives. What fostered positive results? What contributed to negative results? Did the patient learn what was taught?

Efficiency is accomplishing nursing care in the least costly manner. Nurses are accountable to the organization where they work, the nursing profession, and themselves. It is important not to squander resources. This means not wasting time, energy, supplies, or being careless with equipment.

Quality includes looking at the care provided in terms of whether it was appropriate and whether it conformed to professional standards. Freeman and Heinrich indicated that quality is an elusive goal but that care should be examined in terms of comprehensiveness, sensitivity, responsible stewardship, and continued updating of skills. Quality implies a well-defined sense of priorities, since resources are limited.[59]

Quality can be evaluated in terms of *structure, process,* and *outcome*.[60] This evaluation framework can be applied to any health setting. Donabedian stressed that quality of care is not a unitary concept. It involves multiple dimensions. *Structure* refers to the environment in which care is given. Dimensions of structure include "referring to and formulating criteria for adequate physical facilities, good administrative processes, well-qualified staff, good communications, and staff development processes."[61] The assumption is that these are necessary to the provision of good care.

Process refers to what the nurse, as care-giver, does for the client. This includes both technical and interpersonal skills. Dimensions of process evaluation include interactions between the nurse and clients and decisions made in relation to clients. It also includes the interaction between the client and other health-care providers. Categories for rating within the process category include information related to knowledge, organizational skills, skills in human relations, observational ability, and technical skills. Process may refer to activities the client must perform to achieve a certain level of wellness. Other authors prefer to put client behavior under outcomes.

Outcome in the structure-process-outcome model refers primarily to alterations on the health–illness continuum for the client. Changes may occur in the areas of attitude, learning, physiological parameters, developmental milestones, prevention, maintenance, and rehabilitation. Other common outcome measures include death, disease, disability, discomfort, and dissatisfaction. It is important to know the weaknesses of these measures. For example, in using client records to evaluate quality of care, mortality statistics may be available, but the records may be incomplete. In using disease as a measure, it is important to consider the accuracy of the diagnosis. Disease categories don't identify level of discomfort. Disability denotes the inability to perform one's normal activities. Such data may be obtained by self-report and may be subject to bias. Measures of discomfort and dissatisfaction are both obtained by self-report and may be subject to bias.[62]

It is often difficult to know if outcome is related to process or other extraneous factors. Although writers in the field have stressed the importance of linking structure, process, and outcome criteria, results to date have been less than conclusive.[63, 64]

Part of the evaluation of care entails not only what to measure, but how to measure it. Sources of data include the client's record, incident reports, reports from third-party payers, staff interviews and observations, morbidity reports, and client surveys. Tests, interviews, reports, observations, and samples of a product can also be included as data sources.

Data may be obtained while the client is still being served, concurrently, or after the client has been discharged from care, retrospectively. Concurrent data may be obtained from the client's chart, from client interview and inspection, and from staff conferences, interviews, or observation (Fig. 31–6). Retrospective data may be obtained from the client's chart, client interview or questionnaire, and staff conferences.

The nursing process provides a framework for a rational, systematic approach to client care. In community health nursing, this approach is applied to individuals as well as families, groups, and whole communities. Careful, accurate, population-based assessment, planning, implementation, and evaluation are necessary in striving for optimal community health.

SUMMARY

This chapter has introduced concepts of community tools used in community health, the purpose of community health nursing, roles and settings of community health nurses, and the nursing process in community health. The concept of community was defined and highlighted as a system with its own inputs, throughputs, outputs, and feedback. Community systems were described according to emotional, structural, and functional communities. Community health was defined. Epidemiology and biostatistics were described in terms of knowledge they provide in analyzing community health, aiding the community health nurse in looking at the community as a whole and highlighting

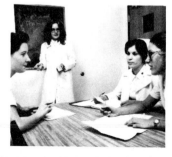

Figure 31–6. Chart audits are one way to strive for excellence.

groups needing particular interventions. The purpose of community health nursing was discussed as was the setting for practice. Roles of community health nurses working in local and state health departments, occupational health, and school health settings were depicted. The nursing process as it applies to community health nursing was described.

Community health nursing demands all that the nurse can bring to it in terms of commitment, intellectual integrity, skill, and caring. The health problems affecting not only the nation's, but also the world's population are great and reflect a need for skilled nurses who can promote maximum physical, social, and emotional health.

Study Questions

1. Traffic accidents are a major killer in the United States today. Describe primary, secondary, and tertiary prevention efforts that might be effective in reducing mortality from this cause.

2. Using your nursing school as an example of a community, describe suprasystem and subsystem influences that affect its health status. In what ways would you describe your school as an emotional community? A structural community? A functional community?

3. A number of individuals in your caseload have hypertension. Using the nursing process and the concept of host-agent-environment, describe the application of these concepts to the nursing care of this particular population group.

4. In a community for which you are developing a health plan, TB and diabetes are the chief causes of morbidity and mortality. If you only had limited resources, what principles of health planning would you use to attack these problems? What rates would you use in assessing the scope of the problem?

5. In conducting a childbirth education class for pregnant women, how would you go about evaluating the effectiveness of your nursing care? What health status indicators would you use? Why?

References

1. Evelyn Benson and Joan McDevitt, *Community Health and Nursing Practice* (Englewood Cliffs, N.J.: Prentice-Hall, 1980), 256.
2. Effie Hanchett, *Community Health Assessment: A Conceptual Tool Kit* (New York: John Wiley & Sons, 1979), 10.
3. Sarah E. Archer, "Selected concepts for community health nurses," in Sarah E. Archer and Ruth P. Fleshman, eds., *Community Health Nursing—Patterns and Practices,* 2nd ed. (North Scituate, Mass.: Duxbury Press, 1979), 23–24.
4. Ibid., 24–27.
5. Ibid., 27–29.
6. John Hanlon and George Pickett, *Public Health—Administration and Practice,* 7th ed. (St. Louis: C.V. Mosby Co., 1979), 4.
7. Ilse R. Lesser, "The community as a patient," in Ilse R. Lesser, Claire Tuchalski, and Rosine Carotenuto, *Community Health Nursing* (Flushing, N.Y.: Medical Examination Publishing Co., 1975), 89.
8. Sarah E. Archer and Ruth P. Fleshman, "Epidemiology and some applications to primary prevention," in S.E. Archer and R.P. Fleshman, *Community Health Nursing-Patients and Practices,* 2nd ed. (North Scituate, Mass.: Duxbury Press, 1979), 219.
9. Benson and McDevitt, *Community Health and Nursing Practice,* 62.
10. Barbara Spradley, *Community Health Nursing; Concepts and Practices* (Boston: Little, Brown & Co., 1981), 207.
11. Lesser, "The community as a patient," 90.
12. Benson and McDevitt, *Community Health and Nursing Practice,* 69.
13. Ruth B. Freeman and Janet Heinrich, *Community Health Nursing Practice,* 2nd ed. (Philadelphia: W.B. Saunders Co., 1981), 145.
14. Phillip E. Sartwell and John M. Last, "Epidemiology," in John M. Last, ed., *Public Health and Preventive Medicine,* 11th ed. (New York: Appleton-Century-Crofts, 1980), 47.
15. Grace Wyshak, "Epidemiology," in Margot J. Fromer, *Community Health Care and the Nursing Process* (St. Louis: C.V. Mosby Co., 1979), 215–221.
16. Ibid., 224.

17. Archer and Fleshman, "Epidemology and Some Applications," *Community Health Nursing,* 224.
18. Benson and McDevitt, *Community Health and Nursing Practice,* 81.
19. Sartwell and Last, "Epidemiology," 21.
20. Benson and McDevitt, *Community Health and Nursing Practice,* 83–84.
21. Ibid., 84.
22. Ibid.
23. U.S. Department of Health, Education and Welfare, *Healthy People—The Surgeon General's Report on Health Promotion and Disease Prevention.* DHEW Publication No. 79–55071 (Washington, D.C.: U.S. Government Printing Office, 1979), 14.
24. Spradley, *Community Health Nursing, Concepts and Practices,* 30.
25. "Nurses today—A statistical portrait," *Am J Nurs* 82, (March 1982); 448–51.
26. Freeman and Heinrich, *Community Health Nursing Practice,* 1.
27. The Executive Committee and the Standards Committee of the American Nurses' Association Division on Community Health Nursing Practice, *Standards of Community Health Nursing Practice* (Kansas City, Mo.: American Nurses' Association, 1974), 10.
28. Ibid., 15.
29. Steven Jonas, "Provisions of public health services," in John M. Last, ed., *Public Health and Preventive Medicine,* 11th ed. (New York: Appleton-Century-Crofts, 1980), 16.
30. Leahy, Cobb, and Jones, *Community Health Nursing,* 17.
31. Jonas, "Provisions of public health services," 1626.
32. John Hanlon, *Public Health Administration and Practice,* 6th ed. (St. Louis: C.V. Mosby Co., 1974), 243.
33. Marjorie J. Keller, "Health needs and nursing care of the labor force," in Margot J. Fromer, *Community Health Care and the Nursing Process* (St. Louis: C.V. Mosby Co., 1979), 413.
34. Carol A. Silbertstein, "Nursing role in occupational health," in Linda Jarvis, ed., *Community Health Nursing: Keeping the Public Healthy* (Philadelphia: F.A. Davis Co., 1981), 127.
35. National Safety Council, *Accident Facts—1982 Preliminary Condensed Edition* (Chicago, Ill.: National Safety Council, March 1982).
36. Kim Maisenbacher, "Prenatal preparation: an industrial application," *Occup Health Nurs,* 29, (February 1981): 19–20.
37. Freeman and Heinrich, *Community Health Nursing Practice,* 514.
38. Anna Mae Tichy, "Wellness, the workers, and the nurse," *Occup Health Nurs* 29, (February 1981):22.
39. Freeman and Heinrich, *Community Health Nursing Practice,* 489.
40. Dorothy S. Oda, "A viewpoint of school nursing," *Am J Nurs* 81, (September 1981):1677.
41. Freeman and Heinrich, *Community Health Nursing Practice,* 490.
42. Marilyn Stember. "Nursing role in school health," in Linda Jarvis, ed., *Community Health Nursing* (Philadelphia: F.A. Davis Co., 1981), 143.
43. Carl D. Helvie, *Community Health Nursing* (Philadelphia: Lippincott, 1981), 136.
44. Ibid.
45. Hanchett, *Community Health Assessment,* 35.
46. William Shonick, "Health Planning," in John M. Last, ed., *Public Health and Preventive Medicine,* 11th ed. (New York: Appleton-Century-Crofts, 1980), 1604.
47. Barry I. Castleman and Manuel J. Vera Vera, "Impending proliferation of asbestos," *Int J Health Serv* 10, (1980):389–403.
48. Russell W. Peterson, "Health and ecological effects of energy systems: An overview," *Envir Health Perspect* 32 (1979):235–39.
49. Victor Fuchs, "Economics, health and post industrial society," *Milbank Mem Fund Q* 52, (Spring 1979); 153–82.
50. John M. Last, ed, *Public Health and Preventive Medicine,* 11th ed. (New York: Appleton-Century-Crofts, 1980), 27.
51. Ibid., 29.
52. Hanlon and Pickett, *Public Health—Administration and Practice,* 280–91.
53. Ibid., 280.
54. Sarah E. Archer, "Selected community health processes," in S.E. Archer and R.P. Fleshman, *Community Health Nursing—Patterns and Practices,* 2nd ed. (North Scituate Mass.: Duxbury Press, 1979), 73.
55. Ibid., 79.
56. Hanlon and Pickett, *Public Health—Administration and Practice,* 285.
57. Freeman and Heinrich, *Community Health Nursing Practice,* 72.
58. George James, "Evaluation in public practice," in Herbert Schulberg, Alan Sheldon, and Frank Baker, eds., *Program Evaluation in the Health Fields* (New York: Behavioral Publications, 1969), 29.
59. Freeman and Heinrich, *Community Health Nursing Practice,* 83.
60. Avedis Donabedian, "Evaluating the quality of medical care," in H.C. Sculberg, A. Sheldon, and

F. Baker, eds., *Program Evaluation in the Health Fields* (New York: Behavioral Publications, 1969), 186–89.

61. Marlene A. Mayers, Ronald B. Norby, and Anita Watson, *Quality Assurance for Patient Care* (New York: Appleton-Century-Crofts, 1977), 6.
62. Allen D. Spiegel and Herbert Hyman, *Basic Health Planning Methods* (Germantown, Md.: Aspen Systems Corp., 1978), 340–41.
63. William E. McAuliffe, "Measuring the quality of medical care: Process versus outcome, *Millbank Mem Fund Q* 57, (Winter 1979):118–52.
64. Robert Brook, Kathleen Williams, and Allyson Avery, "Quality assurance today and tomorrow: Forecast for the Future," *Ann Intern Med*, 85, (1976):809–17.

Annotated Bibliography

Freeman, R.B., Heinrich, J. 1981. *Community Health Nursing Practice*. Philadelphia: Saunders. This is a classic textbook on community health nursing that provides a systematic approach to community assessment and risk assessment of families. It provides methodologies for data collection including a tool for identifying nursing needs of families.

Hall, J.E., Weaver, B.R., 1985. Distributive Nursing Practice: A Systems Approach to Community Health, 2nd ed. Philadelphia: Lippincott. A comprehensive textbook on community health nursing using a systems theory approach throughout. Separate chapter on general systems theory concepts.

Hanlon, J.J., Pickett, G. 1984. *Public Health—Administration and Practice,* 8th ed. St. Louis: C.V. Mosby. This classic textbook is a very comprehensive resource on the field of public health. The many dimensions of health in the community setting are explored in depth. Selected topics include historical roots, international health issues, public health analysis and planning, ecology and health, epidemiology, and health-care delivery services.

Jarvis, L.L. 1985. *Community Health Nursing: Keeping the Public Healthy,* 2nd ed. Philadelphia; F.A. Davis. This text presents a comprehensive view of the community, community health nursing, and many specific social and environmental issues that impact upon public health and nursing. Selected nursing roles in the community are defined and discussed with examples.

Warren, R.L. 1965. *Studying Your Community*. New York: The Free Press. This book presents practical descriptions of community concepts. Selected sections include the economic structure of communities, community planning, housing, recreation, and communication in communities. It is comprehensive in its coverage of recommended topics to consider in community assessment.

Chapter 32

Environmental Concepts

Phyllis B. Heffron
Janet-Beth McCann Flynn

Chapter Outline

- Objectives
- Glossary
- Introduction
    The Ecological Model
    Environmental Pollution
- Ecological Issues and the Nursing Process
- Environmental Control in the Hospital Setting
    The Hospital Environment and the Nurse
    A Safe Environment for Nursing Practice
- Summary
- Study Questions
- References
- Annotated Bibliography

Objectives

At the completion of this chapter, the reader will be able to:

- Define the ecological model
- Discuss the relationship between air pollution and human health
- Discuss the effects of water pollution on health and safety
- List the health effects of at least six toxic substances in the environment
- List three sources of ionizing radiation in the environment
- State at least four ways nurses can assist clients in controlling noise pollution
- Describe the role of the occupational health nurse in reducing environmentally induced health effects
- Describe a safe hospital environment
- List factors needed to make a comfortable hospital environment
- Describe nursing actions that can be carried out to protect individuals from environmental injury

Glossary

Air Pollution. The presence of contaminant substances in the air that do not disperse properly and interfere with human health.

Carcinogenic. Cancer producing.

Decibel. A unit of relative sound measurement.

Decomposition. The breakdown of matter by bacteria; change in the chemical makeup and physical appearance of materials.

Ecology. The study of the relationships of living things to one another and to their environment.

Ecosystem. The interacting system of a biological community and its nonliving surroundings.

Electrical Threshold. The minimum amount of current to which the human body responds.

Environment. In ecological terms, the sum of all external conditions affecting the life, development, and survival of an organism.

Hazardous Waste. Waste materials that by their nature are inherently dangerous to handle or dispose of, such as old explosives, radioactive materials, some chemicals, and some biological wastes; usually produced in industrial operations.

Humidity. The amount of moisture in the air.

Infections. Disease processes caused by infectious agents, such as bacteria, viruses, or other micro-organisms.

Mutagenic. Causing a change in the genetic structure of an organism in subsequent generations.

Noise. Any undesired sound.

Nosocomial Infections. Infections originating in medical facilities, such as hospitals; includes infections with symptoms that may not show up until after the client's discharge, and infections that occur among staff members.

Pesticides. Any substances used to control pests ranging from rats, weeds, and insects to algae and fungi.

Pollutants. Any introduced substances that adversely effect the usefulness of a resource.

Pollution. The presence of matter or energy whose nature, location, or quality produces undesired environmental effects.

Radiation. The emission of particles or rays by the nucleus of an atom.

Radioactive. Substances that emit rays either naturally or as a result of scientific manipulation.

Radioisotopes. Radioactive forms of chemical compounds, such as cobalt-60, used in the diagnosis and treatment of diseases.

Recycling. Converting solid waste into new products by using the resources contained in discarded materials.

Smog. Air pollution associated with oxidants.

Solid Waste Disposal. The final placement of refuse that cannot be salvaged or recycled.

Thermal Pollution. Discharge of heated water from industrial processes that can affect the life processes of aquatic plants and animals.

Teratogenic. Substances that are suspected of causing nonheritable malformations or serious deviations from the normal in or on animal embryos or fetuses.

Toxic Substances. Chemicals or mixtures that may produce an unreasonable risk of injury to health or the environment.

Water Pollution. The addition of enough harmful or objectionable material to damage or contaminate water quality.

INTRODUCTION

The term **environment** is one of those elusive words that can be defined in a multitude of ways. In relation to human beings, the environment most commonly refers to the physical surroundings—air, water, sunlight, noise, and organic and inorganic objects. In a systems framework, the external environment is whatever exists outside the identified system boundary and includes other systems and subsystems. The internal environment exists inside the system's boundary. The immediate environment may be a community, a neighborhood, a house, room, or other enclosure. Environment may refer to social or psychological atmosphere. In actuality, the human environment includes everything that affects humans.

Throughout the ages, human beings have been adapting to the natural environment and have made many attempts to control and shape it.[1] These attempts have resulted in a wide base of knowledge about the complex relationships that exist among living systems. One of the major characteristics of the human–environment relationship is reciprocity. We act on the environment and receive from the environment.[2] In recent years, the effects of human acts on the environment, e.g., industrialization and biomedical and engineering technology, have become increasingly evident and widely studied in terms of ecology, environmental hazards, and human health.

The immediate environment of humankind in terms of community and city planning, institutional design and safety, and environmentally induced psychosocial stressors has received increasing attention as related to the quality of life and individual health status.[3,4]

The nursing profession has been concerned with aspects of the human environment since the days of Florence Nightingale.[5] Basic nursing texts always have emphasized the importance of safety, cleanliness, air quality, and temperature control as integral aspects of total client care and nursing responsibility. Community health nurses extend environmental concerns to areas of preventive health care and maintenance of general public health. Ecological issues impact individuals, families, and communities.[6] Nurses need to be sensitive to and have a basic understanding of these issues as they affect health and the environment. It is natural for clients to seek out the nurse to provide facts, answers, and opinions on a variety of these issues.[7]

The focus of this chapter is the human relationship to the environment and how it relates to nursing and health. An emphasis on human external physical environment requires two major areas of discussion: ecology and the general quality of life, and the immediate environments of humans as related to health-care settings and the home.

The Ecological Model

The condition of the environment in which we live—the air, water, buildings, and grounds—determines to a large extent how we live, what we eat, which diseases we are likely to contract, our state of health, and ability to adapt (Fig. 32–1). The science of **ecology** is primarily a biological science that studies the environment and environmental factors affecting humankind. Of primary concern to ecologists are the dynamic relationships between living things and their surroundings.[8]

This ecological model gives us a broad and suitable framework from which to view environmental issues as they affect clients and the practice of nursing. Ecology encompasses a holistic, systems theory approach that can provide insights into environmental hazards and stresses that affect health adaptation.[9]

Human ecology is concerned very specifically with the human–environment relationship. In addition to the biological and physical inter-relationship that come immediately to mind, cultural, technological, social, and behavioral aspects of human adaptive responses are also included.[10] An important concept of basic ecology is the ecosystem. An **ecosystem** is a total collection of adapted organic and inorganic parts that support a chain of life within a selected area.[11] More simply, an ecosystem is the home or habitat where groups of plants and animals live together in harmonious balance. Our earth is well endowed with ecosystems of a wide variety of sizes, shapes, and content. The entire earth is actually one giant ecosystem, as are ponds, rivers, deserts, forests, and caves. These ecosystems are all physically and biologically different, but they function in the same general way: predictably and in a chainlike fashion.

Radiant energy from the sun sets the chain in motion as the process of photosynthesis allows solar energy to become fixed and stored in green plants. The energy stored by plants is passed along through the ecosystem in a series of steps that involve eating and being eaten, **decomposition,** and recycling back into green plants.[12] In ecology, the living parts of an ecosystem work together in what is called a food chain and are divided into producers (the green plants), consumers (plant eaters and meat eaters), and decomposers (primarily bacteria) (Fig. 32–2). Plant and animal growth within these food chains is dependent on the nonliving materials in the ecosystem, such as water, carbon dioxide, oxygen, and minerals dissolved in the water. These nonliving materials have their own cycles that also occur predictably and interdependently. The water cycle, for example, involves evaporation and condensation. Water vapor in the earth's atmosphere is distributed and moves via air currents, then cools and forms clouds. Rain falls on the earth, soaks into the soil, and fills the springs, rivers, and oceans. Surface water from these open bodies of water evaporates when the sun shines and returns water vapor to the atmosphere. Other cycles that are highly inter-related within the ecosystem are the carbon and oxygen cycle and the nitrogen cycle. These elements and other nonliving materials are constantly recycled through the ecosystem from soil, atmosphere, and water to plants, animals, decomposers, and back again.[13]

Ecosystem functioning is important to understand when studying human health and the environment. Manmade interferences, such as

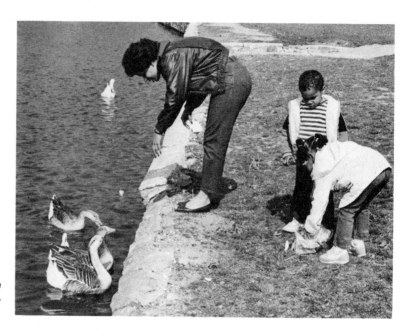

Figure 32–1. The quality of the environment affects individuals, families, and communities.

chemical substances introduced into the environment, can profoundly disturb ecosystems and their equilibrium. "It is because of this biogeochemical cycling that DDT sprayed in an Indian hut to kill the *Anopheles* mosquitoes, or laid down on a California farm to kill cotton pests, appears in penguins in Antarctica and in human mother's milk in New York City."[14] Another example that illustrates a direct "cause and effect" disruption to ecosystems involves the disposal of water used to cool nuclear reactors. When this waste water is discharged into streams or lakes in its heated state, it causes irreversible damage to fish and plant life.[15]

When considering the total human environment, ecological issues are germane to the interest of professional nurses. The list is virtually endless when one considers all the possible hazards, adverse effects, and stresses with which we come in contact. Several of these health-related issues have been selected for further discussion.

Environmental Pollution

Pollution is described in the dictionary as a state or act of uncleanliness, defilement, or impurity. Environmental pollution refers primarily to the pollution of the human physical environment, the atmosphere, the waterways, and the land. The menace of such pollution—smog, garbage heaps of plastic containers, bottles, and pop-top cans, and stagnant pools of foul water—has been growing over the past years, particularly after the postwar period of abundance and high-technology achievement.[16]

Air Pollution. **Air pollution** began to receive a great deal of attention when urban **smog** surfaced as a major public health problem in the early 1960s. Smog, an innovative term meaning the chemical pollution that occurs when automobile exhaust emissions react with sunlight, was particularly evident in cities with high concentrations of cars and aircraft, such as Chicago and Los Angeles.[17] Large industrial cities like Pittsburgh, Pennsylvania, and Newark, New Jersey, were characterized by a pall of sooty, murky air that tended to build up during periods of low wind velocity and certain other atmospheric conditions. People breathing this contaminated air were subject to a variety of respiratory ailments and, in some cases, the smog was directly related to morbidity and mortality.[18]

As general concern for the environment escalated, special interest groups formed to study,

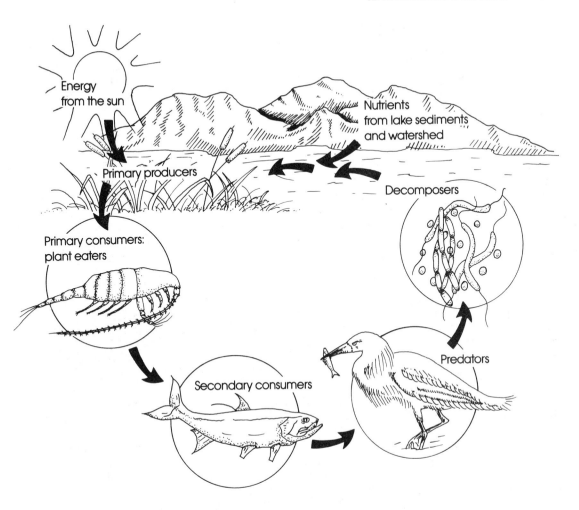

Figure 32–2. The components of an ecosystem are in dynamic equilibrium with their environment.

support, and lobby to clear up the air. It became evident that air pollution affected humans indirectly as well as directly by damaging plants, materials, and other animals.[19] Crops were destroyed by smog and fluoride in the air, wild and domestic animals died from airborne dioxin, and stone on buildings crumbled from the presence of acid in the air.[20]

The leading cause of air pollution is from industrial manufacturing, and the second major cause is automobile exhaust.[21] The smoky by-products of combustion, particularly the burning of coal to generate electricity, disperse large amounts of solid and liquid particles, such as dust, ash, soot, and various metals and chemi-

cals.[22] Poisonous gases, such as sulfur dioxide from industrial processes and hydrocarbons and nitrogen oxide from motor vehicle exhaust, account for numerous adverse health effects that include irritation of the eyes, nose, and throat, respiratory irritation, impairment of cardiac function, and possible **mutagenic** and **carcinogenic** effects.[23]

In 1970, Congress passed the Clean Air Act of 1970, which governs all types of air pollution. This act, administered by the Environmental Protection Agency (EPA), required automobile and industrial manufacturers to reduce poisonous emissions from car exhausts and industrial smokestacks over a 10-year period.[24] Amended again in 1977, the Clean Air Act gave even broader power to the EPA to set standards for any category of industry whose air pollution causes or contributes to the endangerment of public health.[25] Although fraught with political pressures and red tape within and outside the government, this legislation has proved worthwhile, and there is evidence that our air quality has improved. It is recognized increasingly, however, that governmental regulations that impose restrictions, controls, and fines are only one way to attack the problem of air pollution.[26] Knowledge about atmospheric chemistry, air transport, and control are also imperative in understanding and solving the problem.[27]

Water Pollution. Over the ages, various forms of **water pollution** have plagued humankind and the environment. In this country, early laws regarding water pollution were aimed at the prevention of waterborne diseases, such as typhoid fever, cholera, and others. In 1914, the first drinking water standards were enacted, and in 1948 Congress passed the Water Pollution Act.[28] Since that time and increasingly in the past decade, water pollution has come to mean contamination from a number of sources other than infection-causing organisms. With the onset of the industrial revolution in America, the industrial and manufacturing needs shifted from power to the need for water as an agent for cooling and processing. It was this shift that resulted in the release of highly toxic pollutants into our streams and rivers. The quantity of pollutants exceeded the capacity of the water to be naturally cleansed through recycling, and water pollution occurred on a massive scale. In addition, the rapid population growth in the United States also had an effect on water pollution. Many local water treatment plants have been unable to purify water fast enough, and there is greater risk of contamination. Water runoff from mines, farms, construction sites, and city streets have resulted in an increase of both toxic and nontoxic pollutants entering the nation's waterways.[29]

Water pollution can be categorized according to its source. The major sources of water pollution are common organic sewage, bacteria, organic and chemical plant nutrients, earth sediments from soil erosion, **radioactive** materials,

and **thermal pollution** (waste heat from nuclear power plants).[30] Water pollution also can be expanded to include the presence of unsightly garbage and litter thrown into our rivers and lakes.[31]

The effects of water pollution on human health can range from minor skin irritation to death and can affect us directly or indirectly. We can become sick or injured from drinking or coming into skin contact with contaminated water. We are also affected directly by shortages of drinking water or by food shortages caused by diminished growth. Indirectly, we can become ill from eating foods or green plants that have come into contact with polluted water. Water pollution can affect psychological health as well, when water looks bad, smells bad, or tastes bad, regardless of its safety. Water pollution can affect people economically, such as fisherman who have lost their livelihood because of fish contamination with mercury.[32] Thermal pollution, which results when heated water is discharged into rivers or streams, can significantly upset ecological relationships. Clams, snails, crabs, and worms have totally disappeared from much of Florida's Biscayne Bay because of thermal pollution from two power plants.[33]

The responsibility for reducing pollution of our waterways rests with local, state, and Federal agencies as well as with the public at large. On the Federal level, the EPA administers a number of water pollution control programs under the auspices of the Clean Water Act of 1972 and the Safe Drinking Water Act of 1974.[34] The effects of water pollution must continue to be looked at in terms of the total quality of life of individuals.[35]

Toxic Substances. Human beings and the environment are being exposed each year to a large number of chemical substances. In addition to the air we breathe, almost everything we touch, eat, or drink contains them. Among the chemical substances and mixtures being developed and produced, there are some whose manufacture, use, or method of disposal presents unreasonable risks of injury to health or the environment.[36] The term **toxic substances** commonly refers to those chemicals or mixtures of chemicals that produce adverse health effects to humans or animals, either directly or indirectly.

Toxic substances include a number of manufactured chemicals, as well as naturally occurring substances, such as mercury or lead, that are mined and released into the environment. It is estimated that nearly 60,000 chemicals are in use in the United States today, and approximately 800 new chemical substances are proposed each year for manufacture.[37]

In 1976, the Toxic Substances Control Act (TSCA) was enacted by Congress. This Act, administered by the EPA, mandates protection of public health and the environment from chemical risks. The EPA gathers information on chemical substances and tests them for various health effects, including carcinogenicity, mutagenicity, **teratogenicity,** and behavioral toxicity. Regulations can then be passed by the EPA; these may range from a complete ban of the substance to a minor relabeling modification.[38]

The EPA also has responsibility for the Federal Insecticide, Fungicide, and Rodenticide Act (FIFRA). **Pesticides** are chemical or biological substances used to control pests, such as rats, weeds, insects, and fungi. Misuse of pesticides can contaminate the environment and result in their accumulation in ecological food chains.[39]

Additional toxic substances, such as drugs, food, food additives, and cosmetics, are regulated within various other government agencies, like the Food and Drug Administration and the Department of Agriculture.

Health effects from all of these toxic substances vary tremendously and persons can be exposed to them in many ways. Table 32–1 summarizes some of the most significant toxic substances in the environment, their principal characteristics, uses, and health effects.

Solid Waste Disposal. One of the most indisputable environmental problems is the accumulation of garbage, litter, and other unwanted materials known as solid wastes. Solid waste refers to garbage, dead animals, demolition waste (bricks, masonry, piping, and lumber), sewage treatment residue, industrial wastes, and other refuse.[40]

Solid waste disposal in communities always has been a problem. In recent times, the United States has experienced a tremendous increase in the problem. Residential and commercial sources generate solid waste at the rate of 132 million metric tons per year.[41] Industrial waste is more than double that amount, totaling 350 million metric tons a year, of which approximately 41 million metric tons is **hazardous waste.**[42] Economic and population growth and the production of plastic, glass, aluminum, and other disposables all contribute to the problem. In 1970, nearly 73,000 cars were abandoned in New York City.[43]

The problems of solid waste disposal, particularly of toxic hazardous wastes, constitute a number of public health and environmental dangers. The health effects of toxic chemical wastes are summarized in Table 32–1, and sewage disposal problems were discussed earlier in this chapter. The control and eradication of solid waste problems has been mandated to the EPA, which is responsible, among other things, for cleaning up old and abandoned toxic waste sites.[44]

It is beyond the scope of this chapter to discuss the specifics of solid waste disposal and to compare methods. For many years "the old attitude towards solid waste disposal has been to dump it, burn it, or bury it."[45] This attitude still prevails among many people who are not concerned with environmental issues or who are not aware of all the complexities and hazards. With the help of government agencies on all levels and various private interest groups, there are continuing, concerted efforts to deal with solid waste management problems, its treatment, storage, transportation, and disposal.

Radiation. **Radiation** is yet another form of pollution in our environment. It occurs naturally in the atmosphere as well as from man-made sources, such as nuclear reactions and x-rays.

Radiation was first described by Henri Becquerel, a French scientist who accidentally discovered that one element can spontaneously change into another.[46] An element or material is said to be *radioactive* when energy or particles are emitted from the nucleus of its atoms. The actual particles or "rays" that are emitted are called *radiation.*[47]

There are three types of radiation: alpha, beta, and gamma. Each is associated with the

TABLE 32–1. SELECTED TOXIC SUBSTANCES IN THE ENVIRONMENT

Toxic Substance	Characteristics and Use	Principal Health Effects
Arsenic	Highly toxic poison Occurs naturally in coal and oil Formerly used in pesticides and herbicides Currently has very limited agricultural uses and as a weed killer Used in paint, glass, and ceramic industries Large quantities produced from smelting of lead and other metals, from cotton gins, and coal burning Compounds of arsenic are the most toxic	Severity of toxic reaction depends on concentration and type of compounds Acute systemic poisoning with gastrointestinal inflammation, nausea, vomiting, diarrhea, cardiac toxicity, and death Acute occupational exposure can lead to nasal cancer and teratogenic effects Chronic exposure can lead to muscle weakness, anorexia, gastrointestinal symptoms and mucous membrane irritation A carcinogen in the workplace
Asbestos	A widely naturally occurring fiber Used in road building and construction, insulation, cement, floor tiles, pipes, filters, and numerous other sources Can be a source of pollution in drinking water Acid rain component	Occupational exposure to airborne asbestos can cause asbestosis (lung fibrosis), lung cancer, pleural and peritoneal mesothelioma, and gastrointestinal cancer Waterborne asbestos poorly understood but some connection with generalized mesothelioma in the public
Beryllium	A highly toxic nonradioactive metal Used in copper alloys and machine manufacture Significant use in fluorescent light industry discontinued in 1949 because of high incidence of occupational disease: berylliosis Used today primarily in industrial settings that refine it or use it in alloying, e.g., machine shops, ceramic and propellant plants, and foundries	Route of entry through lungs Acute poisoning symptoms include multiple respiratory system problems, weakness, weight loss, anemia Chronic exposure leads to degeneration and death Berylium poisoning can affect people living near beryllium factories
Cadmium	Soft, heavy metal similar to zinc and mercury A harmful toxin in the form of sulfides of carbonate in zinc, copper, and lead ores 50 percent of all the cadmium in United States is used by electroplating industries Used to manufacture batteries, plastics, paints, metal alloys, photographic supplies, glass and rubber products Present as a fine mist during burning of products containing cadmium Food contamination an important source of exposure	Route of entry through inhalation, ingestion, and absorption Occupational exposure produces general malaise, nervousness, dry mouth, impaired sense of smell, shortness of breath, sore throat, chest cramps, back pain, and anorexia Long-term exposure may produce emphysema, liver and kidney symptoms, central nervous system impairment and adverse cardiovascular effects Suspected correlation with hypertension Carcinogenic implications
Chlorine	Dense green-yellow gas Strong oxidizing agent Used in the preparation, processing, and liquification of chlorine Also used in chemical, pulp, and paper processes	Pulmonary edema Pneumonitis Bronchitis
Chromium	A hard metal Contaminates the environment as an aerosol or dust Used in electroplating, manufacturing stainless steel, tanning and photographic supplies, combustion of coal and refuse	Carcinogenic Direct contact causes dermatitis, skin ulcers
Fluoride	A highly reactive gas as hydrogen fluoride	Accumulates more readily in children

(continued)

TABLE 32–1. (Continued)

Toxic Substance	Characteristics and Use	Principal Health Effects
	A corrosive, poisonous, and gaseous chemical element as a compound of fluorine Used to produce phosphate fertilizers, aluminum, brick, tile, steel, and glass By-product of coal combustion Ocean dumping of waste fluoride can cause air pollution	In areas subjected to fluoride pollution from industry, the following symptoms have been reported: polycythemia, fluoride in teeth, nails, urine, and hair of children Chronic exposure of high doses can lead to depression of collagen formation and bone resorption
Mercury	A heavy metal Occurs naturally from erosion and weathering Pollution results from mining, refining of mercury, combustion of fuels and refuse, use of pesticides containing mercury, use as a fungicide, use in paper and pulp industry, and numerous other sources Can cause water pollution from industrial waste and agricultural runoff	Greatest risk to general population is from consumption of contaminated fish Route of entry often inhalation in occupational sites Health effects are mostly neurotoxic with progression to deafness, blindness, paralysis, kidney failure, and death
Nickel	A hard metal Occurs most commonly in oil and coal deposits Used in manufacture of stainless steel and other metal processes Found in nickel-aluminum compounds associated with many industrial uses Used as fuel additive Found in asbestos, coal, and crude oil Air pollution comes from burning of coal and petroleum products	Contact dermatitis Atmospheric nickel can be inhaled or absorbed through the skin; foods contaminated in processing can be ingested Gaseous nickel carbonyl is very toxic and can produce lung cancer; acute poisoning produces chest pain, vertigo, and vomiting Disease from chronic occupational exposure may take up 20 years to develop
Chlorinated hydrocarbons (pesticides)	Man-made chemical compounds including DDT, benzene hexachloride, heptachlor, and others Used as pesticides Do not break down into nontoxic substances in the environment Nearly all uses of DDT and other similarly highly toxic compounds have been banned in the United States	DDT widely studied in terms of its health effects Early symptoms of poisoning include headache, dizziness, and anorexia; some evidence of changes in liver function Major documented effects of DDT poisoning are neurotoxic and include hyperactivity and muscle tremors Carcinogenicity and genetic changes documented in animals Enzyme changes, e.g., can cause a drop in certain hormone levels, such as estrogen
Organophosphates (pesticides)	A group of synthetic pesticides that largely have replaced chlorinated hydrocarbon pesticides such as DDT Some common compounds in this group include atrazine, simazine, parathion, Malathion, and others Can be highly toxic, but do not persist in the environment as long as chlorinated hydrocarbons Very poisonous to both harmful and beneficial insects	Heavy occupational exposure can cause headache, nausea and vomiting, stomach cramps Several deaths reported each year from acute occupational exposure Parathion most toxic to humans Chronic exposure to agricultural workers often misdiagnosed as food poisoning, heat stroke, or gastroenteritis Long-term health effects not known
Herbicides	Defoliant compounds used to destroy noxious weeds and shrubs along highways and for lawn and garden use	Generally of low toxicity when exposure occurs; may cause some irritation and discomfort

(continued)

TABLE 32–1. (Continued)

Toxic Substance	Characteristics and Use	Principal Health Effects
Herbicides (cont.)	Include chlorophenoxy acids, urea derivatives, fenuron and diuron, triazines, acylanilides	Indirect health effects more important; may destroy food supplies for animals, disrupts plant and waste ecosystems by using O_2 in water and affecting fish life Teratogenic and carcinogenic effects in lab animals
Fungicides	Two widely used fungicides are captan and folpet (phthalimides)	Have been shown to be carcinogenic, teratogenic, and mutagenic to experimental animals
Nitrosamines	Include any of a series of organic compounds derived from amines (derivatives of ammonia) and containing the divalent = N:NO radical Occur throughout the environment in food, drugs, tobacco, drinking water, and air Principal sources: direct discharges from industrial processes; formed when natural amines in food (amino acids) combine with polluted air containing nitrogen compounds; formed in human stomach when nitrates (found in some meat and poultry products) are ingested	Laboratory tests have shown these substances to be carcinogenic and mutagenic
Polychlorinated biphenyls (PCBs)	Widely used in industrial compound, chemically similar to DDT Very prevalent in the environment; a partial listing of uses includes electrical equipment, lumber, metal, concrete, paint, printing ink, solvents, varnishes, and floor tile Released in industrial wastes Does not break down readily and is passed along through the food chain, e.g., found in fish and wild animals	Correlated to lethal effects in game birds and reduced reproductive capacity in fish eating mammals, minks, and seals Etiologic agent in "Yusho Disease" (first reported in Japan after accidental ingestion of high concentration of PCBs) characterized by severe skin disorders, eye discharge, loss of hair, numbness of extremities, headaches, gastrointestinal symptoms, deformed nails, joints, and bones Aftereffects of disease can include permanent central nervous system damage Carcinogenic in rodents Occupationally exposed persons have experienced nausea, vertigo, eye and nasal irritation, asthmatic bronchitis, dermatitis, fungus, and acne
Vinyl chloride (VC)	A plasticizer used in the production of polyvinyl chloride (PVC), the most commonly used clear plastic Escapes in air and water as a pollutant Occupational exposure occurs in polyvinyl chloride plants General public is exposed via aerosol containers, plastic wraps on foods, and drinking water; also used widely in industry, home and medical science, in wall coverings, upholstery, appliances, cosmetics, and perfumes Polyvinyl chloride releases hydrochloric acid when burned	Affects calcium metabolism and shows an increase in abortion and fetal abnormalities when given to lab animals at relatively low doses Associated with liver cancer and other carcinomas Studies have also suggested increased rates of birth defects in communities where PVC manufacturing plants are located
Polybrominated biphenyls (PBBs)	Highly toxic flame retardant	Long-term toxicity unknown

(continued)

TABLE 32–1. (Continued)

Toxic Substance	Characteristics and Use	Principal Health Effects
	It is persistent in the environment and bioaccumulates Added to fibers and plasticized materials, such as typewriter and calculator casings, shavers, and hand tools Released to environment during manufacturing process	Short-term toxicity studies show impaired reproductive and liver function, nervous disorders, and teratogenic effects
Kepone	Highly poisonous chlorinated organic compound Long life in the environment, and bioaccumulates Used as fire retardants, plasticizers, and pesticides Released in waste water and atmosphere during manufacture Seafood contamination another threat to humans	Has produced serious illness among workers in Kepone manufacturing plants; symptoms include neurologic disorders, skin changes, muscle spasms, sterility, liver lesions, cancer, and others Has produced adverse reproductive effects in rats

Adapted from William J. Baumol and Wallace E. Oates, Economics, Environmental Policy, and the Quality of Life *(Englewood Cliffs, N.J.: Prentice-Hall, 1979), 48–57: a compilation of many sources.*

type of energy ray or particle emitted from the nucleus. Alpha particles are actually changed nuclei, such as a helium nucleus being emitted from a uranium isotope. Beta particles are electrons emitted from the nucleus, and gamma rays are emissions of high-energy light.

Ionizing radiation refers to the ability of radiation to make molecular changes and is of most concern to human health. It can disrupt molecules within the body cells and cause destruction leading to cell death or other abnormal deviations.

Of the three types of radiation, gamma radiation is the most damaging to the human body.[48] It has a relatively low ionization capability, is high in its ability to penetrate body tissues, and has a cumulative effect in the body. Small doses over a long period of time can be devastating. Alpha particles, such as uranium and plutonium, are dangerous to human health because they can be ingested through food and water or inhaled into the lungs. Once in the body, these heavy metals have a tendency to concentrate in the bones; subsequent damage to bone marrow and blood forming cells can occur and lead to leukemia.[49]

Beta particles have a moderate ability to ionize and are low in penetration. Health effects from this type of exposure are primarily skin and surface abnormalities, such as eye cataracts.

Everyone is subject to a certain amount of radiation from natural sources in the environment. These natural sources include cosmic radiation from the sun, radiation in the soil and rocks, and small amounts of radiation that are emitted within the body.[50] Other sources are from man-made sources, such as fallout from nuclear bomb tests, exposure and leakage from nuclear power plants and from x-rays in medicine and dentistry.

The use of radiation in medical and dental practice is well established. There are applications in both diagnosis and therapy, such as the use of **radioisotopes**, e.g., cobalt-60. A complete discussion of radiation in health-care settings follows in the next section.

The use of nuclear power plants and the degree to which they are hazardous to health has been a running public and political debate for some time. There are currently over 60 operating nuclear plants in the United States.[51] These nuclear plants, or reactors, use radioactive isotopes like uranium or plutonium as their fuel source. By a process of fission (splitting of the atom, which produces heat and radiation), steam is produced from water, and electricity is generated.[52] The process is technical and complex, but the major concerns for health and safety center around leakage of radiation from these reactors, exposure to workers, and contamination from toxic wastes.

The world has witnessed two disasters in recent times, the most serious occurring in 1986 at the Soviet Union's Chernobyl nuclear reactor near the city of Kiev. An explosion and fire at this site resulted in numerous deaths and untold cases of radiation sickness, as well as a range of contaminated food and water supplies in dozens of nearby countries.

Radioactive pollutants from these reactors can be in the form of liquids, solids, and gases.[53] Waste disposal, particularly of highly radioactive used fuel elements and fission products, is a critical problem. At present these wastes are buried in cement drums or million-gallon stainless steel tanks under the sea or 14 feet underground.[54]

The concern regarding adverse effects of man-made nuclear energy has prompted a number of national and international efforts to control environmental and population contamination.

At present, a number of Federal agencies are responsible for protecting the public from unnecessary radiation exposure. The EPA, for example, is developing standards for disposal of radioactive wastes and working on guidelines for nuclear accident prevention.[55]

Noise. Unwanted sound, loud or soft, makes us nervous, irritable, angry, listless, or unable to sleep. The amount and intensity of environmental **noise** is a growing problem in the United States. Noise is considered a pollutant because of its ability to permanently damage the ear and contribute to a variety of other physical and mental ills.

Sources of excessive noise are frequently associated with urban areas and include general industrial activity, building construction, motor vehicles, and jet airplanes.[56] Building construction, in particular, is a major environmental problem. In the home, electrical appliances are a major contributor of noise pollution: radios, TVs, stereos, typewriters, vacuum cleaners, dishwashers, blenders, exhaust fans, hair dryers, and power tools.

The major health effects of excessive noise are summarized below[57,58]:

- Permanent inner ear damage ranging from slight impairment to total deafness
- Temporary inner ear damage, leading to chronic hearing losses
- Masking of warning signals (e.g., vehicular horns) that can lead to industrial and domestic accidents
- Disturbance of sleep, rest, and relaxation
- Interference with speech communication
- Annoyance, frayed nerves, and other psychological disturbances
- Reduction of the opportunity for privacy
- Constriction of blood flow throughout the body[57]

The ear is very vulnerable to harm from noise because it cannot close itself like an eyelid; it is designed by nature always to be alert.[59] The **decibel** is the most commonly used measure of sound. Environmental readings can be taken on a standard noise meter in units of decibels. A reading of zero represents the threshold of audible sound for normal human hearing.[60] The higher the decibel level, the louder the noise. Scientists believe that continuous 8-hour exposure to levels of 85 decibels can result in permanent hearing loss.[61] Some common environmental sources of noise and their associated decibel levels appear in Figure 32–3.

Noise control is one of the most difficult environmental problems because it involves virtually everyone in all the activities of daily living. The EPA and other organizations, such as the American Speech-Learning-Hearing Association, are working toward preventing noise induced hearing impairment and reducing environmental noise. In addition, local governments and community organizations are developing noise standards and educating the public about the health hazards of noise pollution and its prevention.

The EPA's Office of Noise Abatement and Control recommends the following actions for noise reduction in the home[62]:

- Install exhaust fans on rubber mounts

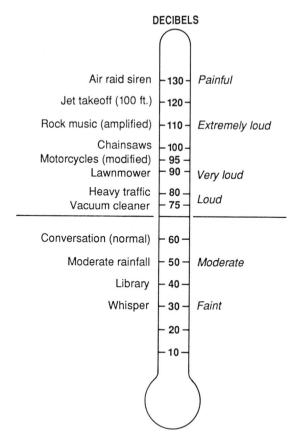

DECIBELS

Air raid siren — 130 — *Painful*

Jet takeoff (100 ft.) — 120 —

Rock music (amplified) — 110 — *Extremely loud*

Chainsaws — 100 —
Motorcycles (modified) — 95 —
Lawnmower — 90 — *Very loud*

Heavy traffic — 80 —
Vacuum cleaner — 75 — *Loud*

Conversation (normal) — 60 —

Moderate rainfall — 50 — *Moderate*

Library — 40 —

Whisper — 30 — *Faint*

— 20 —

— 10 —

Figure 32–3. Some common decibel levels in everyday life.

- Caulk windows and install storm windows to cut down outside noise and conserve energy
- Use vinyl flooring or thick linoleum in kitchens and bathrooms
- Use wall-to-wall and stair carpeting with felt or rubber padding to dampen noise
- Use drapes to help absorb noise
- Keep radios, televisions, and stereos at a lower volume
- Use vibration mounts under large electrical appliances such as washers, dryers, and dishwashers
- Place foam pads or towels under electric typewriters, blenders, and other small appliances
- Replace metal garbage cans with plastic ones

ECOLOGICAL ISSUES AND THE NURSING PROCESS

Nurses traditionally have been concerned about various environmental issues that affect our immediate surroundings. Safety and comfort measures within the home and hospital have been well-documented as major health determinants and important components of nursing care. Occupational health nurses, particularly in industrial manufacturing settings, have taken an active role in promoting the importance of job safety and the prevention of illness associated with the workplace environment.

As nurses continue to view health and illness in a holistic fashion, concerns about health and the environment are accentuated in importance and broadened in scope. The ecological perspective of the human–environment relationship provides nurses with additional knowledge about acute and chronic health effects, methods of illness prevention, and influences on the general quality of life.

The ways in which nurses can apply their understanding of environmental issues to the nursing process include research, client and community assessment, health teaching, and other methods of therapeutic intervention that promote client adaptation.

Certain aspects of a client's environment need to be considered when taking a nursing history or conducting a general assessment. These include type and location of housing, specifics of employment—e.g., where employed, known occupational hazards, and length of employment—leisure activities, and personal habits.

Occupational health nurses have a primary responsibility in assessment of environmental hazards and conditions that influence health status. Under the Occupational Health and Safety Act of 1970 (OSHA) health professionals who work in occupational health settings are mandated to seek information and facilitate detection of relationships between the physical and mental ill health of workers and their job environment.[63] OSHA requires that all employers provide workplaces that will not endanger the safety or health of employees. Catherine Tinkham, a community health nurse leader and author, has developed a data-collection tool for use by nurses in setting up industrial nursing services. Some of the assessment questions contained in this tool are[64]:

- Types of industry?
  Centralized or decentralized?
  How many buildings?
  Are the buildings close together or far apart?
- What product is produced?
- What operations and activities are carried out?
- What occupational hazards are present that could affect health, e.g., gases, radiation, weather, noise?
- What kinds of illnesses and injuries are reported among the employees?
- Number of workers who have chronic illnesses?
- Number of workers with physical handicaps including visual and learning conditions?

Another part of the environmental assessment process is direct observation. Community health nurses must be alert for health hazards in the home and look for potential environmental pollution problems that might exist in the geographic area. Occupational health nurses need to make visual inspections of the work site and watch workers as they carry out tasks. Periodic screening of persons at high risk for environmentally induced illnesses is another assessment method that nurses can use. Blood tests to determine levels of lead and chemical substances and routine chest x-rays for miners are examples.

It is also important for nurses to identify aspects of the environment that influence health positively and to encourage adaptive behaviors that help people cope with the environment.[65] Citizen participation in community efforts to reduce pollution and conserve our natural resources is one way people attempt to adapt. Carpooling and **recycling** of solid waste are also examples.

Nursing interventions associated with environmental problems vary according to the knowledge and position of the nurse and the nature of the problem. Direct nursing care for acute illnesses caused by environmental problems is carried out by occupational health nurses, emergency room nurses, and hospital nurses. In these settings, familiarity with causative agents, e.g., toxic substances, and their treatments is crucial.

In the long run, efforts directed toward primary prevention of environmentally induced health problems are the most effective nursing intervention. Educating the public about the effects and prevention of noise, pollution, cancer-causing agents, radiation exposure, and lead poisoning can be done through various mass media techniques and one-to-one communication. Health education is not a panacea for eliminating environmental health effects or guaranteeing major changes in peoples' health behaviors, but it can serve to provide clients with enough information for them ultimately to make rational decisions on their own.

ENVIRONMENTAL CONTROL IN THE HOSPITAL SETTING

Healthy individuals are capable of adapting to or adjusting their environment by controlling heating, lighting, ventilation, coloring, and many other things. Individuals create a pleasant environment in which they feel comfortable. When individuals become ill and enter the hospital, they can no longer control or manipulate their surroundings as they wish.

Loss of control over the environment can affect how people adapt to hospitalization. Because of this, nurses must serve as advocates and assist individuals to adapt to the environment, as well as adapt the environment so that it is safe and comfortable.

A safe environment is one that is free from electrical hazards, thermal hazards, radiation, fire, drug and chemical hazards, pollution, microorganisms, and psychological trauma. A comfortable environment is one in which unpleasant stimuli, such as extremes of temperature, color, odors, and noise, are controlled. A comfortable environment is also one in which there is adequate space and privacy. Many hospital departments are involved in protecting clients from hazards and unpleasant surroundings. Examples include: the maintenance department, houskeeping department or environmental control department, and the nurse epidemiologists. Other agencies monitor radiation and building safety.

All clients are at risk for injury, and nurses should assess carefully the environment with safety in mind. There are clients, however, who are at risk to environmental hazards. These include: the elderly, children, the handicapped, the emotionally disturbed, individuals with low resistance to disease, and the client experiencing sensory alterations.

The Hospital Environment and the Nurse

Air quality refers to the adequacy and cleanliness of air available. Mechanisms should be available to circulate the air in the room. Air conditioners with air circulation devices are useful. Large circulating fans are also available from the housekeeping department.

Humidity is the amount of moisture present in the air. Geographic location, weather, and time of the year can contribute to the amount of humidity.

Air that is too dry, or too low in humidity, can cause excessive drying of the skin and may cause skin to crack or break down. The mucous membranes dry as well, and this may cause irritation to the nose and throat, inability to cough up secretions, and excessive drying of the mouth and tongue. Conversely, environments that have high humidity can cause joint pain and other feelings of discomfort. This discomfort may be caused because the body regulates its temperature partly by perspiring. High humidity air affects the rate at which perspiration evaporates and makes individuals uncomfortable.

Room *temperature* contributes to feelings of comfort. Room temperature is a personal preference. A room temperature of 68 to 72°F (20 to 22°C) is considered comfortable by most people, although babies and older people may require a warmer room temperature.

Many odors in the hospital environment are unpleasant. Odors may come from trash cans, body wastes, strong chemicals, cigarette smoke, body odors, and many other things. Even strong perfumes on hospital personnel or visitors can be overwhelming for persons who are ill. All units should be kept free of body waste, trash, dirty linens, and other objects that have strong or disturbing odors.

Other factors related to an adequate environment for respiration include assessment of any *allergens* present. Several things contribute to "interior pollution." Air **pollutants** include plants, flowers, dust, perfumes, and cigarette smoke. These all can be controlled by eliminating them from the unit.

Many agencies now have policies against smoking. Smoking is only permitted in designated smoking areas.

The amount and quality of *lighting* contributes to comfort and safety. When lighting is not adequate, eyestrain, headaches, irritability, and altered visual perceptions may occur. Conversely, when light is too bright or is turned on for 24 hours a day, it is difficult for clients to get high-quality rest and sleep. Nurses should regulate light so that it duplicates nature's day–night cycle by turning lights on during the waking hours and turning them down or off during the sleeping hours. Lighting during the daylight hours should support outdoor lighting, not replace it. Ideally, clients should have access to windows to help keep their spirits up and to keep them oriented to the day–night cycle.

Children and older people may find night lights comforting, but this is a personal preference. Night lights serve to orient clients to strange surroundings at night and adds a safety feature if clients use the bathroom at night.

Noise, as an environmental hazard, recently has been classified by some authorities as a pollutant. Surprisingly, hospitals very often are guilty of noise pollution. One would like to think of hospitals as quiet places where the sick go to get well. Hospitals are large action-oriented agencies that employ hundreds of people to care for clients. Whenever hundreds of human beings are engaged in action-oriented tasks, a great deal of noise is created.

Loud noises can be irritating and fatiguing to well individuals and even more so to individuals who are ill or in pain. Persons who are ill and hospitalized may be disturbed by noises that would not normally bother them. Loud talking or a television, for example, may disturb their rest and even produce complaints or outbursts of anger.

Some noises tend to be more irritating than others. Sudden loud noises, such as a metal item being dropped, cause a fright response. Squeaking wheels and doors are another. Telephones disturb people, as do loud talking and laughing. Some of these things can be expected and tolerated during the day, but at night they can be particularly troublesome.

If nurses realize the extent to which loud noises are disturbing, they can begin to be more aware and assess noise levels on their units. It then becomes possible to eliminate, control, or correct the noise level.

Decor and Other Factors. Environmental decor can be manipulated to provide a pleasant atmosphere. Research has demonstrated that use of colors can contribute to the way people feel.

Soft *colors* tend to contribute to feelings of comfort. Blues, greens, pale yellows, and soft pinks are restful and can be used in and around patient units. Bright colors, such as red and canary yellow, are stimulating colors and are best used in lounges and corridors located away from units. Grays, blacks, and browns are depressing, somber colors and, unless used on floors and baseboards, are not good choices.

Many agencies are now using more color in room divider curtains, draperies, bedspreads and blankets, on walls, ceilings, and floors. Well-selected colors brighten the environment and make it more cheerful.

Most hospital *furnishings* are quite different from home furnishings; their purpose and use should be explained on admission. Special care should be given to explaining how the call bell and communication unit work. Clients also should be oriented to their room, the rest of the floor, and shown where the toilet and bath facilities are located. Finally, newly admitted clients should be introduced to roommates and the staff who will be caring for them.

Individuals who are hospitalized have, to some extent, lost control over their *privacy.* Nurses need to be aware of this and assess this need. Closed doors, drawn curtains, and appropriate drapings are several means for meeting this need.

Nurses also need to be aware of the legal aspects of invasion of privacy. Avoid this problem by knocking before entering a client's room, asking permission to go into the closet or bedside cabinet, and so forth.

Clutter is always unappealing, and this is true in the hospital as well as other settings. Nothing makes a unit more unattractive than yesterday's newspaper, remnants of breakfast, and medical supplies and equipment littering the top of every surface. The client's permission, however, should be obtained before disposing of personal items.

Although nurses do not have much control over the amount of *space* available, they usually are able to provide clients with some space that is defined as their own. The concept of space, like privacy, requires that nurses assess the need for personal space and respect it. Many of the same actions used to ensure privacy are employed to provide clients with the feeling of their own territory. Boundaries should be assessed and respected and permission asked before entering a client's space. Some hospitals, for example, have rules about staff members sitting on the edge of clients' beds. This may or may not be appropriate, but it is a good example of what it means to invade a client's space.

The need for *safety* at the bedside is another component of the general environmental assessment. The most common injuries that bedfast clients sustain are related to burns and falls.

Fire dangers are the most frightening. Burns from fire generally result from smoking in bed. If clients are permitted to smoke in their rooms, ashtrays should be provided, and smoking should be monitored to prevent this hazard. Prevention is the best defense against burns. Should a fire start, prompt, safe, and efficient actions must be taken by hospital staff. The first step in the procedure is to remove clients from immediate danger. The second step is to attempt to contain the fire by using fire extinguishers and closing windows and fire doors. All accredited hospitals are required to have detailed fire plans and hold regularly scheduled drills and educational sessions.

Burns can be caused by scalding liquids, chemicals, radiation, light bulbs used for heat treatments, hot-water bottles, heating pads, electric blankets, and lamps. Careful testing of bath water and other solutions with thermometers will help prevent injury from scalding liquids. Safe storage of caustic chemicals and radioactive materials will decrease that type of burn. Monitor clients undergoing heat-lamp treatment and position lamps carefully to reduce the chance of injuring them. Wrapping a hot-water bottle in several layers of towels and placing it in a securely fastened pillow case will reduce chances for this type of burn. Eliminating the use of electric heating pads and electric blankets is the most effective way of controlling this type of injury.

Falls are the next most common injury sustained by hospital clients. Most falls occur when clients get up too fast and faint, stay up too long and become weakened, or attempt to function independently before they are strong enough. Some of the reasons these falls occur are because health-care providers do not respond quickly enough to call lights, clients do not understand how to call the nurse, they overestimate the amount of strength they have, and they are confused or disoriented. Nurses need to assess their clients' abilities and strengths, and the various hazards to safety.

Specific actions can be taken by nurses to provide a more secure environment. These include:

- Keeping the bed in the low position
- Raising all side rails when clients are in bed
- Raising the furthest side rail when clients are out of bed
- Encouraging clients to wear slippers with firm nonskid surfaces or shoes when out of bed
- Keeping floors free of trash, electric cords, and water
- Ensuring that walking devices, such as canes and crutches, have intact rubber tips
- Ensuring that all beds, wheelchairs, and stretchers have locked wheels before transferring clients
- Providing adequate personnel to move clients
- Keeping all medications locked in medicine room
- Placing safety caps on lotions and powders
- Assessing clients for suicide potential and taking appropriate actions
- Using restraints such as posey jackets and wrist restraints as needed

No body system or component is immune to the risk of becoming infected. For infections to begin, a series of six factors must be present:

- Infectious agent
- Reservoirs
- Exit from reservoir
- Mode of transmission
- Portal of entry
- Susceptible person

Infections that are acquired by hospitalized clients are called **nosocomial infections.** All clients and health-care providers are at risk for developing nosocomial infections, but certain groups can be identified as high risk. These include infants and young children, the elderly, the chronically ill, the debilitated, the poorly nourished, the burned, the postoperative, the immunosuppressed, the client with a low white blood count, and the extremely anxious. Staff members who work continually with infected clients or contaminated equipment are also at high risk for nosocomial infections.

Means of spread of infection must be assessed by nurses and nursing actions employed to decrease the chance of nosocomial infections. These methods are quite diverse and depend on the means of transmission. The most important of these is employing careful hand-washing techniques after having any contact with clients or their supplies and equipment. All clients with identified contagious infections should be placed in isolation rooms, and correct isolation procedures in caring for them should be observed. All health-care providers or visitors who have infections should be kept away from clients, especially those designated as high risk. If this is not possible or practical, they should wash their hands carefully and put on a mask and, if appropriate, a gown. Dirty laundry in hampers should be disposed of often and not allowed to sit on the unit since it can serve as a medium for bacteria growth. Trash also should be discarded frequently, as it provides a good medium for the growth of microorganisms.

Careful techniques of food storage in hospital kitchens and on hospital units can reduce this type of infection. It is not pleasant to suffer from food poisoning when well, and it can be very harmful for those debilitated by illness.

Food never should be stored on hospital units for longer than 24 hours. All foodstuffs placed in the refrigerator should have a time and a date. Any foods or liquids that do not smell or look appropriate should be discarded. Foodstuffs should be kept in pest-resistant containers to keep down vermin. Pests such as mice, flies, and other insects must be exterminated. If all of these factors are assessed and controlled, the number of nosocomial infections can be reduced.

All health-care providers in direct contact with clients should be aware of the safe use of *electricity*, electrical equipment, and the hazards of using electricity. Understanding how to use electrical equipment safely is particularly important in instances where more than one piece of electrical equipment is being used for one client.[66] It is even more important when it is used for clients who are especially vulnerable to electrical injury, such as those with indwelling catheters or wet dressings.[67]

According to Ohm's law (of electricity), anyone in contact with an electrical appliance can become a part of the electrical circuit.[68] This can occur because of a mechanical defect in the electrical equipment or because of normal leakage of current from equipment. The insulating material must be sufficient to reduce the level of electrical leakage so that it is kept below threshold. The **electrical threshold** is the minimum amount of current to which the human body responds. Threshold levels vary depending on whether the skin is intact or wet.

Protecting clients from electrical hazards is one of the nurse's roles (Table 32–2). Once the needs are assessed, client units and other spaces should be kept free of electrical hazards.

Mechanical pacemakers that stimulate the heart are frequent in hospitalized individuals. Many of these pacemakers are known as demand pacemakers and function only on the absence of an electrical impulse from the heart. If microwave pulses are present in the environment, the pacemaker will not perceive the absence of the electrical impulse from the heart, and ventricular contractions will not occur. It is, therefore, vitally important for nurses to assess the potential threat to client safety.

Although *radiation* does not fall directly within the practice of nursing, it is used exten-

TABLE 32–2. ELECTRICAL HAZARDS

Overloaded circuits
Defective wiring
Inadequate or overloaded fuses
Excessive current
Inadequate grounding
Damaged plugs
Frayed cords
Insecure sockets
Handling electrical equipment with hands
Excessive use of extension cords

sively in the health-care system as a means of diagnosis and treatment. Because of the use of radioactive materials, in the form of x-rays, scans, and radioactive implants, nurses need to assess their hazards and take steps to assure safety for clients, staff, visitors, and for themselves.

Radioactive materials are supplied in sealed sources (radioactive chemicals sealed in a coating), unsealed sources (radioactive chemicals not sealed in a coating), and x-rays.[69] Clients who are treated with x-rays or other radioactive materials receive treatment in specially designed rooms, and there should be no radioactivity outside of these treatment rooms. The United States Government has designed regulations to guide the installation of x-ray equipment.

Health-care agencies have specially trained personnel who work in the x-ray and radiotherapy departments. These personnel control their exposure to radioactive material by:

- Reducing the time spent in contact with radiation
- Increasing distance from the source of radiation
- Wearing lead aprons, gloves, or drapes
- Standing behind lead barriers
- Wearing metered tags that are sent periodically for exposure analysis

Nurses can use the above methods in practice as well as when assisting clients who are being treated with radiation or who are receiving radioactive materials as a part of the diagnostic process. Even if the duration of the exposure to the radioactive material is brief, nurses should keep in mind that brief exposures to radiation over long periods of time may be equal to one long dose of radiation and may be hazardous to their health. Women who are pregnant should not be exposed to radiation, if possible.

Clients who have received temporary radioactive material as implants act as another source of radiation in the environment. Limits should be set on the amount of time nurses spend with these clients, and nurses should wear lead aprons and gloves when in contact with them. Clients should have private bathrooms when in this type of isolation, and all radioactive body discharges (feces, urine, vomitus, etc.) must be dealt with safely. In most instances, nurses should wear rubber gloves.

Obviously, persons undergoing treatment with radioactive material and subsequent isolation experience anxiety, fear, and stress. Nurses need to be supportive to clients and their families during the duration of the treatment.

Hospitals have numerous *toxic substances* and chemicals in the form of drugs, medications, and strong disinfectants. Nurses always should ensure that these substances are labeled properly, stored in secure areas designated for the purpose, and are in safe containers with child-proof tops. The latter is especially true in areas of the hospital where children and confused or disoriented clients are diagnosed and treated.

A potential danger from drugs or chemicals arises from the use of outdated or deteriorated substances. Any drug or chemical that has changed in its appearance, texture, or odor, or has passed its expiration date should be discarded or returned to the pharmacy, since it may no longer be safe to use. Should any altered drug or chemical be administered accidently, a physician should be notified immediately and the hospital procedure for such instances followed.

Building safety entails keeping everything in good repair and well lighted. Fire exits should be clearly marked and have easy access. In addition, stairwells should be well-marked, unlocked, and well-lighted.

Discovery of loose tiles, faulty equipment, burned out lights, etc., should be reported to the appropriate department immediately.

A Safe Environment for Nursing Practice

Nurses are also exposed to environmental hazards. Part of the nursing responsibility is to follow good health practices and maintain a high level of wellness.

Maintaining good nutrition is one of the most basic areas in which nurses can set an example, as well as keeping themselves alert and healthy. Nurses are busy people, and those who work in acute-care settings often have long hours of duty, irregular shift assignments, and overloaded client care responsibilities. These very problems, which often make it difficult to observe good nutritional habits, are some of the reasons why adequate nutrition is so necessary.

Another basic area of good health practice is obtaining adequate rest, relaxation, and sleep. An adequate number of hours of sleep should be obtained every 24 hours and relaxing activities planned for off hours. Activities such as jogging, yoga, or exercise may be very helpful in reducing stress as will pursuing hobbies or other special interests.

Dental and health checkups should be at least yearly and immunizations kept up-to-date. Another important and frequently overlooked health behavior is staying home when ill. Illness needs to be treated with rest, and nurses should remain home when ill.

In maintaining a high level of wellness, nurses are able to function at their best and serve as a role model for clients and the general public.

Nurses can observe specific behaviors based on scientific principles in order to *prevent disease or injury* to themselves. These include the use of proper body mechanics, good personal hygiene and hand washing, proper treatment of contaminated materials, correct use of equipment, and careful manipulation of toxic substances.

Good *personal hygiene* habits and good hand-washing techniques reduce the chance of cross contamination. Nurses always should wash their hands after touching clients, bed linens, bedpans, secretions, and toxic substances. Soap, friction, and running water should be used, and the fingernails, knuckles, and wrists should be washed as well.

Nurses frequently are called upon to prepare medications or manipulate toxic substances. Studies have shown links between the use of anticancer drugs and subsequent precancerous lesions or new primary growth.[70] The risk for nurses handling such drugs has not yet been identified, but it has been shown that nurses working with drugs to treat cancer have mutagens in their urine.[71]

Extensive research to validate these hypotheses has not been conducted, so there is little to support the banning of these drugs. It is vital for nurses to know about the dangers of handling such drugs.

Other more common drugs can produce allergic dermatitis. Some of these drugs include aminophylline, benzocaine, cytoxics, the "mycin" drugs (such as streptomycin), penicillin, and phenothiazines. Nurses should take special care when manipulating the above drugs.

Nurses handle a variety of chemicals as well as drugs. The chemicals encountered include antiseptics, detergents, alcohol, dyes, bacteriostatic agents, and other chemicals such as anaesthetic liquids and gases. In addition to being harmful to skin and mucous membrances, many chemicals and gases are highly flammable and increase the chances for fire.

For protection from drugs and chemicals, nurses should know:

- Chemical names of substances
- Trade names
- Hazards
- Poison antidotes
- Precautions for storage
- Precautions for use

By observing simple safety precautions, nurses can avoid side effects from manipulating strong or harmful substances in the work environment.

SUMMARY

The human environment includes everything that affects us: the physical environment, the social and psychological environment, and the internal environment. Our relationship with the environment is interdependent and reciprocal. This give and take relationship is central to the adaptation process of which all living things are a part. The characteristics and consequences of the human–environment relationship have a direct effect on human health, survival, and the quality of life. The nursing profession is interested in what these relationships are, how their characteristics are manifested, and what the consequences of selected human–environment actions are.

Ecology is the science that studies the dynamic relationships of living things to one another and to their environment. The ecological model encompasses a holistic approach that can provide insights into environmental hazards and stresses that can affect human health and the ability to adapt. An important concept within ecology is the ecosystem. The ecosystem is very simply a collection of adapted living organisms within a particular environment. Knowledge about environmental conditions and hazards comes from studying these ecosystems and how they relate with natural cycles such as the water cycle, nitrogen cycle, atmospheric movements, and so forth.

There are many conditions within the human environment that affect health status and the general quality of life. Some of the major ecological issues that have been identified include air pollution, water pollution, toxic substances, solid waste accumulation, ionizing radiation, and noise. Each of these issues has some unique health effects, and many have related and overlapping consequences. Radiation, for example, can pollute air and water as well as result in a hazardous waste disposal problem.

Nurses can use their knowledge about ecology and environmental hazards as they carry out the nursing process. Knowledge about environmentally induced acute illnesses, e.g., chemical poisoning and waterborne diseases, can assist them in the assessment process and in choosing appropriate interventions, including health education and other methods of prevention.

Community health nurses and occupational health nurses have assessment responsibilities in the home and work setting. Occupational health nurses have an opportunity to reach large numbers of people within education programs that emphasize hazard identification and prevention of industrial accidents and work-related illnesses. Nurses in the community are engaged in other forms of primary prevention, too, such as mass screening programs.

Nurses are also concerned about effects of the immediate environment on the hospitalized client. Hospitalized clients, to some extent, lose control over their environment. This can affect how they feel, behave, and adapt. Nurses are in a good position to serve as advocates in this area and assist clients by providing a safe and comfortable environment.

A safe environment is free from electrical hazards, physical barriers that contribute to falls, thermal hazards, radiation, fire, drug and chemical hazards, pests, pollution, harmful microorganisms, and psychological trauma. A comfortable environment is free from unpleasant stimuli, such as extremes of temperature, color, unpleasant or strong odors, and excessive noise. In addition, a comfortable environment attends to space and privacy needs.

Nurses who work in institutional settings are exposed to many of the same environmental hazards as clients. Repeated radiation exposure and frequent contact with toxic substances and microorganisms are occupational hazards that nurses need to be aware of. The responsibility to identify these hazards and take action to eliminate them rests with each individual and the institution. Nurses and other health professionals have an additional responsibility to maintain their own personal health status and serve as role models in the promotion of good nutrition and other beneficial health practices.

Study Questions

1. List the various causes of air pollution in your community. What evidence, if any, do you see that indicates that people are concerned about it and its health effects?

2. Identify a major river or other body of water in your area. What are some actual or potential sources of water pollution affecting it?

3. Contact your city or county health department to learn what environmental health services are offered. How do these services affect such things as solid waste disposal and noise pollution? Are radiation levels in the area monitored?

4. Visit the office of an occupational health nurse and describe the nurse's role. List areas where primary prevention might lessen or

eliminate health effects of environmental hazards.

5. Interview a hospitalized patient about the hospital environment. Identify nursing measures that could improve or enhance the quality of this particular environment.

6. List at least four occupational hazards that can affect the health of nursing personnel. How can the ill effects of these hazards be prevented?

References

1. James M. Fitch, *American Building: The Environmental Forces that Shape It.* (New York: Schocken Books, 1975), 4.
2. Ibid.
3. Ibid, 4–14.
4. Jack Smolensky, *Principles of Community Health,* 4th ed. (Philadelphia: W.B. Saunders Co., 1977), 1.
5. Lillian DeYoung, *Dynamics of Nursing* (St. Louis: C.V. Mosby Co., 1981), 12–13.
6. Linda Jarvis, *Community Health Nursing: Keeping the Public Healthy* (Philadelphia: F.A. Davis Co., 1982), 621.
7. Ruth Murray and Judith Zentner, *Nursing Concepts for Health Promotion* (Englewood Cliffs, N.J.: Prentice-Hall, 1975), 250.
8. Smolensky, *Principles of Community Health,* 25.
9. Jeannette Lancaster, *Community Mental Health Nursing* (St. Louis: C.V. Mosby Co., 1980), 22.
10. Ibid., 10.
11. Smolensky, *Principles of Community Health,* 26.
12. Robert Leo Smith, *The Ecology of Man: An Ecosystem Approach* (New York: Harper & Row, 1972), 3, 5.
13. Ibid., 14, 15.
14. Osborn Segerberg, Jr., *Where Have All the Flowers, Fishes, Birds, Trees, Water and Air Gone?* (New York: David McKay Co. 1971), 54.
15. Evelyn Rose Benson and Joan Quinn McDevitt, *Community Health and Nursing Practice,* 2nd ed. (Englewood Cliffs, N.J.: Prentice-Hall, 1980), 58.
16. Ibid., 53.
17. William J. Baumol and Wallace E. Oates, *Economics, Environmental Policy, and the Quality of Life* (Englewood Cliffs, N.J.: Prentice-Hall, 1979), 46.
18. Barbara Ward and René Dubos, *Only One Earth* (New York: W.W. Norton & Co., 1972), 57.

19. Parker C. Reist, "Air pollution," in L. Jarvis, *Community Health Nursing* (Philadelphia: F.A. Davis Co., 1981), 642.
20. Ibid., 644.
21. Ibid., 434.
22. Baumol and Oates, *Economics, Environmental Policy*, 47.
23. Ibid., 45–47.
24. William O. Douglas, *The Three Hundred Year War* (New York: Random House, 1972).
25. Reist, "Air pollution," 645.
26. Ibid.
27. Ibid.
28. Murray and Zentner, *Nursing Concepts for Health Promotion*, 251.
29. U.S. Environmental Protection Agency, *Your Guide to the U.S. Environmental Protection Agency* (Washington, D.C.: Office of Public Affairs A-107, 1982), 7.
30. Edgar W. Butler, *Urban Sociology* (New York: Harper & Row, 1976), 448.
31. Melvin A. Bernarde, *Our Precious Habitat* (New York: W.W. Norton & Co., 1973), 149.
32. David P. Spath "Water pollution," in L. Jarvis, *Community Health Nursing* (Philadelphia: F.A. Davis Co., 1981), 660.
33. *As We Live and Breathe: The Challenge of Our Environment* (Washington, D.C.: The National Geographic Society, 1971), 96.
34. U.S. Environmental Protection Agency, *Your Guide*, 8, 9.
35. Spath, "Water pollution," 660.
36. U.S. Environmental Protection Agency, *Your Guide*, 17.
37. "Toxic Substances Control Act," Public Laws 94–669, October 11, 1976, p. 90 Stat. 2003.
38. Ibid.
39. "The Federal Insecticide, Fungicide, and Rodenticide Act," Public Law 92–516, p. 86 STAT 973–999.
40. Bernarde, *Our Precious Habitat*, 179.
41. U.S. Environmental Protection Agency Statistics, Office of Public Affairs (Washington, D.C.: 1982).
42. Ibid.
43. Bernarde, *Our Precious Habitat*, 178.
44. U.S. Environmental Protection Agency Reports, Office of Public Affairs (Washington, D.C.: 1982).
45. Bernarde, *Our Precious Habitat*, 183.
46. Leo J. Malone, *Basic Concepts of Chemistry* (New York: John Wiley & Sons, 1981), 54–59.
47. Ibid.
48. Ibid.
49. Ibid.
50. Carol A. Silberstein, "Ionizing radiation and community health," in L. Jarvis, *Community Health Nursing* (Philadelphia: F.A. Davis Co., 1981), 682.
51. Ralph Nader and John Abbott, *The Menace of Atomic Energy* (New York: W.W. Norton & Company, 1979), 10.
52. Ibid., 38.
53. Richard W. Wagner, *Environment and Man* (New York: W.W. Norton & Co., 1971), 213.
54. Ibid., 214.
55. U.S. Environmental Protection Agency, *Your Guide*, 19.
56. Joseph J. Seneca and Michael K. Taussig, *Environmental Economics*, 2nd ed. (Englewood Cliffs, N.J.: Prentice-Hall, 1979), 191.
57. Ibid., 194.
58. James D. Miller, *Effects of Noise on People* (Washington, D.C.: U.S. Environmental Protection Agency, 1971).
59. Henry Still, *In Quest of Quiet* (Harrisburg, Pa.: Stackpole Books, 1970), 13.
60. Seneca and Taussig, *Environmental Economics*, 191.
61. *Noise From Heavy Construction* (Washington, D.C.: U.S. Environmental Protection Agency, 1972).
62. U.S. Environmental Protection Agency, Office of Noise Abatement and Control (Washington, D.C., 1978).
63. Mary Louise Brown "The quality of the work environment," *Am J Nurs* 75, (October 1975): 1756–57.
64. Catherine W. Tinkham "The plant as the patient of the occupational health nurse," *Nurs Clin North Am* 7, (March 1972): 100–102.
65. Evelyn R. Benson and Joan Q. McDevitt, *Community Health Nursing Practice* (Englewood Cliffs, N.J.: Prentice-Hall, 1980), 59.
66. I.M. Meth, "Electrical safety in the hospital," *Am J Nurs* 80 (1980):1344–48.
67. Ibid., 1344.
68. Nurse Action Group, "Protection is better than Curie," *Nurs Mirror* 152, (1981): 26–30.
69. Nurse Action Group "Beware of the drug," *Nurs Mirror* 152, (1981): 34–38.
70. Ibid.
71. Ibid.

Annotated Bibliography

Campbell, E.B., M.A. Williams and S.M. Mlynarczyk. After the fall—confusion *Am J Nurs* 86(2):151–154. The authors of this article describe risk factors that may contribute to confusion following a fall and a change in environment.

Clark, C.C. 1981. *Enhancing Wellness: A Guide for Self-Care.* New York: Springer. Included in this text are self-assessment tools for personal living, work, and play environments. Discusses high-risk groups related to harmful substances and protective measures.

Dickey, L.D. 1976. *Clinical Ecology.* Springfield, Ill.: Chas. C. Thomas. This is a basic textbook on the clinical study of the effects of chemicals, food, allergenic substances, and other environmental agents on the individual.

Kirkis J. 1982. Tactics to hold microbes at bay. *RN* 45(6):81. This brief article summarizes how infection spreads and tells how to reduce it.

Lee, P.S. and B.J. Pash. 1983. Preventing patient falls. *Nurs 83* 13(2):118–20. This article gives several reasons why falls occur and suggests a nursing checklist to prevent falls.

Maddocks G. 1981. A childproof environment: Careful—don't touch. *Nurs Mirror* 152(21):i–xiv. This series of articles discusses how children are injured and the types of injuries most frequently encountered. Age groups range from infants through adolescents.

Mattia, M.A. 1983. Hazards in the hospital. The sterilants: Ethylene oxide and formaldehyde. *Am J Nurs* 83(2):240–43. This article discusses the hazards of selected toxic chemicals and suggests ways of reducing these hazards.

Meth, I.M. 1980. Electrical safety in the hospital. *Am J Nurs* 80(7):1344–48. This excellent article discusses the concept of electricity and applies it to environmental safety.

National Study Commission on Cytotoxic Exposure. 1984. *Consensus to Unresolved Questions Concerning Cytotoxic Agents.* Rockville, Md.: U.S. Department of Health and Human Services. This pamphlet provides information regarding safe handling and administration of cytotoxic drugs.

Nurse Action Group. 1981. Beware of the drug. *Nurs Mirror* 152(6):34–38. This article discusses chemical and drug hazards present in the work environment and steps to take to avoid injury.

Nurse Action Group. 1981. Protection is better than Curie. *Nurs Mirror* 152(8):26–30. This article discusses radiation, treatment, and relevant nursing action.

Odum, E.P. 1971. *Fundamentals of Ecology,* 3rd ed. Philadelphia: Saunders. A basic ecology textbook that stresses ecosystem dynamics.

Witte, N.S. 1979. Why the elderly fall. *Am J Nurs* 79(11):1950–52. Falls are the second leading cause of death in the United States, and the elderly are susceptible to falling for a variety of reasons. This article explains the reasons, give examples, and suggests actions to prevent falls.

Index

AANA. *See* American Association of Nurse Anesthetists

AARP. *See* American Association of Retired Persons

Abortion, 275

Absolute moral principles, 268

Academic health centers, 115, 128–129

Access to care, 115, 667
  as output measure, 131

Accommodation, 395
  in decision making, 630
  in learning theory, 404

Accountability, 231
  continuing education, 250–255
  credentials, 238–243
  moral judgement, development of, 270–272
  nurse as moral agent, 269–270
  for nursing practice, 220–223
  and nursing research, 361
  professional literature and, 243–250
  quality assurance, 236–238

Accreditation, 230
  concept and purpose, 240–241
  continuing education, 253–254
  criteria and standards, 242–243
  overview, 241–242
  process, 243
  types, 242

Accreditors, 115, 122–123

ACNM. *See* American College of Nurse Midwives

ACSN. *See* Association of Collegiate Schools of Nursing

Active change, 351, 353

Activity, 182
  assessment guidelines for, 193–194

Acupuncture, 534

ADAMHA. *See* Alcohol, Drug Abuse, and Mental Health Administration

Adaptation, 100, 105–106. *See also* General adaptation syndrome (GAS)
  aging process and, 443
  anthropological, 108–109, 112
  biological, 106
  educational models, 111
  in family processes, 631
  human nature and, 109–110
  physiological, 106–107
  psychosocial, 107–108, 112
  in Roy's nursing theory, 80
  stress and, 107

Adaptation theory, 100, 105–109

Adaptive system, nursing as, 110

A.D.N. programs. *See* Associate degree nursing (A.D.N.) programs

Adolescence. *See also* Children
  behavioral stage of, 201
  learning in, 332–333
  perception of death, 568–570
  teaching in, 340

Adulthood
  behavioral stages, 201
  learning in, 332–333
  teaching in, 340

Adventitious crisis, 581, 585

Advocacy, 261, 269

Aeration, 181
  assessment guidelines for, 190–191

Affective domain, 329
  learning and, 331

Agape, 261, 266

Age. *See also* Aging assessment and, 200–201
  grief response and, 568
  pain and, 527
  sleep patterns and, 481
Agency, 205, 211–212
  for community health nursing
    official, 661–662
    voluntary, 662–663
  for interpreters for hearing-impaired, 470
Agent, 653, 656
  of change. *See* Change agent
  in epidemiology, 655–656
  moral, nurse as, 269–270
Aging, 433, 434–435. *See also* Age; Gerontological
      nursing
  attitudes towards, 437–438
  current research, 441–442
  demographics, 435–436
  health assessment and, 201, 448–450
  health status and, 442–444
  nursing process and, 446–452
  theories of, 434, 438
    biological, 438–439, 440
    psychological, 439
    sociological, 439–441
Agism, 434
Air pollution, 675, 678–680
AJN. *See American Journal of Nursing*
Alcohol, Drug Abuse, and Mental Health Adminis-
      tration (ADAMHA), 662
Alcohol abuse, altered sleep patterns from, 483
Altruism, 262, 267
AMA. *See* American Medical Association
America, nursing in
  early leaders, 13–19
  history of, 10–12
  landmark studies, 19–22
American Association of Nurse Anesthetists
      (AANA), 240
American Association of Retired Persons (AARP),
      437
American Child Health Association, 662
American College of Nurse Midwives (ACNM),
      240
American Diabetes Association, 662
American Heart Association, 662
American Journal of Nursing (AJN), 14–18, 244,
      248–249, 251
American Nurses' Association (ANA)
  community health nursing definition, 661
  continuing education, 253–254
  gerontological nursing standards, 444–446
  nursing definition of, 38
  quality assurance model, 237, 238
  quality of care model, 236
  standardized qualifications, 40–41
American Nurses' Association (ANA) Code, 221,
      222, 234. *See also Code for Nurses*
  and informed consent, 218
American Public Health Association (APHA), ac-
      creditation and, 242
ANA. *See* American Nurses' Association
Analgesic, 519, 531
  action sites, 536
Analyses of variance (ANOVA), 385
Annual age-specific mortality rate, 659
Annual case-specific death rate, 659
Anorexia, 489, 501
ANOVA. *See* Analyses of variance
Anthropological adaptation, 108–109, 112
Anticipatory grief, 559, 564
Anticipatory guidance, 581
Anxiety, 395, 543, 544–545, 581–582
  behavioral responses, 547
    adaptive and maladaptive, 547–549
    internal and external, 547, 549
  Caplan's phases of, 583
  coping/defense mechanisms, 197, 549–550
  in interpersonal theory, 401
  levels, 545–546
  nursing considerations, 550
  nursing process in, 555–556
  physiological response, 546–547
  psychoanalitic theory and, 399
  theories, 545
APHA. *See* American Public Health Association
Apnea. *See* Sleep apnea
Applied research, 360, 363
Archives of Psychiatric Nursing, 250
Army and Navy Nurse Corps, 25
Aspiration, 489, 493
Assault, 205, 213
Assessing, 137. *See also* Health assessment
  client needs, in teaching process, 343–344
  in nursing process, 144–150
Assimilation, 395
  in learning theory, 404
Associate degree nursing (A.D.N.) programs,
      29–30
Association of Collegiate Schools of Nursing
      (ACSN), 16
Atelectasis, 489
  prevention and treatment of, 510–511
Attitude, 307
  in SMCR model, 313
Audiovisual (AV) aids, 343
Auscultation, 191
Automated data processing (ADP), 56
Autonomy, 262
AV aids. *See* Audiovisual (AV) aids

AVLINE, 246
Avoidance, 395
  in learning theory, 403

Baccalaureate nursing
  programs, 29–30, 38–41
  research skills expected in, 363
Bargaining, in decision making, 630
Barriers
  to change, 351, 352, 353–354
  to learning, 329
    internal and external, 333–334
Basic research, 360, 363
Battery, 205, 213
Bed equipment, 508
Bed-wetting. See Enuresis
Bedrest. See Therapeutic bedrest
Bedsores. See Decubitus ulcers
Behavior
  anxiety and, 547–549
  control, ethical issues in, 276
  developmental level and, 200–201
  and stress, 554
Behavioral objectives, 335–336
  ways to write, 337
Behavioral science theory, and human communica-
    tion theory, relationship to, 309–311
Behavioral systems, 69
  Johnson's model of, 75
Belief systems, 62
  and philosophy-of-life umbrella, 63
Beneficence, 262, 269
Bereavement, 559, 563
Berlo's source–message–channel–receiver (SMCR)
    model of communication, 312–315
Berne, Eric, 400–401
Bias, 360
BIOETHICS, 246
Biological adaptation, 106
Biological sexuality, 419, 422
Bion, Wilfred
  group definition, 602
  and small group theory, 603
Biostatistics, in epidemiology, 657–659
Birth rate, 657–658
Bisexuals, 419, 423
Body alignment, of client on bedrest, 506–509
Body image, 409, 412–413
Body maintenance, 181
  assessment guidelines for, 195, 196
Body movement, 315–316
Boundary, 100
  in family processes, 626–627

maintaining, 627
  of group, 601, 604, 605
  in systems theory, 102
Brown Report, 21–22
  nursing education, 28
Budget and Emergency Deficit Control Act (1985),
    131
Budget Reconciliation Act (1981), 131, 132
Bundge, Helen L., 18
Burnout, 35
  syndrome, 54–55
Burns, prevention of, 690–691

Cadet Nursing Corps, 23–24
Cancer registries, 666
Caplan, Gerald, 582–583
Carcinogenic, defined, 675
Cardiovascular system, effect of immobility on,
    493–494
Case mix, 115, 121
Case-specific fatality rate, 659
Case study, 360
  research design, 375–376
  in research process, 372
Catholic University of America, nursing process
    phases of, 170
CATLINE, 246
CDC. See Center for Disease Control
Celibacy, 419, 423
Center for Disease Control (CDC), 662
Central tendency, 360
Centrality concept, 605–606
Certification, 116, 222, 230, 239–240
  frameworks for, 121, 122
CEU. See Continuing Education Unit
Change, 351
  components of, 352
  overt, 351, 353
  passive, 351, 353
  planned, 351, 352
  revolutionary, 351, 353
  spontaneous, 352, 353
  target for, 352
  types, 353
Change agent, 329, 351, 352
  nurses as, 330
Change theory, 351, 352
  and nursing process, 354–356
Channel, in SMCR model, 314
Charting. See Record-keeping
Chi-square test, 360, 384, 386
Children. See also Adolescence; Infancy; School-age
    children
  grief response in 568

Children *(cont.)*
  pain assessment in, 528–530
  pain reaction in, 528
  perception of death, 568–570
China, early health care in, 4–5
Circadian cycle, 477, 478
Circulation, 181
  assessment guidelines for, 191–192
Civil law, 206
Civil legal process, 212
Civil war
  health care during, 11
  nursing education and, 27
Clean Air Act (1970), 679
Clean Water Act (1972), 680
Client
  case study, 151–152
    nursing care plan for, 153–164
  developmental level of, 200–201
  health assessment by, 185
  in health-care system
    as input, 116–118
    as output, 130
    as throughput, 124–127
  and hospital environment, 688–689
  needs of, 145
  rights of. *See Patient's Bill of Rights;* Right(s)
Clinical specialists, 45
Closed-ended question, 360
Closed system, 100
  in systems theory, 103
Co-leader model, 606
  advantages and disadvantages of, 607
Code for Nurses, 139, 264, 265. *See also* American
    Nurses' Association (ANA) Code
  moral principles and values, 269
Coefficient alpha, 360, 381
Coercive power, 630
Cognitive ability, 182
  assessment guidelines for, 196–197
Cognitive domain, learning and, 331
Cohesiveness, of group, 601, 610
Committee on the Grading of Nursing Schools,
    20–21, 234
Common law, 206, 208
Common-law couples, 626
Communes, 626
Communication. *See also* Human communication
    theory
  components in 308–309
  consummatory, 307, 317
  cultural aspects in health assessment, 296–297
  dysfunctional, 307, 317–318
    between couples, 638–639
  effective, 307, 318
  facilitating, 318–319

  in family processes, 631
  instrumental, 308, 316–317
  interpersonal, 309
  intrapersonal, 309
  nurse–client relationship, 322–325
  in nursing process, 325, 326
  patterns
    in family under stress, 638
    within groups, 605–606
  presymbolic, 308
  public, 309
  of research results, 387
  techniques, 319–322
  therapeutic, 308, 318
  types, 315–318
Communities of solution, 654
Community
  and community health concept, 655
  and epidemiology, 655–659. *See also* Epidemiol-
    ogy
  of identifiable need, 655
  nursing role in, 660–661
  of problem ecology, 654
  resources, 640
  as a system, 656
  types, 654–655
Community assessment, 653, 664–665
  health and illness data, 665–667
  observation, 665
  statistical use, 665
Community health. *See also* Public health
  concept, 655
  rates used in, 657–659
Community health nursing, 653
  agencies for
    official, 661–662
    voluntary, 662–663
  and group work, 602
  and illness prevention, 659–660
  and nursing process, 664–670
  purposes, 659
  role determination, 660–661
  in schools, 664
  in work setting, 663–664
Community Mental Health Centers Act (1983),
    583
Community resources, in family assessment,
    640
Complementarity, 69
  in Rogers' nursing theory, 78
Complexes, 395
  in psychoanalytic theory, 400
Compromise, in decision making, 630
Computer technology, 55–56
Concept, 61, 64–65
  in nursing, 65

Confidentiality, 273, 274, 360
  in health records, 217–218
  invasion of privacy, 213–214
  privileged communication, 213
  in research process, 378–379
Congruence, 395
  in interpersonal theory, 401
Conscious, 395
  in psychoanalytic theory, 399
Consciousness, levels of. *See* Levels of consciousness (LOC)
Consensus, 630
Consent, 206. *See also* Informed consent
Conservation, in Levine's nursing theory, 81–82
Constitutional law, 206, 215–216
Construct, 360, 381
  validity, 360, 381
Consummatory communication, 307, 317
Contact hour, 230
Contemporary nursing, 36
Content validity, 360, 381
Contextual stimuli, 69
Continuing education, 250–251
  accreditation of, 253–254
  defined, 230
  mandatory, 254–255
  professional associations and, 253
  trends, 251–252
  unit (CEU), 252
Continuing Education Unit (CEU), 230, 252
Continuing Nursing Education, 251
Contract, 206, 214–215
Contracture, 489
Control, 360
  in research process, 372
Core values, 283
  in American culture, 287–288
Correlation coefficient, 360, 383–384
Correlation research, 360, 363
Court system, 208
Covert change, 351, 353
Credentials, 230, 238–243. *See also* Accreditation; Certification; Licensure; Registration
Criminal law, 215
Crisis, 582
  adventitious, 581, 585
  Caplan's characteristics of, 583
  developmental, 582, 584–585
  identifying individuals in, 586
  model, 590
    example, 590
  nursing process and, 588–596
  predicting, 585–586
  prevention, 587–588
  sequence diagram, 584
  situational, 582, 585

suicide as response to, 586–587
  theory, 582–584
  types, 584–585
Crisis intervention, 582
  theoretical development, 582–584
Critical defining characteristics, 169
  in P-E-S format, 174
Critical mass community, 655
Cronbach's alpha, 360, 381
Cross-examination, 206, 216
Cross-sectional design, 360
Crude birth rate, 657–658
Crude death rate, 657–658
Cultural assessment tool, 298–299
Cultural relativism, 283, 290
Culture, 283. *See also* Ethnicity
  American, characteristics of, 286–288
  biocultural perspectives, 285–286
  components, 284
  and cultures, 288–290
  disease and illness and, 294–296
  in family assessment, 639
  food and, 292–293
  grief response and, 569
  impact on nursing, 284–285
  nursing process and, 296–302
  pain and, 527
  religion and, 293–294
  social roles and, 290–292
Culture shock, 289–290
Cultures, 283–284
  culture and, 288–290
Cumulative Index to Nursing and Allied Health Literature, The, 245, 250

Data, 360
  analysis, in research process, 382–386
  collection of. *See* Data collection
Data bases, access to, 246–247
Data collection
  in dimensions of human beings, 188–200
  in research process, 379–382
    measuring instrument selection, 381–382
  techniques, 186–188
DDST. *See* Denver Developmental Screening Test
Deaconess Institute at Kaiserworth, 8–9
Death
  child's and adolescent's perception of, 570
  and suicide, 587
Death rate, 657–658
  annual case-specific, 659
  fetal, 658
Decibels, 675
  levels in everyday life, 687
Decision making, in family processes, 630–631

Decomposition, 675
  in ecosystem, 677
Decubitus ulcers, 489, 494–496, 511–512
Deductive reasoning, 63
Defacto decision making, 630
Defamation, 213
Defendant, 206, 211
Defense mechanism, 543, 550, 551
  Freud and, 399
Degrees of freedom, 386
Demonstration, as teaching method, 342
Denver Developmental Screening Test (DDST), 200
Department of Health and Human Services (HHS), 662
Dependent nursing actions, 35
  in episodic care, 44–45
Dependent variable, 360
  in research process, 371
Depression, American nursing during the, 23
Descriptive research, 360, 363
Descriptive statistics, 360, 382–383
Developmental crisis, 584, 586–587
Developmental intervention, 668
Developmental self-care, 77
Dewey, John, 331
Diagnosis, medical versus nursing, 170. *See also* Nursing diagnosis
Diagnosis-related groups (DRGs), 116
  home care and, 127
Diagnostic statement, 169
  guidelines for, 175–176
  and nursing care plan, 175
Diaphragmatic excursion, 191
Differentiation
  in family processes, 631–632
  in systems theory, 105
Directional hypothesis, 360
  in research process, 372
Discrimination Act, 438
Disease
  culture and, 294–296
  prevention, levels, 654, 659
Distributive care, 35
  nursing role in, 46, 47–48
Division of Nursing, 662
Dix, Dorothea L., 11
Dock, Lavinia L., 15
Doctoral level nursing programs, 42–43
Dream sleep, 478–479
DRGs. *See* Diagnosis-related groups
Drives, 396
  in psychoanalytic theory, 400
Drug abuse, altered sleep patterns from, 483
Due process, 206, 208
Duvall, E. M., family life cycle of, 634

Dyads
  in group communication network, 606
  nuclear, 620
Dynamic equilibrium, 100
  in systems theory, 103–104
Dysfunctional communication, 307, 317–318
  between couples, 638–639

Ecology, 675
  and model of environment, 677–678, 679
Ecomap, 619, 641–642
Ecosystem, 675, 677, 679
Education
  associate degree programs, 30
  collegiate, 28–31
  continuing. *See* Continuing education
  early schemes, 26–27
  enrollment trends, 42
  entry into practice, 38, 40–42
  graduate, 30–31, 42–43. *See also* Graduate education
  in health-care system
    client–family, 127
    professionals, 127
  Hospital Diploma Schools, 27–28
  inservice, 230, 251
  Lysaught Report, 29–30
  Nurse Training Act (1979), 52
  programs overview, 40–41, 128
  systems theory and adaptation models in, 111
Education of Nursing Technicians, 30
EEG. *See* Electroencephalogram
Effective communication, 307, 318
Ego, 396
  development, 200
  in psychoanalytic theory, 399
Egoism, 262, 267
Elder Abuse Law, 438
Electrical hazards, in hospital environment, 692
Electrical threshold, 675, 692
Electroencephalogram (EEG), 477
  pattern changes during sleep, 479–480
  in sleep/wakefulness studies, 479
Elimination, 182
  assessment guidelines for, 193
  defecation, 489
  effect of immobility on, 499–500
Embolus, 490, 493–494
Emotional communities, 654
Emotional environment, in family assessment, 638–639
Emotional status, 182
  assessment guidelines for, 197

Empathy, 307
  in nurse–client relationship, 323–324
Employer, 206
  responsibility of, 211
Endorphins, 519, 534
Energy, 100
  in family processes, 627
  in systems theory, 105, 112
Enrollment, in nursing education programs, 42
Enterostomal therapy, 45–46
Entropy, 100
  in systems theory, 105
Enuresis, 477, 482
Environment, 676
  in community, 665
  ecological model, 677–678
  emotional, 638–640
  in epidemiology, 656
  home, 640
  hospital. *See* Hospital environment
  human adaptation to, 676
  nursing interests in, 677, 687–688
  pollution of, 678–687. *See also* Pollution
  toxic substances in, 680–681, 682–685. *See also* Pollution; Toxic substances
Environmental Protection Agency (EPA)
  air pollution and, 679–680
  Office of Noise Abatement and Control, 686–687
  radioactive pollutants and, 686
  toxic substances and, 681
  water pollution and, 680
EPA. *See* Environmental Protection Agency
Epidemic, 653
Epidemiology, 653, 655
  disease transmission, chain of causation, 656
  host, agent, and environment in, 655–656
  methods, 657
  terminology, 657–659
Episodic care, 36
  nursing role in, 43–46
    and practice areas, 45
Equifinality, 100
  in systems theory, 104–105
Erikson, Erik
  behavioral stages, 200–201
  eight stages of man, 585
  existential-humanistic theory, 402
Ethics, 139, 262. *See also* Accountability; American Nurses' Association (ANA) Code; *Code for Nurses*
  importance to nursing, 263–264
  justice-based, 268–269
  love-based, 265–266
  major orientations, 264–269

placebo and, 537
  of teaching, 338–339
Ethnicity. *See also* Culture
  in family assessment, 639
  pain and, 527–528
Ethnocentrism, 284, 290
Etiology, 169
  in P-E-S format, 174
Evaluation, 138, 230, 236, 653
  of community health nursing, 669–670
  cultural aspects, 302
  in nursing process, 144, 164–166
  in teaching process, 347
Evaluation research, 360
Evolutionary change, 351, 353
Existential-humanistic theory, 401–403
Existentialism, in Paterson and Zderad's nursing theory, 81
Expanded role, 36, 46, 48–49
Experimental research, 360, 363
  designs, 374–375
Expert power, 630
Expert witness, 206, 212
Extended family, 619, 624
Extroversion, 396
  in psychoanalytic theory, 400
Eye disease, danger signals for, 467. *See also* Vision

F-test. *See* Analyses of variance
Facilitators
  of change, 351, 352, 353
  of learning, 329
    external and internal, 334
Falls, prevention of, 691
False imprisonment, 213
Family. *See also* Family assessment; Kinship system
  assessment of
  concepts and assumptions, 620
  cultural aspects in health assessment, 300–301
  extended, 619, 624
  functions, 632–633
  historical perspectives, 621
    early, 621
    industrial revolution, 621–623
    space age, 623
  life cycle, 633–634
  nuclear, 620, 624
  and nursing process, 634–647
  organizational types, 624–626
  of orientation, 619
  as primary group, 602
  processes, 626–632

Family (cont.)
  single-parent, 620, 624–625
  social roles in, 290–292
  systems/adaptation approach to, 624–632
  theoretical approaches to study of, 623–624,
    625
Family assessment, 635
  community resources, 640
  emotional environment, 638–639
  family strengths, 640–641
  health picture, 636–637
  home environment, 640
  home visit, 635–636
  household roster, 635–636
  income, 639–640
  information sources, 635
  nursing diagnosis, 643–644
  nutrition, 637
  recreation, 639
  safety, 637
  sleep and rest provisions, 638
  social influences, 639
  tools in, 641–643, 644
Family life cycle, 646
Family strengths, in family assessment, 640–641
Fatality rate, case-specific, 661
FDA. See Food and Drug Administration
Fear, 543, 544, 550
  nursing process in, 555–556
  responses to, 550–552
Fecal impaction, 490, 499
Federal Depository Library System, 247
Feedback, 100
  in health-care system, 131–132
  in systems theory, 104
Fetal death rate, 658
Fight or flight response, 543, 546
Fluid imbalances, immobility and, 501
Food, culture and, 292–293. See also Nutrition
Food and Drug Administration (FDA), 664
Frail elderly, 434
Framework, 61, 65
  for family study, 623–624, 625
  theoretical, in research process, 361, 370–371
Franklin, Martha M., 15
Freud, Sigmund, 399
Fromm, Erich, 402–403
Functional community, 655

Gagné, Robert, 331
Games, in teaching, 340, 341. See also Communi-
  cation; Play
GAS. See General adaptation syndrome
Gate-control theory, of pain, 520–523
Gender identity, 419, 422

Gender role, 419, 422–423
General adaptation syndrome (GAS), 100, 544
  psychosocial assessment and, 107
  in stress theory, 552–553
General systems theory, 100
  adaptation in. See Adaptation; Adaptation theory
  educational models of, 111
  energy in, 105, 112
  overview and significance, 101. See also Sys-
    tem(s)
Genogram, 619, 643, 644
Geopolitical communities, 654
Geriatrics, 434, 436–437. See also Aging
  nurse specialists, 46
Gerontological nursing, 434, 436–437
  ANA standards in, 444
  as specialty, 444–446
Gerontology, 434, 436–437
Glasgow Coma Scale, 467
Goal(s), 138, 329
  in group functions, 608–609
  in nursing process, 144
  in teaching process, 335–337
Goldmark Report, 19–20
  nursing education, 27
  standards of care, 234
Good Samaritan Acts, 216
Goodrich, Annie W., 16
Goostray, Stella, 17–18
Grading Committee Report. See Committee on the
  Grading of Nursing Schools
Graduate education, 30–31
  doctoral, 42–43
  masters, 42
    study areas, 43
Gramm–Rudman. See Budget and Emergency Defi-
  cit Control Act 1985
Gray Panthers, 437
Grief, 559, 562–563
  anticipatory, 559, 563
  factors influencing, 567–670
  maladaptive, 560–568
Grieving, 582
Group discussion, as teaching method, 341
Group dynamics, 602, 603
Group process, 602
  in group structure, 609–611
  personal goals and, 608
Group psychotherapy, 603
Group roles, 605
Group(s), 601, 602
  boundary, 601, 604, 605
  communication networks, 605–606
  concepts, theoretical foundations of, 603
  equilibrium, 604
  functions, 608–609

in general population, 602
holistic character, 603–604
leadership, 606–608
nursing process and, 611–615
open versus closed systems, 604
planning for, 613–614
primary and secondary, 602
process. *See* Group process
role network, 605
social roles in, 290–292
structural forms, 605
types, 611, 612
Growth
and development, 200–201, 395–406
in ecosystem, 677
in family processes, 631–632
Guidelines for Implementing the Code for Nurses,
    221

Hall, Lydia W., 18–19
Hazardous waste, 676, 681
Healers, 295–296
Healing, 295–296
HEALTH, 247
Health
biocultural perspectives, 285–286
defined, 36
perception, cultural aspects in health assessment,
    297
views of
    holistic, 37–38
    traditional, 37
WHO definition of, 37
Health assessment, 181
community. *See* Community assessment
cultural aspects, 296–301
data collection techniques in, 186–188
developmental level in, 200–201
in dimensions of human beings, 188–200
in elderly client, 446–450
in family situations. *See* Family assessment
framework for, 182–184
for group intervention, 612–613
human resources for, 185
in immobility, 503–505
nurse versus other health-care providers, 184
of pain, 531–533
sexual, 427–428
Health care
access to, 115, 131
American nursing and
    history of, 10–19
    in twentieth century, 22–26
in antiquity, 3–8
common needs, 125

in eighteenth century, 8
and holism, 110–111. *See also* Holistic health
    care
landmark studies, 19–22
in nineteenth century, 8–10
nursing education and, 26–31
Health-care center
and access to care, 131
classification scheme for, 121
Health-care financing legislation, 124. *See also*
    Medicaid; Medicare
Health-care plans, 131
Health-care practices, 182
assessment guidelines for,199
Health-care system, 116
components, 117
feedback in, 131–132
inputs, 116–124
outputs, 130–131
throughputs, 124–130
Health-care team, 116
health assessment by, 185
    nurse versus, 184
in health-care system, 119–120
Health-deviation self-care, 70
Orem's components of, 77
Health for All by the Year 2000, 130
Health-illness continuum, 36, 37
Health-illness practices, cultural aspects in health
    assessment, 297
Health Laws, 131. *See also* Legislation; Public Law
    (PL)
Health maintenance organization (HMO), 116,
    123
as primary care provider, 126
Health Resources and Services Administration
    (HRSA), 662
Health services legislation, 124
Hearing
alterations in, 464
assessment, 467–468
Hearing impaired client
care plan for, 469, 470
nurse–client relationship, 472
Helicy, 70
in Rogers' nursing theory, 78
Henderson, Virginia, nursing theory of, 71–72,
    88–89
Heterosexual, 420, 423
HHS. *See* Department of Health and Human Ser-
    vices
High-fiber diet, 512–513
High technology medicine, 116, 121
Hill–Burton Act, 122
Hippocrates,5
HISTLINE, 246

Historical research, 360, 363
  design, 376
History of Nursing, The, 14
HMO. *See* Health maintenance organization
Holism, 100
  Adler's concept of, 400
  health care and, 110–111
  in systems and adaptation theory, 109–110
Holistic health care 100
  stress and, 110–111
  terminology, 110
Holistic health model, 37–38
Holmes, T., 553
Home environment, in family assessment, 640
Home health agency, 116, 126–127
Home visit, in family assessment, 635–636
Homeodynamics, 100, 104
Homeostasis, 104. *See also* Ecology
  model, 677–678
Homosexual relationships, 423
Hormone, 420, 422
Hospice nurses, 46
Hospital environment
  air quality in, 689
  client's lack of control over, 688–689
  decor and other factors in, 690
  electrical hazards in, 694
  infections in, 691–692
  noise in, 689–690
  radiation in, 692–693
  safety in, 690–691
    of building, 693
    for nursing practice, 693–694
  temperature in, 689
  toxic substances in, 693
Hospital information systems (HIS), 56
Hospitalization
  effect on sexual integrity, 425–426
  and sleep deprivation, 483
Host, 654, 656
Household roster, in family assessment, 636
HRSA. *See* Health Resources and Services Administration
Human communication theory. *See also* Communication
  behavioral science theory and, relationship to, 309–311
  models, 311–315
Human need theory, 141–142
Humanism, 100
  in systems and adaptation theory, 109–110
Humanistic Nursing, 80
Hypersomnia, 477, 481–482
Hypnosis, 538
Hypostatic pneumonia, 490, 492

Hypothesis
  definitions of, 360–361
  statement formulation, 371–372, 373

ICN. *See* International Council of Nurses
Id, 396
  in psychoanalytic theory, 399
Illness, 36
  biocultural perspectives, 285–286
  culture and, 294–296
  holistic view of, 37–38
  Lipowski's concept of, 530
  sexuality and, 425
Immobility, 490. *See also* Therapeutic bedrest
  assessment, 503–505
  forms of, 491
  metabolism and nutrition and, 500–501
  nursing process in, 503–515
  physical problems of, 491–500
  psychological aspects of, 501–503
Implementation, 138, 230, 236
  of community health nursing, 668–669
  cultural aspects, 301–302
  in nursing process, 144, 152–164
  in teaching process, 346–347
Incidence, 654
Independent nursing actions, 36
  in episodic care, 44
Independent nursing practice, 36, 49
Independent variable, 360
  in research process, 371
Index Medicus, 370
Inductive reasoning, 63
Industrial revolution, family history during, 621–623
Infancy. *See also* Children
  behavioral stage of, 200
  learning in, 331–332
  teaching in, 339
Infant mortality rate, 658
Infection, 676
  nosocomial, 676, 691–692
Infection control nurses, 46
Infectious Diseases: Cases, Deaths, and Vaccinations, 666
Inferential statistics, 360, 384–385
Informational power, 630
Informed consent, 206, 360
  record-keeping and, 218–219
  in research process, 378–379
Input, 100
  in health-care system, 116–124
  in systems theory, 103
Inservice education, 230, 251

Insomnia, 477, 481
Institute of Medicine (IOM), nurse supply and, 52–53
Instrumental communication, 308, 316–317
Insurers, in health-care system, 123
Integrity, conservation of, in Levine's nursing theory, 81–82
Intellectual skill, 143
Intensive care unit (ICU), environmental stimuli and, 460, 461
Intercultural variability, 284, 289
Interdependent nursing actions, 36
  in episodic care, 44
International Council of Nurses (ICN), 16
International nursing, 49
  opportunities for, 50
International Nursing Index, 245, 250, 370
International Statistical Classification of Diseases, Injuries, and Causes of Death (ICD), 666
Interpersonal communication, 309
Interpersonal Relations in Nursing, 72
Interpersonal skills, 143
Interpersonal theory, 400–401
Interviewing, 182
  as data collection technique, 186–187
Intracultural variability, 284, 289
Intrapersonal communication, 309
Introversion, 396
  in psychoanalytic theory, 400
Invasion of privacy, 206, 213–214. See also Privacy
IOM. See Institute of Medicine
Ionizing radiation, as pollutant, 685

JCAH. See Joint Commission on Accreditation of Hospitals
Johnson, Dorothy E., nursing theory of, 70, 75, 90–91
Johnson, V.E., 424
Joint Commission on Accreditation of Hospitals (JCAH), 123, 242
Jourard, Sidney, 401–402
Journals, professional nursing, 248–250
Jung, Carl, 399–400
Jurisdiction, 206
Justice-based ethics, 268–269

Kant, I., 268
Kidney
  effect of body positions on, 500
  stones, as therapeutic bedrest hazard, 500
Kinesics, 308
King, Imogene M., nursing theory of, 76, 92–93

Kinship systems, 291
  in U.S., characteristics of, 626
Kohlberg, L., 270–272
Korean war, American nursing during, 25–26

Law, 206. See also Legislation
  affecting nursing practice, 208–216
  "natural," 266–267
  philosophy and religion, distinctions between, 263
  sources of, 207–208
Law witness, 206, 212–213
Leadership, 351
  of group
    effective, 607–608
    models, 606–607
    styles, 607
  process, 143
Learning, 329
  barriers to, 329
    external, 333, 334
    internal, 333–334
  domains, 331
  facilitators of, 329, 334
  and nursing process, 343–347
  principles of, 330, 331, 332
  theories, 330–331
  throughout life span, 331–333
Learning theory, personhood and, 403–404
Lecture, as teaching method, 341–342
Legislation, 216. See also *individually named Acts; Public Law (PL)*
  health-care system and, 123–124
Legitimate power, 629
Lethality assessment, 582, 587
Levels of consciousness (LOC), 459
  alterations in, 463
  assessment, 466, 467
Levine, Myra E., nursing theory of, 81–82, 96–97
Lewin, Kurt
  group definition, 602
  group dynamics research of, 603
  and learning theory, 404
Liability, 206
  determining, 211
Libertarianism, 262, 265
Libraries, 245–246
  federal depository, 247
  national. See National Library of Medicine (NLM)
  regional, 247
Licensed practical nurses (L.P.N.s), 25
Licensure, 239
  and accountability for practice, 220–222

Life cycle
   of family, 633–634, 646
   social roles in, 290–292
Life expectancy, aging and, 442–443
Life-style, 182
   assessment guidelines for, 198
Life tasks, 72
Lindemann, Erich, 582–583
Lippincott's Guide to Nursing Literature, 249
Literature review, in research process, 369–370.
     See also Professional literature
Litigation, 206
Living systems, 109, 112. *See also* Equifinality
Living wills, 276
LOC. *See* Levels of consciousness (LOC)
Local health department, community health nurs-
   ing through, 661
Looking-glass self, 409, 410
Loss, 560–562
   categories, 561–562
   common reactions to, 563
   coping with, 562–567
   defined, 559–560
   nursing process and, 570–577
Love-based ethics, 265–266
L.P.N.s. *See* Licensed practical nurses
Lysaught Report, 29–30

Maass, Clara L., 15–16
Mahoney, Mary E., 13
Maintenance functions, 602
   of group, 609, 610
Maintenance roles, 605
Maladaptive grief, 568
Malpractice, 206
   common acts of, 210–211
   legal principles of, 209–210
Mandatory Retirement Act, 438
Manpower legislation, 124
Maslow, Abraham, 402
Masters, W.H., 424
Master's level nursing programs, 42–43
Materia Medica for Nurses, 15
Maternal mortality rate, 658–659
May, Rollo, 401
McGill–Melzack Pain Questionnaire, 532
Mean, defined, 361, 382–383
Measurement, 182
   as data collection technique, 187–188
   instrument selection, in research process,
     381–382
Media, influence on health-care system, 118
Median, defined, 361, 383

Medicaid, 123, 124
   growth of, 125
Medical diagnosis, nursing diagnosis versus, 170
Medical information systems (MIS), 56
Medical model
   defined, 36
   and health assessment, 184
Medical orders, management of, 219–220
Medical record, 206
Medicare, 123, 124
   growth of, 125
MEDLARS, 246
MEDLINE, 246
Melzack, R., 520–522
Metabolism, immobility and, 500–501
Middle ages, health care in, 5–7
Mobility, 490. *See also* Immobility
   alterations in, 490
Mode, defined, 361, 383
Model, 61, 65
   medical, 36
Modesty, cultural aspects in health assessment, 300
Monogamy, 620, 626
Moral agent, nurse as, 269–270
Moral judgement, development of, 270–272
Morality
   absolute principles, 268
   models in nursing practice, 266
Morals, 262
   in nursing, 269
Morbidity, aging and, 442–443
Morbidity rate, in community assessment, 665–666
Mortality, aging and, 442–443
Mortality rate
   annual age-specific, 659
   in community assessment, 665–666
   infant, 658
   maternal, 658–659
   perinatal, 658
Mourning, 560, 563
   stages, 563–567
Musculoskeletal system, effect of immobility on,
   496–499
Myths, sexual, 421

NANDA. *See* North American Nursing Diagnosis
    Association
Narcissism, 396
   in psychoanalytic theory, 400
Narcolepsy, 477, 482
National Association of Colored Graduate Nurses
    (NACGN), 15
National Center for Health Statistics (NCHS), 666
National Center for Nursing Research, 128, 662

National Commission for the Study of Nursing and Nursing Education (NCSNNE), 29
National Institutes of Health (NIH), 56, 662
National League for Nursing (NLN)
    accreditation and, 242
    standardized qualifications, 40–41
National League for Nursing Education (NLNE), 16, 234, 242
National Library of Medicine (NLM), 245
    data bases available through, 246–247
National Organization for Public Health Nursing (NOPHN), 233
National Safety Council, 663
National Technical Information Service (NTIS), 247–248
"Natural law," 266–267
Needs
    assessment of, nursing diagnosis based on, 147–149
    of client, 145
Negentropy, 100
    in systems theory, 105
Negligence
    common acts of, 210–211
    legal principles of, 209–210
Neonatal mortality rate, 658
Neuman, Betty M., nursing theory of, 82, 96–97
Nightingale, Florence, 9–10
    as nursing theorist, 71
    pledge, 12
NIH. See National Institutes of Health
NLN. See National League for Nursing
Noise, 676
    and decibel levels, 687
    EPA reduction recommendations, 686–687
    excessive, effects of, 686
    in hospital environment, 689
Non-rapid eye movement (NREM) sleep, 479–481
Nondirectional hypothesis, 361
    in research process, 372
Nonmaleficence, 262, 269
Nonparametric statistical tests, 386
Nonverbal communication, 315–316
    and assessment, 185
Norms, 230, 232, 602
    in decision making, 631
North American Nursing Diagnosis Association (NANDA), 140, 171
Nosocomial infection, 676, 691–692
Nuclear dyad, 620
    as family type, 624
Nuclear family, 620, 624
Nuclear power plants, 685–686
Null hypothesis, 360
    in research process, 372

Nurse
    baccalaureate, research skills expected of, 363
    as change agent, 330
    code for. See American Nurses' Association (ANA) Code; *Code for Nurses*
    and group work, 602–603
    health assessment by, 185
        versus health-care team, 184
    hospital environment and, 689–693
    as moral agent, 269–270
    Nightingale pledge for, 12
    population ratios, by region, 53
    rights and responsibilities, of, 223, 225–226
Nurse anesthetists, 45
Nurse–client relationship
    communication and, 322–325
    in Travelbee's nursing theory, 79
Nurse practitioner, 36, 46, 48–49
Nurse Training Act (1979), 52
Nursing. See also Health care
    definitions of, 38, 39, 143, 182
    Division of, 662
    gerontological. See Gerontological nursing
    specialization. See Specialty areas
Nursing: A Social Policy Statement, 183
Nursing actions
    automatic, 69, 73
    deliberative, 69, 73
    examples, 44
Nursing audit, 230, 238, 251
Nursing care plan
    case example, 153–164
    diagnostic statement and, 175
    sexual integrity and, 428, 429
Nursing Classification System Committee, purpose, goals, and tasks of, 611
Nursing diagnosis, 138, 140, 169
    approved list, 173
    case study, 176–178
    diagnostic statement and, 175–176
    in family assessment, 643–644
    guidelines for using, 177
    in immobility, 505
    needs assessment and, 147–149
    and nursing process, 170–171
    versus medical diagnosis, 170
Nursing diagnostic process, 169
    NANDA formalization of, 171–178. *See also* P-E-S format
Nursing Economics, 250
Nursing Economics Business Perspectives for Nurses, 250
Nursing function, King's levels of, 76
Nursing Home Project, 125
Nursing information system, 36, 56

Nursing orders, 170
Nursing practice
  accountability for, 220–223
  defined, Maryland and Delaware, 221
  laws affecting, 208–216
  morality models in, 266
  safe environment for, 693–694
Nursing Practice Acts, 233
  and accountability for practice, 220–222
Nursing process, 135, 138–139
  in anxiety, fear and stress, 555–556
  change theory and, 354–356
  communication in, 325–326
  community health nursing in, 664–670
  components, 143
  in crisis, 588–596
  culture and, 296–302
  cyclical nature of, 144
  environmental issues and, 687–688
  family in, 634–648. See also Family assessment
  in gerontology, 446–452
  and group intervention, 611–615
  in immobility, 503–515
  loss and, 570–577
  nursing diagnosis and, 170–171
  pain and, 531–539
  and personhood, 404–405
  philosophical base, 144
  in sensory deprivation, 465–473
  sexuality and, 424–429
  sleep and, 483–485
  in suicide, 588–596
  teaching–learning process in, 343–347
  theoretical–conceptual frameworks, 139–140
    human need, 141–142
    perception, 142–143
Nursing Research, 18, 248
Nursing Research Index, 370
Nursing Studies Index, 71, 245–246, 250, 370
Nursing Theorists and their Work, 83
Nursology, 70
  in Paterson and Zderad's nursing theory, 81
Nutrition, 182
  assessment guidelines for, 192–193
  for client on bedrest, 513–514
  cultural aspects in health assessment, 297, 300
  in family assessment, 639
  immobility and, 500–501
Nutting, Mary A., 14

Objective words, 337
Objectives, 230, 330
  taxonomies of, 338
  in teaching process, 335–337. See also Behavioral objectives

Observation, 182
  as data collection technique, 187
Occupational Health, 250
Occupational health, 663–664
Occupational Health and Safety Act (1970)
    (OSHA), 687–688
Office of the Chief Nurse, 662
Ohm's law, 692
Ombudsman Act, 438
Oncology nurse specialists, 46
Open-ended question, 361
Open system, 100
  in systems theory, 103
Operational definitions, 361
  in research process, 372
Orders
  medical, management of, 219–220
  nursing, 170
Orem, Dorothea E., nursing theory of, 76–77,
    92–93
Orientation, 230
  programs, 251
Orlando, Ida J., nursing theory of, 73–74, 90–91
Orthostatic hypotension, 490, 491, 494
OSHA. *See* Occupational Health and Safety Act
    (1970)
Osteoporosis, 490, 497–498
Otto, Herbert A., 641
Outcome criteria, 138
  in nursing process, 144
Output, 100. *See also* Outcome criteria
  in health-care system, 130–131
  in systems theory, 103
Overt change, 351, 353
Overt sexual behavior, nursing process and,
    426–427

P-E-S format. *See* Problem-Etiology-Signs and
    Symptoms format
Pain, 520
  characteristics and classification, 523–527
  Copp's meaning of, 530
  intervening variables, 527–530
  and nursing process, 531–539
  persons at risk, 530
  response to, 530–531
  theories, 520–523
Pain reaction, 519, 523
  in children, 528
  in ethnic groups, 527–528
Pain scales, 533
Pain sensation, 519, 523
Pain threshold, 520, 523
Pain tolerance, 520, 523
Paradoxical sleep, 478–479

Parasomnias, 477, 482
Parenting, as family function, 632–633
Passive change, 351, 353
Paterson, Josephine G., nursing theory of, 80–81, 96–97
Patient. *See* Client
Patient's Bill of Rights, 222–223, 224, 272, 273, 330
Pattern theory, of pain, 520
Pavlov, Ivan, 330
Pediatric Nurse Practitioner, The, 250
Pediatric Nursing, 250
Peer review, 230
Peplau, Hildegard E., nursing theory of, 72–73, 88–89
Perception theory, 142–143
Percussion notes, 191
Perinatal mortality rate, 658
Periodicals, 248–250. *See also* individually named publications
Peripheral nervous system, effect of immobility on, 496–499
Personality, 396–397
Personhood, 397
   nursing process and, 404–405
   theories of, 398–404
      benefits from learning about, 397–398
Pesticide, 676, 681
Philosophy, 61, 62, 330
   and personal belief system, 62, 63
   religion and law, distinctions between, 263
   in teaching process, 335
Philosophy-of-life umbrella, 63
Physical assessment, for elderly patient, 448–450. *See also* Health assessment
Physiological adaptation, 106–107
Physiological dimension, 182, 183–184
   data collection in, 188–195
Piaget, J., 403
Pilot study, 361
   in research process, 379
Placebo, 520, 537
Plan for Implementation of Standards of Nursing Practice, 236
Planned change, 351, 352
Planned Parenthood, 662
Planners, 116
   in health-care system, 122–123
Planning, 138, 654
   cultural aspects, 301
   literature on, 247–248
   in nursing process, 144, 150–152
   in teaching process, 344–346
   Play, learning through, 332, 333. *See also* Games
Pledge, Florence Nightingale, 12
Pneumonia, hypostatic, 490, 492

Politics of Nursing, 244
Pollution, 676, 678
   of air, 678–680
   by noise, 686, 687
   from radiation, 681, 685–686
   from solid waste disposal, 681
   thermal, 676
   by toxic substances, 680–681, 682–685
   of water, 676, 680
Polyandry, 620, 626
Polygamy, 620, 626
Polygyny, 620, 626
Population
   nurse ratios, by region, 53
   specifying, in research process, 376–377
   study definition, 361
Positioning, of client on bedrest, 506–509
Power
   and decision making, 631
   in family processes, 629–630
   police, 206
PPO. *See* Preferred Provider Organization
Practice
   nursing. *See* Nursing practice
   as teaching method, 342
Preferred Provider Organization (PPO), 123
Preschooler, behavioral stage of, 200
Presymbolic communication, 309
Prevalence, defined, 654, 657
Prevention
   crisis, 587–588
   of disease, levels, 654, 659
   primary and secondary, 582, 588, 654, 659
   suicide, 594, 596
   tertiary, 654
Preverbal sounds, 315
Primary care, 36
   aging process and, 443
   elements of, 126
   expanded nursing role in, 48
Primary group, 602
Primary nursing, 36
   in episodic care, 45–46
Primary prevention, 582, 588, 654, 659
Principles of learning, 330, 331, 332
Privacy
   cultural aspects in health assessment, 300
   in hospital environment, 690
   invasion of, 206, 213–214
   for teaching, 342
Privileged communication, 206, 213
Problem, 170
   identification of. *See* Nursing diagnosis
   in P-E-S format, 172
   in research process, 368–369
   taxonomy for, 172–174

Problem-Etiology-Signs and Symptoms (P-E-S) format, 171–174
    diagnostic statement and, 175–176
    different approaches to, 174–175
Problem-solving, research process versus, 362–366. *See also* Nursing process
Process, 61
    in nursing, 66, 143–144. *See also* Nursing process
    perception of, 65–66
    in theory, 63–64
Professional associations
    and continuing education, 253
    in health-care system, 121, 122
Professional literature, 243–244
    access to, 245–248
    to encourage accountability, 244–245
    journals and periodicals, 248–250
    purposes, 244
    review in research process, 369–370
Professional Standards Review Organization (PSRO), 236
Prospective Payment Act (1983), 123, 131
Prospective reimbursement, 116
PSRO. *See* Professional Standards Review Organization
Psychiatric nursing, family system and, 620–621
Psychoanalytic theory, 398–400
Psychodynamic nurse–client relationship, phases of, 72
Psychomotor domain, 330
    learning and, 331
Psychosocial adaptation, 107–108, 112
Psychotherapy, group, 603
Public communication, 309
Public health. *See also* Community health
    association for, (APHA), 242
    Winslow definition of, 655
Public Health Nurse Quarterly, 251
Public Health Nursing Manual, 233
Public Health Service. *See* United States Public Health Service (USPHS)

Quality assurance, 230, 236
    concept and purpose, 236–237
    methodology, 237
    in nursing, 237–238
Quality Patient Care Scale, 238
Quasi-experimental research designs, 375

Radiation
    in hospital environment, 692–693
    as pollutant, 676, 681, 685–686
    radioactive definition, 676

Radioisotopes, 676, 685
Rahe, R., 553
Random numbers, 377, 378
Random sample, 361, 377–378
Range, defined, 361, 383
Rapid eye movement (REM) sleep, 479–481
Rapport, in Travelbee's nursing theory, 79
Rates, used in community health, 657–659
Rational paternalism, 265
Reactive hyperemia, 490, 494–495
Reality shock, 36, 53–54
Reasonable care, 206–207, 210
Reasonably prudent person doctrine, 207, 209
Receiver, in SMCR model, 314–315
Record-keeping
    and access to records, 217–218
    common errors in, 219
    informed consent and, 218–219
    responsibility for, 216–217
Recreation, in family assessment, 639
Recycling, 676
Referred pain, 524
Referrent power, 629
"Reflected appraisals", 410
Reformation, health care during the, 7–8
Regional Medical Programs (RMPs), 251
Registered nurse (RN), 41
    regional distribution, 52–53
    supply and demand for, 51–52
Registration, of nurses, 232–233
Regulators, 116
    in health-care system, 122–123, 129–130
Reimbursement
    policies, 116, 131
    prospective, 116
Relaxation, 535
    and anxiety, 546–547
    in family life, 633
    the nurse and, 55
Reliability, research process and, 361, 381
Religion. *See also* Spiritual dimension
    cultural aspects in health assessment, 296–297
    culture and, 293–294
in family assessment, 639
    grief response and, 569
    pain and, 528
    philosophy and law, distinctions between, 263
REM. *See* Rapid eye movement (REM) sleep
Res ipsa loquitur, 207
Research, 360
    accountability, 361
    classification, 363
    evaluation, 386, 387
        for clinical application, 389
    evolution, 364, 365–366
    future directions, 366, 367

in health-care system, 128–129
hypothesis. *See* Hypothesis
process. *See* Research process
question. *See* Research question
social relevancy, 361–362
trends, 364, 366
Research process, 143–144
steps in, 366, 368–387
versus problem-solving, 362–366
Research question
criteria for determining, 368, 369
formulation, 368, 369
variables within, 372
Research skills, expected levels of, 363–364
Residual stimuli, 70
Respiratory system, effect of immobility on,
492–493
Respondeat superior, 207, 211
Rest, 182
assessment guidelines for, 193–194
provisions for, in family assessment, 638
Reticular activating system (RAS), 459, 461, 462,
477
wakefulness and, 478–479
Reticular formation, 459, 461, 477
and wakefulness, 478–479
Review of systems (ROS), in elderly client,
446–447. *See also* Health assessment
Revolutionary change, 351, 353
Reward power, 630
Right(s), 207, 208
of client, 222–223, 224
accountability for practice, 222–223
as ethical issue, 272, 273
to end life, 275–276
to life, 274–275
of nurse, 223, 225–226
as ethical issue, 272, 274
RN Magazine, 248
Robb, Isabel A. H., 13–14
Robert Wood Johnson Foundation, 125
Rogers, Carl
and existential-humanistic theory, 401–402
and interpersonal theory, 401
Rogers, Martha E., nursing theory of, 77–78,
94–95
Role complementarity, 629
Role enactment, 628
Role playing, as teaching method, 342
Roles
in family processes
formal and informal, 629
types, 628–629
variations, 629
in group, 605
in nursing, 43–47

Rotating leader model, 606
advantages and disadvantages of, 607
Roy, Sr. Callista
nursing theory of, 80, 94–95
self-concept model, 411–412

Safe Drinking Water Act (1974), 680
Safety
in family assessment, 637
in legislation for, 123–124
and occupational health, 663
Sample, 361
specifying, in research process, 376–377
Sampling, procedure for, 377–378
Scale(s), 361. *See also individually named scales*
for pain, 533
in research process, 371
School-age children. *See also* Children
behavioral stage of, 200–201
learning in, 332
teaching of, 339–340
School health, 664
Screening programs, 659
Secondary care facilities, 116
client care in, 124–125
Secondary group, 602
Secondary prevention, 582, 588, 654, 659
Secondary sex characteristics, 420, 422
Self, components, 412–413
Self-care, 70
activities, for client on bedrest, 509–51
health-deviation, 70, 77
Orem's nursing systems for, 77
types, 77
universal, 70, 77
Self-concept, 409, 410
development, 410–412
grief response and, 567
nursing process and, 412–4
theorists, 410
Self-disclosure, 396
in existential-humanistic
Self-esteem, 409
characteristics, 411
physical appearance
Selye, Hans, 552
Sensation, 182
assessment guid
Sensory alteratior
deprivation,
overload, 46
Sensory defic
hearing,
smell ar
tactile,

"S
Sig
"Si
in
Signs
in
Single
Single
adva
Single-p
Situation
Skin, effe
Skinner, E
and stin
Sleep, 477,
amounts
assessmen
cycle of, 4
nursing pro
provisions f
stages, 479–

Sensory deficit *(cont.)*
  visual, 464
Sensory deprivation, 459, 462–463
  nursing process in, 465–473
Sensory overload, 459, 463
  assessment of, 465–466
Sensory perception, 459, 460
Sensory process, 460–461
Sensory reception, 460–461
Sex identity. *See* Gender identity
Sex role. *See* Gender role
Sexual differentiation, 420, 422
Sexual dysfunctions, 427
Sexual integrity, 420
  effect of hospitalization on, 425–426
  in nursing process, 424–425
  and overt sexual behavior, 426–427
Sexual myths, 421
Sexual orientation, 420, 423
Sexual response, 423–424
Sexuality, 182, 420
  assessment guidelines for, 194–195
  basic assumptions about, 424
  components, 422–423
  concept, 422
  and family function, 632
  and illness, 425
  and nursing process, 424–429
  professional interest in, 420–421
Shannon–Weaver model of communication, 311–312
Shortages, of nurses, 49, 51–53
  nurse:population ratios, 53
ick role, 284
  cultural aspects, 295
ick role theory", 118
nificance, level of, 385–386
nificant others", 410
  fluence on self-concept, 412
  and symptoms, 170, 308
  -E-S format, 174
  adults, as family form, 625–626
  eader model, 606
  ntages and disadvantages of, 607
  arent family, 620, 624, 625
  al crisis, 582, 585
  ct of immobility on, 494–496
  . F., 331
  ulus-response interaction, 403
  478
  needed, 478
  tool, 484
  78. *See also* Circadian cycle
  cess and, 483–485
  or, in family assessment, 638
  481

Sleep apnea, 477, 482
  and REM sleep, 481
Sleep cycle schema, 481
Sleep patterns, alterations in, 481–483
Sleep-walking. *See* Somnambulism
Small group theory, 603
SMCR. *See* Berlo's source–message–channel–receiver (SMCR) model of communication
Smell, altered sense of, 464
  assessment, 468
  care plan for client with, 469–470
  nurse–client relationship, 472
Social readjustment rating scale, 553
Social relevancy, or nursing research, 361–362
Social roles, 284
  in family, group and life cycle, 290–292
Social Security Act, 131
Social welfare, aging process and, 443–444
Sociocultural dimension, 182, 183–184
  data collection in, 197–199
Sociometric isolate, in group communication network, 606
Sociometric star concept, in group communication network, 606
Somatotyping, 398
Somnambulism, 477, 482
Source, in SMCR model, 312–313
Space
  in communication, 316, 317
  in hospital environment, 690
  for teaching, 342
Space age, family history in, 623
Speciality areas, 45–46
  certification programs, 223, 241
  gerontology, 46, 445. *See also* Gerontological nursing
  standards of practice, 235–236
Specificity theory, of pain, 520, 521
Spiritual dimension, 182, 183–184
  data collection in, 199–200
Spiritual responses, assessment guidelines for, 200. *See also* Religion
Spontaneous change, 352, 353
St. Thomas Aquinas, 265–267
  abortion, 275
  paradigm case argument and, 269
Staff development. *See* Inservice education
Standard deviation, 361, 383
Standards, 207, 230, 231
  agencies that establish, 129–130
  of care. *See* Standards of care
  characteristics of, 232
  as output measure, 131
  of practice. *See* Standards of practice
Standards of care, 207, 231–236
  determination of, 210

Standards of Nursing Practice, 330
  Operating Rooms, 236
Standards of practice, 221–222
  in gerontological nursing, 444–446
Standing orders, 219–220
State Boards of Nursing, 220–221
State health department, community health nursing
      through, 661–662
Stater Nursing Competencies Rating Scale, 238
Statistics
  in community assessment, 665
  in epidemiology, 657–659. *See also* Birth rate;
      Death rate; Fatality rate; Mortality rate
  in research process, 360, 385
    ANOVA, 385
    Chi-square, 386
    correlation measures, 383–384
    degrees of freedom, 386
    elementary descriptive, 382–383
    inferential, 384
    level of significance, 385–386
    nonparametric, 386
    t-Test, 384
Statute(s), 207
  of limitations, 207
Steady state, 100
  in systems theory, 103–104
Stereotyping, 284, 290
Stewart, Isabel M., 16–17
Stimson, Julie C., 17
Stimuli
  contextual, 69
  focal, 70
  residual, 70
Stimulus-response, 396
  in learning theory, 403
Stress, 100, 544, 552. *See also* Burnout; Reality
      shock
  and adaptation, 107
  aging process and, 443
  and holistic health care, 110–111
  nursing process in, 555–556
  responses to
    adaptive, 554–555
    behavioral, 554
    maladaptive, 555
    physiological, 548, 554
  theories, 552–553
Stressor, 100, 544
Structural communities, 654
Subcultures, 284
Subgroups, in group communication network, 606
Subpoena, 207, 213
Suicide
  intervention, 595–596
  myths about, 586–587

prevention, 594, 596
risk
  assessment of, 591–592
  circumstances related to, 594
  survivors of, 582, 587
Sullivan, Harry S., 400, 410
Superego, 396
  in psychoanalytic theory, 399
Supplemental intervention, 668
Supplies, for teaching, 342
Support, in loss, 574–575
Support networks, 182
  assessment guidelines for, 198–199
Surgery, for pain relief, 537–538
Survey research designs, 372–374
Survivors, of suicide, 582, 587
"Susto", 294
Sympathy, 308
  in nurse–client relationship, 323–324
Symptoms. *See* Signs and symptoms
Syndrome, 544
  burnout, 54–55
  cubital tunnel compression, 499
  general adaptation. *See* General adaptation syn-
      drome (GAS)
  stress, 552
System(s), 101–102. *See also* Ecosystem
  adaptive, nursing as, 110
  behavioral, 69, 75
  belief, 62, 63
  boundaries in, 102
  community as, 654
  energy in, 105
  entropy in, 105
  equifinality in, 104–105
  feedback in, 104
  general theory. *See* General systems theory
  health-care. *See* Health-care system
  hierarchy, 102
  input, output, and throughout in, 103
  living, 109, 112. *See also* Equifinality
  negentropy in, 105
  nursing information, 36, 56
  open and closed, 103
  open versus closed, in groups, 604
  of retrieval, access to, 246–247
  Review of (ROS), 446–447
  steady state/dynamic equilibrium in 103–104

T-group. *See* Training group
T-cell, 520
  in pain theories, 520–522
t-test, 384–385
Taft–Hartley Act (1974), 121
Targets for change, 352

Task functions, 602
  of group, 609, 610
Task group, 611, 612
Task roles, 605
Taste, altered sense of, 464
  assessment, 468
  care plan for client with, 469–470
  nurse–client relationship, 472
Tax Equity and Fiscal Responsibility Act (TEFRA), 123, 131
Taxonomy, 170
  of nursing diagnoses, 172–174
Teaching, 330, 334–338
  ethics of, 338–339
  instructional methods, 340–342
  and nursing process, 343–347
  space, time, supplies, and privacy in, 342
  throughout lifespan, 339–340
  tools or aids, 342–343
Team concept. *See also* Health-care team of *Charaka-Samhita*, 4
  development of, 25
Technical skill, 143
Technology
  computerized, 55–56
  ethical issues in, 276–277
  in health-care system, 120–121
TEFRA. *See* Tax Equity and Fiscal Responsibility Act
Telephone order (T.O.), 219
Temperature, in hospital environment, 689
TENS. *See* Transcutaneous electrical nerve stimulation
Territoriality, cultural aspects in health assessment, 300
Tertiary care facilities, 116
  client care in, 124–125
Tertiary prevention, 582, 588, 654, 659
Testimony, 207, 216
Textbook of the Principles and Practice of Nursing, 72
Thanotologist, 46
Theoretical framework, 361
  in research process, 370–371
Theory, 61, 62
  adaptation, 100, 105–109
  concepts and, 70
  construction, 70
  nurse-authors of, 70–71
    Henderson, 71–72
    Johnson, 75
    King, 76
    Levine, 81–82
    Neuman, 82
    Orem, 76–77
    Orlando, 73–74

others, 82–83
    Paterson and Zderad, 80–81
    Peplau, 72–73
    Rogers, 77–78
    Roy, 80
    summary comparison, 88–97
    Travelbee, 78–79
    Wiedenbach, 74–75
  in nursing, 63
  processes in, 63–64
  for professional stature, 70
  purpose, 63
  of systems. *See* General systems theory; System(s)
Therapeutic bedrest, 490
  hazards, 492
  uses, 490–491
Therapeutic communication, 308, 317–318
Therapeutic group, 611, 612
Therapy group, 611, 612
Thermal pollution, 676, 680
Thoracic expansion, 190
Thorndike, Edward L., 330–331
Thrombophlebitis, 490, 493–494
Thrombus, 490, 493
Throughput, 100
  in health-care system, 124–130
  in systems theory, 103
Time
  in communication, 316
  for teaching, 342
Time orientation, cultural aspects in health assessment, 300
T.O. *See* Telephone order
Toddler, behavioral stage of, 200
Tort, 207
  affecting nursing practice, 209–214
Touch
  altered sense of, 464–465
    assessment, 468
    care plan for client with, 470
    nurse–client relationship, 472
  cultural aspects in health assessment, 300
Toxic substances, 676, 680–681, 682–685
  in hospital environment, 693
Toxic Substances Control Act (TSCA) (1976), 681
Training group, 603, 611, 612
Transcultural nursing, 49
Transcutaneous electrical nerve stimulation (TENS), 524, 538–539
Travelbee, Joyce, nursing theory of, 78–79, 94–95
Truth, Sojourner, 13
TSCA. *See* Toxic Substances Control Act (1976)
Tubman, Harriet, 13
Turning, 509
Twentieth century, American nursing during, 22–26

Ulcers, decubitus, 489, 494–496
Umbrella, philosophy-of-life, 63
Unconscious, 396
  in psychoanalytic theory, 399
Unions, in health-care system, 121
United States of America. *See* America; entries under *American*
United States Public Health Service (USPHS)
  community health nursing with, 662
  statistics from, 666
Universal self-care, 70
  Orem's components of, 77
Urinary incontinence, 490
Urinary retention, 490, 500
Urinary stasis, 490, 500
USPHS. *See* United States Public Health Service
Utilitarianism, 262, 267
Utility, 262

VA. *See* Veterans Administration
Validity, research process and, 361, 381
Valsalva maneuver, 490, 494
Value(s), 230, 262. *See also* Core values
  American, 286–288
  middle-class, 286–288
  in nursing, 269
Variables
  measurement levels for, 380
  in research process, 371
  statistical tests and, 385
Vedas, The, 4
Venous stasis, 490, 493
Verbal communication, 315–316
Verbal order (V.O.), 219
Verdict, 207
Veterans Administration (VA), 662
Vietnam war, American nursing during, 26
Vision
  alterations in, 464
  assessment, 466–467

Visiting Nurse Association, 126, 665
Visiting Nurse Manual, 233
Visually impaired client
  care plan for, 469
  nurse–client relationship with, 471–472
Vocal fremitus, 190–191

Wakefulness, and reticular formation, 478–479.
  See also Sleep
Wald, Lillian D., 14–15
Wall, P. D., 520–522
Water pollution, 676, 680
Watson, John, 330
Weekly Epidemiological Reports, 666
Wellness, defined, 36, 37
Weltanschauung, 64
WHO. *See* World Health Organization
WHO Statistics Annual, 666
Wiedenbach, Ernestine, nursing theory of, 74–75, 90–91
Witness, expert and lay, 206, 212–213
Works Progress Administration (WPA), 23
World Health Organization (WHO)
  and health-care outcomes, 130
  health definition, 37
  statistical reports from, 666
World War I, American nursing during, 22
  postwar, 22–23
World War II, American nursing during, 23–25
  postwar, 25
WPA. *See* Works Progress Administration

Yin and Yang, 294

Zborowski, M., 527
Zderad, Loretta T., nursing theory of, 80–81
Zeitgeist, 64